PAIN IN WOMEN

PAIN IN WOMEN

EDITORS

May L. Chin

PROFESSOR OF ANESTHESIOLOGY AND CRITICAL CARE MEDICINE
GEORGE WASHINGTON UNIVERSITY
WASHINGTON, DC

Roger B. Fillingim

PROFESSOR, UNIVERSITY OF FLORIDA COLLEGE OF DENTISTRY
DIRECTOR, UF PAIN RESEARCH AND INTERVENTION CENTER OF EXCELLENCE
GAINESVILLE, FL

Timothy J. Ness

PROFESSOR OF ANESTHESIOLOGY
UNIVERSITY OF ALABAMA AT BIRMINGHAM
BIRMINGHAM, AL

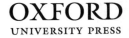

OXFORD
UNIVERSITY PRESS

OXFORD
UNIVERSITY PRESS

Oxford University Press is a department of the University of Oxford.
It furthers the University's objective of excellence in research, scholarship,
and education by publishing worldwide

Oxford   New York
Auckland   Cape Town   Dar es Salaam   Hong Kong   Karachi
Kuala Lumpur   Madrid   Melbourne   Mexico City   Nairobi
New Delhi   Shanghai   Taipei   Toronto

With offices in
Argentina   Austria   Brazil   Chile   Czech Republic   France   Greece
Guatemala   Hungary   Italy   Japan   Poland   Portugal   Singapore
South Korea   Switzerland   Thailand   Turkey   Ukraine   Vietnam

Oxford University Press © 2013

Published in the United States of America by
Oxford University Press
198 Madison Avenue, New York, New York 10016

Oxford is a registered trademark of Oxford University Press in the UK
and certain other countries

Library of Congress Cataloging-in-Publication Data
Pain in women / edited by May L. Chin, Roger B. Fillingim, Timothy J. Ness.
p. ; cm.
Includes bibliographical references and index.
ISBN 978-0-19-979641-0 (hardback : alk. paper) – ISBN 978-0-19-979653-3 (e-book)
I. Chin, May L.   II. Fillingim, Roger B., 1962-   III. Ness, Timothy J.
[DNLM: 1. Pain.   2. Analgesics—therapeutic use.   3. Pain Management.   4. Sex Factors.
5. Women. WL 704]

616'.0472 —dc23
2012022536

1 3 5 7 9 8 6 4 2
Printed in the United States of America
on acid-free paper

PREFACE

AS RECENTLY detailed in an Institute of Medicine Report, pain represents one of the most costly and prevalent public health conditions in the United States, and the burden of pain is substantially greater for women than men.[1] Women make up half of the world's population. Yet the overall treatment of pain in women remains challenging to this day. The differences between men and women are anatomical, physiological, and psychosocial in nature. Consequently, several unique features come to mind when discussing pain as experienced by women, such as pain related to pregnancy, pain related specifically to female organs, and chronic painful conditions that have a higher prevalence in the female population.

The purpose of this book is to address the current understanding of mechanisms related to sex differences, and the clinical management of common acute and chronic painful conditions in women, using up-to-date evidence-based information. The painful conditions discussed include those that are specific to female anatomy and physiology and conditions that have a higher female prevalence.

The book is divided into three sections. The first section covers basic science topics related to sex differences in pain. The epidemiology of painful conditions with female prevalence; sex differences in response to pain and to analgesics; the role of sex hormones and genotype in pain perception and analgesia; sex differences in cerebral responses to pain revealed by brain imaging; and the role of psychosocial factors, including psychological interventions, will be discussed in this section.

The second and third sections are clinically directed. The second section focuses on pain specific to female patients. Topics include the management of labor pain; the management of painful conditions during pregnancy; and the management of pain in the opioid-tolerant pregnant patient. The latter includes discussion on the impact of pain management on the fetus in utero and on the newborn who is breastfed. Chronic pain specific to females, including dysmenorrhea, chronic pelvic pain, and vulvodynia, will be discussed in this section. Cancer-related pain issues in women will be addressed in the chapter on persistent pain after breast cancer treatment and the chapter on interventional management of pelvic cancer pain.

The third section covers painful conditions with high female prevalence. These include fibromyalgia, chronic fatigue syndrome, and neuropathic pain in complex regional pain syndrome. Visceral pain with female prevalence such as irritable bowel syndrome and chronic pelvic pain of undetermined etiology will also be addressed in this section. This section also includes chapters on the presentation of cardiac pain in women; headaches including migraine; and temporomandibular joint disorders and orofacial pain.

The book is intended for a wide readership, including physicians and allied health care professionals who encounter female patients with acute or chronic painful conditions. In addition, residents and medical students in training as well as graduate students in health sciences will benefit greatly from this book as they continue to learn about and manage difficult and complex issues related to pain in female patients.

May L. Chin, MD
Roger B. Fillingim, PhD
Timothy J. Ness, MD, PhD

REFERENCE

1. IOM Committee on Advancing Pain Research, Care, and Education. *Relieving Pain in America: A Blueprint for Transforming Prevention, Care, Education, and Research*. Washington, DC: National Academies Press, 2011.

CONTENTS

CONTRIBUTORS

Leon Aarts, MD PhD
Department of Anesthesiology
Leiden University Medical Center
Leiden, The Netherlands

Kenneth Geving Andersen, MD
Section for Surgical Pathophysiology &
Department of Breast Surgery
Rigshospitalet, University of Copenhagen
Copenhagen, Denmark

Kari Kopko Bancroft, MD
Resident in Anesthesiology
University at Buffalo, School of Medicine
Buffalo, NY

**Andrew Baranowski, BSc Hons, MBBS,
    FRCA, MD, FFPMRCA**
The Centre for Uro-genital, Pelvic and Visceral
    pain, The National Hospital for Neurology
    and Neurosurgery, Queen Square
University College London Hospitals
NHS Foundation Trust
London, United Kingdom

May L. Chin, MD
Professor, Department of Anesthesiology and
    Critical Care Medicine
CoDirector, GW Pain Center
George Washington University
Washington, DC

Daniel Clauw, MD
University of Michigan
Ann Arbor, MI

Rebecca Craft, PhD
Department of Psychology
Washington State University
Pullman, WA

Peter Czakanski, MD PhD
Assistant Professor, Departments of
    Anesthesiology and Obstetrics &
    Gynecology
University of Alabama at Birmingham School
    of Medicine
Birmingham, AL

Albert Dahan, MD PhD
Department of Anesthesiology
Leiden University Medical Center
Leiden, The Netherlands

Margaret D. Eugenio, MD
Fellow, Department of Internal Medicine
Division of Gastroenterology
School of Medicine
University of Washington
Seattle, WA

Roger B. Fillingim, PhD
Professor, University of Florida College of
    Dentistry
Director, UF Pain Research and Intervention
    Center of Excellence
Gainesville, FL

Eileen Handberg, PhD, ARNP
Research Associate Professor of Medicine
Division of Cardiovascular Medicine
University of Florida College of Medicine
Gainesville, FL

Margaret M. Heitkemper, PhD
Department of Biobehavioral
Nursing and Health Systems
University of Washington
Seattle, WA

Frank J. P. M. Huygen, MD, PhD
Department of Anesthesiology
Erasmus MC
Rotterdam, The Netherlands

Monica E. Jarrett, PhD
Professor, Department of Internal Medicine
Division of Gastroenterology
School of Medicine
University of Washington
Seattle, WA

Maryam Jowza, MD
Fellow in Pain Medicine
Department of Anesthesia, Critical Care, and
    Pain Medicine
Massachusetts General Hospital
Boston, MA

Henrik Kehlet, MD, PhD
Section for Surgical Pathophysiology
Rigshospitalet, University of Copenhagen
Copenhagen, Denmark

Edmund Keogh, BSc, MSc, PhD
Centre for Pain Research &
    Department of Psychology
University of Bath,
Bath, United Kingdom

Asma A. Khan, BDS, PhD
Center for Neurosensory Disorders
University of North Carolina
Chapel Hill, NC

Christopher D. King
University of Florida, College of Dentistry
Gainesville, FL

Oscar A. de Leon-Casasola, MD
Professor of Anesthesiology and Medicine
Vice-Chair for Clinical Affairs
Dept. of Anesthesiology, University at
    Buffalo, School of Medicine
Chief, Pain Medicine and Professor of
    Oncology
Roswell Park Cancer Institute
Buffalo, NY

Linda LeResche, ScD
Professor, Department of Oral Medicine
University of Washington
Seattle, WA

Pei Feng Lim, BDS, MS
Center for Neurosensory Disorders
University of North Carolina
Chapel Hill, NC

Marian Limacher, MD
Senior Associate Dean for Faculty Affairs and
    Professional Development
AHA Endowed Professor of Cardiovascular
    Research
University of Florida College of Medicine
Gainesville, FL

William Maixner, DDS, PhD
Center for Neurosensory Disorders
University of North Carolina
Chapel Hill, NC

Jeffrey S. Mogil
Department of Psychology and Centre for
  Research on Pain
McGill University
Montreal, Canada

Marissa de Mos, MD, PhD
Department of Anesthesiology
Erasmus MC
Rotterdam, The Netherlands

Geeta Nagpal, MD
Fellow in Pain Medicine
Department of Anesthesia, Critical Care, and
  Pain Medicine
Massachusetts General Hospital
Boston, MA

Timothy J. Ness, MD, PhD
Professor, Department of Anesthesiology
University of Alabama at Birmingham
Birmingham, AL

Marieke Niesters, MD, MS
Department of Anesthesiology
Leiden University Medical Center
Leiden, The Netherlands

Satnam S. Nijjar, MD
Department of Neurology
Johns Hopkins University School of
  Medicine
Baltimore, MD

B. Lee Peterlin, DO
Department of Neurology
Johns Hopkins University School of Medicine
Baltimore, MD

Andrea J. Rapkin, MD
Professor, Department of Obstetrics and
  Gynecology
David Geffen School of Medicine at the
  University of California, Los Angeles
Los Angeles, CA

James P. Rathmell, MD
Vice Chair and Chief, Division of Pain
  Medicine
Department of Anesthesia, Critical Care and
  Pain Medicine
Massachusetts General Hospital
Henry Knowles Beecher Professor of
  Anaesthesia
Harvard Medical School
Boston, MA

Margarete Ribeiro-Dasilva
University of Florida, College of Dentistry
Gainesville, FL

Meredith T. Robbins, PhD
Associate Professor, Department of
  Anesthesiology
University of Alabama at Birmingham
Birmingham, AL

Jason Rosenberg, MD
Department of Neurology
Johns Hopkins University School of Medicine
Baltimore, MD

Nilda E. Salaman, MD
Assistant Professor, Department of
  Anesthesiology and Critical Care
  Department
George Washington University
Washington, DC

Elise Sarton, MD, PhD
Department of Anesthesiology
Leiden University Medical Center
Leiden, The Netherlands

Alethia Baldwin Sellers, MD
University of Alabama at Birmingham
Birmingham, AL

Amy Stenson, MD, MPH
Assistant Professor, Department of Obstetrics
  and Gynecology
David Geffen School of Medicine at the
  University of California, Los Angeles
Los Angeles, CA

Irene Tracey, PhD
Centre for Functional Magnetic Resonance
    Imaging of the Brain
Nuffield Department Clinical Neurosciences
Nuffield Division Anaesthetics
University of Oxford
Oxford, United Kingdom

Katy Vincent, MRCOG, PhD
Centre for Functional Magnetic Resonance
    Imaging of the Brain
Nuffield Department Clinical Neurosciences
Nuffield Division Anaesthetics
Nuffield Department of Obstetrics and
    Gynaecology
University of Oxford
Oxford, United Kingdom

Christopher M. Viscomi, MD
Professor of Anesthesiology
University of Vermont
College of Medicine
Burlington, VT

Ursula Wesselmann, MD, PhD
Professor, Departments of Anesthesiology and
    Neurology
University of Alabama at Birmingham School
    of Medicine
Birmingham, AL

Cynthia A. Wong, MD
Professor and Vice Chair
Department of Anesthesiology
Northwestern University Feinberg School of
    Medicine
Chicago, IL

SECTION ONE

SEX DIFFERENCES IN PAIN

EPIDEMIOLOGY, PAIN PERCEPTION, AND ANALGESIC RESPONSES

1

EPIDEMIOLOGY OF PAIN CONDITIONS WITH HIGHER PREVALENCE IN WOMEN

Linda LeResche

INTRODUCTION

Epidemiology is the study of the distribution, determinants, and natural history of diseases or conditions in populations.[1] This chapter focuses on the population distribution of pain conditions that occur more frequently in women than in men, as well as known and suspected risk factors for these conditions. Data on pain duration and natural history are scarcer, but they are discussed if available. I first provide a framework for understanding epidemiologic data on gender differences in pain, including special issues that need to be addressed when studying symptomatic conditions such as pain. Next, I summarize available data on prevalence, incidence, duration, and risk factors for specific pain conditions that are more prevalent in women and in men, that is, fibromyalgia, complex regional pain syndrome, irritable bowel syndrome, interstitial cystitis, chronic pelvic pain, cardiac pain, migraine, and orofacial pain. Finally, I address the similarities and differences among pain conditions that differentially affect women, shared risk factors for these pain problems, and whether these pain conditions co-occur more often than would be expected by chance.

FRAMEWORK FOR UNDERSTANDING GENDER DIFFERENCES IN THE EPIDEMIOLOGY OF PAIN

Epidemiologic Measures

Epidemiologic studies assess disease in a population, providing information on the full spectrum of the condition, not only the cases that come to clinical attention. Thus, epidemiologic studies are able to differentiate risk factors associated with disease mechanisms from those associated with treatment seeking. Epidemiologic studies can also provide comprehensive information to assess the burden of specific conditions on society. The basic measures epidemiologists use to describe the distribution, determinants, and natural history of diseases and conditions in populations are prevalence, incidence, duration, and risk.

Prevalence is defined as the proportion of persons in the population with a disease or condition at a particular time. Both the number of persons with the condition (i.e., the numerator of the prevalence rate) and the total population at risk of having the condition (i.e., the denominator) have to be known to calculate a prevalence rate. If the assessment of number of cases and number of persons at risk is done at a single point in time (or approximates this kind of measure), the resulting measure is called point prevalence. Other kinds of prevalence rates include period prevalence (e.g., number of cases in the population over a 1-year time period) or lifetime prevalence (number of persons who experience the condition at some time during the life span).

The most appropriate time periods for assessing the prevalence of a given pain condition may differ, depending on the nature of the condition. Many conditions that are more prevalent in women are chronic, recurrent conditions, with repeated episodes lasting weeks or months. Point prevalence assesses the presence of pain on the day of the interview. Thus, a point prevalence measure might not capture significant pain problems that are frequent or persistent, if they are not present at the time of the survey. For this reason, period prevalence is probably the most appropriate type of prevalence measure for such kinds of pain conditions. The best time period for determining period prevalence is likely to vary with aims of the study. If the subject is to be asked about nontrivial pain, a period of 3 to 6 months generally is chosen because this period is long enough to capture recent cases but not so long that it taxes the subject's memory and hence diminishes the quality of the data.

Incidence is defined as the rate of onset of the condition over a defined time period (usually 1 year). To calculate an incidence rate, one needs to be able to count the number of new cases appearing in a population over the time period (numerator of the incidence rate) as well as the number of persons at risk of developing the condition (the denominator). It is important to remember that persons at risk include all those capable of developing the condition for the first time. This excludes current cases as well as those who already have a history of the condition. One of the issues in calculating incidence rates for pain conditions that are recurrent (e.g., migraine and temporomandibular disorders) is that people who appear not to have the condition at the initial (baseline) assessment of the study may, in fact, have a history of the condition. Thus, cases that appear to be new onsets of the problem between the baseline and the follow-up survey may actually be recurrent cases.

Duration is simply the length of time the condition lasts. For episodic or recurrent conditions, the total duration is the sum of the durations of individual episodes.

Prevalence, incidence, and duration are related, such that *Prevalence = Incidence × Mean Duration*. (For episodic or recurrent conditions, a variation on this equation holds, i.e., *Prevalence = Incidence × Mean Episode Duration × Mean Number of Episodes*).[2] Thus, it is sometimes possible to calculate an estimate of incidence from data on prevalence and duration or to estimate duration if both prevalence and incidence are known. Knowing or being able to calculate all three measures is important, as this information can provide insight on reasons for gender differences in rates of pain. For example, if a condition is twice as prevalent in women as in men, but incidence rates for the two sexes are similar (implying that the duration of the condition is twice as long in women), research might be directed less toward understanding risk of initial onset and more toward understanding the factors associated with continuation of the pain condition in women.

Risk is defined as the likelihood that persons who do not have a specific condition (but who have particular attributes or are exposed to certain "risk factors") will develop the condition.

Case Definition

Because the aims of epidemiology are to estimate prevalence, to enumerate onsets (i.e., incidence), or to discover risk factors for a condition, deciding who should be counted as a case is central to conducting epidemiologic studies. For some conditions, case definition is relatively straightforward and relies on testing a biological sample or on observing a highly specific clinical sign (e.g., a characteristic rash). However, for conditions with pain as a central defining characteristic, a number of issues related to case definition must be considered, including issues related to measuring pain by self-report and deciding on thresholds for symptom severity and duration.

The International Association for the Study of Pain (IASP) defines pain as "an unpleasant sensory and emotional experience associated with actual or potential tissue damage or described in terms of such damage."[3] Since experience is, by definition, individual, case definitions of pain conditions must rely, at least to a certain extent, on self-report measures. Despite the misgivings of some scientists who dismiss self-report measures as subjective and unreliable, evidence indicates[4] that many such measures, including simple verbal descriptor scales and numerical rating scales, have acceptable degrees of reliability (reproducibility). Researchers can enhance the reliability of pain measurement by increasing the clarity and specificity of the questions asked. This is accomplished by using standardized questions that are easily understood by people of all educational levels and that are highly specific in terms of pain location, pain severity, frequency and duration, and/or the functional outcomes of pain. The Rose Questionnaire for angina[5] is one such questionnaire.

Case definitions for other pain conditions rely on a combination of standardized questions and standardized clinical assessment (e.g., the Research Diagnostic Criteria for Temporomandibular Disorders[6] or the American College of Rheumatology [ACR] criteria for fibromyalgia[7]). An additional advantage of standardized diagnostic criteria, be they based solely on questionnaires or on a combination of questionnaires and examination measures, is that they facilitate both comparison across studies and the combining of data in meta-analyses.

Gender-Related Issues in Pain Epidemiology

Despite the fact that self-report is, by definition, a valid measure of pain, self-report also reflects the experience of the individual as a gendered being living within a given social context. Thus, if prevalence rates, incidence rates, or pain duration differ by gender, these differences could be due to a range of factors that influence the complex experience of pain in women and men. Evidence, some reviewed in subsequent chapters, suggests there are sex differences in the biological substrates that transmit and modulate pain signals; that men and

women differ in their ability to detect and discriminate various stimuli, including nociceptive stimuli; and that cognitive and emotional responses to pain differ by gender.[8] Gender differences may occur also in pain-related behaviors, including willingness to report pain. In assessing epidemiologic data on pain, we are, of necessity, assessing the cumulative effect of all these sex- and gender-related factors on the outcome of pain report.

PAIN CONDITIONS WITH HIGHER FEMALE PREVALENCE

Fibromyalgia

Fibromyalgia is a chronic, widespread musculoskeletal pain condition in which muscles are tender upon palpation. The condition is usually defined according to the 1990 ACR criteria,[7] which require a 3-month history of chronic widespread pain at the time of the interview (defined as pain on both the right and left side of the body and pain both above and below the waist, as well as pain in the axial skeleton). Upon examination, 11 of 18 specific body sites must also be tender to palpation in order to meet diagnostic criteria for fibromyalgia.

Although chronic widespread pain as defined by the ACR criteria is not uncommon, affecting 15%–22% of women and 3%–9% of men,[9] the prevalence of fibromyalgia is much lower. Large studies of fibromyalgia prevalence in the population that have used strict ACR 1990 criteria and studied both sexes over the adult life span are summarized in Table 1.1.

Prevalence rates in these studies ranged from 3.4% to 4.9% in women and 0.2% to 1.6% in men. Although female-to-male prevalence ratios can be calculated from these data, they are inherently unstable for the US[10] and Spanish[11] studies because of the very small number of men with the condition. The best estimate of the female-to-male ratio (about 3 to 1) comes from the Canadian study,[12] where the confidence intervals on prevalence are relatively tight. The age of peak prevalence in women varies from study to study, with highest rates among women in middle age or older age groups.

Table 1.1 Population-Based Prevalence Studies of Fibromyalgia Using American College of Rheumatology 1990 Criteria

REFERENCE	STUDY SITE	NO. OF SUBJECTS	AGES STUDIED	PREVALENCE IN WOMEN PERCENT (95% CI)	PREVALENCE IN MEN PERCENT (95% CI)	AGE OF PEAK PREVALENCE, WOMEN
White et al., 1994[12]	London Ontario, Canada	3,395* 2,090 ♀ 1,290 ♂	18+ years	4.9 (4.7, 5.1)	1.6 (1.3, 1.9)	55–64 years
Wolfe et al., 1995[10]	Wichita Kansas, USA	3,006**	18+ years	3.4 (2.3, 4.6)	0.5 (0.0, 1.0)	70–79 years
Carmona et al., 2001[11]	Spain	2,192 1,178 ♀ 1,014 ♂	20+ years	4.2	0.2	40–49 years

*Fifteen subjects refused to answer the question asking their gender.

**Sex distribution of the sample not reported.

COMPLEX REGIONAL PAIN SYNDROME

Complex regional pain syndrome (CRPS), previously called reflex sympathetic dystrophy, is a chronic pain problem characterized by the presence of diffuse pain, associated with allodynia (pain response to usually nonpainful stimuli) and autonomic disturbances (changes in skin color, temperature, and/or sweating). Impaired motor function may also be present. CRPS may appear spontaneously (Type I), or it may be precipitated by injury (Type II).[13]

Only a handful of population-based studies of CRPS exist. Because it is assumed that virtually all cases of CRPS come to treatment, either in primary or specialty care, these studies are done by reviewing medical records in geographical areas where these records are available for an entire population. An early study in Olmsted County, Minnesota,[14] using IASP criteria[3] to define cases, found an incidence rate of 5.46 per 100,000 person years at risk for CRPS Type I—the more common type, where no obvious nerve injury is present. Incidence rose with age up to 50 years and peaked in the 50–59-year-old age group, declining thereafter for both men and women. The sex ratio was approximately four women for one man. A study conducted a few years later in the Netherlands[15] found a much higher incidence rate using the same IASP criteria to define cases (16.8 per 100,000 person years at risk). The age peak in this study was somewhat higher than that found in the Minnesota study (60–69 years), but the sex ratio was similar (3.4 to 1). The Minnesota study also calculated a 1-year period prevalence rate, which was found to be 20.57/100,000 persons or approximately 0.02%. Interestingly, although there was no significant sex difference in the rate of eventual recovery, the sex ratio among prevalent cases was approximately 7 to 1 (i.e., 1.75 times the sex ratio for incidence), suggesting that the duration of the condition may be longer for women than men.

IRRITABLE BOWEL SYNDROME

Irritable bowel syndrome (IBS) is a functional gastrointestinal disorder involving diarrhea, constipation, or both, as well as abdominal pain. Several sets of diagnostic criteria have been used to define IBS over the past three decades, and prevalence and incidence rates, as well as gender ratios, differ depending on the criteria used. The most recent international criteria are the Rome II (1999)[16] and Rome III (2006)[17] criteria, which differ from each other primarily in the time frame and frequency of symptoms. The Rome II criteria are considered stricter, as they require that symptoms have been present for a total of at least 12 weeks in the prior year, whereas the Rome III criteria only require that symptoms have been present for 3 days/month over the last 3 months. Because fewer studies have been done using the newer Rome III criteria, we focus on studies that have employed the stricter Rome II criteria.

Studies of adults of both sexes conducted in the Canada and the United States using Rome II criteria have found prevalence rates of 12.1%[18] and 6.7%,[19] respectively. However, both studies used methods that involved random-digit-dialed telephone interviews, and the response rates were low (less than 35%). It is probable that the survey respondents were more interested in the subject matter than those who did not agree to participate, and thus more likely to have IBS. Under these circumstances, the resulting prevalence rates are likely overestimates. In another US study that surveyed only women,[20] the response rate was higher (74.8%), and the prevalence rate was 5.4%. This latter figure is similar to that found in a birth cohort from New Zealand[21] (5.3% in women, 3.3% in men) as well as that calculated in a systematic review[22] of studies from European Union countries, where the mean weighted overall population (both sexes) prevalence for the six studies that used Rome II criteria was 3.76%. In those studies from Western countries where prevalence rates are reported for both sexes, reported prevalence rates are 1.6 to 2.0 times higher in women than in men.

Interestingly, the picture in Asian countries is different. In reports reviewed by Choung and Locke[23] (see ref. 23, Table 2), prevalence rates using the Rome II criteria to diagnose IBS in Asian countries were in general higher than in Western countries, ranging from 5.7% to 22.1% across seven studies, with a median prevalence of 8.6%. Furthermore, gender differences in rates of IBS were much less apparent in population-based studies conducted in Asia, ranging from 0.84 (i.e., more men than women meeting criteria for the disorder) to 1.26, with a median across five studies of 1.04.

The reasons for the discrepancies between Western and Asian countries in prevalence and gender ratios are not clear. Perhaps Asian men are more attentive to or more willing to report gastrointestinal symptoms than men in Western countries; dietary differences might affect the diarrhea and constipation symptoms; or genetic differences across populations might account for the observed differences.

The age distribution of IBS differs across studies, with some investigations (e.g., Ref. 19) showing a peak in the 25–44-year-old age group and others (e.g., Refs. 24,25) showing little variability across the adult life span. Because of the often insidious onset of IBS symptoms, as well as the changing criteria used to define cases of IBS in various iterations of the Rome Criteria, incidence rates and duration are difficult to estimate. Choung and Locke[23] report incidence rate estimates of 200 to 400 new onset cases per 100,000 person years (0.2% to 0.4% per year) based on studies in Western countries. If this incidence rate is accurate, average duration of IBS would be approximately 10–20 years.

Painful Bladder Syndrome/Interstitial Cystitis/Chronic Pelvic Pain

Chronic pelvic pain is an overarching term that can include persistent pain originating in the reproductive organs, the bladder, or any other structure in the pelvic region. Painful bladder syndrome (PBS) is a subtype of chronic pelvic pain characterized by suprapubic pain. Although there are a great many definitions of painful bladder syndrome,[26] most of the definitions require the presence of some combination of urinary frequency, urgency, and/or nocturia (awakening with need to urinate more than once during the night). Other definitions also include the requirement that pain increases as the bladder fills and/or is relieved upon emptying the bladder. Research diagnostic criteria for interstitial cystitis (IC) developed in the late 1980s by the National Institute of Diabetes and Digestive and Kidney Diseases (NIDDK) included not only pain and urgency but also findings of glomerulations or ulcers on cystoscopic examination. Cystoscopic examinations are often not feasible in large epidemiologic studies. In addition, many experts consider the

NIDDK criteria too strict to describe the spectrum of disease seen in clinical practice.[27] Thus, the terms *interstitial cystitis* and *painful bladder syndrome* are sometimes used interchangeably in epidemiologic studies. Further complicating the issues of symptom-based case definition is the recent realization that many of the symptoms of chronic prostatitis are similar or identical to those of interstitial cystitis/painful bladder syndrome,[27] although different questionnaires may be used to assess symptoms in the two sexes.[28] Because prostatitis is a disease of men, and interstitial cystitis has been traditionally considered a "woman's disease," changes in case definition and use of specific questionnaires can have major implications for assessing gender differences in the epidemiology of these pain problems.

Excellent data on rates of PBS in the community come from the Boston Area Community Health Survey (BACH Survey).[26,29] The BACH sample included 2,301 men and 3,205 women aged 30 to 79 years from the Boston area, and it was purposely constructed to include approximately equal numbers of persons in three racial/ethnic groups: black, white, and Hispanic. PBS was operationally defined as pain increasing as the bladder fills (fairly often, usually, or almost always) and/or pain relieved by urination (fairly often, usually, or almost always), with symptoms lasting for at least 3 months. Using this definition, the prevalence of PBS was 1.3% in men and 2.6% in women, with peak prevalence in women 40 to 60 years of age, and in men 50 to 80 years old. Prevalence was higher among those of low socioeconomic status, but rates did not differ by racial/ethnic group when analyses were controlled for socioeconomic status. In addition to age, sex, and socioeconomic status, factors associated with PBS in women include being physically inactive, worry about a sibling, worry about paying for basics (transportation, housing, food, health care), depression, and a history of physical, emotional, or sexual abuse.[29]

Recent incidence estimates for IC come from a study conducted in a managed care population in the Portland, Oregon, metropolitan area.[30] Incident cases were identified based on newly coded ICD-9 diagnoses of IC in the medical record. No cases were identified in men. The estimated incidence rate was 15 per 100,000 women per year, with a mean age at diagnosis of 51 years.

Chronic pelvic pain in women may also be caused by endometriosis, pelvic inflammatory disease, urethral syndrome, and pelvic congestion syndrome.[31] However, in many cases a specific disease cannot be diagnosed, and pain is characterized by site and triggering factors as either dysmenorrhea (painful menses), dyspareunia (deep pain during intercourse), or noncyclic pelvic pain. A systematic review of chronic pelvic pain studies worldwide[32] summarized data from 106 studies on chronic dysmenorrhea, 54 studies on dyspareunia, and 18 studies on chronic, noncyclic pelvic pain. Tens of thousands of women contributed data for each condition, but there were few studies from developing countries. Rates of all three conditions varied greatly across studies. Even in studies rated to be of high quality, prevalence rates varied substantially, ranging from 16.8% to 81% for dysmenorrhea, 8% to 21.8% for dyspareunia, and 2.1% to 24% for noncyclical pain. These variable rates are likely explained in great part by variability in case definitions. However, true population differences may also explain some of the differences in rates.

Cardiac Pain

It is well known that myocardial infarction is more common in men than in women, although symptoms of myocardial infarction differ by gender.[33] The epidemiology of angina pectoris (chest pain on exertion), a common initial presentation of coronary disease, presents a different picture, however. Hemingway and colleagues[34] conducted a systematic review and meta-analysis of 74 studies in which comparisons could be made between angina prevalence rates in men and women. The studies covered 31 countries and included data on over 13,000 female and 11,000 male angina cases in populations of approximately 200,000 women and 200,000 men. All studies used the Rose questionnaire to assess for presence of angina.[5] The weighted mean prevalence rates varied substantially from country to country, but if rates were high in men in a given country, they were also high in women in the same population. Overall angina prevalence rates were higher among women in 55 of the 74 studies. The pooled female-to-male sex ratio across all the studies was 1.20 (95% confidence interval, 1.14 to 1.28, $p < .00001$). Stratified analyses showed that the sex ratio did not differ significantly according to participant age or birth cohort, the year the survey was started, or the sex ratio for myocardial infarction in the country where the study was conducted. The excess in women also did not differ by study methodological factors, including language of the questionnaire, administration method, or survey response rate. The female excess was higher in American studies (1.40) and higher among nonwhites than whites. The only geographic area where the prevalence rates for angina were higher in men than in women was India and Sri Lanka.

Migraine

The epidemiology of migraine has been studied throughout the world. A meta-analysis[35] conducted in 1999 found 18 studies that provided age- and sex-specific prevalence estimates using International Headache Society Criteria[36] for migraine, and several large population-based studies have been conducted since that time. Gender prevalence ratios for migraine (F:M) are typically found to be around 3:1, with prevalence peaking in the 30–39-year-old age group.[35] For example, data from three large U.S.-based studies[37-39] conducted using almost identical methods over a 15-year period are shown in Table 1.2. In addition to showing stable gender prevalence ratios, these results suggest that rates of migraine have not changed much over this time.

Race, as well as age and gender, is associated with migraine prevalence; specifically, migraine rates in the United States are higher in whites than in African Americans, and rates are lower in Africa than in North America.[35,37] In the United States, risk of migraine is also inversely related to household income, after adjusting for age, sex, race, region of the country, and household size.[39]

Of specific interest in the context of this book, about half of women with migraine experience menstrual migraine (i.e., migraine attacks in the period 2 days before to 2 days after the start of menses) and between 3.5% and 21% of women with migraine experience migraine only during this time frame.[40] In clinical migraine populations, menstrual migraines also appear to be more severe than migraines occurring at other times of the month.[40]

Table 1.2   Three US Population-Based Prevalence Studies of Migraine Using International Headache Society Criteria

STUDY/ REFERENCE	NO. OF SUBJECTS*	PREVALENCE IN WOMEN (PERCENT)	PREVALENCE IN MEN (PERCENT)	GENDER PREVALENCE RATIO (F:M)	AGE OF PEAK PREVALENCE
American Migraine Study I (1989)[37]	10,808 ♀ 9,660 ♂	17.6	5.7	3.1	30–39 years (both sexes)
American Migraine Study II (1999)[38]	15,467 ♀ 14,260 ♂	18.2	6.5	2.8	30–39 years (both sexes)
American Migraine Prevalence and Prevention Study (2004)[39]	85,571 ♀ 77,185 ♂	17.1	5.6	3.1	30–39 years (both sexes)

*All studies based on random samples of the US population; all studied individuals 12 years of age and older and assessed 1-year period prevalence.

Using sophisticated statistical modeling techniques, Stewart and colleagues[41] derived estimates of migraine incidence across the life span in males and females. These estimates, modeled using data from a very large cross-sectional study,[39] are consistent with those found in smaller longitudinal studies conducted in specific age groups. Cumulative lifetime incidence (including cases that remitted) was 43% in women and 18% in men. Median age of onset was 25 years of age among women and 24 years among men. Incidence rates appear to be 2.5 to 3 times higher than prevalence rates. These very high incidence rates (i.e., indicating that more than 4 in 10 women will experience at least one episode of migraine in their lifetime) suggest that research could profitably be directed toward identifying factors that are associated with the continuation of migraine, rather than focusing solely on risk factors for onset.

Temporomandibular Disorders/ Orofacial Pain

Temporomandibular muscle and joint disorders (referred to collectively as "TMJD" or more simply as "TMD") are musculoskeletal conditions characterized by pain in the temporomandibular (jaw) joint and/or the associated masticatory muscles. TMD pain is the most prevalent of the chronic orofacial pain conditions, and it is similar to back pain in its intensity, persistence, and psychological impact.[42] TMD pain is uncommon in children before puberty.[43] Table 1.3 lists several studies that provide estimates of the prevalence TMD in adult populations.[42,44–47] All studies used similar but not identical case definitions, inquiring into ongoing pain in the temporomandibular region. Prevalence rates range from 9% to 15% for women and from 3% to 10% for men. These rates are remarkably consistent, given that investigators used somewhat different case definitions and assessed different populations. TMD pain was found to be 1.5–2 times more common in women than in men in nearly every study. Also, in all studies where the pattern of age-specific prevalence was clear, the peak age was around 35–45 years. Although standardized research diagnostic criteria for TMD are now available,[6] few studies have yet used these criteria to examine the prevalence of specific subtypes of TMD such as myalgia (pain in the masticatory muscles) and/or arthralgia (pain in the temporomandibular joint) in the general adult population.

Table 1.3   Population-Based Prevalence Studies of Pain in the Temporomandibular Region

REFERENCE	STUDY SITE	NO. OF SUBJECTS	AGES STUDIED	PREVALENCE IN WOMEN (PERCENT)	PREVALENCE IN MEN (PERCENT)	GENDER PREVALENCE RATIO (F:M)	AGE OF PEAK PREVALENCE
Helkimo, 1974[44]	Finland (Lapps)	600	15–65 years	14.0	10.0	1.4	35–44 years
Locker and Slade, 1988[45]	Toronto, Ontario, Canada	377 ♀ 300 ♂	18+ years	9.5	5.0	1.9	<45 years
Von Korff, et al., 1988[42]	Seattle, Washington, USA	593 ♀ 423 ♂	18–75 years	15.0	8.0	1.9	25–44 years
Goulet et al., 1995[46]	Quebec, Canada	497 ♀ 400 ♂	18+ years	9.0	5.0	1.8	35–54 years
Matsuka et al., 1996[47]	Okayama City, Japan	368 ♀ 304 ♂	20+ years	11.7	9.9	1.2	20–39 years

Estimates of onset rates of TMD pain from a number of studies are also very consistent, indicating that incidence rates of TMD pain are on the order of 2%–3% per year.[48–52] This fairly low incidence rate suggests that the high prevalence of TMD pain in the population is due to its relatively long duration, rather than high rates of onset.

Both age and sex are associated with TMD pain prevalence, suggesting that some factor in women of reproductive age may increase risk. TMD pain prevalence increases dramatically in girls during the first 5 years after menarche,[53] and some research has found that use of hormone replacement therapy is associated with increased risk for TMD pain[54,55] or for orofacial pain in general,[56] although other work[57] has found no association. Additional research[58,59] suggests that estrogen may serve as a pain modulator in women with TMD pain. Although research on race is not as extensive for TMD as it is for migraine, rates of TMD pain appear to lower in African Americans than in whites,[60,61] and age-specific prevalence patterns have also been found to differ by race and ethnicity.[62] Two well-designed studies found that persons with pain in other body sites (e.g., back pain, abdominal pain) were at increased risk for developing TMD.[45,48] Several studies indicate that, as with other chronic pain conditions, depression and psychosocial distress are likely important risk factors. Genetic factors also appear to play a role in the TMD etiology.[63]

The epidemiologic evidence base is not as extensive for the less prevalent chronic orofacial pain conditions as it is for TMD. However, there is some evidence to suggest that female gender is also a risk factor for many of these rarer conditions, including burning mouth pain,[61] atypical facial pain/atypical odontalgia,[64] and trigeminal neuralgia.[65]

COMORBIDITY OF PAIN CONDITIONS WITH HIGH FEMALE PREVALENCE

The New Oxford American Dictionary defines comorbidity as the simultaneous presence of two chronic diseases or conditions in a patient. Two (or more) chronic pain conditions could occur in the same person for a number of possible reasons. First, the co-occurrence could simply be due to chance, especially if the conditions are frequent. For example, if the prevalence of TMD pain in women is 14% and the prevalence of migraine in women is 18%, we would expect that 3% of women in the population (.14 × .18) would have both conditions purely by chance. However, co-occurrence rates for pain conditions that occur preferentially in women appear to be higher than would be expected by chance. If rates of co-occurrence are higher than chance expectations, it is possible that the conditions are different manifestations of the same underlying disease process. (This could be particularly likely if the conditions share common symptoms.) It is also possible that the conditions share common risk factors (e.g., genetic, hormonal, behavioral, or social factors), that having one condition increases the risk of acquiring the other, or that the first condition is even a direct cause of the second condition. It is also possible that *treatment* of one condition increases risks for acquiring a second. For example, use of opioid medications may bring about increased pain sensitivity (opioid-induced hyperalgesia),[66] which could place a patient at greater risk for additional pain problems.

Although there are quite a number of studies documenting comorbidity of pairs or groups of the pain conditions discussed in this book, most of these studies have taken place in treatment settings. Such studies, while valuable, need to be interpreted carefully, because cases in treatment settings—especially in tertiary care settings—are likely to have more severe pain than those in the general population, to be concerned enough about their health problems to seek care, and, by seeking care, to be more likely to be examined by a physician, who may find conditions that the person might not otherwise have viewed as a problem. Thus, these studies may be very useful in documenting treatment needs, but perhaps not as useful as population-based studies for untangling questions of etiology. A few of the findings from population-based studies on comorbidities are described next.

Studies show greater-than-expected rates of overlap of pain conditions in the same region of the body, including chronic pelvic pain and

IBS[67,68] and TMD/orofacial pain and headache.[69] It is possible that some of these findings are attributable to shared and overlapping symptoms, leading to difficulties in diagnosis, but it is also possible that having one pain condition results in local sensitization of the nociceptive system and/or focuses attention on other symptoms in the same body region.

Comorbidities of conditions in disparate body regions (albeit possibly linked by functional system) have also been shown to occur in population-based studies. For example, a recent meta-analysis found a link between migraine with aura and ischemic stroke, especially in women; however, the same study found no link of migraine with myocardial infarction or death due to cardiovascular disease.[70] A history of migraine has also been linked with CRPS,[71] and fibromyalgia has been found to be associated more often than chance expectation with headache (not specified as migraine or nonmigraine) and IBS.[72] Fibromyalgia in this study was also strongly associated with depression,[72] possibly indicating that depression is a shared risk factor for both FM and IBS. Overall, having multiple existing pain conditions, regardless of site, is associated with onset of new pain problems in longitudinal studies,[49,52] suggesting that dysregulation of central pain modulation systems may contribute to the overall problem of pain comorbidity in women.

SUMMARY

In summary, epidemiologic studies show that women are more likely than men to experience a wide range of pain problems in a variety of body sites and systems. It appears that women are also vulnerable to experiencing combinations of these pain problems at rates beyond the level of chance. The time is ripe for research to address the epidemiology of specific pain conditions where good data are lacking. In addition, research is badly needed concerning the epidemiology of comorbidity among those pain conditions that are more prevalent in women than men. These studies carry costs and complexities, but they have the potential to yield valuable information about etiologic factors and thus to lead to more effective preventive and management interventions.

REFERENCES

1. Lilienfeld AM, Lilienfeld DE. *Foundations of Epidemiology*. 2nd ed. New York: Oxford University Press; 1980.
2. Von Korff M, Parker RD. The dynamics of the prevalence of chronic episodic disease. *J Chron Dis* 1980;33:79–85.
3. Task Force on Taxonomy, International Association for the Study of Pain. *Classification of Chronic Pain*. (Mersky H, Bogduk N eds.). Seattle, WA: IASP Press; 1994.
4. Turk DC, Melzack R, eds. *Handbook of Pain Assessment*. 3rd ed. New York: Guilford Press; 2011.
5. Rose GA. The diagnosis of ischaemic heart pain and intermittent claudication in field surveys. *Bull World Health Org* 1962;27:645–58.
6. Dworkin SF, LeResche L. Research Diagnostic Criteria for Temporomandibular Disorders: Review, criteria, examinations and specifications, critique. *J Craniomandib Disord Facial Oral Pain* 1992;6:301–55.
7. Wolfe F, Smythe HA, Yunus MB, et al. The American College of Rheumatology 1990 Criteria for the Classification of Fibromyalgia. Report of the Multicenter Criteria Committee. *Arthritis Rheum* 1990;33(2):160–72.
8. LeResche L. Sex, gender and clinical pain. In: Flor H, Kalso E, Dostrovsky JO, eds. *Proceedings of the 11th World Congress on Pain*. Seattle, WA: IASP Press; 2006: 543–54.
9. Gran JT. The epidemiology of chronic generalized musculoskeletal pain. *Best Pract Res Clin Rheumatol* 2003;17(4):547–61.
10. Wolfe F, Ross K, Anderson J, Russell IJ, Hebert L. The prevalence and characteristics of fibromyalgia in the general population. *Arthritis Rheum* 1995;38(1):19–28.
11. Carmona L, Ballina J, Gabriel R, Laffon A; EPISER Study Group. The burden of musculoskeletal diseases in the general population of Spain: results from a national survey. *Ann Rheum Dis* 2001;60(11):1040–5.
12. White KP, Speechley M, Harth M, Ostbye T. The London Fibromyalgia Epidemiology Study: the prevalence of fibromyalgia syndrome in London, Ontario. *J Rheumatol* 1999;26(7):1570–6.
13. Maihöfner C, Seifert F, Markovic K. Complex regional pain syndromes: new pathophysiological concepts and therapies. *Eur J Neurol* 2010;17(5):649–60.
14. Sandroni P, Benrud-Larson LM, McClelland RL, Low PA. Complex regional pain syndrome type I: incidence and prevalence in Olmsted County, a population-based study. *Pain* 2003;103(1–2):199–207.

15. de Mos M, de Bruijn AG, Huygen FJ, Dieleman JP, Stricker BH, Sturkenboom MC. The incidence of complex regional pain syndrome: a population-based study. *Pain* 2007;129(1–2):12–20.
16. Thompson WG, Longstreth GF, Drossman DA, Heaton KW, Irvine EJ, Müller-Lissner SA. Functional bowel disorders and functional abdominal pain. *Gut* 1999;45(Suppl 2):II43–7.
17. Longstreth GF, Thompson WG, Chey WD, Houghton LA, Mearin F, Spiller RC. Functional bowel disorders. *Gastroenterol* 2006;130(5):1480–91.
18. Thompson WG, Irvine EJ, Pare P, Ferrazzi S, Rance L. Functional gastrointestinal disorders in Canada: first population-based survey using Rome II criteria with suggestions for improving the questionnaire. *Dig Dis Sci* 2002;47(1):225–35.
19. Hungin AP, Chang L, Locke GR, Dennis EH, Barghout V. Irritable bowel syndrome in the United States: prevalence, symptom patterns and impact. *Aliment Pharmacol Ther* 2005;21(11):1365–75.
20. Chey WD, Olden K, Carter E, Boyle J, Drossman D, Chang L. Utility of the Rome I and Rome II criteria for irritable bowel syndrome in U.S. women. *Am J Gastroenterol* 2002;97(11):2803–11.
21. Talley NJ, Howell S, Poulton R. The irritable bowel syndrome and psychiatric disorders in the community: is there a link? *Am J Gastroenterol* 2001;96(4):1072–9.
22. World Gastroenterology Organisation Advisory Board. Systematic review on the management of irritable bowel syndrome in the European Union. *Eur J Gastroenterol Hepatol* 2007;19(Suppl 1):S11–37.
23. Choung RS, Locke GR 3rd. Epidemiology of IBS. *Gastroenterol Clin North Am* 2011;40(1):1–10.
24. Hillilä MT, Färkkilä MA. Prevalence of irritable bowel syndrome according to different diagnostic criteria in a non-selected adult population. *Aliment Pharmacol Ther* 2004;20(3):339–45.
25. Mearin F, Badía X, Balboa A, et al. Irritable bowel syndrome prevalence varies enormously depending on the employed diagnostic criteria: comparison of Rome II versus previous criteria in a general population. *Scand J Gastroenterol* 2001;36(11):1155–61.
26. Clemens JQ, Link CL, Eggers PW, et al. Prevalence of painful bladder symptoms and effect on quality of life in black, Hispanic and white men and women. *J Urol* 2007;177(4):1390–4.
27. Hanno PM. Interstitial cystitis-epidemiology, diagnostic criteria, clinical markers. *Rev Urol* 2002;4(Suppl 1):S3–8.
28. Marszalek M, Wehrberger C, Temml C, Ponholzer A, Berger I, Madersbacher S. Chronic pelvic pain and lower urinary tract symptoms in both sexes: analysis of 2749 participants of an urban health screening project. *Eur Urol* 2009;55(2):499–507.
29. Link CL, Pulliam SJ, Hanno PM, et al. Prevalence and psychosocial correlates of symptoms suggestive of painful bladder syndrome: results from the Boston area community health survey. *J Urol* 2008;180(2):599–606.
30. Patel R, Calhoun EA, Meenan RT, O'Keeffe Rosetti MC, Kimes T, Clemens JQ. Incidence and clinical characteristics of interstitial cystitis in the community. *Int Urogynecol J Pelvic Floor Dysfunct* 2008;19(8):1093–6.
31. Grace VM, Zondervan KT. Chronic pelvic pain in New Zealand: prevalence, pain severity, diagnoses and use of the health services. *Aust NZ J Public Health* 2004;28(4):369–75.
32. Latthe P, Latthe M, Say L, Gülmezoglu M, Khan KS. WHO systematic review of prevalence of chronic pelvic pain: a neglected reproductive health morbidity. *BMC Public Health* 2006;6:177.
33. Kirchberger I, Heier M, Kuch B, Wende R, Meisinger C. Sex Differences in patient-reported symptoms associated with myocardial infarction (from the Population-Based MONICA/KORA Myocardial Infarction Registry). *Am J Cardiol* 2011;107(11):1585–9.
34. Hemingway H, Langenberg C, Damant J, Frost C, Pyörälä K, Barrett-Connor E. Prevalence of angina in women versus men: a systematic review and meta-analysis of international variations across 31 countries. *Circulation* 2008;117(12):1526–36.
35. Scher A, Stewart W, Lipton RB. Migraine and headache: a meta-analytic approach. In: Crombie IK, Croft PR, Linton SJ, LeResche L, Von Korff M, eds. *Epidemiology of Pain*. Seattle, WA: IASP Press; 1999: 159–70.
36. Headache Classification Committee of the International Headache Society. Classification and diagnostic criteria for headache disorders, cranial neuralgias and facial pain. *Cephalalgia* 1988; 8(Suppl 7):1–96.
37. Stewart WF, Lipton RB, Celentano DD, Reed ML. Prevalence of migraine headache in the United States. Relation to age, income, race, and other sociodemographic factors. *JAMA* 1992;267(1):64–9.
38. Lipton RB, Stewart WF, Diamond S, Diamond ML, Reed M. Prevalence and burden of migraine in the United States: data from the American Migraine Study II. *Headache* 2001;41(7):646–57.

39. Lipton RB, Bigal ME, Diamond M, Freitag F, Reed ML, Stewart WF; AMPP Advisory Group. Migraine prevalence, disease burden, and the need for preventive therapy. *Neurology* 2007;68(5):343–9.

40. Martin VT, Lipton RB. Epidemiology and biology of menstrual migraine. *Headache* 2008;48(Suppl 3):S124–30.

41. Stewart WF, Wood C, Reed ML, Roy J, Lipton RB; AMPP Advisory Group. Cumulative lifetime migraine incidence in women and men. *Cephalalgia* 2008;28(11):1170–8.

42. Von Korff M, Dworkin SF, LeResche L, Kruger A. An epidemiologic comparison of pain complaints. *Pain* 1988;32(2):173–83.

43. Drangsholt M, LeResche L. Temporomandibular disorder pain. In: Crombie IK, Croft PR, Linton SJ, LeResche L, Von Korff M, eds. *Epidemiology of Pain*. Seattle, WA: IASP Press; 1999: 203–33.

44. Helkimo M. Studies on function and dysfunction of the masticatory system. IV. Age and sex distribution of symptoms of dysfunction of the masticatory system in Lapps in the north of Finland. *Acta Odontol Scand* 1974;32(4):255–67.

45. Locker D, Slade G. Prevalence of symptoms associated with temporomandibular disorders in a Canadian population. *Community Dent Oral Epidemiol* 1988;16(5):310–3.

46. Goulet J-P, Lavigne GJ, Lund JP. Jaw pain prevalence among French-speaking Canadians in Quebec and related symptoms of temporomandibular disorders. *J Dent Res* 1995;74(11):1738–44.

47. Matsuka Y, Yatani H, Kuboki T, Yamashita A. Temporomandibular disorders in the adult population of Okayama City, Japan. *Cranio* 1996;14(2):158–62.

48. Heikinheimo K, Salmi K, Myllärniemi S, Kirveskari P. Symptoms of craniomandibular disorder in a sample of Finnish adolescents at the ages of 12 and 15 years. *Eur J Orthod* 1989;11(4):325–31.

49. Von Korff M, LeResche L, Dworkin SF. First onset of common pain symptoms: A prospective study of depression as a risk factor. *Pain* 1993;55(2):251–8.

50. Kitai N, Takada K, Yasuda Y, Vernonck A, Carels C. Pain and other cardinal TMJ dysfunction symptons: a longitudinal survey of Japanese female adolescents. *J Oral Rehab* 1997;24(107):741–8.

51. Nilsson I-M, List T, Drangsholt M. Incidence and temporal patterns of temporomandibular disorder pain among Swedish adolescents. *J Orofac Pain* 2007;21(2):127–32.

52. LeResche L, Mancl LA, Drangsholt M, Huang G, Von Korff M. Predictors of onset of facial pain and temporomandibular disorders in early adolescence. *Pain* 2007;129(3):269–78.

53. LeResche L. Gender and hormonal effects on clinical TMJD pain. In: McNamara JA Jr, Kapila SD, eds. *Temporomandibular Disorders and Orofacial Pain: Separating Controversy from Consensus*. Monograph 46, Craniofacial Growth Series, Ann Arbor: Department of Orthodontics and Pediatric Dentistry and Center for Human Growth and Development, University of Michigan; 2009: 107–23.

54. LeResche L, Saunders K, Von Korff M, Barlow W, Dworkin SF. Use of exogenous hormones and risk of temporomandibular disorder pain. *Pain* 1997;69(1–2):153–60.

55. Wise EA, Riley JL III, Robinson ME. Clinical pain perception and hormone replacement therapy in postmenopausal women experiencing orofacial pain. *Clin J Pain* 2000;16(2):121–6.

56. Macfarlane TV, Blinkhorn AS, Davies RM, Kincey J, Worthington HV. Association between female hormonal factors and orofacial pain: study in the community. *Pain* 2002;97(1–2):5–10.

57. Hatch JP, Rugh JD, Sakai S, Saunders MJ. Is the use of exogenous estrogen associated with temporomandibular signs and symptoms? *J Am Dent Assoc* 2001;132(3):319–26.

58. LeResche L, Mancl L, Sherman JJ, Gandara B, Dworkin SF. Changes in temporomandibular pain and other symptoms across the menstrual cycle. *Pain* 2003;106(3):253–61.

59. LeResche L, Sherman JJ, Huggins KH, et al. Musculoskeletal orofacial pain and other signs and symptoms of temporomandibular disorders during pregnancy: a prospective study. *J Orofac Pain* 2005;19(3):193–201.

60. Plesh O, Crawford PB, Gansky SA. Chronic pain in a biracial population of young women. *Pain* 2002;99(3):515–23.

61. Lipton JA, Ship JA, Larach-Robinson D. Estimated prevalence and distribution of reported orofacial pain in the United States. *J Am Dent Assoc* 1993;124(4):115–21.

62. Isong U, Gansky SA, Plesh O. Temporomandibular joint and muscle disorder-type pain in U.S. adults: the National Health Interview Survey. *J Orofac Pain* 2008;22(4):317–22.

63. Diatchenko L, Slade GD, Nackley AG, et al. Genetic basis for individual variations in pain perception and the development of a chronic pain condition. *Hum Mol Genet* 2005;14(1):135–43.

64. Marbach JJ, Hulbrock J, Hohn C, Segal AG. Incidence of phantom tooth pain: an atypical facial neuralgia. *Oral Surg Oral Med Oral Pathol* 1982;53(2):190–3.

65. Katusic, S, Beard CM, Bergstralh E, Kurland L. Incidence and clinical features of trigeminal neuralgia, Rochester, Minnesota, 1945–1984. *Ann Neurol* 1990;27(1):89–95.

66. Angst MS, Clark JD. Opioid-induced hyperalgesia: a qualitative systematic review. *Anesthesiol* 2006;104(3):570–87.

67. Choung RS, Herrick LM, Locke GR 3rd, Zinsmeister AR, Talley NJ. Irritable bowel syndrome and chronic pelvic pain: a population-based study. *J Clin Gastroenterol* 2010;44(10):696–701.

68. Barry MJ, Link CL, McNaughton-Collins MF, McKinlay JB; Boston Area Community Health (BACH) Investigators. Overlap of different urological symptom complexes in a racially and ethnically diverse, community-based population of men and women. *BJU Int* 2008;101(1):45–51.

69. Plesh O, Adams SH, Gansky SA. Temporomandibular joint and muscle disorder-type pain and comorbid pains in a national US sample. *J Orofac Pain* 2011;25(3):190–8.

70. Schürks M, Rist PM, Bigal ME, Buring JE, Lipton RB, Kurth T. Migraine and cardiovascular disease: systematic review and meta-analysis. *BMJ* 2009;339:b3914. doi: 10.1136/bmj.b3914.

71. de Mos M, Huygen FJ, Dieleman JP, Koopman JS, Stricker BH, Sturkenboom MC. Medical history and the onset of complex regional pain syndrome (CRPS). *Pain* 2008;139(2):458–66.

72. Weir PT, Harlan GA, Nkoy FL, et al. The incidence of fibromyalgia and its associated comorbidities: a population-based retrospective cohort study based on International Classification of Diseases, 9th Revision codes. *J Clin Rheumatol* 2006;12(3):124–8.

2

SEX DIFFERENCES IN EXPERIMENTAL PAIN RESPONSES

Christopher D. King, Margarete Ribeiro-Dasilva, and Roger B. Fillingim

INTRODUCTION

Research addressing sex and gender differences in pain has proliferated in recent years. Indeed, as we previously reported, published articles regarding sex, gender, and pain have increased at a substantially higher rate over the past 25–30 years compared to the growth of publications for the pain field in general.[1] This increased interest reflects not only greater attention to clinical and nonhuman animal research but also extends to human laboratory studies that explore sex and gender differences in response to experimentally induced pain. Experimental pain models represent a group of standardized and controlled methods for probing the functioning of the pain system in humans. Other chapters in this volume address the substantial sex and gender differences that have been documented in the prevalence and severity of clinical pain, which represents the public health impetus for the increase in research regarding sex, gender, and pain. More specific to the topic of this chapter, one rationale for investigating sex differences in experimental pain responses is to test the hypothesis that sex differences in nociceptive processing may contribute to the increased burden of clinical pain among women.[2,3] The clinical relevance of experimental pain models has been previously reviewed,[4,5] and increasing evidence supports the assertion that enhanced pain sensitivity represents a preexisting risk factor for increasingly severe acute pain as well as for new onset of chronic pain.[6–8] Thus, if women possess greater pain sensitivity (operationalized using experimental pain models) than men, this may be associated with increased risk for future development of clinical pain in women. Another goal in studying experimental pain responses is to reveal potential sex differences in the functioning of the pain system, which could enhance understanding of mechanisms contributing to pain in a sex-specific manner (for more details, see Chapter 5).

Several recent reviews of the literature regarding sex and gender differences in experimental pain responses are available,[1,9,10] and we will not attempt to reproduce these efforts here. Rather, this chapter endeavors to provide a brief summary of the findings regarding sex differences in experimental pain responses, followed by a discussion of potential biopsychosocial mechanisms contributing to these differences. We will conclude with a summary of the findings and a discussion of clinical relevance and potential future directions.

SEX-RELATED DIFFERENCES IN EXPERIMENTAL PAIN

An abundance of studies has examined sex differences in experimentally induced pain.

Previous qualitative and quantitative reviews by members of our research group[1,3,11] concluded that females display greater sensitivity than males across a range of experimental pain models. Sex differences in experimental pain have been evaluated using a wide range of stimulus modalities, including pressure, electrical, ischemic, thermal, and other models of experimental pain (e.g., chemical). Dynamic models of experimental pain have been used to engage systems underlying facilitation and inhibition of pain. Pain sensitivity has been assessed by a number of different measurement outcomes, including behavioral indices of threshold (defined by time or intensity to the first sensation of pain) and tolerance, and subjective self-report measures of pain intensity and unpleasantness. This section will summarize our recent review,[1] which reported a representative sample of studies published after 1995 regarding sex differences across several pain modalities. Additional studies published since that review have also been added.

Mechanical Pain Stimuli

Mechanical pain includes a family of stimuli, the most common of which are blunt pressure applied to the skin overlying a muscle and punctate (i.e., pinprick) cutaneous mechanical pain. Pressure pain is commonly assessed with pressure algometry, which typically involves applying increasing blunt pressure to a body site and assessing a perceptual endpoint (e.g., the amount of pressure required to first produce pain—the pain threshold). Cutaneous mechanical pain can be assessed with monofilaments (e.g., Von Frey hairs) or with weighted metal probes.[12,13] A previous meta-analytic review found that pressure pain produced the largest and most consistent sex differences.[11] The current list of studies in Table 2.1 supports this observation. Overall, females had lower threshold and tolerance levels, suggesting higher pressure pain sensitivity compared to males with the exception of the study by Nie et al.[14] Two studies found that females provided higher ratings of suprathreshold pressure pain than males, with the sex difference increasing in magnitude with greater stimulus intensity,[15,16] while two studies showed no such sex differences in

suprathreshold pressure pain ratings.[14,17] In contrast, sex differences in cutaneous mechanical pain thresholds have been generally nonsignificant,[18,19] with the exception of one recent study with a very large sample size.[12] In summary, the recent literature continues to provide strong support for the hypothesis that females are more sensitive to pressure pain, though cutaneous mechanical pain thresholds show inconsistent sex differences.

Electrical Pain Stimuli

Pain threshold and tolerance for cutaneous electrical stimuli were significantly lower in healthy females compared to males (Table 2.1). These recent findings present a more consistent picture than the five studies in a previous review,[11] which found that electrical stimuli produced inconsistent findings and a moderate effect size for the sex difference. In addition to perceptual responses, studies of electrical stimuli often assess the nociceptive flexion reflex (NFR), a spinal pain–related muscle reflex, which represents a neurophysiological measure of electrical nociceptive sensitivity.[20] Some studies have demonstrated that lower levels of electrical stimulation are require to elicit an NFR in women than men[21,22]; however, others have shown no sex difference in this reflex.[23–25]

Ischemic Pain Stimuli

Overall, a majority of the studies reported no differences in behavioral or subjective measures of pain during the submaximal effort tourniquet test between males and females (Table 2.1). Two studies reported that males displayed higher pain threshold and/or tolerance.[26,27] Despite large sample sizes for several studies,[27–30] sex differences in ischemic pain have not been statistically significant due to their small effect sizes.

Cold Pain Stimuli

Most studies support the hypothesis that cold pain sensitivity during cold water immersion is more pronounced in females (Table 2.1). Females typically required less time to reach pain threshold and/or tolerance and were more likely to

Table 2.1 Studies Reporting Sex Differences in Experimental Pain Models of Pressure, Electrical, Ischemic, and Thermal Pain

	BEHAVIORAL MEASURES		SUBJECTIVE RATINGS	
	DIFFERENCE	NO DIFFERENCE/MIXED(*)	DIFFERENCE	NO DIFFERENCE
Pressure/ mechanical	Chesterton et al. (2003)[132] Fillingim et al. (2005)[98] Garcia et al. (2007)[136] Kindler et al. (2011)[137] Komiyama & De Laat (2005)[17] Komiyama et al. (2007)[16] Komiyama et al. (2009)[138] Neziri et al. (2011)[139] Wang et al. (2010)[140]	*Ayesh et al. (2007)[133] *Binderup et al. (2010)[135] Nie et al. (2005)[14] Sarlani & Greenspan (2002)[18] Sarlani et al. (2004)[19]	Ellermeir & Westphal (1995)[15] Komiyama et al. (2007)[16]	Komiyama & De Laat (2005)[134] Nie et al. (2005)[14]
Electrical	al' Absi et al. (2006)[141] Ashina et al. (2006)[142] Komiyama et al. (2009)[138] Nyklicek et al. (1999)[143] Rhudy et al. (2010)[144] Goffaux, et al. (2011)	Ayesh et al. (2007)[133]		
Ischemic	Girdler et al. (2005)[27]	Bragdon et al. (2002)[50] Edwards et al. (2004)[28] *Fillingim & Maixner (1996)[26] Fillingim et al. (2005)[98]	Fillingim & Maixner (1996)[26] Girdler et al. (2005)[27]	

Cold	*Jones et al. (2003)[127]	Dixon et al. (2004)[145]	al' Absi et al. (2002)[146]	Baad-Hansen et al. (2005)[39]
	*Keogh et al. (2000)[147]	Edwards et al. (2004)[28]	al' Absi et al. (2003)[148]	Dixon et al. (2004)[145]
	*Neziri et al. (2011)[139]	George et al. (2006)[149]	al' Absi et al. (2004)[150]	Mitchell et al. (2004)[151]
	Pud et al. (2006)[59]	Bento et al. (2010)[152]	Bento et al. (2010)[152]	Ruscheweyh et al. (2010)[153]
		Jackson et al. (2005)[154]	Jackson et al. (2005)[154]	Zimmer et al. (2003)[155]
		Keogh et al. (2005)[156]	Jones et al. (2003)[127]	
		Kim et al. (2004)[157]	Kim et al. (2004)[157]	
		Lowery et al. (2003)[158]	Lowery et al. (2003)[158]	
		Mitchell et al. (2004)[151]	Neziri et al. (2011)[139]	
		Myers et al. (2001)[107]	Nielsen et al. (2008)[159]	
		Thompson et al. (2008)[160]	Pud et al. (2006)[59]	
		Weisenberg et al. (1995)[161]	Sarlani et al. (2003)[162]	
		Zimmer et al. (2003)[155]		
Heat	*Defrin et al. (2009)[163]	al' Absi et al. (2004)[150]	al' Absi et al. (2004)[150]	Fillingim et al. (1998)[164]
	Fillingim & Maixner (1996)[26]	Bragdon et al. (2002)[50]	Fillingim & Maixner (1996)[26]	Nielsen et al. (2008)[159]
	*Fillingim et al. (1998)[164]	Edwards et al. (1999)[165]	Fillingim et al. (2005)[98]	
	*George et al. (2007)[34]	Edwards et al. (2004)[28]	Jensen & Petersen (2006)[166]	
	Jensen & Petersen (2006)[166]	Fillingim et al. (1999a)[167]	Kim et al. (2004a)[157]	
	*Jones et al. (2003)[127]	Fillingim et al. (1999b)[168]	Paulson et al. (1998)	
	*Kindler et al. (2011)[137]	Fillingim et al. (2005)[98]	Sarlani et al. (2003)[162]	
		Girdler et al. (2005)[27]	Treister et al. (2010)[169]	
		Neziri et al. (2011)[139]	Tousignant et al. (2005)[170]	
		Thompson et al. (2008)[160]	Tousignant et al. (2008)[171]	
		Wise et al. (2002)[172]		

Notes: Studies are listed as reporting a significant difference in experimental pain sensitivity.

*Indicates studies reported sex differences on one measure, which was usually tolerance for behavioral measures of pain.

report higher continuous or retrospective pain ratings. Based on the present set of studies, it appears that sex differences in cold pain are consistent, particularly for suprathreshold measures such as tolerance and pain ratings.

Heat Pain Stimuli

The vast majority of studies reported that females were more sensitive to heat pain than males during contact heat or hot water immersion (Table 2.1). Despite the previous conclusion that heat pain produced less consistent sex differences compare to other stimulus modalities,[11] more recent findings consistently demonstrate greater heat pain sensitivity differences among females versus males.

SEX-RELATED DIFFERENCES IN DYNAMIC MODELS OF EXPERIMENTAL PAIN

A number of investigators have used more dynamic models of pain to evaluate sex differences. One could argue that such pain assays, including temporal summation of pain and

tonic pain induced via intramuscular administration of chemical stimuli, may provide more clinically relevant information. These studies also support the previous suggestion that sex differences will be more noticeable with painful stimuli that produce deep, tonic pain.[3]

Temporal Summation of Pain

In general, studies of temporal summation of heat and mechanical pain (Table 2.2) reveal more pronounced temporal summation of pain than males; however, four studies observed no sex differences in temporal summation of heat[31,32] or mechanical[14,33] pain. Sex differences in temporal summation have also been demonstrated in patients with low back pain[34] and temporomandibular disorders.[35] Thus, on balance, the evidence supports the conclusion that temporal summation is greater among females than males.

Spatial Summation

Unlike temporal summation, no differences have been observed between males and females with spatial summation of heat[36,37] or cold

Table 2.2 Studies Reporting Sex Differences in Experimental Pain Models of Temporal Summation Chemical and Muscle Pain, and Pain Inhibition

	DIFFERENCE	NO DIFFERENCE
Temporal summation (Heat)	George et al. (2007)[34] Fillingim et al. (1998)[59] Kindler et al. (2011)[137] Robinson et al. (2004)[112]	Staud et al. (2003)[32] Cathcart et al. (2009)[31]
Temporal summation (Mechanical)	Sarlani & Greenspan (2002)[18] Sarlani et al. (2004)[19] Sarlani et al. (2007)[35]	Nie et al. (2005)[14] Lautenbacher et al. (2008)[33]
Spatial summation		Defrin et al. (2008)[173] Lautenbacher et al. (2001)[37] Martikainen et al. (2004)[38]
Chemical pain	†Baad-Hansen et al. (2005)[39] Gazerani et al. (2005)[40] Gazerani et al. (2007)[174] Frot et al. (2004)[175]	Jensen & Petersen (2006)[166]

(continued)

Table 2.2 *(Continued)*

	DIFFERENCE	NO DIFFERENCE
Muscle pain	Cairns et al. (2001)[176]	
	Cairns et al. (2003)[177]	
	Falla et al. (2008)[178]	
	Gazerani et al. (2006)[179]	
	Ge et al. (2004)[43]	
	Ge et al. (2005a)[180]	
	Ge et al. (2005b)[181]	
	Ge et al. (2006)[182]	
	Svensson et al. (2003)[183]	
Diffuse noxious Inhibitory control	Arendt-Nielson et al. (2008)[184]	Baad-Hansen et al. (2005)[39]
	Ge et al. (2004)[43]	Cathcart et al. (2009)[31]
	Goodin et al. (2009)[48]	Edwards et al. (2003)[185]
	Granot et al. (2008)[44]	France & Suchowiecki (1999)[21]
	Serrao et al. (2004)[25]	France & Suchowiecki (2001)[186]
	Staud et al. (2003)[32]	Lautenbacher et al. (2008)[33]
	Weissman-Fogel et al. (2008)[45]	Martikainen et al. (2004)[38]
		Oono et al. (2008)[187]
		Pud et al. (2005)[188]
		Quiton & Greenspan (2007)[189]
		Rosen et al. (2008)[190]
		Treister et al. (2010)[169]
		Tousignant-Laflamme et al. (2008)[171]
		Wang et al. (2010)[140]
Stress-induced Analgesia	Bragdon et al. (2002)[50]	al' Absi et al. (2003)[148]
	*Girdler et al. (2005)[27]	
	*Koltyn et al. (2001)[49]	
	*Rhudy et al. (2001)[191]	
	Sternberg et al. (2001)[51]	
Habituation	*Hashmi & Davis (2009)[53]	
	*Hashmi & Davis (2010)[192]	
Placebo	Aslaksen et al. (2008)[55]	Olofsen et al. (2007)[60]
	Aslaksen et al. (2011)[57]	
	Compton et al. (2003)[58]	
	Flaten et al. (2006)[56]	
	Pud et al. (2006)	

†Lower pain sensitivity among females than males.

*Greater pain inhibition among females.

pain[38] (Table 2.2). Thus, the current studies do not support sex differences in spatial summation of pain, though additional studies with larger sample sizes would increase confidence in this conclusion.

Capsaicin

Responses to the TRPV1 agonist, capsaicin, have been compared across sexes, and three of these five studies reveal significant sex-related differences in subjective pain ratings, suggesting higher sensitivity in females due to increased activation of C-fibers among females, though one study reported higher ratings of capsaicin pain in males[39] (Table 2.2). However, these observations appear to be dependent on the menstrual cycle, as women were found to report less pain during the luteal phase.[40]

Hypertonic Saline and Glutamate Muscle Injections

These models of chemical pain induction in muscle are likely to provide greater response in females due to their tonic or prolonged duration. All nine of the identified studies involving intramuscular injections of glutamate and hypertonic saline found that females reported more pain compared to males, providing strong support for the hypothesis that females are more sensitive to muscle pain (Table 2.2).

MODULATION OF EXPERIMENTAL PAIN

The experience of pain is influenced by endogenous modulation, which can be assessed in the laboratory setting using different experimental paradigms. Perhaps the most frequently implemented model that represents a dynamic form of endogenous inhibition is diffuse noxious inhibitory controls (DNIC), more recently referred to as conditioned pain modulation.[41] Another form of pain inhibition is stress-induced analgesia (SIA), in which a physical or psychosocial stressor is administered and its effects on experimental pain are measured. In addition, placebo analgesia has been increasingly investigated as an active pain inhibitory process, and several recent studies

have addressed sex differences in placebo analgesia. Finally, two studies examining sex differences in habituation to pain are described later. Sex differences in both basal pain sensitivity and clinical pain may reflect the activity of endogenous pain modulatory systems, which suggests that females and males likely differ in their ability to modulate pain. The available evidence addressing this possibility is reviewed later.

Diffuse Noxious Inhibitory Controls

DNIC refers to a form of endogenous pain modulation in which the perception of one painful stimulus (the test stimulus) is attenuated by a heterotopically applied conditioning stimulus at a remote site. Some investigators have speculated that DNIC may be of substantial clinical relevance because dysfunction in endogenous pain inhibitory systems is believed to contribute to certain chronic pain conditions.[32,42] Over half of the studies (Table 2.2) failed to find significant sex differences in endogenous pain modulation. A few of the studies suggest that DNIC is more pronounced in males than females based on psychophysical[32,43–45] and neurophysiological[25] studies. Based on the available studies, conclusions related to sex-related differences in DNIC remain tentative pending additional studies. A recent meta-analysis of sex differences in DNIC reported that males had more efficient DNIC compared to females on both behavioral and subjective measures of pain based on calculated ratios of percent changes scores.[46] Future research investigating sex differences in DNIC should attend to characteristics of pain induction (e.g., stimulus intensity, duration), stimulation site, and possible role of biological[47] and psychological[48] mediators.

Stress-Induced Analgesia

A majority of studies of SIA indicate that females exhibit more efficient pain inhibitory responses compared to males (Table 2.2). For example, using an isometric handgrip exercise, pressure pain threshold was elevated in females but not males, suggesting that SIA was greater in females.[49] However, sex-related differences in SIA are dependent on the type of stressor and pain modality. In response to a simulated argument stressor, no sex differences in males in stress-induced analgesia emerged, but greater blood pressure the stressor was associated with lower pain sensitivity only among men.[50] Sternberg et al[51] reported that cold pain was reduced during stress associated with competition in males that engaged more cognitive aspects (e.g., video game), while pain was reduced by physical exercise (e.g., treadmill running) in females.

Habituation

Sex differences in the attenuation of pain following repeated painful stimulation have received little attention. In a series of studies by Hashmi and Davis,[52,53] the repeated application of a 30-second thermal pulse produces a greater reduction in females compared to males. Further research is needed to allow definitive conclusions regarding the magnitude and meaning of sex differences in pain habituation.

Placebo Analgesia

As noted in a recent review,[54] data regarding sex differences in placebo analgesia are limited with only a handful of studies comparing responses between males and females. In experimental studies, the magnitude of placebo analgesia appears to be greater in males compared to females during ratings of pain intensity[55,56] and unpleasantness.[57] Clinical studies that compared placebo and drug responses between males and females have given mixed results, and no definitive conclusion can be made. One study reported that males exhibited a greater increase of cold pressor test tolerance with placebo compared to females.[58] Another study reported greater placebo and morphine responses in females as indicated by increased cold pressor test thresholds and lower pain ratings compared to men.[59] Placebo responses were similar across sex in two psychophysical studies comparing alfentanyl[60] and topical lidocaine to placebo,[61] and one clinical study evaluating nalbuphine and placebo on postoperative pain.[62] A meta-analysis by Averbuch and Katzper[63] revealed no sex differences in placebo responses during a clinically relevant pain model (e.g.,

third molar extraction model). Overall, additional studies are needed to determine whether the ability to reduce pain via placebo is comparable between males and females.

Summary of Experimental Pain Findings

A large number of studies using widely varying methodologies have investigated sex differences in experimental pain sensitivity. Based on the overall findings, it can be concluded that females are more sensitive to painful stimulation as assessed in the laboratory. From the pattern of results it is difficult to pinpoint any specific mechanism(s), because the sex differences appear relatively consistently across multiple stimulus modalities. However, the recently developed literature on pain in response to intramuscular injections of algesic substances reveals robust and consistent differences, suggesting that deep, tonic stimuli that mimic clinical musculoskeletal pain may be particularly sensitive to sex differences. Sex differences in endogenous pain modulation have received more limited attention, but the available evidence suggests that males and females may differ in this regard as well, though the direction and magnitude of the effects are quite variable. The mechanisms and practical importance of these sex differences merit further investigation in future studies.

BIOPSYCHOSOCIAL MECHANISMS UNDERLYING SEX DIFFERENCES IN EXPERIMENTAL PAIN RESPONSES

The studies described earlier clearly demonstrate sex differences in responses to experimentally evoked pain, including evidence not only that men and women differ in baseline pain sensitivity but also in measures of endogenous pain modulation. However, the mechanisms responsible for these sex differences are complex and not well understood. Inevitably, multiple factors contribute to sex and gender differences in pain, and for convenience we will describe them as either psychosocial or biological. We recognize the artificiality of this dualistic conceptualization, which refers principally to the level of analysis rather than the actual mechanism of action. For example, stereotypical gender roles are typically represented as a psychosocial variable that contributes to sex differences in pain, based on the assumption that gender roles are learned and therefore reflect the influences of psychosocial processes. However, substantial evidence indicates that gender roles are also influenced by hormonal and neurobiological factors[64] and may therefore represent proxies for these underlying biological processes, which could ultimately account for sex differences in nociceptive responses. Thus, when discussing the putative mechanisms underlying sex differences in pain, the categories "psychosocial" versus "biological" are used for convenience with full knowledge that these terms may actually refer to the same underlying processes described at different levels of analysis. Potential "biological" and "psychosocial" contributions to sex differences in pain have been previously reviewed[3,65–73] and are discussed in more detail elsewhere in this volume (see Chapters 6 and 7). Next, we briefly discuss several biopsychosocial mechanisms that may underlie sex differences in pain sensitivity.

BIOLOGICAL MECHANISMS UNDERLYING SEX DIFFERENCES IN PAIN SENSITIVITY

Sex Hormones

The influence of gonadal hormones extends beyond their reproductive actions and includes effects on memory, emotion, motor coordination, and pain sensitivity. As reviewed elsewhere, abundant evidence indicates that hormonal factors (e.g., menstrual cycle effects, exogenous hormone use) can influence experimental pain responses in humans.[1,68] Estrogens, the most studied gonadal hormones in pain, can potentially affect pain sensitivity via multiple pathways, including influences on the peripheral nervous system and central nervous system, effects on the skeletal system, and immune and cardiovascular influences.[74] Regarding peripheral nervous system and central nervous system pathways, estrogen receptors alpha and beta (ERα and/or ERβ) are located in numerous nervous system structures involved in nociception, including dorsal root

ganglia,[75] the dorsal horn of the spinal cord,[76] the periaqueductal gray,[77] hypothalamus,[78] limbic system,[79] several cortical areas,[80] hippocampus, and basal forebrain.[81] Although abundant evidence supports the influence of estrogens in pain, the exact mechanisms by which estrogens contribute to sex differences in pain responses remain unknown.

Estrogen exerts its effects by binding to extra or intracellular nuclear ERα and ERβ.[82] Some evidence suggests that the effects of estrogens on pain processing may depend on which estrogen receptor subtype is being activated. For example, in mice, estrogen binding to ERβ exerted a pro-nociceptive effect, and binding to ERα produced anti-nociceptive effects during the first phase of the formalin test.[83] In contrast, selective activation of the ERα in the spinal cord of rats was pro-nociceptive in visceral pain.[84] Also, while wild-type female mice showed lower mechanical nociceptive thresholds than males, females lacking either ERα or ERβ did not differ from males in mechanical nociception, either at baseline or after inflammation.[85] This suggests that both estrogen receptor subtypes are important for sex differences in mechanical hyperalgesia. These conflicting findings likely result from differences in the pain models and species used; nonetheless, these data implicate both ER subtypes in altering nociceptive responses. However, additional research is needed to determine the roles of the estrogen receptor subtypes in pain processing.

In addition to estrogens, the functions of other sex steroid hormones, including progesterone and testosterone, differ substantially between the sexes at different life stages and may produce diverse effects on the peripheral and central nervous system. Progesterone receptors are expressed in the central nervous system,[86] including the spinal cord.[87] Progesterone maintained the thermal and tactile hypersensitivity ovariectomized female rats both in the noninjured state and following L5 nerve root ligation.[88] In male rats, testosterone administration has been found to decrease nociceptive responses following inflammatory manipulations, such as formalin- or complete Freund's adjuvant-induced pain.[89,90] In humans, an uncontrolled trial of testosterone supplementation in hypogonadal men with chronic pain showed improvement on one of the included measures of pain intensity.[91]

In summary, gonadal hormones can substantially affect pain processing due to their broad spectrum of action, and they can be a key factor underling sex difference in pain responses. However, understanding of the specific pathways whereby sex hormones produce their effects on pain processing remains limited. Additional research is needed to illuminate the complex mechanisms mediating hormonal contributions to sex differences in pain.

Opioid Mechanisms

The endogenous opioid neurotransmitters and opioid receptors are centrally implicated in responses to stress, in the suppression of pain, and in the action of opiate analgesic drugs.[92] Abundant preclinical evidence demonstrates sex-related differences in functioning of the opioid system. For example, sex differences in antinociceptive responses to opioid compounds have been widely reported,[66,93] and females show lower mu opioid receptor density in the periaqueductal gray compared to males.[94] Human studies examining sex differences in opioid analgesia are discussed elsewhere in this volume (see Chapter 4), and limited data have addressed sex differences in endogenous opioid function in humans. Zubieta and colleagues[95] demonstrated that greater pain-induced activation of brain μ-opioid receptors among men than women, suggesting that the endogenous opioid system may play a more active role in pain modulation for males than females. Such sex differences in opioid system function may be influenced by gonadal hormones; women showed greater baseline μ-opioid receptor availability and higher pain-induced receptor binding in a high-estrogen compared to a low-estrogen state, such that responses of women in the high-estrogen state were comparable to the basal responses observed in men.[96]

Genetic Contributions

As noted elsewhere in this volume (see Chapter 5), sex-dependent genetic contributions to nociceptive responses have been extensively observed in preclinical models, and these genetic influences represent additional mechanisms that could mediate sex differences in pain responses. In a large twin study, the heritability of neck pain was found to be higher among females than males, suggesting a sex difference in the genetic contribution to this pain phenotype.[97] Regarding experimental pain, we previously demonstrated a genetic association of a μ-opioid receptor gene (OPRM1) A118G polymorphism with pressure pain sensitivity, which was significant for males but not females.[98] Moreover, a sex x genotype interaction emerged for heat pain ratings, such that the rare allele conferred reduced heat pain sensitivity in men but increased heat pain sensitivity in women. These human findings suggest the possibility that genetic factors differentially influence pain responses in females and males; however, additional research is needed to further define this important issue.

Brain Mechanisms

Sex differences in cerebral processing of pain-related information may also contribute to differences in pain perception (see Chapter 3). For example, during tonic muscle pain, males displayed signal changes in the dorsolateral prefrontal cortex (DLPFC), whereas females displayed signal changes in the mid-cingulate cortex.[99] In response to nociceptive visceral afferent stimulation, female patients with irritable bowel syndrome show greater activation of areas related to emotional processing (including the ventromedial prefrontal, anterior and infragenual cingulate cortices, and amygdala), whereas males showed greater activation in cognitive areas (e.g., the DLPFC, insular cortex, and dorsal pons).[100] More recently, Goffaux and colleagues[23] found similar spinal reflex responses to electrical pain in males and females; however, females reported greater pain and showed a reduced N150 evoked potential response generated by the medial prefrontal cortex and potentially dampened by negative affect, including anxiety. These findings may suggest a greater cortically mediated emotional response that may contribute to increased pain in women. These sex differences were mediated by trait anxiety, and the authors concluded that increased activation of the medial prefrontal cortex produced increased anxiety leading to greater pain among women. Thus, sex differences in cerebral processing of pain likely contribute to differences in pain sensitivity.

Anatomical Differences

Some investigators have suggested that sex differences in body size may contribute to sex differences in pain perception, based on the notion that density of peripheral nociceptors would be inversely related to body size. In support of this possibility, body weight was positively correlated with the threshold for electrical "annoyance," and controlling for body weight rendered the sex difference in electrical annoyance thresholds nonsignificant.[101] In contrast, Lautenbacher and Strian[102] found no association between body size or sex and heat pain thresholds. These researchers subsequently reported greater electrical pain sensitivity in women but found no association between body size and electrical pain responses within males or females.[103] In a recent study, height was associated with cold pain thresholds in women but not men, and women and men of similar heights appeared not to differ in their pain responses.[104] Selim et al[105] reported greater epidermal nerve fiber density (ENFD) in women than men, even after controlling for body mass index, and also greater mechanical pain sensitivity in women. ENFD was weakly correlated with mechanical pain responses, raising the possibility that greater ENFD in women may contribute to their higher mechanical pain sensitivity, though this was not directly addressed. Taken together, these findings provide some evidence that anthropometric factors, such as weight and height, should be accounted for when examining sex differences in pain.

PSYCHOSOCIAL MECHANISMS UNDERLYING SEX DIFFERENCES IN PAIN SENSITIVITY

As described by Keogh in this volume (Chapter 7) and by us previously,[1] multiple psychosocial processes are thought to influence sex differences in pain, including stereotypical gender roles, cognitive processes (e.g., coping, catastrophizing), and affective responses (e.g., anxiety,

depression). Regarding gender roles, several studies have explored the relationship of masculinity and femininity to pain sensitivity (see ref. 70 for a review). For example, higher masculinity relative to femininity predicted lower mechanical[106] and cold pain sensitivity[107,108]; however, sex differences in pain typically remained significant even after controlling for these gender role measures. In addition to these general measures of masculinity and femininity, others have found that pain-related gender roles are also associated with experimental pain responses.[109–112] Also, several studies have reported that experimenter gender influences pain responses, such that males have been found to report less pain in the presence of a female experimenter,[113–116] while other investigators have failed to show any effect of experimenter gender on pain responses.[106,107,117,118] Thus, some evidence relates gender-related constructs (e.g., femininity, masculinity) to pain responses; however, stereotypical gender roles do not typically account for sex differences in pain perception.

Cognitive/affective factors significantly influence pain responses and represent potential determinants of sex differences in pain.[71,72] Regarding cognitive processes, sex differences in pain coping and catastrophizing have been widely reported.[1] Indeed higher levels of catastrophizing have been found among healthy women versus men,[28,119,120] and in one study catastrophizing mediated sex differences in recent daily pain but not the sex difference in heat pain sensitivity.[28] More recently, women were found to report higher catastrophizing and lower challenge appraisals (i.e., they were less likely to conceptualize the experimental pain task as a challenge), and catastrophizing but not challenge appraisals mediated sex differences in experimental pain responses.[121] Regarding affective processes, both anxiety and depression are more common among women than men,[122–125] and both of these affective constructs are strongly associated with pain. Interestingly, anxiety appears to be more strongly related to experimental pain responses among men than women,[126–128] while limited information has addressed whether depression is differentially related to experimental pain responses across sexes.[1] The "psychosocial" factors appear to contribute importantly to sex differences in pain sensitivity, and additional information regarding the association of psychological factors with experimental pain responses can be found elsewhere in this volume (see Chapter 7).

CONCLUSIONS AND FUTURE DIRECTIONS

This chapter summarizes recent research regarding sex differences in responses to experimentally evoked pain and discusses biological and psychosocial factors that may account for such differences. The evidence reviewed generates several overarching conclusions, including the following: (1) Across most experimental pain modalities, the direction of sex differences in basal pain sensitivity is remarkably consistent, with women exhibiting greater sensitivity (e.g., lower threshold and tolerance and higher pain ratings) than men; (2) using dynamic pain models (e.g., temporal summation of pain), which may be more clinically relevant, a similar pattern of results emerges; (3) studies of DNIC, a measure of endogenous pain inhibitory capacity, show more robust pain inhibition among men than women; (4) other assays of endogenous pain modulation show less consistent sex differences; and (5) a multitude of biopsychosocial variables have been found to contribute to sex differences in experimental pain responses.

Moving beyond these general conclusions, there are several important questions to be addressed by future research. First, to what extent are sex differences in experimental pain responses associated with sex differences in clinical pain? Increasing evidence demonstrates that laboratory measures of pain sensitivity and endogenous pain inhibition predict the severity of subsequent clinical pain[8] and the future development of chronic pain.[129-131] However, whether increased pain sensitivity among women explains sex differences in their greater incidence or severity of future clinical pain has not been directly investigated. If experimental pain sensitivity were found to mediate sex differences in clinical pain development, this would support additional research to further elucidate the mechanisms underlying sex differences in

pain sensitivity, since these mechanisms would likely contribute to sex differences in clinical pain. Second, to what extent are sex differences in experimental pain mediated by response biases (e.g., stoicism in men vs. pain expression in women)? This issue is particularly relevant to the influence of gender roles on pain responses because one interpretation of these findings is that women and men do not experience pain differently; women simply express pain more openly, whereas men deny it. An alternative hypothesis is that the biological mechanisms that in part drive gender roles, including both genetic and early hormonal influences, also influence nociceptive sensitivity. Moreover, the cognitive and affective correlates of gender roles are able to directly influence pain responses by engaging pain modulatory processes. In other words, while there may be sex differences in willingness to report pain, this may actually reflect rather than produce sex differences in pain responses. Thus, an important target for future research is to better understand interactions between "biological" and "psychological" factors. Elucidating the biological pathways whereby psychological processes exert their influences on pain, and vice versa, could lead to novel pain treatments for both women and men.

REFERENCES

1. Fillingim RB, King CD, Ribeiro-Dasilva MC, Rahim-Williams B, Riley JL, III. Sex, gender, and pain: a review of recent clinical and experimental findings. *J Pain* 2009;10(5):447–85.
2. Cairns BE. The influence of gender and sex steroids on craniofacial nociception. *Headache* 2007;47(2):319–24.
3. Fillingim RB, Maixner W. Gender differences in the responses to noxious stimuli. *Pain Forum* 1995;4(4):209–21.
4. Edwards RR. Individual differences in endogenous pain modulation as a risk factor for chronic pain. *Neurology* 2005;65(3):437–43.
5. Edwards RR, Sarlani E, Wesselmann U, Fillingim RB. Quantitative assessment of experimental pain perception: multiple domains of clinical relevance. *Pain* 2005;114:315–9.
6. Diatchenko L, Nackley AG, Slade GD, Fillingim RB, Maixner W. Idiopathic pain disorders—pathways of vulnerability. *Pain* 2006;123(3):226–30.

7. Yarnitsky D, Crispel Y, Eisenberg E, et al. Prediction of chronic post-operative pain: pre-operative DNIC testing identifies patients at risk. *Pain* 2008;138(1):22–8.

8. Kehlet H, Jensen TS, Woolf CJ. Persistent post-surgical pain: risk factors and prevention. *Lancet* 2006;367(9522):1618–25.

9. Hurley RW, Adams MC. Sex, gender, and pain: an overview of a complex field. *Anesth Analg* 2008;107(1):309–17.

10. Paller CJ, Campbell CM, Edwards RR, Dobs AS. Sex-based differences in pain perception and treatment. *Pain Med* 2009;10(2):289–99.

11. Riley JL, Robinson ME, Wise EA, Myers CD, Fillingim RB. Sex differences in the perception of noxious experimental stimuli: a meta-analysis. *Pain* 1998;74:181–7.

12. Greenspan JD, Slade GD, Bair E, et al. Pain sensitivity risk factors for chronic TMD: descriptive data and empirically identified domains from the OPPERA case control study. *J Pain* 2011;12:T61–74.

13. Rolke R, Magerl W, Campbell KA, et al. Quantitative sensory testing: a comprehensive protocol for clinical trials. *Eur J Pain* 2006;10(1):77–88.

14. Nie H, Arendt-Nielsen L, Andersen H, Graven-Nielsen T. Temporal summation of pain evoked by mechanical stimulation in deep and superficial tissue. *J Pain* 2005;6(6):348–55.

15. Ellermeier W, Westphal W. Gender differences in pain ratings and pupil reactions to painful pressure stimuli. *Pain* 1995;61:435–9.

16. Komiyama O, Kawara M, De Laat A. Ethnic differences regarding tactile and pain thresholds in the trigeminal region. *J Pain* 2007;8(4):363–9.

17. Komiyama O, De Laat A. Tactile and pain thresholds in the intra- and extra-oral regions of symptom-free subjects. *Pain* 2005;115(3):308–15.

18. Sarlani E, Greenspan JD. Gender differences in temporal summation of mechanically evoked pain. *Pain* 2002;97(1–2):163–9.

19. Sarlani E, Grace EG, Reynolds MA, Greenspan JD. Sex differences in temporal summation of pain and aftersensations following repetitive noxious mechanical stimulation. *Pain* 2004;109(1–2):115–23.

20. Rhudy JL, France CR. Defining the nociceptive flexion reflex (NFR) threshold in human participants: a comparison of different scoring criteria. *Pain* 2007;128(3):244–53.

21. France CR, Suchowiecki S. A comparison of diffuse noxious inhibitory controls in men and women. *Pain* 1999;81(1–2):77–84.

22. Mylius V, Kunz M, Schepelmann K, Lautenbacher S. Sex differences in nociceptive withdrawal reflex and pain perception. *Somatosens Mot Res* 2005;22(3):207–11.

23. Goffaux P, Michaud K, Gaudreau J, Chalaye P, Rainville P, Marchand S. Sex differences in perceived pain are affected by an anxious brain. *Pain* 2011;152(9):1065–73.

24. Neziri AY, Andersen OK, Petersen-Felix S, et al. The nociceptive withdrawal reflex: normative values of thresholds and reflex receptive fields. *Eur J Pain* 2010;14(2):134–41.

25. Serrao M, Rossi P, Sandrini G, et al. Effects of diffuse noxious inhibitory controls on temporal summation of the RIII reflex in humans. *Pain* 2004;112(3):353–60.

26. Fillingim RB, Maixner W. The influence of resting blood pressure and gender on pain responses. *Psychosom Med* 1996;58:326–32.

27. Girdler SS, Maixner W, Naftel HA, Stewart PW, Moretz RL, Light KC. Cigarette smoking, stress-induced analgesia and pain perception in men and women. *Pain* 2005;114(3):372–85.

28. Edwards RR, Haythornthwaite JA, Sullivan MJ, Fillingim RB. Catastrophizing as a mediator of sex differences in pain: differential effects for daily pain versus laboratory-induced pain. *Pain* 2004;111(3):335–41.

29. Fillingim RB, Hastie BA, Ness TJ, Glover TL, Campbell CM, Staud R. Sex-related psychological predictors of baseline pain perception and analgesic responses to pentazocine. *Biological Psychology* 2005;69:97–112.

30. Fillingim RB, Kaplan L, Staud R, et al. The A118G single nucleotide polymorphism of the mu-opioid receptor gene (OPRM1) is associated with pressure pain sensitivity in humans. *J Pain* 2005;6(3):159–67.

31. Cathcart S, Winefield AH, Rolan P, Lushington K. Reliability of temporal summation and diffuse noxious inhibitory control. *Pain Res Manage* 2009;14(6):433–8.

32. Staud R, Robinson ME, Vierck CJ, Jr., Price DD. Diffuse noxious inhibitory controls (DNIC) attenuate temporal summation of second pain in normal males but not in normal females or fibromyalgia patients. *Pain* 2003;101(1–2):167–74.

33. Lautenbacher S, Kunz M, Burkhardt S. The effects of DNIC-type inhibition on temporal summation compared to single pulse processing: does sex matter? *Pain* 2008;140(3):429–35.

34. George SZ, Wittmer VT, Fillingim RB, Robinson ME. Sex and pain-related psychological variables are associated with thermal pain sensitivity

for patients with chronic low back pain. *J Pain* 2007;8(1):2–10.

35. Sarlani E, Garrett PH, Grace EG, Greenspan JD. Temporal summation of pain characterizes women but not men with temporomandibular disorders. *J Orofac Pain* 2007;21(4):309–17.

36. Defrin R, Benstein-Sheraizin A, Bezalel A, Mantzur O, Arendt-Nielsen L. The spatial characteristics of the painful thermal grill illusion. *Pain* 2008;138(3):577–86.

37. Lautenbacher S, Nielsen J, Andersen T, Arendt-Nielsen L. Spatial summation of heat pain in males and females. *Somatosens Mot Res* 2001;18(2):101–5.

38. Martikainen IK, Narhi MV, Pertovaara A. Spatial integration of cold pressor pain sensation in humans. *Neurosci Lett* 2004;361(1–3):140–3.

39. Baad-Hansen L, Poulsen HF, Jensen HM, Svensson P. Lack of sex differences in modulation of experimental intraoral pain by diffuse noxious inhibitory controls (DNIC). *Pain* 2005;116(3):359–65.

40. Gazerani P, Andersen OK, Arendt-Nielsen L. A human experimental capsaicin model for trigeminal sensitization. Gender-specific differences. *Pain* 2005;118(1–2):155–63.

41. Yarnitsky D, Arendt-Nielsen L, Bouhassira D, et al. Recommendations on terminology and practice of psychophysical DNIC testing. *Eur J Pain* 2010;14(4):339.

42. King CD, Wong F, Currie T, Mauderli AP, Fillingim RB, Riley JL, III. Deficiency in endogenous modulation of prolonged heat pain in patients with irritable bowel syndrome and temporomandibular disorder. *Pain* 2009;143(3):172–8.

43. Ge HY, Madeleine P, Arendt-Nielsen L. Sex differences in temporal characteristics of descending inhibitory control: an evaluation using repeated bilateral experimental induction of muscle pain. *Pain* 2004;110(1–2):72–8.

44. Granot M, Weissman-Fogel I, Crispel Y, et al. Determinants of endogenous analgesia magnitude in a diffuse noxious inhibitory control (DNIC) paradigm: do conditioning stimulus painfulness, gender and personality variables matter? *Pain* 2008;136:142–9.

45. Weissman-Fogel I, Sprecher E, Pud D. Effects of catastrophizing on pain perception and pain modulation. *Exp Brain Res* 2008;186(1):79–85.

46. Popescu A, LeResche L, Truelove EL, Drangsholt MT. Gender differences in pain modulation by diffuse noxious inhibitory controls: a systematic review. *Pain* 2010;150(2):309–18.

47. Tousignant-Laflamme Y, Marchand S. Excitatory and inhibitory pain mechanisms during the menstrual cycle in healthy women. *Pain* 2009;146(1–2):47–55.

48. Goodin BR, McGuire L, Allshouse M, et al. Associations between catastrophizing and endogenous pain-inhibitory processes: sex differences. *J Pain* 2009;10(2):180–90.

49. Koltyn KF, Trine MR, Stegner AJ, Tobar DA. Effect of isometric exercise on pain perception and blood pressure in men and women. *Med Sci Sports Exerc* 2001;33(2):282–90.

50. Bragdon EE, Light KC, Costello NL, et al. Group differences in pain modulation: pain-free women compared to pain-free men and to women with TMD. *Pain* 2002;96(3):227–37.

51. Sternberg WF, Bokat C, Kass L, Alboyadjian A, Gracely RH. Sex-dependent components of the analgesia produced by athletic competition. *Journal of Pain* 2001;2:65–74.

52. Hashmi JA, Davis KD. Effects of temperature on heat pain adaptation and habituation in men and women. *Pain* 2010;151(3):737–43.

53. Hashmi JA, Davis KD. Women experience greater heat pain adaptation and habituation than men. *Pain* 2009;145(3):350–7.

54. Klosterhalfen S, Enck P. Neurophysiology and psychobiology of the placebo response. *Curr Opin Psychiatry* 2008;21(2):189–95.

55. Aslaksen PM, Flaten MA. The roles of physiological and subjective stress in the effectiveness of a placebo on experimentally induced pain. *Psychosom Med* 2008;70(7):811–8.

56. Flaten MA, Aslaksen PM, Finset A, Simonsen T, Johansen O. Cognitive and emotional factors in placebo analgesia. *J Psychosom Res* 2006;61(1):81–9.

57. Aslaksen PM, Bystad M, Vambheim SM, Flaten MA. Gender differences in placebo analgesia: event-related potentials and emotional modulation. *Psychosom Med* 2011;73(2):193–9.

58. Compton P, Charuvastra V, Ling W. Effect of oral ketorolac and gender on human cold pressor pain tolerance. *Clin Exp Pharmacol Physiol* 2003;30(10):759–63.

59. Pud D, Yarnitsky D, Sprecher E, Rogowski Z, Adler R, Eisenberg E. Can personality traits and gender predict the response to morphine? An experimental cold pain study. *Eur J Pain* 2006;10(2):103–12.

60. Olofsen E, Romberg R, Bijl H, et al. Alfentanil and placebo analgesia: no sex differences detected in models of experimental pain. *Anesthesiology* 2005;103(1):130–9.

61. Robinson ME, Riley JL, Brown FF, Gremillion H. Sex differences in response to cutaneous anesthesia—a double blind randomized study. *Pain* 1998;77(2):143–9.

62. Gear RW, Miaskowski C, Gordon NC, Paul SM, Heller PH, Levine JD. The kappa opioid nalbuphine produces gender- and dose-dependent analgesia and antianalgesia in patients with postoperative pain. *Pain* 1999;83(2):339–45.

63. Averbuch M, Katzper M. Gender and the placebo analgesic effect in acute pain. *Clin Pharmacol Ther* 2001;70(3):287–91.

64. Hines M. Gender development and the human brain. *Annu Rev Neurosci* 2011;34:69–88.

65. Aloisi AM, Bonifazi M. Sex hormones, central nervous system and pain. *Horm Behav* 2006;50(1):1–7.

66. Craft RM, Mogil JS, Aloisi AM. Sex differences in pain and analgesia: the role of gonadal hormones. *Eur J Pain* 2004;8(5):397–411.

67. Craft RM. Modulation of pain by estrogens. *Pain* 2007;132(Suppl 1):S3–12.

68. Fillingim RB, Ness TJ. Sex-related hormonal influences on pain and analgesic responses. *Neuroscience and Biobehavioral Reviews* 2000;24:485–501.

69. Craft RM. Sex differences in drug- and non-drug-induced analgesia. *Life Sci* 2003;72(24): 2675–88.

70. Bernardes SF, Keogh E, Lima ML. Bridging the gap between pain and gender research: a selective literature review. *Eur J Pain* 2008;12(4):427–40.

71. Myers CD, Riley JL, III, Robinson ME. Psychosocial contributions to sex-correlated differences in pain. *Clin J Pain* 2003;19(4):225–32.

72. Robinson ME, Riley JL, III, Myers CD. Psychosocial contributions to sex-related differences in pain responses. In: Fillingim RB, ed. *Sex, Gender, and Pain*. Seattle, WA: IASP Press; 2000: 41–68.

73. Jones A, Zachariae R. Gender, anxiety, and experimental pain sensitivity: an overview. *J Am Med Womens Assoc* 2002;57(2):91–4.

74. Craft RM. Modulation of pain by estrogens. *Pain* 2007;132(Suppl 1):S3–12.

75. Patrone C, Andersson S, Korhonen L, Lindholm D. Estrogen receptor-dependent regulation of sensory neuron survival in developing dorsal root ganglion. *Proc Natl Acad Sci USA* 1999;96(19):10905–10.

76. Amandusson A, Hermanson O, Blomqvist A. Estrogen receptor-like immunoreactivity in the medullary and spinal dorsal horn of the female rat. *Neurosci Lett* 1995;196(1–2):25–8.

77. Vanderhorst VG, Schasfoort FC, Meijer E, van Leeuwen FW, Holstege G. Estrogen receptor-alpha-immunoreactive neurons in the periaqueductal gray of the adult ovariectomized female cat. *Neurosci Lett* 1998;240(1):13–6.

78. Mori H, Matsuda K, Pfaff DW, Kawata M. A recently identified hypothalamic nucleus expressing estrogen receptor alpha. *Proc Natl Acad Sci USA* 2008;105(36):13632–7.

79. Ter Horst GJ. Estrogen in the limbic system. *Vitam Horm* 2010;82:319–338.

80. Kritzer MF. Regional, laminar, and cellular distribution of immunoreactivity for ER alpha and ER beta in the cerebral cortex of hormonally intact, adult male and female rats. *Cereb Cortex* 2002;12(2):116–28.

81. Blurton-Jones M, Tuszynski MH. Estrogen receptor-beta colocalizes extensively with parvalbumin-labeled inhibitory neurons in the cortex, amygdala, basal forebrain, and hippocampal formation of intact and ovariectomized adult rats. *J Comp Neurol* 2002;452(3):276–87.

82. Laflamme N, Nappi RE, Drolet G, Labrie C, Rivest S. Expression and neuropeptidergic characterization of estrogen receptors (ERalpha and ERbeta) throughout the rat brain: anatomical evidence of distinct roles of each subtype. *J Neurobiol* 1998;36(3):357–78.

83. Coulombe MA, Spooner MF, Gaumond I, Carrier JC, Marchand S. Estrogen receptors beta and alpha have specific pro- and anti-nociceptive actions. *Neuroscience* 2011;184:172–82.

84. Ji Y, Tang B, Traub RJ. Spinal estrogen receptor alpha mediates estradiol-induced pronociception in a visceral pain model in the rat. *Pain* 2011;152(5):1182–91.

85. Li L, Fan X, Warner M, Xu XJ, Gustafsson JA, Wiesenfeld-Hallin Z. Ablation of estrogen receptor alpha or beta eliminates sex differences in mechanical pain threshold in normal and inflamed mice. *Pain* 2009;143(1–2):37–40.

86. Warembourg M, Logeat F, Milgrom E. Immunocytochemical localization of progesterone receptor in the guinea pig central nervous system. *Brain Res* 1986;384(1):121–31.

87. Labombarda F, Guennoun R, Gonzalez S, et al. Immunocytochemical evidence for a progesterone receptor in neurons and glial cells of the rat spinal cord. *Neurosci Lett* 2000;288(1):29–32.

88. LaCroix-Fralish ML, Tawfik VL, Nutile-McMenemy N, DeLeo JA. Progesterone mediates gonadal hormone differences in tactile and thermal hypersensitivity following L5 nerve root ligation in female rats. *Neuroscience* 2006;138(2):601–8.

89. Aloisi AM, Ceccarelli I, Fiorenzani P, De Padova AM, Massafra C. Testosterone affects formalin-induced responses differently in male and female rats. *Neurosci Lett* 2004;361(1–3): 262–4.

90. Harbuz MS, Perveen-Gill Z, Lightman SL, Jessop DS. A protective role for testosterone in adjuvant-induced arthritis. *Br J Rheumatol* 1995;34(12):1117–22.

91. Aloisi AM, Ceccarelli I, Carlucci M, et al. Hormone replacement therapy in morphine-induced hypogonadic male chronic pain patients. *Reprod Biol Endocrinol* 2011;9:26.

92. Bodnar RJ. Endogenous opiates and behavior: 2009. *Peptides* 2010;31(12):2325–59.

93. Craft RM. Sex differences in opioid analgesia: from mouse to man. *Clin J Pain* 2003;19:175–86.

94. Bernal SA, Morgan MM, Craft RM. PAG mu opioid receptor activation underlies sex differences in morphine antinociception. *Behav Brain Res* 2007;177(1):126–33.

95. Zubieta JK, Smith YR, Bueller JA et al. mu-opioid receptor-mediated antinociceptive responses differ in men and women. *J Neurosci* 2002;22(12):5100–7.

96. Smith YR, Stohler CS, Nichols TE, Bueller JA, Koeppe RA, Zubieta JK. Pronociceptive and antinociceptive effects of estradiol through endogenous opioid neurotransmission in women. *J Neurosci* 2006;26(21):5777–85.

97. Fejer R, Hartvigsen J, Kyvik KO. Sex differences in heritability of neck pain. *Twin Res Hum Genet* 2006;9(2):198–204.

98. Fillingim RB, Kaplan L, Staud R, et al. The A118G single nucleotide polymorphism of the mu-opioid receptor gene (OPRM1) is associated with pressure pain sensitivity in humans. *J Pain* 2005;6(3):159–67.

99. Henderson LA, Gandevia SC, Macefield VG. Gender differences in brain activity evoked by muscle and cutaneous pain: a retrospective study of single-trial fMRI data. *Neuroimage* 2008;39(4):1867–76.

100. Naliboff BD, Berman S, Chang L et al. Sex-related differences in IBS patients: central processing of visceral stimuli. *Gastroenterology* 2003;124(7):1738–1747.

101. Larkin WD, Reilly JP, Kittler LB. Individual differences in sensitivity to transient electrocutaneous stimulation. *IEEE Trans Biomed Eng* 1986;33:495–04.

102. Lautenbacher S, Strian F. Sex differences in pain and thermal sensitivity: the role of body size. *Percept Psychophys* 1991;50:179–83.

103. Lautenbacher S, Rollman GB. Sex differences in responsiveness to painful and non-painful stimuli are dependent upon the stimulation method. *Pain* 1993;53:255–64.

104. Tashani OA, Alabas OA, Johnson MI. Cold pressor pain responses in healthy Libyans: effect of sex/gender, anxiety, and body size. *Gend Med* 2010;7(4):309–19.

105. Selim MM, Wendelschafer-Crabb G, Hodges JS, et al. Variation in quantitative sensory testing and epidermal nerve fiber density in repeated measurements. *Pain* 2010;151(3):575–81.

106. Otto MW, Dougher MJ. Sex differences and personality factors in responsivity to pain. *Percept Mot Skills* 1985;61:383–90.

107. Myers CD, Robinson ME, Riley JL, III, Sheffield D. Sex, gender, and blood pressure: contributions to experimental pain report. *Psychosom Med* 2001;63(4):545–50.

108. Thorn BE, Clements KL, Ward LC, et al. Personality factors in the explanation of sex differences in pain catastrophizing and response to experimental pain. *Clin J Pain* 2004;20(5):275–82.

109. Nayak S, Shiflett SC, Eshun S, Levine FM. Culture and gender effects in pain beliefs and the prediction of pain tolerance. *Cross-Cultural Res* 2000;34(2):135–51.

110. Pool GJ, Schwegler AF, Theodore BR, Fuchs PN. Role of gender norms and group identification on hypothetical and experimental pain tolerance. *Pain* 2007;129(1–2):122–9.

111. Robinson ME, Riley JL, III, Myers CD, et al. Gender role expectations of pain: relationship to sex differences in pain. *J Pain* 2001;2:251–7.

112. Robinson ME, Wise EA, Gagnon C, Fillingim RB, Price DD. Influences of gender role and anxiety on sex differences in temporal summation of pain. *J Pain* 2004;5(2):77–82.

113. Aslaksen PM, Myrbakk IN, Hoifodt RS, Flaten MA. The effect of experimenter gender on autonomic and subjective responses to pain stimuli. *Pain* 2007;129(3):260–8.

114. Gijsbers K, Nicholson F. Experimental pain thresholds influenced by sex of experimenter. *Percept Mot Skills* 2005;101(3):803–7.

115. Kallai I, Barke A, Voss U. The effects of experimenter characteristics on pain reports in women and men. *Pain* 2004;112(1–2):142–7.

116. Levine FM, De Simone LL. The effects of experimenter gender on pain report in male and female subjects. *Pain* 1991;44:69–72.

117. Bush FM, Harkins SW, Harrington WG, Price DD. Analysis of gender effects on pain perception and symptom presentation in temporomandibular joint pain. *Pain* 1993;53:73–80.

118. Essick G, Guest S, Martinez E, Chen C, McGlone F. Site-dependent and subject-related variations in perioral thermal sensitivity. *Somatosens Mot Res* 2004;21(3–4):159–75.

119. Fillingim RB, Wilkinson CS, Powell T. Self-reported abuse history and pain complaints among healthy young adults. *Clin J Pain* 1999;15: 85–91.

120. Osman A, Barrios FX, Gutierrez PM, Kopper BA, Merrifield T, Grittmann L. The Pain Catastrophizing Scale: further psychometric evaluation with adult samples. *J Behav Med* 2000;23(4):351–65.

121. Forsythe LP, Thorn B, Day M, Shelby G. Race and sex differences in primary appraisals, cata-strophizing, and experimental pain outcomes. *J Pain* 2011;12(5):563–72.

122. Bekker MH, van Mens-Verhulst J. Anxiety dis-orders: sex differences in prevalence, degree, and background, but gender-neutral treat-ment. *Gend Med* 2007;4(Suppl B):S178–93.

123. Toufexis DJ, Myers KM, Davis M. The effect of gonadal hormones and gender on anxi-ety and emotional learning. *Horm Behav* 2006;50(4):539–49.

124. Munce SE, Stewart DE. Gender differences in depression and chronic pain conditions in a national epidemiologic survey. *Psychosomatics* 2007;48(5):394–9.

125. Silverstein B. Gender differences in the preva-lence of somatic versus pure depression: a rep-lication. *Am J Psychiatry* 2002;159(6):1051–2.

126. Fillingim RB, Keefe FJ, Light KC, Booker DK, Maixner W. The influence of gender and psy-chological factors on pain perception. *J Gender Cult Health* 1996;1:21–36.

127. Jones A, Zachariae R, Arendt-Nielsen L. Dispositional anxiety and the experience of pain: gender-specific effects. *Eur J Pain* 2003;7(5):387–95.

128. Jones A, Zachariae R. Investigation of the interactive effects of gender and psychological factors on pain response. *Br J Health Psychol* 2004;9(Pt 3):405–18.

129. Diatchenko L, Slade GD, Nackley AG, et al. Genetic basis for individual variations in pain perception and the development of a chronic pain condition. *Hum Mol Genet* 2005;14(1): 135–143.

130. Kasch H, Qerama E, Bach FW, Jensen TS. Reduced cold pressor pain tolerance in non-recovered whiplash patients: a 1-year pro-spective study. *Eur J Pain* 2005;9(5):561–9.

131. Yarnitsky D, Crispel Y, Eisenberg E, et al. Prediction of chronic post-operative pain: pre-operative DNIC testing identifies patients at risk. *Pain* 2008;138(1):22–8.

132. Chesterton LS, Barlas P, Foster NE, Baxter GD, Wright CC. Gender differences in pressure pain threshold in healthy humans. *Pain* 2003;101(3): 259–66.

133. Ayesh EE, Jensen TS, Svensson P. Somatosensory function following painful repetitive electrical stimulation of the human temporomandibular joint and skin. *Exp Brain Res* 2007;179(3):415–25.

134. Meagher MW, Arnau RC, Rhudy JL. Pain and emotion: effects of affective picture modula-tion. *Psychosom Med* 2001;63(1):79–90.

135. Binderup AT, Arendt-Nielsen L, Madeleine P. Pressure pain sensitivity maps of the neck-shoulder and the low back regions in men and women. *BMC Musculoskelet Disord* 2010;11:234.

136. Garcia E, Godoy-Izquierdo D, Godoy JF, Perez M, Lopez-Chicheri I. Gender differ-ences in pressure pain threshold in a repeated measures assessment. *Psychol Health Med* 2007;12(5):567–79.

137. Kindler LL, Valencia C, Fillingim RB, George SZ. Sex differences in experimental and clini-cal pain sensitivity for patients with shoulder pain. *Eur J Pain* 2011;15(2):118–23.

138. Komiyama O, Wang K, Svensson P, Arendt-Nielsen L, Kawara M, De LA. Ethnic differences regarding sensory, pain, and reflex responses in the trigeminal region. *Clin Neurophysiol* 2009;120(2):384–9.

139. Neziri AY, Scaramozzino P, Andersen OK, Dickenson AH, Arendt-Nielsen L, Curatolo M. Reference values of mechanical and thermal pain tests in a pain-free population. *Eur J Pain* 2011;15(4):376–83.

140. Wang K, Svensson P, Sessle BJ, Cairns BE, Arendt-Nielsen L. Painful conditioning stimuli of the craniofacial region evokes diffuse nox-ious inhibitory controls in men and women. *J Orofac Pain* 2010;24(3):255–61.

141. al'Absi M, France C, Harju A, France J, Wittmers L. Adrenocortical and nociceptive responses to opioid blockade in hypertension-prone men and women. *Psychosom Med* 2006;68(2):292–8.

142. Ashina S, Bendtsen L, Ashina M, Magerl W, Jensen R. Generalized hyperalgesia in patients with chronic tension-type headache. *Cephalalgia* 2006;26(8):940–8.

143. Nyklicek I, Vingerhoets AJ, Van Heck GL. Hypertension and pain sensitivity: effects of gender and cardiovascular reactivity. *Biol Psychol* 1999;50(2):127–42.

144. Rhudy JL, Bartley EJ, Williams AE, et al. Are there sex differences in affective modula-tion of spinal nociception and pain? *J Pain* 2010;11(12):1429–41.

145. Dixon KE, Thorn BE, Ward LC. An evaluation of sex differences in psychological and physiological responses to experimentally-induced pain: a path analytic description. *Pain* 2004;112(1–2): 188–96.

146. al'Absi M, Petersen KL, Wittmers LE. Adrenocortical and hemodynamic predictors of pain perception in men and women. *Pain* 2002;96(1–2):197–204.

147. Keogh E, Hatton K, Ellery D. Avoidance versus focused attention and the perception of pain: differential effects for men and women. *Pain* 2000;85(1–2):225–30.

148. al'Absi M, Petersen KL. Blood pressure but not cortisol mediates stress effects on subsequent pain perception in healthy men and women. *Pain* 2003;106(3):285–95.

149. George SZ, Dannecker EA, Robinson ME. Fear of pain, not pain catastrophizing, predicts acute pain intensity, but neither factor predicts tolerance or blood pressure reactivity: an experimental investigation in pain-free individuals. *Eur J Pain* 2006;10(5):457–65.

150. al'Absi M, Wittmers LE, Ellestad D, et al. Sex differences in pain and hypothalamic-pituitary-adrenocortical responses to opioid blockade. *Psychosom Med* 2004;66(2):198–206.

151. Mitchell LA, MacDonald RA, Brodie EE. Temperature and the cold pressor test. *J Pain* 2004;5(4):233–7.

152. Bento SP, Goodin BR, Fabian LA, Page GG, Quinn NB, McGuire L. Perceived control moderates the influence of active coping on salivary cortisol response to acute pain among women but not men. *Psychoneuroendocrinology* 2010;35(6):944–8.

153. Ruscheweyh R, Stumpenhorst F, Knecht S, Marziniak M. Comparison of the cold pressor test and contact thermode-delivered cold stimuli for the assessment of cold pain sensitivity. *J Pain* 2010;11(8):728–36.

154. Jackson T, Iezzi T, Chen H, Ebnet S, Eglitis K. Gender, interpersonal transactions, and the perception of pain: an experimental analysis. *J Pain* 2005;6(4):228–36.

155. Zimmer C, Basler HD, Vedder H, Lautenbacher S. Sex differences in cortisol response to noxious stress. *Clin J Pain* 2003;19(4):233–9.

156. Keogh E, Bond FW, Hanmer R, Tilston J. Comparing acceptance- and control-based coping instructions on the cold-pressor pain experiences of healthy men and women. *Eur J Pain* 2005;9(5):591–8.

157. Kim H, Neubert JK, Rowan JS, Brahim JS, Iadarola MJ, Dionne RA. Comparison of experimental and acute clinical pain responses in humans as pain phenotypes. *J Pain* 2004;5(7): 377–84.

158. Lowery D, Fillingim RB, Wright RA. Sex differences and incentive effects on perceptual and cardiovascular responses to cold pressor pain. *Psychosom Med* 2003;65(2):284–91.

159. Nielsen CS, Stubhaug A, Price DD, Vassend O, Czajkowski N, Harris JR. Individual differences in pain sensitivity: genetic and environmental contributions. *Pain* 2008;136:21–9.

160. Thompson T, Keogh E, French CC, Davis R. Anxiety sensitivity and pain: generalisability across noxious stimuli. *Pain* 2008;134(1–2): 187–96.

161. Weisenberg M, Tepper I, Schwarzwald J. Humor as a cognitive technique for increasing pain tolerance. *Pain* 1995;63(2):207–12.

162. Sarlani E, Farooq N, Greenspan JD. Gender and laterality differences in thermosensation throughout the perceptible range. *Pain* 2003;106(1–2):9–18.

163. Defrin R, Shramm L, Eli I. Gender role expectations of pain is associated with pain tolerance limit but not with pain threshold. *Pain* 2009;145(1–2):230–36.

164. Fillingim RB, Maixner W, Kincaid S, Silva S. Sex differences in temporal summation but not sensory-discriminative processing of thermal pain. *Pain* 1998;75(1):121–7.

165. Edwards RR, Fillingim RB, Yamauchi S, et al. Effects of gender and acute dental pain on thermal pain responses. *Clin J Pain* 1999;15(3):233–7.

166. Jensen MT, Petersen KL. Gender differences in pain and secondary hyperalgesia after heat/capsaicin sensitization in healthy volunteers. *J Pain* 2006;7(3):211–17.

167. Fillingim RB, Maddux V, Shackelford JM. Sex differences in heat pain thresholds as a function of assessment method and rate of rise. *Somatosensory Motor Res* 1999;16(1):57–62.

168. Fillingim RB, Edwards RR, Powell T. The relationship of sex and clinical pain to experimental pain responses. *Pain* 1999;83:419–25.

169. Treister R, Eisenberg E, Gershon E, Haddad M, Pud D. Factors affecting—and relationships between-different modes of endogenous pain modulation in healthy volunteers. *Eur J Pain* 2010;14(6):608–14.

170. Tousignant-Laflamme Y, Rainville P, Marchand S. Establishing a link between heart rate and pain in healthy subjects: a gender effect. *J Pain* 2005;6(6):341–7.

171. Tousignant-Laflamme Y, Page S, Goffaux P, Marchand S. An experimental model to

measure excitatory and inhibitory pain mechanisms in humans. *Brain Res* 2008;1230:73–9.

172. Wise EA, Price DD, Myers CD, Heft MW, Robinson ME. Gender role expectations of pain: relationship to experimental pain perception. *Pain* 2002;96(3):335–42.

173. Defrin R, Pope G, Davis KD. Interactions between spatial summation, 2-point discrimination and habituation of heat pain. *Eur J Pain* 2008;12(7):900–9.

174. Gazerani P, Andersen OK, Arendt-Nielsen L. Site-specific, dose-dependent, and sex-related responses to the experimental pain model induced by intradermal injection of capsaicin to the foreheads and forearms of healthy humans. *J Orofac Pain* 2007;21(4):289–02.

175. Frot M, Feine JS, Bushnell MC. Sex differences in pain perception and anxiety. A psychophysical study with topical capsaicin. *Pain* 2004;108(3):230–6.

176. Cairns BE, Hu JW, Arendt-Nielsen L, Sessle BJ, Svensson P. Sex-related differences in human pain and rat afferent discharge evoked by injection of glutamate into the masseter muscle. *J Neurophysiol* 2001;86(2):782–91.

177. Cairns BE, Wang K, Hu JW, Sessle BJ, Arendt-Nielsen L, Svensson P. The effect of glutamate-evoked masseter muscle pain on the human jaw-stretch reflex differs in men and women. *J Orofac Pain* 2003;17(4):317–25.

178. Falla D, Arendt-Nielsen L, Farina D. Gender-specific adaptations of upper trapezius muscle activity to acute nociceptive stimulation. *Pain* 2008;138(1):217–25.

179. Gazerani P, Wang K, Cairns BE, Svensson P, Arendt-Nielsen L. Effects of subcutaneous administration of glutamate on pain, sensitization and vasomotor responses in healthy men and women. *Pain* 2006;124(3):338–48.

180. Ge HY, Arendt-Nielsen L, Farina D, Madeleine P. Gender-specific differences in electromyographic changes and perceived pain induced by experimental muscle pain during sustained contractions of the upper trapezius muscle. *Muscle Nerve* 2005;32(6):726–33.

181. Ge HY, Madeleine P, Arendt-Nielsen L. Gender differences in pain modulation evoked by repeated injections of glutamate into the human trapezius muscle. *Pain* 2005;113(1–2):134–40.

182. Ge HY, Madeleine P, Cairns BE, Arendt-Nielsen L. Hypoalgesia in the referred pain areas after bilateral injections of hypertonic saline into the trapezius muscles of men and women: a potential experimental model of gender-specific differences. *Clin J Pain* 2006;22(1):37–44.

183. Svensson P, Cairns BE, Wang K, et al. Glutamate-evoked pain and mechanical allodynia in the human masseter muscle. *Pain* 2003; 101(3):221–7.

184. Arendt-Nielsen L, Sluka KA, Nie HL. Experimental muscle pain impairs descending inhibition. *Pain* 2008;140(3):465–71.

185. Edwards RR, Fillingim RB, Ness TJ. Age-related differences in endogenous pain modulation: a comparison of diffuse noxious inhibitory controls in healthy older and younger adults. *Pain* 2003;101(1–2):155–65.

186. France CR, Suchowiecki S. Assessing supraspinal modulation of pain perception in individuals at risk for hypertension. *Psychophysiology* 2001;38(1):107–13.

187. Oono Y, Fujii K, Motohashi K, Umino M. Diffuse noxious inhibitory controls triggered by heterotopic CO_2 laser conditioning stimulation decreased the SEP amplitudes induced by electrical tooth stimulation with different intensity at an equally inhibitory rate. *Pain* 2008;136(3):356–65.

188. Pud D, Sprecher E, Yarnitsky D. Homotopic and heterotopic effects of endogenous analgesia in healthy volunteers. *Neurosci Lett* 2005;380(3):209–13.

189. Quiton RL, Greenspan JD. Sex differences in endogenous pain modulation by distracting and painful conditioning stimulation. *Pain* 2007;132(Suppl 1):S134–49.

190. Rosen A, Feldreich A, Dabirian N, Ernberg M. Effect of heterotopic noxious conditioning stimulation on electrical and pressure pain thresholds in two different anatomical regions. *Acta Odontol Scand* 2008;66(3):181–8.

191. Rhudy JL, Meagher MW. Noise stress and human pain thresholds: divergent effects in men and women. *Journal of Pain* 2001;2:57–64.

192. Hashmi JA, Davis KD. Noxious heat evokes stronger sharp and annoying sensations in women than men in hairy skin but not in glabrous skin. *Pain* 2010;151(2):323–9.

3

BRAIN IMAGING

SEX DIFFERENCES IN CEREBRAL RESPONSES TO PAIN

Katy Vincent and Irene Tracey

INTRODUCTION

A significant body of evidence suggests that sex differences exist in the response to experimental pain.[1] However, as discussed in other chapters of this book, the factors underlying these differences are varied and multiple factors may contribute at any one time, even in a well-designed study. Brain imaging techniques that assess the cerebral response to pain allow a mechanistic interpretation of any observed differences compared to behavioral studies.[2] Additionally, they provide a more objective measure of the pain experience than that obtained from subjective reports alone. This is particularly pertinent when sex differences are being investigated, as gender role expectations and social factors both play a part.[1]

While the use of brain imaging techniques allows us to identify the important factors contributing to sex differences in the response to pain, it is important to remember that sex differences occur in a number of physiological processes.[3] In some instances this may be the underlying variable of interest; however, sex differences in the physiological processes used by the imaging techniques may potentially interfere with a valid interpretation of the results. Therefore, in this chapter we will initially briefly review the sex differences in anatomy and physiology that could impact on the imaging techniques that are currently in use. We will also consider how the variation in endogenous and exogenous hormones in women may affect these results. Bearing these factors in mind, we will then consider the results of studies specifically addressing sex differences in the cerebral response to pain in healthy subjects and how these and other findings might be extrapolated into patients with chronic pain conditions.

SEX DIFFERENCES IN BRAIN ANATOMY AND PHYSIOLOGY: IMPLICATIONS FOR THE INTERPRETATION OF CEREBRAL RESPONSES TO PAIN

Anatomy

Knowledge of brain anatomy is clearly crucial for the interpretation of brain imaging data. However, brain structure is also important in the analysis of the data, and for some techniques, such as electroencephalogram (EEG) or cortical evoked potentials (CEPs), for accurate electrode placement prior to data collection. When analyzing brain imaging data, the individual's functional data are usually registered to a standard brain template,[4] allowing conclusions to be drawn about a population response or comparisons to be made between groups. This standard brain can be a representative brain from the sample, an average brain of the whole sample, or a reference template such as Montreal Neurological Institute 152 (MNI 152) as is used in the two main analysis packages, SPM and FSL (http://www.fil.ion.ucl.ac.uk/spm; http://www.fmrib.ox.ac.uk/fsl). When a reference template is used, specific brain regions can be identified by their coordinates in three-dimensional space, these coordinates can then be used to identify the location of functional activations after analysis of the data or to define a priori regions of interest (ROIs) to restrict the analysis.[5] The original reference atlas used was that of Talairach and Tournoux,[6] but MNI coordinates are reported with increasing frequency.[4]

It is well known that women have smaller brains than men[7]; however, as long as the proportional sizes of the major subdivisions are similar, then the techniques by which they are transformed should be reasonably accurate.[8] Although some studies have suggested that this would be a valid assumption,[7] other work disagrees, with women having been shown to have a thicker cortex in many regions,[9] smaller white matter volume (both absolute and relative to intracranial volume),[10] but a higher gray:white matter volume ratio.[11] For example, in one study where brain volume was matched between the sexes, no difference in gray:white matter volume ratio was found; however, women did have higher regional gray matter volumes in the caudate and left orbitofrontal region, left superior temporal gyrus, and left superior frontal gyrus.[12] Other studies have identified increased cortical thickness in similar regions in women.[9,13,14] Additionally, a number of anatomical studies have also identified sex differences in the hippocampus and amygdala, with the former being larger in women and the latter in men, after adjusting for total brain volume.[15]

Individual anatomical variation raises issues that need to be considered in the analysis and reporting of brain imaging studies. While these are pertinent to all brain imaging studies, they may be of particular importance in studies comparing different groups where the variation between the groups is likely to be greater than that between individuals, for example men versus women, old versus young, and patients versus controls. First, it is important that the standard space template used registers each subject's data accurately. This process can be improved by initially registering functional data to the subject's own structural scan before then registering to a standard space.[8] Secondly, the advantages of whole-brain versus ROI analyses need to be considered.[4,5] Without strong a priori hypotheses as to which brain regions might differ between groups, whole-brain analyses are necessary; however, subtle differences in the size or location of regions between the groups may dilute the results, potentially producing a false-negative result. If a priori hypotheses exist, then ROI analyses can be performed (though, of course, unexpected differences between the groups will not be identified with this method). However, this leads us to the third point: care needs to be taken in both how ROIs are defined and significant activation patterns located. Of particular relevance to this chapter, the Talairach atlas[6] was based on a single hemisphere (assuming symmetry) of a 60-year-old French woman while the cohort contributing to the MNI 152 consisted of significantly more men than women.[16] Therefore, particularly in regions known to be influenced by sex, it is important to examine the data for each subject to be sure it really lies within the ROI, and when defining ROIs to consider each individual's brain structure rather than transforming ROIs from standard space.[5]

Connectivity

A number of more recent studies have focused on the connectivity between different brain regions, both structurally (using diffusion tensor imaging)[17] and functionally, either at rest (resting state networks)[18] or during a task (functional connectivity).[19] Although to date no studies have examined sex differences in functional connectivity during pain, variation in connectivity may underlie different activation patterns and thus deserves discussion here.

Sexual dimorphisms certainly appear to be significant when considering structural connectivity.[20] However, whether sex differences in the morphology of the corpus callosum (the major white matter tract connecting the two hemispheres of the brain) exist is controversial.[20] Although some studies have suggested a smaller volume of this structure in women,[10,21] others have not found this to be the case,[22] and a recent study suggests that women have a larger relative area of the corpus callosum when adjusted for brain size.[10] Diffusion studies do, however, suggest greater connectivity between the two hemispheres in men.[20] Similarly, sex differences in other white matter diffusion parameters are fairly consistently reported.[20] It appears that, once age and brain volume have been controlled for, women demonstrate an increase in overall cortical connectivity and higher values of both local and global efficiency,[23] perhaps suggesting that women make more efficient use of the available white matter. This hypothesis would be consistent with the finding of a stronger association between cognitive performance and white matter volume in women.[24]

Both positron emission tomography (PET) and functional magnetic resonance imaging (fMRI) have been used to assess for sex differences in resting state functional connectivity; however, again the results have been contradictory.[20,25,27] Of relevance to this chapter, two studies have shown differences in resting functional connectivity of regions particularly associated with the pain experience[26,27]—specifically the amygdala and periaqueductal gray (PAG). Thus, men show greater functional connectivity of the left amygdala, while the right is strongest in women.[26] Moreover, the regions showing strong connectivity to the amygdala differ between the sexes, with the sensorimotor cortex, striatum, and pulvinar being identified in men, but the subgenual cortex and hypothalamus in women.[26] For the PAG, greater connectivity with the dorsal anterior cingulate cortex (ACC) was found in women, whereas in men connectivity was increased with the insula/operculum and prefrontal cortices (PFC).[27] It has been suggested that women focus more on the affective component of pain while men concentrate on the sensory component[1,26]; thus, the finding that a known pain modulatory area (the PAG)[28] is more strongly connected to a brain region associated with the affective component of the pain experience (ACC)[29–31] in women, and to a

region associated with sensory discrimination (insula)[32,33] in men, is of particular interest.

Of course, identification of connectivity between two regions, either structural or functional, requires careful definition of the regions and thus the caveats discussed earlier apply just as much to the identification of ROIs for connectivity studies as for task-related studies.

Physiology

While a detailed review of sex differences in physiology is beyond the scope of this chapter (but can be found elsewhere[3]), it is important to consider how physiological factors may interact with both the noxious stimulus and with the brain imaging techniques used. For example, differences in basal temperature may influence thermal pain sensitivity, while differences in both the distribution and relative volume of body fat might be expected to influence a variety of peripheral stimuli.[1,34] How sex differences in physiology may influence the variables that brain imaging techniques measure is briefly discussed next.

A number of studies have suggested differences in blood pressure, both resting and in response to stress, between the sexes,[35] while others have shown higher global cerebral blood flow in women.[7] Such differences may impact on imaging techniques that rely on cerebral blood flow to provide a signal. [^{15}O]H$_2$O PET and the more recent technique of arterial spin labeling (ASL) quantify absolute blood flow[7,36] and therefore need to take these sex differences into account. Women also appear to have higher metabolic rates of cerebral glucose utilization,[7] and therefore [^{18}F]fluorodeoxyglucose PET studies would need to consider this variable. In view of these findings, it would seem sensible to recommend that PET and ASL studies of pain processing in healthy subjects obtain a baseline measure before commencing the pain paradigm. These factors would not be so easy to control for in pain patients, however. fMRI analysis techniques compare task-related activity to baseline activity[4] and thus might be expected to be influenced by such variables to a lesser extent. However, it is plausible that those subjects with higher basal rates of either blood flow or glucose metabolism may have less additional response to a noxious stimulus and thus these factors may also impact on the results of fMRI studies. More research in this area is necessary to allow an accurate understanding of the influence of these factors on the imaging signal of interest. Furthermore, should sex differences in these variables be found to be region specific, this would be a greater confound than if a global effect were observed.

Chemistry

Sex differences have been identified for a wide variety of neurotransmitter systems within the brain. Thus, for example, cortical γ-aminobutyric acid (GABA) levels are higher[37] and dopaminergic function is enhanced in women,[38] while μ-opioid binding potential is greater in men in specific brain regions.[39] Differences in the rates of synthesis of certain neurotransmitters also occur, with men synthesizing serotonin significantly faster than women.[38] Furthermore, the influence of stress on neurotransmitter levels appears to be sexually dimorphic.[40,41] Although these sex differences in neurochemistry may be the explanation for some of the behavioral and neural differences observed between the sexes in the response to pain, they could also be potential confounding factors, particularly in PET studies. Thus, as a minimum requirement, targeted PET studies investigating sex differences in the response to pain should also consider differences in baseline binding potential in order to accurately interpret their results.

THE CONFOUND OF HORMONAL VARIATION IN WOMEN

Sex steroid hormones exert their influences throughout life: from intrauterine and neonatal effects, through puberty, adulthood, and old age. Organizational effects of these hormones on the developing brain occur via molecular, genetic, and epigenetic mechanisms[42] and determine sexually dimorphic behaviours such as play patterns, spatial learning, and bird song in a variety of species.[43] Thus, it would be reasonable to also expect such effects to underlie a large proportion of the observed sex differences in pain experience. However, sex hormones also exert activational effects,[43] and in

view of the significant differences in hormonal milieu between men and women, these effects are also likely to contribute to sex differences in pain. This hypothesis is supported by epidemiological data demonstrating increasing differences in pain symptoms after puberty,[44] the time at which hormonal profiles begin to differ markedly between the sexes. When considering the results of studies investigating the cerebral response to pain, it is also important to remember that between puberty and menopause, hormone levels fluctuate significantly in women; this variation may alter the response to experimental pain stimuli,[45] but it also may influence brain parameters as discussed next.

Sex steroid hormones have been shown to alter both brain anatomy and connectivity. Recent studies investigating hormonal effects on brain volume have observed a peak gray matter volume at ovulation[46] and suggested that specific effects of circulating hormones underlie the observed sex differences in the volume of the left inferior frontal gyrus (estradiol and testosterone) and the right temporal pole (progesterone).[47] A number of authors have reported effects of sex hormones on the functional coupling of the two hemispheres of the brain (intrahemispheric connectivity)[48,49] and on connectivity between other brain regions.[50] In general, it appears that estradiol and progesterone enhance such coupling, while the effects of testosterone are more varied, appearing to increase connectivity between subcortical brain areas but decrease subcortico-cortical connectivity.[50]

A number of the physiological processes discussed earlier as potentially contributing to sex differences in pain perception have also been shown to vary with the menstrual cycle, including basal body temperature, pulse, and blood pressure.[3,51] A further confound for pain studies, is the well-known influence of the menstrual cycle on mood.[52,53] The interpretation of PET and ASL studies is also complicated by the influence of the menstrual cycle on cerebral glucose metabolism. Not only does this vary with cycle phase, but the effect appears to be region specific. For example, it has been shown that glucose metabolism is significantly higher in the midfollicular phase in the thalamus, PFC, and temporoparietal and inferior temporal regions but significantly higher in the midluteal phase in anterior and superior temporal regions, occipital, cerebellar, cingulate, and anterior insula cortices.[38] Finally, there is good evidence that sex steroids influence neurotransmitter activity, with specific effects of estrogen on the endogenous opioid system[54] and both progesterone (and its metabolites) and estrogen on GABA.[47,55,56]

The widespread use of exogenous hormones, both as contraceptives and postmenopausal hormone replacement therapy (HRT), adds another layer of complexity. These preparations alter the hormonal milieu directly but additionally influence other measures, including receptors for themselves and for other hormones and circulating proteins such as sex hormone binding globulin (SHBG).[57] While there are inconsistencies in the literature, a number of studies suggest that the use of estradiol-containing preparations either increases sensitivity to experimental noxious stimuli[58,59] or predisposes to the development of painful conditions.[44,60–62] Additionally, hormonal therapies are known to influence a variety of physiological factors, including weight, mood, and blood pressure.[57] Investigation of the effects of exogenous hormones on the brains of reproductive age women are relatively limited; however, there is an extensive literature on the central effects of postmenopausal HRT. Much of this work has focused on working memory and verbal fluency, frequently concentrating on the hippocampus in light of the hypothesized neuroprotective effects of estradiol on brain aging/atrophy and the development of Alzheimer's disease.[63–65] The majority of these studies suggest that exogenous estradiol increases both structural and functional connectivity of the brain[50]; however, the effects of progesterone and testosterone appear to be dependent on both brain region and task.[62,66–69]

Thus, although hormonal factors may be the underlying variable of interest, they may also be a significant confound when investigating sex differences in the cerebral response to pain. To gain a better understanding of this complex area, it is imperative that future studies consider hormonal factors in their design. At the very least, only specific groups of women should be investigated, that is, those with naturally fluctuating hormones or using low-dose combined oral contraceptive pills or postmenopausal women with/without HRT. Ideally, however, men should be compared to women in a variety of hormonal states. Unfortunately, the majority of studies to date do not mention the hormonal status of the women investigated or whether those taking exogenous hormones were excluded. The one study that carefully controlled the hormonal milieu elegantly demonstrates the advantage of so doing and is discussed in detail later in this chapter.[54]

BRAIN IMAGING STUDIES SPECIFICALLY ADDRESSING SEX DIFFERENCES IN THE RESPONSE TO PAIN IN HEALTHY SUBJECTS

A number of studies have investigated sex differences in the response to experimental pain using brain imaging techniques. These are discussed in detail next and summarized in Table 3.1. It can be seen from this table that the majority of these studies did identify sex differences in the brain response to pain, even when no behavioral difference was found. Unfortunately, comparisons between these studies are somewhat limited by the variety of different stimuli and body sites stimulated during the experimental paradigms. Furthermore, only three of these studies mentioned the hormonal status of the women investigated and only two of these controlled for this factor.

When assessing for differences in brain imaging response between groups, it is tempting to obtain the mean response for each group and then visually compare these images, but this does not ensure a statistically valid result; therefore, only results obtained via a direct comparison of the sexes will be discussed here.[4]

Somatic Pain Perception

Paulson and colleagues[70] were the first to use a brain imaging technique to investigate sex differences in the response to pain. They applied thermal stimuli of 40°C (warm but painless) and 50°C (painful) to the left volar forearm during PET scans. Female subjects found the higher temperature more intense than males, but there was no difference in ratings for the

Table 3.1 Summary of Studies Investigating Sex Differences in the Cerebral Response to Pain

AUTHORS	TECHNIQUE	SAMPLE SIZE	PAIN STIMULUS	STIMULUS SITE	FIXED PERCEPTION VS. STIMULUS INTENSITY	BEHAVIORAL DIFFERENCE	IMAGING DIFFERENCE	HORMONE CONTROLLED?
Neonates								
Ozawa et al., 2011[87]	NIRS	40	Venous puncture	Dorsum hand	NA	N	N	NA
Reproductive age								
Somatic stimuli								
Paulson et al., 1998[70]	PET Labeled H_2O	10M 10F	Thermal	L forearm	Stimulus	Y	Y	ND
Derbyshire et al., 2002[71]	PET Labeled H_2O	11M 10F	Laser	Dorsum R hand	Perception	N	Y	ND
Moulton et al., 2006[72]	fMRI	11M 17F	Thermal	Dorsum foot	Perception	N	Y	ND
Straube et al., 2009[73]	fMRI	18M 18F[b]	Electrical, sc	L index finger	Perception	Y	Y	ND

Deep/visceral stimuli

Zubieta et al., 2002[39]	PET [11C]carfentanil	14M 14F	Hypertonic saline	masseter	Perception	N	Y	Y[d]
Hobson et al., 2005[92]	MEG/cortical evoked potentials	MEG:8M 8F CEPs: 6M 5F	Electrical	Esophagus	Perception	N	N	ND
Smith et al., 2006[54]	PET [11C]carfentanil	8M 10F	Hypertonic saline	masseter	Perception	N	Y/N[c]	Y[d]
Berman et al., 2006[93]	fMRI	7M 6F	Distension	Rectum	Stimulus	ND	Y	Y[e]

a No difference in ratings but difference in MPQ sensory scores.

b fMRI data only analyzed from 12M and 12F subjects.

c Significant difference between men and women only when women in low estradiol state.

d Hormonal status verified with serum hormone profile.

e Menstrual cycle stage assessed by date of LMP (half follicular, half luteal phase).

F, female; fMRI, functional magnetic resonance imaging; im, intramuscular; L, left; M, male; MEG, magnetoencephalography; N, no; NA, not applicable; ND, not described; NIRS, near-infrared spectroscopy; NS, not significant; PET, positron emission tomography; R, right; sc, subcutaneous; Y, yes.

40°C stimulus. While acknowledging the striking similarities between the sexes in activation patterns in response to painful stimuli, the authors did identify increased activation of the contralateral thalamus and anterior insula in females and found that the left PFC activated in the female subjects, whereas it was in the right PFC where activation was seen in males. One difficulty with interpreting these results is the increased pain intensity ratings given by the female subjects in response to these stimuli; thus, it is plausible that the increased activation of the thalamus and insula observed in the female subjects reflects pain intensity rather than an underlying sex difference.

Derbyshire and colleagues[71] attempted to address this issue by using laser stimuli of fixed pain intensity (warm, mild pain and moderate pain) rather than a fixed energy input. However, their analysis asked a somewhat different question; thus, rather than identifying brain regions that were differentially activated between the sexes in response to the three different stimulus intensities, they instead identified brain regions where activation correlated with pain ratings and where this correlation was different between the sexes (i.e., where stimulus intensity coding was different between the sexes). Despite no sex difference in the energy level required for these three stimulus intensities, there were differences in the brain areas encoding stimulus intensity. Thus, stimulus intensity was encoded more strongly in contralateral primary and secondary somatosensory cortices (S1 and S2), anterior and posterior insula, and PFC and bilateral parietal cortices in men, while the correlation was stronger in the ipsilateral perigenual cingulate in women. The authors suggest that their findings imply a "sensory processing dominance" in male relative to female subjects.

In a subsequent study using laser stimuli on only male volunteers, subjects were instructed to attend to either the localization of the stimulus or its unpleasantness; greater activation of S1 and the inferior parietal cortex occurred during attention to localization, while attention to unpleasantness was associated with greater activation of a number of regions, including bilateral perigenual cingulate cortex.[30] This is in agreement with other studies suggesting

that the anterior cingulate cortex (ACC) plays a role in encoding the unpleasantness of painful stimuli.[29,31] This could be taken as support of Derbyshire's interpretation of their data; however, their results may actually say more about how the different sexes use ratings of painful sensations, suggesting that men rate on the basis of pain intensity while women make an assessment of the pain experience as a whole and thus their ratings combine both sensory and affective components.

One other published study has investigated sex differences in the response to a noxious thermal stimulus, in this instance applied to the dorsum of the foot.[72] Three temperatures were chosen for each subject in this study: 41°C (innocuous), 1°C below pain tolerance (pain 2), and 2°C below pain tolerance (pain 1). Therefore, in fact, the design fixed neither stimulus intensity nor perception between subjects; however, there was no significant difference between the sexes in either pain ratings or temperatures used, and thus the authors consider it to be a fixed perception study. It is hard to know how generalizable their findings are to the general population, however, as almost one third of the subjects recruited were excluded after psychophysical testing (20/61) because the investigators required pain tolerance to be between 45°C and 50°C and both pain stimuli to be experienced as painful, with at least 5 points on a 100-point VAS between them. Their analysis methods were interesting, however, as they assessed the brain response to painful stimuli in terms of both the spatial extent and the amplitude of activations in a number of predefined ROIs, and they considered the directionality of the BOLD change (i.e., increase or decrease). Thus, although they found no sex difference in the spatial extent of activations, men showed greater amplitude of activation in bilateral S1 and mid-ACC, while the response in the DLPFC showed an interaction between sex and stimulus intensity. Interestingly, however, almost all ROIs showed a greater percentage of negative BOLD signals in the women, particularly with the higher stimulus intensity. While the experimental design makes these results hard to generalize, the finding that more deactivations occur in women in response to such stimuli is intriguing and warrants further investigation.

One possible explanation for this finding is a sex difference in resting state activity; however, as discussed, this is still a controversial area.[20,25] Importantly, what this study highlights is the need for careful consideration of the methods used to analyze functional imaging data.

In the most recent study, electrical stimuli were delivered subcutaneously to the tip of the left index finger at four different intensities: not perceived (10% below lowest perceived intensity during intensity determination period), perceived but not painful, mildly painful, and moderately painful.[73] As with the previous study, analysis was restricted to a set of predetermined ROIs: dorsal/pregenual MPFC, anterior insula, ACC, thalamus, S1, and posterior insula/S2.

The women required significantly less intensity to produce painful sensations; however, there was no difference in the stimulus intensity required for the nonpainful stimuli between the sexes. Interestingly, there was no main effect of sex on the brain response independent of stimulus intensity, but differences in activation of the MPFC and left anterior insula were observed when the stimulus intensities were considered separately (Fig. 3.1). In the MPFC, increasing stimulus intensity appeared to be associated with increasing activation in the women but increasing deactivation in the men, such that a significant difference in activation was seen for the most painful of the stimuli. Interestingly, a similar pattern was observed

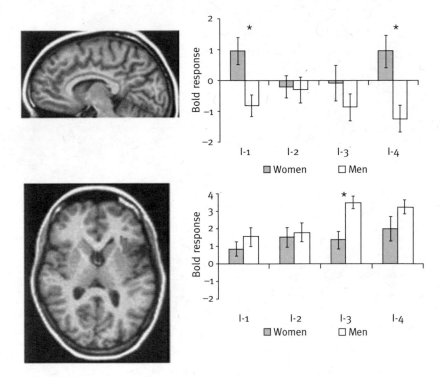

FIGURE 3.1 Effect of stimulus intensity and sex on the brain response to noxious stimulation. Results are shown as both a representative slice with the statistical parametric map overlaid on a T1 scan and as graphs of the parameter estimates (mean + SEM) in response to each stimulus intensity. Asterisks indicate a significant difference between the sexes. (*Left*) Medial prefrontal cortex (MPFC). Increased activation was found in the MPFC in women compared to men in response to moderately painful stimuli and to not perceived stimuli (not shown). (*Right*) Anterior insula. Increased activation was found in the anterior insula for men compared to women in response to the mildly painful stimulus. (Adapted from Straube T, Schmidt S, Weiss T, Mentzel HJ, Miltner WHR. Sex differences in brain activation to anticipated and experienced pain in the medial prefrontal cortex. *Hum Brain Mapp* 2009;30:689–98.)

Table 3.2 Summary of Brain Regions Identified as Showing a Sex Difference in the Amplitude of Response to a Noxious Stimulus

STIMULUS	THERMAL[70]	THERMAL[72]	LASER[71]	ELECTRICAL[73]	ELECTRICAL[92]	DISTENSION[93]	HYPERTONIC SALINE[39]	HYPERTONIC SALINE[54]		
ANALYSIS	ROI	ROI	WB[a]	ROI	ROI	ROI	WB[b]	WB[b]	WOMEN LOW E2	WOMEN HIGH E2
BRAIN REGION										
S1	=	M	M	=	=	x	=	=	=	=
S2	x	=	M	=	=	x	=	=	=	=
AI	W	=	=	M	=	M	=	=	=	=
PI	=	=	M	=	=	x	=	=	=	=
ACC	=	M	W	=	=	=	=	=	=	=
MCC	x	x	=	x	=	M	=	=	=	=
PCC	x	=	=	x	=	x	=	=	=	=
PFC	M/W	M/W	M	W	x	x		=	=	=
Parietal	x	x	M	x	x	x		=	=	=
SMA	x	M	=	x	x	x	=	=	=	=
Thalamus	F	x	=	x	x	M	M	M	=	=
Hypothalamus	x	x	=	x	x	x	=	M	=	=
Amygdala	x	x	=	x	x	=	M	M	=	=
V Striatum	=	x	=	x	x	x	M	=	=	=
D brainstem	x	x	=	x	x	=	=	=	=	=
NAc	x	x	=	x	x	x	=	M	=	=
Premotor	=	x	=	x	x	x	=	=	=	=
Cerebellum	=	x	=	x	x	x	=	=	=	=

[a] Analysis identified regions encoding stimulus intensity rather than areas responding to noxious stimulus.

[b] Analysis identified activation of the endogenous opioid system only.

ACC, anterior cingulate cortex (including perigenual cingulate); AI, anterior insula; D brainstem, dorsal brainstem; M, men; MCC, midcingulate cortex; NAc, nucleus accumbens; PCC, posterior cingulate cortex; parietal, parietal cortex; PI, posterior insula; ROI, ROI analysis; V striatum, ventral striatum; W, women; WB, whole-brain analysis; =, no sex difference observed; x, not considered in analyses.

for the below-perception stimulus, which the authors describe as an anticipation period. All four of the stimulus intensities were associated with activation in the left anterior insula in both sexes; however, this was significantly greater in men for the mildly painful stimulus, and there was a trend toward significance for the moderately painful stimulus as well.

While many differences exist between these four studies, both in terms of experimental design and analysis methods, the somatosensory cortices, PFC, anterior insula, and ACC are consistently identified as the regions most likely to represent sex differences in somatic pain perception (Table 3.2). That the somatosensory cortices, insula, and ACC may represent differences in the sensory and affective components of the pain experience has already been discussed. The PFC, however, are particularly implicated in the top-down modulation of pain,[28] particularly by cognitive and emotional factors, having been demonstrated to play a role in the modulation of pain by expectation (placebo),[74] perceived control,[75] depression,[76-78] catastrophizing,[79] and anticipatory anxiety.[80,81] Given that cognitive and emotional factors are frequently suggested to underlie sex differences in the pain experience,[1] this could explain the identification of sex differences in activation of the PFC in response to pain in all the studies discussed earlier. However, the PFC is also rich in estrogen receptors,[82,83] and a number of studies have demonstrated hormonal influences on prefrontal regions during cognitive, verbal, and memory tasks.[67,84-86] Thus, the observed effects may represent organizational or activational effects of the sex hormones on the PFC rather than the influence of cognitive or emotional factors. Interestingly, a recent study investigating the response of the PFC to pain in neonates between 4 and 6 days old using near-infrared spectroscopy[87] did not demonstrate an effect of gender on pain intensity or on prefrontal activation in response to a painful experience (blood sampling). Thus, it is unlikely that differential PFC activation between the sexes in response to pain reflects an underlying organizational influence of sex hormones on these brain regions. Whether these differences represent the influence of cognitive/emotional factors or activational effects of sex hormones

remains to be elucidated; moreover, the two explanations are not mutually exclusive, as sex steroid hormones (at both physiological and supraphysiological levels) are known to alter mood and emotional state.[88,89]

Deep/Visceral Pain Perception

It is well known that visceral and somatic nociception differ,[90] yet the network of regions recently identified as being involved in the perception of visceral pain[91] is remarkably similar to that classically described for somatic stimuli.[2,33] Two relatively small, brain imaging studies have specifically addressed the question of sex differences in the cerebral response to visceral pain, the first using perception matched electrical stimuli to the esophagus,[92] and the second using rectal distension matched for pressure.[93] It is unlikely that either study was adequately powered to detect behavioral differences, and thus it is unsurprising that no sex differences were found for the mean intensity of electrical stimulation of the esophagus or VAS ratings in response to these stimuli,[92] while unfortunately, the second study did not report behavioral data.[93] The response to esophageal stimulation was investigated using two imaging methods, magnetoencephalography (MEG) and cortical evoked potentials (CEPs).[92] Predefined ROIs (S1, S2, anterior and posterior insula, perigenual cingulate, midcingulate, and posterior cingulate) were used in the analysis of the MEG data, while CEPs were restricted to an investigation of timing and laterality; no sex differences were identified with either imaging modality. As the authors point out, their stimulus was brief and designed to record the early stages of esophageal pain processing and therefore it may not have been the ideal stimulus with which to detect sex differences. Unfortunately, neither this study nor the investigation of the fMRI response to rectal distension[93] examined the response in the PFC. Berman and colleagues[93] used similar analysis methods to Moulton's study investigating thermal stimuli to the foot,[72] assessing both spatial extent and directionality of the BOLD change in response to the distension in a set of predefined ROIs (anterior insula, midcingulate, anterior cingulate, thalamus, amygdala, ventral striatum, and dorsal brainstem).[93] However, in view of the small sample size and the fact that no correction was made for multiple comparisons, these results should be interpreted with caution. Nonetheless, as in the somatic study, women were found to deactivate more voxels than men in almost all ROIs studied in response to the two inflation pressures, and interestingly there was a trend toward this being true during an expectation condition as well. This difference reached significance across all conditions (expectation, 25 mmHg, 45 mmHg) for the midcingulate and thalamus. Interestingly, however, when considering the proportion of activated voxels that showed a decreased BOLD signal in response to the condition, sex-related differences were greatest for the 25 mmHg distension, which was reported as uncomfortable rather than painful.

In terms of obtaining any understanding of the mechanisms underlying sex differences in pain perception, the two studies by Zubieta, Smith, and colleagues[39,54] are by far the most useful. In both these studies they used PET and a μ-opioid receptor specific radiotracer ([11C]carfentanil) to investigate both baseline μ-opioid receptor availability and the activation of this system in response to a sustained noxious stimulus (infusion of hypertonic saline into the masseter muscle) of fixed intensity. In the first study[39] they compared men with women in the follicular phase of their menstrual cycle (2–9 days after the onset of menstruation), confirmed with hormonal profiles. While there were no sex differences in the behavioral responses to the painful stimuli, sex differences in baseline binding potential and activation in response to pain were observed. Specifically, women showed higher μ-opioid binding in the amygdala at baseline, but men had significantly greater pain-related activation of this system in the anterior thalamus, ventral pallidum/substantia innominata, nucleus accumbens, and amygdala, while women had significantly reduced activation in the nucleus accumbens. The second study[54] extended these findings by using a similar experimental design, except that women were scanned at two time points, once in their early follicular phase as in the previous study, and once after 7–9 days of transdermal estradiol, producing a high-estradiol, low-progesterone

state. Data from the men were then compared to that from the women in each hormonal state separately. As in the earlier study, there was no significant difference in the pain intensity ratings or the volume of hypertonic saline required to maintain the pain intensity between the men and the women at either time point. However, baseline μ-opioid receptor availability was significantly greater in the women in the nucleus accumbens/anterior hypothalamus in both the low- and high-estradiol states in this experimental cohort. Interestingly, in response to sustained pain, the men showed significantly greater activation of μ-opioid receptor mediated neurotransmission in the thalamus, nucleus accumbens/hypothalamus, and amygdala compared to women in the low-estradiol state, similar to the previous study, but no differences between men and women in the high-estradiol state (Fig. 3.2). Not only do these studies suggest that at least some of the sex differences in pain arise from differences in the activation of the endogenous opioid system, they also demonstrate different receptor availability (binding potential) at baseline, potentially underlying sex differences in the response to opioid analgesia.[94] Perhaps more important, however, they elegantly demonstrate the need to consider the hormonal status of the women involved. Thus, by only considering women at one point in their cycle conclusions might be drawn that are not true throughout the cycle; alternatively, considering women at any time in the cycle as a homogenous group might conceal differences that do exist at specific times. Although it could be argued that the study by Smith and colleagues was not truly physiological, because they artificially created a high-estradiol, low-progesterone state,[54] such a strategy allowed them to carefully control the hormonal environment to mimic the late follicular/early luteal state. Alternatively, they could have considered the women at two points in their natural cycles; however, individual fluctuations in hormone concentration are quite variable[95] and therefore the division of the menstrual cycle into phases defined by ovarian or endometrial morphology may still not produce a cohort with comparable hormonal profiles.

Interestingly, the sex differences identified in these two studies[39,54] are notably different

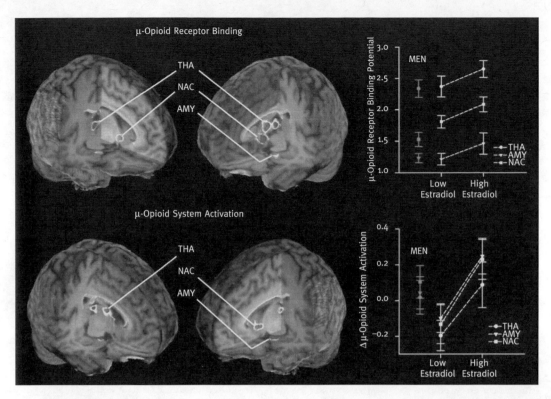

FIGURE 3.2   Effect of estradiol and sex on μ-opioid receptor binding and μ-opioid-receptor-mediated neurotransmission in response to a sustained painful stimulus. (*Top left*) Brain regions where a significant influence of estradiol treatment on μ-opioid receptor binding was identified in women. (*Bottom left*) Brain regions where a significant influence of estradiol treatment on μ-opioid-receptor-mediated neurotransmission in response to a painful stimulus was identified in women. (*Top right*) Baseline μ-opioid receptor binding potential (mean + SEM) in the thalamus (THA), amygdala (AMY), and nucleus accumbens (NAc) in men and women in a low- and high-estradiol state. (*Bottom right*) Change in μ-opioid receptor binding potential in response to a noxious stimulus (mean + SEM) in the thalamus (THA), amygdala (AMY), and nucleus accumbens (NAc) in men and women in a low- and high-estradiol state. (Adapted from Smith YR, Stohler CS, Nichols TE, Bueller JA, Koeppe RA, Zubieta J-K. Pronociceptive and antinociceptive effects of estradiol through endogenous opioid neurotransmission in women. *J Neurosci* 2006;26(21):5777–85.)

from the other studies discussed here. Possible explanations for these discrepancies include the failure of other studies to control for the hormonal status of the women; the differing imaging techniques; the choice of ROIs for analysis; and the pain stimulus used. Thus, brain regions that were identified in other studies but not by Smith and Zubieta may represent mechanisms other than the endogenous opioid system by which pain is modulated. It is interesting, however, that ACC, PFC, and insula were not identified by these PET studies as they have previously been shown to be involved in the modulation of pain by the μ-opioid system[96,97] and were identified by a number of the other studies. It is also surprising that the studies using fMRI or H₂O PET did not consistently identify the thalamus, nucleus accumbens, amygdala and hypothalamus. Both the nucleus accumbens and hypothalamus are small structures and thus might be hard to identify with whole-brain analyses and none of the studies utilizing ROI analysis considered either of these regions. Similarly, the amygdala and striatum were not considered in many of the ROI studies (Table 3.2). Alternatively, a sustained pain stimulus may be more successful at activating the endogenous opioid system than other brief stimuli such as electrical and laser. In support of this explanation, rectal distension was also associated with greater activity in the thalamus in men.[93]

In summary, brain imaging studies in healthy subjects consistently reveal sex differences in the cerebral response to pain, although the specifics of these differences vary between studies. Notably, there is evidence to suggest that women focus on the affective component of the pain experience in response to a somatic stimulus to a greater extent than men and that the PFC appears to play a central role in generating sex differences in pain in adults. Furthermore, it can be seen that without controlling for the hormonal profile of the women, significant differences will be overlooked and inaccurate conclusions drawn. It is particularly intriguing that behavioral responses to pain are often remarkably similar between the sexes despite differences in the neuronal correlates of the experience. Thus, as has been suggested elsewhere,[98] it is plausible that sex differences in the brain exist to prevent rather than to create sexual dimorphisms in behavior.

USING BRAIN IMAGING STUDIES TO INVESTIGATE SEX DIFFERENCES IN THE RESPONSE TO PAIN IN PATIENTS

It is well known that chronic pain conditions show a female predominance,[44,99] and a number of factors have been proposed that may mediate this relationship.[1] Other chronic conditions, including depression and posttraumatic stress disorder, also occur more frequently in women and are associated with an alteration in the response to pain.[78,100,101] It is therefore surprising that, to the best of our knowledge, there are no published studies investigating sex differences in pain perception in patients (chronic pain, psychiatric, or any other patient category) with functional imaging techniques. A few studies have investigated rectal distension

in patients with irritable bowel syndrome; however, while the stimuli were considered aversive, they were not reliably rated as painful.[102–104] Interestingly, these studies also identified the insula and PFC as two of the areas where sex differences in the brain response to distension occurred.

Over and above a purely academic interest, a major aim of pain neuroscience is to increase our understanding of pain such that ultimately the suffering of the millions of patients around the world living with chronic pain conditions is reduced. To this end, brain imaging techniques can be useful in a number of ways: revealing how exogenous pain is processed in these patients[33]; imaging their own pain[105,106]; identifying novel therapeutic targets[107]; understanding the mechanisms of novel therapeutic agents (pharmacologic fMRI)[107]; and identifying why some patients may respond differently to treatments.[108] However, at present, a large proportion of the imaging studies investigating patient responses to experimental pain concentrate on female patients (e.g., in irritable bowel syndrome, fibromyalgia, and major depression[78,109–114]), while studies in healthy subjects, particularly pharmacologic studies[115–117] frequently focus on male subjects. While this is understandable, given both the preponderance of women in chronic pain populations and the difficulties of both controlling for hormonal effects and the need to exclude pregnancy in drug studies, it makes the application of findings from one group of studies to another markedly more difficult.

Sex differences in the response to analgesics have been widely, although not consistently, described.[1,94,118] In addition to the potential factors underlying sex differences in pain perception, physiological differences could also influence both pharmacodynamics and pharmacokinetics.[3] Furthermore, it is plausible that different pathological mechanisms between the sexes produce the same clinical phenotype, similar to the findings in healthy subjects that suggest that different neuronal mechanisms produce the same behavioral outcome. Sex differences are also well established in the response to both acute and chronic stress[41,119] and while both sexes show alterations in the activity of the hypothalamic-pituitary-adrenal axis in association with chronic pain,[120,121] the diurnal variation in cortisol levels is influenced to a greater extent in men.[122] Additionally, serotonin synthesis in the brains of female patients with irritable bowel syndrome differs from that of female controls while there is no difference between male patients and controls.[123] Thus, without considering both sexes separately in both pathology-related and pharmacologic studies, it is unlikely that the optimal treatment strategies will be identified.

CONCLUSIONS

In the current era of individualized, multidisciplinary treatment packages, it is crucial that we understand the sex differences in the response to pain both in health and disease. An understanding of sex differences in endogenous pain modulatory mechanisms, psychology, and the responses to both analgesics and stress are central to this aim. Given the variety of biopsychosocial factors that contribute to sex differences, brain imaging studies are ideally placed to dissect out the influences of these contributory factors. However, to maximize the potential of these studies to produce useful translational data, they need to be carefully designed, not least in terms of controlling for the hormonal status of the women involved.

REFERENCES

1. Fillingim RB, King CD, Ribeiro-Dasilva MC, Rahim-Williams B, Riley, JL, III. Sex, gender, and pain: a review of recent clinical and experimental findings. *J Pain* 2009;10(5):447–85.
2. Tracey I, Mantyh PW. The cerebral signature for pain perception and its modulation. *Neuron* 2007;55(3):377–91.
3. Miller V, Hay M. *Principles of Sex-based Differences in Physiology* Vol 34. London: Elsevier; 2004.
4. Smith SM. Overview of fMRI analysis. *Br J Radiol* 2004;77(Suppl 2):S167–75.
5. Poldrack RA. Region of interest analysis for fMRI. *Soc Cog Affect Neurosci* 2007;2(1):67–70.
6. Talairach J, Tournoux P. *Co-Planar Stereotaxic Atlas of the Human Brain: 3-Dimensional Proprtional System—An Approach to Cerebral Imaging.* New York: Thieme; 1988.
7. Cosgrove KP, Mazure CM, Staley JK. Evolving knowledge of sex differences in brain structure, function, and chemistry. *Biol Psychiatry* 2007;62(8):847–55.
8. Jenkinson M, Bannister P, Brady M, Smith S. Improved optimisation for the robust and accurate linear registration and motion correction of brain images. *Neuroimage* 2002;17:825–41.
9. Luders E, Narr KL, Thompson PM, et al. Gender effects on cortical thickness and the influence of scaling. *Hum Brain Mapp* 2006;27(4):314–24.
10. Leonard CM, Towler S, Welcome S, et al. Size matters: cerebral volume influences sex differences in neuroanatomy. *Cereb Cortex* 2008;18(12):2920–31.
11. Allen JS, Damasio H, Grabowski TJ, Bruss J, Zhang W. Sexual dimorphism and asymmetries in the gray-white composition of the human cerebrum. *Neuroimage* 2003;18(4):880–94.
12. Luders E, Gaser C, Narr KL, Toga AW. Why sex matters: brain size independent differences in gray matter distributions between men and women. *J Neurosci* 2009;29(45):14265–70.
13. Luders E, Narr KL, Thompson PM, et al. Mapping cortical gray matter in the young adult brain: effects of gender. *Neuroimage* 2005;26(2):493–501.
14. Sowell ER, Peterson BS, Kan E, et al. Sex differences in cortical thickness mapped in 176 healthy individuals between 7 and 87 years of age. *Cereb Cortex* 2007;17(7):1550–60.
15. Goldstein JM, Seidman LJ, Horton NJ, et al. Normal sexual dimorphism of the adult human brain assessed by in vivo magnetic resonance imaging. *Cereb Cortex* 2001;11(6):490–7.
16. Collins DL, Neelin P, Peters TM, Evans AC. Automatic 3D intersubject registration of MR volumetric data in standardized Talairach space. *J Comput Assist Tomogr* 1994;18(2):192–205.
17. Johansen-Berg H. Imaging the relationship between structure, function and behaviour in the human brain. *Brain Struct Funct* 2009;213(6):499–500.
18. Greicius MD, Krasnow B, Reiss AL, Menon V. Functional connectivity in the resting brain: A network analysis of the default mode hypothesis. *Proc Natl Acad Sci USA* 2003;100(1):253–8.
19. Friston KJ, Buechel C, Fink GR, Morris J, Rolls E, Dolan RJ. Psychophysiological and modulatory interactions in neuroimaging. *Neuroimage* 1997;6(3):218–29.
20. Gong G, He Y, Evans AC. Brain connectivity: gender makes a difference. *Neuroscientist* 2011;17(5):575–91.
21. Westerhausen R, Kreuder F, Dos Santos Sequeira S, et al. Effects of handedness and gender on macro- and microstructure of the

corpus callosum and its subregions: a combined high-resolution and diffusion-tensor MRI study. *Brain Res Cogn Brain Res* 2004;21(3):418–26.

22. Luders E, Rex DE, Narr KL, et al. Relationships between sulcal asymmetries and corpus callosum size: gender and handedness effects. *Cereb Cortex* 2003;13(10):1084–93.

23. Gong G, Rosa-Neto P, Carbonell F, Chen ZJ, He Y, Evans AC. Age- and gender-related differences in the cortical anatomical network. *J Neurosci* 2009;29(50):15684–93.

24. Gur RC, Turetsky BI, Matsui M, et al. Sex differences in brain gray and white matter in healthy young adults: correlations with cognitive performance. *J Neurosci* 1999;19(10):4065–72.

25. Weissman-Fogel I, Moayedi M, Taylor KS, Pope G, Davis KD. Cognitive and default-mode resting state networks: do male and female brains "rest" differently? *Hum Brain Mapp* 2010;31(11):1713–26.

26. Kilpatrick LA, Zald DH, Pardo JV, Cahill LF. Sex-related differences in amygdala functional connectivity during resting conditions. *Neuroimage* 2006;30(2):452–61.

27. Kong J, Tu PC, Zyloney C, Su TP. Intrinsic functional connectivity of the periaqueductal gray, a resting fMRI study. *Behav Brain Res* 2010;211(2):215–9.

28. Bingel U, Tracey I. Imaging CNS modulation of pain in humans. *Physiol* 2008;23:371–80.

29. Rainville P, Duncan GH, Price DD, Carrier B, Bushnell MC. Pain affect encoded in human anterior cingulate but not somatosensory cortex. *Science* 1997;277(5328):968–71.

30. Kulkarni B, Bentley DE, Elliott R, et al. Attention to pain localization and unpleasantness discriminates the functions of the medial and lateral pain systems. *Eur J Neuroscience* 2005;21(11):3133–42.

31. Tolle TR, Kaufmann T, Siessmeier T, et al. Region-specific encoding of sensory and affective components of pain in the human brain: a positron emission tomography correlation analysis. *Ann Neurol* 1999;45(1):40–7.

32. Brooks JC, Zambreanu L, Godinez A, Craig AD, Tracey I. Somatotopic organisation of the human insula to painful heat studied with high resolution functional imaging. *Neuroimage* 2005;27(1):201–9.

33. Apkarian AV, Bushnell MC, Treede RD, Zubieta JK. Human brain mechanisms of pain perception and regulation in health and disease. *Eur J Pain* 2005;9(4):463–84.

34. Greenspan JD, Craft RM, LeResche L, et al. Studying sex and gender differences in pain and analgesia: a consensus report. *Pain* 2007; 132(Suppl 1):S26–45.

35. Fillingim RB, Maixner W. The influence of resting blood pressure and gender on pain responses. *Psychosom Med* 1996;58(4):326–32.

36. Tjandra T, Brooks JC, Figueiredo P, Wise R, Matthews PM, Tracey I. Quantitative assessment of the reproducibility of functional activation measured with BOLD and MR perfusion imaging: implications for clinical trial design. *Neuroimage* 2005;27(2):393–401.

37. Sanacora G, Mason GF, Rothman DL, et al. Reduced cortical gamma-aminobutyric acid levels in depressed patients determined by proton magnetic resonance spectroscopy. *Arch Gen Psychiatry* 1999;56(11):1043–7.

38. Reiman EM, Armstrong SM, Matt KS, Mattox JH. The application of positron emission tomography to the study of the normal menstrual cycle. *Hum Reprod* 1996;11(12):2799–805.

39. Zubieta JK, Smith YR, Bueller JA, et al. mu-opioid receptor-mediated antinociceptive responses differ in men and women. *J Neurosci* 2002;22(12):5100–7.

40. Curtis AL, Bethea T, Valentino RJ. Sexually dimorphic responses of the brain norepinephrine system to stress and corticotropin-releasing factor. *Neuropsychopharmacology* 2006;31(3):544–54.

41. Kajantie E, Phillips DI. The effects of sex and hormonal status on the physiological response to acute psychosocial stress. *Psychoneuroendocrinology* 2006;31(2):151–78.

42. Jazin E, Cahill L. Sex differences in molecular neuroscience: from fruit flies to humans. *Nat Rev Neurosci* 2010;11(1):9–17.

43. Cooke B, Hegstrom CD, Villeneuve LS, Breedlove SM. Sexual differentiation of the vertebrate brain: principles and mechanisms. *Front Neuroendocrinol* 1998;19(4):323–62.

44. LeResche L. Epidemiologic perspectives on sex differences in pain. In: Fillingim RB, ed. *Sex, Gender and Pain*. Seattle, WA: IASP Press; 2000: 233–49.

45. Sherman JJ, LeResche L. Does experimental pain response vary across the menstrual cycle? A methodological review. *Am J Physiol Regul Integr Comp Physiol* 2006;291(2):R245–56.

46. Hagemann G, Ugur T, Schleussner E, et al. Changes in brain size during the menstrual cycle. *PLoS One* 2011;6(2):e14655.

47. Witte AV, Savli M, Holik A, Kasper S, Lanzenberger R. Regional sex differences in grey matter volume are associated with sex hormones in the young adult human brain. *Neuroimage* 2010;49(2):1205–12.

48. Weis S, Hausmann M, Stoffers B, Vohn R, Kellermann T, Sturm W. Estradiol modulates functional brain organization during the menstrual cycle: an analysis of interhemispheric inhibition. *J Neurosci* 2008;28(50):13401–10.

49. Hausmann M, Gunturkun O. Steroid fluctuations modify functional cerebral asymmetries: the hypothesis of progesterone-mediated interhemispheric decoupling. *Neuropsychologia* 2000;38(10):1362–74.

50. Peper JS, van den Heuvel MP, Mandl RC, Pol HE, van Honk J. Sex steroids and connectivity in the human brain: A review of neuroimaging studies. *Psychoneuroendocrinology* 2011;36(8):1101–13.

51. Pfleeger M, Straneva PA, Fillingim RB, Maixner W, Girdler SS. Menstrual cycle, blood pressure and ischemic pain sensitivity in women: a preliminary investigation. *Int J Psychophysiol* 1997;27(2):161–6.

52. Metcalf MG, Livesey JH, Wells JE, Braiden V. Mood cyclicity in women with and without the premenstrual syndrome. *J Psychosom Res* 1989;33(4): 407–18.

53. Rubinow DR, Schmidt PJ. Gonadal steroid regulation of mood: the lessons of premenstrual syndrome. *Front Neuroendocrinol* 2006;27(2):210–6.

54. Smith YR, Stohler CS, Nichols TE, Bueller JA, Koeppe RA, Zubieta J-K. Pronociceptive and antinociceptive effects of estradiol through endogenous opioid neurotransmission in women. *J Neurosci* 2006;26(21):5777–85.

55. Harada M, Kubo H, Nose A, Nishitani H, Matsuda T. Measurement of variation in the human cerebral GABA level by in vivo MEGA-editing proton MR spectroscopy using a clinical 3 T instrument and its dependence on brain region and the female menstrual cycle. *Hum Brain Mapp* 2011;32(5):828–33.

56. Epperson CN, Haga K, Mason GF, et al. Cortical gamma-aminobutyric acid levels across the menstrual cycle in healthy women and those with premenstrual dysphoric disorder: a proton magnetic resonance spectroscopy study. *Arch Gen Psych* 2002;59(9):851–8.

57. Guillebaud J. *Contraception*. 4th ed. Philadelphia, PA: Churchill Livingstone; 2004.

58. Goolkasian P. Cyclic changes in pain perception: an ROC analysis. *Percep Psychophys* 1980;27(6):499–504.

59. Bohm-Starke N, Johannesson U, Hilliges M, Rylander E, Torebjèork E. Decreased mechanical pain threshold in the vestibular mucosa of women using oral contraceptives: a contributing factor in vulvar vestibulitis? *J Reprod Med* 2004;49(11):888–92.

60. LeResche L, Saunders K, Von Korff MR, Barlow W, Dworkin SF. Use of exogenous hormones and risk of temporomandibular disorder pain. *Pain* 1997;69(1–2):153–60.

61. Grushka M, Ching V, Epstein J. Burning mouth syndrome. *Adv Oto Rhin Laryng* 2006;63:278–87.

62. Allais G, Bussone G, Airola G, et al. Oral contraceptive-induced menstrual migraine. Clinical aspects and response to frovatriptan. *Neurol Sci* 2008;29:186–90.

63. Smith YR, Zubieta JK. Neuroimaging of aging and estrogen effects on central nervous system physiology. *Fertil Steril* 2001;76(4):651–9.

64. Wise PM. Estrogen therapy: does it help or hurt the adult and aging brain? Insights derived from animal models. *Neuroscience* 2006;138(3): 831–5.

65. Wise PM, Dubal DB, Rau SW, Brown CM, Suzuki S. Are estrogens protective or risk factors in brain injury and neurodegeneration? Reevaluation after the women's health initiative. *Endocr Rev* 2005;26(3):308–12.

66. van Wingen G, Mattern C, Verkes RJ, Buitelaar J, Fernandez G. Testosterone reduces amygdala-orbitofrontal cortex coupling. *Psychoneuroendocrinology* 2010;35(1):105–13.

67. van Wingen G, Mattern C, Verkes RJ, Buitelaar J, Fernandez G. Testosterone biases automatic memory processes in women towards potential mates. *Neuroimage* 2008;43(1):114–20.

68. van Wingen G, van Broekhoven F, Verkes RJ, et al. How progesterone impairs memory for biologically salient stimuli in healthy young women. *J Neurosci* 2007;27(42):11416–23.

69. van Wingen GA, van Broekhoven F, Verkes RJ, et al. Progesterone selectively increases amygdala reactivity in women. *Mol Psychiatry* 2008;13(3):325–33.

70. Paulson PE, Minoshima S, Morrow TJ, Casey KL. Gender differences in pain perception and patterns of cerebral activation during noxious heat stimulation in humans. *Pain* 1998;76(1–2): 223–9.

71. Derbyshire SWG, Nichols TE, Firestone L, Townsend DW, Jones AKP. Gender differences in patterns of cerebral activation during equal experience of painful laser stimulation. *J Pain* 2002;3(5):401–11.

72. Moulton EA, Keaser ML, Gullapalli RP, Maitra R, Greenspan JD. Sex differences in the cerebral BOLD signal response to painful heat stimuli. *Am J Physiol Regul Integr Comp Physiol* 2006;291(2):R257–67.

73. Straube T, Schmidt S, Weiss T, Mentzel HJ, Miltner WHR. Sex differences in brain

activation to anticipated and experienced pain in the medial prefrontal cortex. *Hum Brain Mapp* 2009;30:689–98.

74. WagerTD,RillingJK,SmithEE,etal.Placebo-induced changes in FMRI in the anticipation and experience of pain. *Science* 2004;303(5661):1162–7.

75. Wiech K, Kalisch R, Weiskopf N, Pleger B, Stephan KE, Dolan RJ. Anterolateral prefrontal cortex mediates the analgesic effect of expected and perceived control over pain. *J Neurosci* 2006;26(44):11501–9.

76. Berna C, Leknes S, Holmes E, Edwards RR, Goodwin G, Tracey I. Induction of depressed mood disrupts emotion regulation neurocircuitry and enhances pain unpleasantness. *Biol Psychiatry* 2010;67(11):1083–90.

77. Schweinhardt P, Kalk N, Wartolowska K, Chessell I, Wordsworth P, Tracey I. Investigation into the neural correlates of emotional augmentation of clinical pain. *Neuroimage* 2008;40(2):759–66.

78. Bär K-J, Wager G, Koschke M, et al. Increased prefrontal activation during pain perception in major depression. *Biol Psychiatry* 2007;62(11):1281–7.

79. Gracely RH, Geisser ME, Giesecke T, et al. Pain catastrophizing and neural responses to pain among persons with fibromyalgia. *Brain* 2004;127(4):835–43.

80. Ploghaus A, Tracey I, Gati JS, et al. Dissociating pain from its anticipation in the human brain. *Science* 1999;284(5422):1979–81.

81. Kalisch R, Wiech K, Critchley HD, et al. Anxiety reduction through detachment: subjective, physiological, and neural effects. *J Cogn Neurosci* 2005;17(6):874–83.

82. Perlman WR, Matsumoto M, Beltaifa S, et al. Expression of estrogen receptor alpha exon-deleted mRNA variants in the human and non-human primate frontal cortex. *Neurosci* 2005;134(1):81–95.

83. Montague D, Weickert CS, Tomaskovic-Crook E, Rothmond DA, Kleinman JE, Rubinow DR. Oestrogen receptor alpha localisation in the prefrontal cortex of three mammalian species. *J Neuroendocrinol* 2008;20(7):893–903.

84. Craig MC, Fletcher PC, Daly EM, et al. Gonadotropin hormone releasing hormone agonistsalterprefrontalfunctionduringverbalencoding in young women. *Psychoneuroendocrinology* 2007;32(8–10):1116–27.

85. Craig MC, Fletcher PC, Daly EM, et al. Physiological variation in estradiol and brain function: a functional magnetic resonance imaging study of verbal memory across the follicular phase of the menstrual cycle. *Horm Behav* 2008;53(4):503–8.

86. Berman KF, Schmidt PJ, Rubinow DR, et al. Modulation of cognition-specific cortical activity by gonadal steroids: a positron-emission tomography study in women. *Proc Natl Acad Sci USA* 1997;94(16):8836–41.

87. Ozawa M, Kanda K, Hirata M, Kusakawa I, Suzuki C. Effect of gender and hand laterality on pain processing in human neonates. *Early Hum Dev* 2011;87(1):45–48.

88. Steiner M, Dunn E, Born L. Hormones and mood: from menarche to menopause and beyond. *J Affect Disord* 2003;74(1):67–83.

89. Oinonen KA, Mazmanian D. To what extent do oral contraceptives influence mood and affect? *J Affect Dis* 2002;70(3):229–40.

90. Robinson DR, Gebhart GF. Inside information: the unique features of visceral sensation. *Mol Interv* 2008;8(5):242–53.

91. Moisset X, Bouhassira D, Denis D, Dominique G, Benoit C, Sabat JM. Anatomical connections between brain areas activated during rectal distension in healthy volunteers: a visceral pain network. *Eur J Pain* 2010;14(2):142–48.

92. Hobson AR, Furlong PL, Worthen SF, et al. Real-time imaging of human cortical activity evoked by painful esophageal stimulation. *Gastroenterol* 2005;128(3):610–9.

93. Berman SM, Naliboff BD, Suyenobu B, et al. Sex differences in regional brain response to aversive pelvic visceral stimuli. *Am J Physiol Regul Integr Comp Physiol* 2006;291(2):R268–76.

94. Fillingim RB, Gear RW. Sex differences in opioid analgesia: clinical and experimental findings. *Eur J Pain* 2004;8(5):413–25.

95. Alliende ME. Mean versus individual hormonal profiles in the menstrual cycle. *Fertil Steril* 2002;78(1):90–5.

96. Zubieta JK, Smith YR, Bueller JA, et al. Regional mu opioid receptor regulation of sensory and affective dimensions of pain. *Science* 2001;293(5528):311–5.

97. Zubieta JK, Bueller JA, Jackson LR, et al. Placebo effects mediated by endogenous opioid activity on mu-opioid receptors. *J Neurosci* 2005;25(34):7754–62.

98. De Vries GJ. Minireview: sex differences in adult and developing brains: compensation, compensation, compensation. *Endocrinology* 2004;145(3):1063–8.

99. Unruh AM. Gender variations in clinical pain experience. *Pain* 1996;65(2–3):123–67.

100. Blackburn-Munro G, Blackburn-Munro RE. Chronic pain, chronic stress and depression: coincidence or consequence? *J Neuroendocrinol* 2001;13(12):1009–23.

101. Strigo IA, Simmons AN, Matthews SC, Craig AD, Paulus MP. Association of major depressive disorder with altered functional brain response during anticipation and processing of heat pain. *Arch Gen Psychiatry* 2008;65(11):1275–84.

102. Labus JS, Naliboff BN, Fallon J, et al. Sex differences in brain activity during aversive visceral stimulation and its expectation in patients with chronic abdominal pain: a network analysis. *Neuroimage* 2008;41(3):1032–43.

103. Naliboff BD, Berman S, Chang L, et al. Sex-related differences in IBS patients: central processing of visceral stimuli. *Gastroenterology* 2003;124(7):1738–47.

104. Berman S, Munakata J, Naliboff BD, et al. Gender differences in regional brain response to visceral pressure in IBS patients. *Eur J Pain* 2000;4(2):157–72.

105. Apkarian AV, Krauss BR, Fredrickson BE, Szeverenyi NM. Imaging the pain of low back pain: functional magnetic resonance imaging in combination with monitoring subjective pain perception allows the study of clinical pain states. *Neurosci Lett* 2001;299(1–2):57–60.

106. Foss JM, Apkarian AV, Chialvo DR. Dynamics of pain: fractal dimension of temporal variability of spontaneous pain differentiates between pain States. *J Neurophysiol* 2006;95(2):730–6.

107. Schweinhardt P, Bountra C, Tracey I. Pharmacological FMRI in the development of new analgesic compounds. *NMR Biomed* 2006;19(6):702–11.

108. Woolf CJ. Central sensitization: implications for the diagnosis and treatment of pain. *Pain* 2011;152(3 Suppl):S2–15.

109. Berman SM, Naliboff BD, Suyenobu B, et al. Reduced brainstem inhibition during anticipated pelvic visceral pain correlates with enhanced brain response to the visceral stimulus in women with irritable bowel syndrome. *J Neurosci* 2008;28(2):349–59.

110. Bonaz B, Baciu M, Papillon E, et al. Central processing of rectal pain in patients with irritable bowel syndrome: an fMRI study. *Am J Gastroenterol* 2002;97(3):654–61.

111. Elsenbruch S, Rosenberger C, Bingel U, Forsting M, Schedlowski M, Gizewski ER. Patients with irritable bowel syndrome have altered emotional modulation of neural responses to visceral stimuli. *Gastroenterol* 2010;139(4):1310–19.

112. Cook DB, Lange G, Ciccone DS, Liu WC, Steffener J, Natelson BH. Functional imaging of pain in patients with primary fibromyalgia. *J Rheumatol* 2004;31(2):364–78.

113. Jensen KB, Kosek E, Petzke F, et al. Evidence of dysfunctional pain inhibition in Fibromyalgia reflected in rACC during provoked pain. *Pain* 2009;144(1–2):95–100.

114. Wood PB, Schweinhardt P, Jaeger E, et al. Fibromyalgia patients show an abnormal dopamine response to pain. *Eur J Neurosci* 2007;25(12):3576–82.

115. Iannetti GD, Zambreanu L, Wise RG, et al. Pharmacological modulation of pain-related brain activity during normal and central sensitization states in humans. *Proc Natl Acad Sci USA* 2005;102(50):18195–200.

116. Borras MC, Becerra L, Ploghaus A, et al. fMRI measurement of CNS responses to naloxone infusion and subsequent mild noxious thermal stimuli in healthy volunteers. *J Neurophysiol* 2004;91(6):2723–33.

117. Wise RG, Rogers R, Painter D, et al. Combining fMRI with a pharmacokinetic model to determine which brain areas activated by painful stimulation are specifically modulated by remifentanil. *Neuroimage* 2002;16(4):999–1014.

118. Craft RM, Mogil JS, Aloisi AM. Sex differences in pain and analgesia: the role of gonadal hormones. *Eur J Pain* 2004;8(5):397–411.

119. McLaughlin KJ, Baran SE, Conrad CD. Chronic stress- and sex-specific neuromorphological and functional changes in limbic structures. *Mol Neurobiol* 2009;40(2):166–82.

120. Gaab J, Baumann S, Budnoik A, Gmünder H, Hottinger N, Ehlert U. Reduced reactivity and enhanced negative feedback sensitivity of the hypothalamus-pituitary-adrenal axis in chronic whiplash-associated disorder. *Pain* 2005;119(1–3):219–24.

121. Fries E, Hesse J, Hellhammer J, Hellhammer DH. A new view on hypocortisolism. *Psychoneuroendocrinol* 2005;30(10):1010–6.

122. Turner-Cobb JM, Osborn M, da Silva L, Keogh E, Jessop DS. Sex differences in hypothalamic-pituitary-adrenal axis function in patients with chronic pain syndrome. *Stress* 2010;13(4):292–300.

123. Nakai A, Kumakura Y, Boivin M, et al. Sex differences of brain serotonin synthesis in patients with irritable bowel syndrome using alpha-[11C]methyl-L-tryptophan, positron emission tomography and statistical parametric mapping. *Can J Gastroenterol* 2003;17(3):191–6.

4

SEX DIFFERENCES IN ANALGESIC RESPONSES

CLINICAL AND EXPERIMENTAL STUDIES

Marieke Niesters, Albert Dahan, Leon Aarts, and Elise Sarton

INTRODUCTION

Humans rely on potent analgesic agents to obtain relief from severe pain. The most important agents include the opioids, with morphine as the prototypical μ-opioid receptor agonist, and are still considered the gold standard for treatment of severe acute pain and chronic cancer and noncancer pain that is unresponsive to nonopioid analgesics. Animal studies indicate that responses to analgesics are dependent on many, often interacting, factors such as nociceptive sensitivity, genetics, age, and sex. Indeed, the presence of sexual dimorphism in antinociceptive responses to opioid agents has been well established in mice and rats.[1-4] Also in humans the presence of sex as a possible determining factor in analgesic efficacy is increasingly appreciated and studied.[3] In this chapter we discuss the current literature reporting quantitative data on responses to analgesic agents in the two sexes. The emphasis of our systematic review will be on a recently performed meta-analysis of human experimental and clinical studies on μ- and mixed action μ/κ-opioids.[5] Next, we will discuss data on nonopioid analgesics, including nonsteroidal anti-inflammatory drugs, the N-methyl-D-aspartate antagonist ketamine, and local anesthetics. This review is restricted to experimental studies in adult

human volunteers (i.e., studies in persons without preexisting pain and in which painful responses are elicited in a specific nociceptive assay) and clinical studies in patients (i.e., studies in patients with pain).

OPIOIDS

Pooled Quantitative Data

While numerous studies on opioid efficacy have been performed in both clinical and experimental settings, the number of studies systematically exploring sex effects in opioid analgesia or antinociception is rather limited. We recently searched the literature (the following electronic databases were searched: PubMed, EMBASE, WOS, Cochrane Library, CIAHL, PsycINFO, Academic Search premier) for studies assaying acute opioid analgesia in men and women and were able to collect 47 unique published reports that generated quantitative data on at least one opioid analgesic (or antinociceptive) efficacy in adult humans (18 years or older).[5-44] The initial search produced about 2,400 papers of which most reported data on abuse characteristics of opioids in males versus females ($n > 1,500$) or did not present original data ($n \approx 400$). The remaining studies were either not performed in humans, were on chronic pain, were studies in children, or did not provide sufficient detail to enable us to extract qualitative data on a sex effect of the opioids tested. Finally, one unpublished report on three opioids was added (Zacny JP. Gender differences in opioid analgesia in human volunteers: morphine, butorphanol and nalbuphin. 2008, unpublished observation).

An initial meta-analysis (using the random effects model) on the total pooled data set (*n* = 50 studies on single opioids testing 6,459 men and 6,979 women) yielded a standardized difference in means (± standard error) of 0.21 ± 0.05 (*p* < .01), favoring analgesic efficacy of opioids in women (Fig. 4.1),[5-44] although the estimated additional beneficial effect in women is small (a standardized difference in means of 0.2 is small, 0.35 moderate, 0.5 intermediate, 0.6 appreciable, 0.8 large). The heterogeneity between studies was large (I^2 = 91), but this was expected taking into account the fact that the 50 studies included data on full μ-agonists (tested opioids were morphine, morphine-6-

glucuronide, meperidine, fentanyl, alfentanil, -endorphin, and hydromorphone), partial μ-agonists (buprenorphine), and mixed action μ/κ-opioids (pentazocine, nalbuphine, butorphanol) and were performed either in clinical (postsurgical analgesia or analgesia in the emergency department) or experimental settings (i.e., antinociceptive studies in healthy volunteers without pain). With the large variations within the experimental designs of the 50 studies, further subanalyses were carried out with more homogeneous data sets.

FULL OR PARTIAL μ-AGONISTS

Thirty-six of the studies retrieved from the literature were performed on full or partial μ-agonists (testing 6,216 men and 6,740 women).[6-35] Performing a meta-analysis on these data, a standard difference in means of 0.10 ± 0.08 (*p* = .20) failed to yield a difference between the sexes as was observed in the total

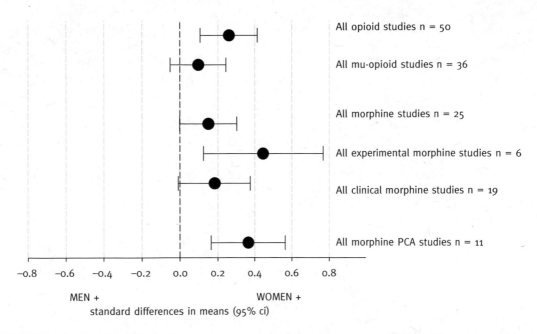

FIGURE 4.1   Opioid effect in men versus women. Results of a meta-analysis on 50 papers retrieved from the literature on analgesic or antinociceptive efficacy. (Data are from Niesters M, Dahan A, Kest B, et al. Do sex differences exist in opioid analgesia? A systematic review and meta-analysis of human experimental and clinical studies. *Pain* 2010;151:61–8.) Analysis on the total data set (μ and mixed μ/κ opioids; *n* = 50 studies) and subanalyses (μ-agonists and morphine studies) are shown. Significant greater opioid analgesia was observed in women in the whole data set, experimental studies on μ-agonists and patient controlled analgesia (PCA) morphine studies. MEN+ indicates greater analgesic opioid effect in men; WOMEN+ indicates greater opioid analgesic in women.

pooled data. The absence of any clear difference in effect between the sexes may still be explained by the pooling of different opioids in the data set (one μ-agonist may show sex dependency while another does not). Most of the studies were performed on morphine. Pooling the morphine data ($n = 27$) irrespective of setting (clinical or experimental) yielded a standard difference in means of 0.15 ± 0.09 ($p = .09$), indicating absence of sex effect (see Table 4.1 for the studies used in the analysis). No meaningful subanalysis was possible on any of the other μ-opioids tested due to small number of studies per distinct opioid. Alternatively, the lack of sex differences in this data set may be related to the pooling of experimental and clinical data.

A subanalysis on experimental studies ($n = 11$) on μ-opioids (irrespective of the opioid tested) yielded a significant sex effect with a standardized difference in means of 0.35 ± 0.05 ($p = .047$),[18,29-35] favoring greater opioid antinociception in women. Still, the sex difference in effect is moderate in magnitude. Six of the studies were on morphine, which pooled together yielded a significant standardized difference in means of 0.45 ± 0.04 ($p = .04$), indicating that women respond with greater antinociception than men when given morphine in an experimental setting (Table 4.1). However, the data were dominated by one study (Sarton et al.).[34] Removal of that study caused the loss of a significant sex difference (standard difference in means = 0.28 ± 0.16, $p = .10$, $n = 5$).

Clinical studies on μ-agonists could be divided into two distinct groups.[6-28] Group A: Fifteen studies were on postoperative pain relief for a variety of surgeries using patient controlled analgesia (PCA) for 17 to 72 h postsurgery using mostly morphine ($n = 11$, Table 4.1). The measured endpoint in these studies was opioid consumption. Group B: Ten studies examined the effect of single- or multiple-opioid doses, either postoperatively or in the emergency department, and measurements were made in a short time span following drug administration (minutes to hours). The measured endpoints were numerical pain score or dose required to attain full pain relief (Table 4.1).

An analysis on all clinical studies (Groups A + B) revealed an absence of a sex effect: standardized difference in means 0.09 ± 0.09 ($p = .29$).[6-28] Since the majority of studies were on morphine ($n = 19$), a subanalysis was performed (irrespective of method of pain relief), still yielding no significant sex effect: standardized difference in means 0.18 ± 0.13 ($p = .06$). Restricting the analysis to PCA morphine (a subset derived from Group A, Table 4.1) did yield a sex effect with greater morphine analgesia in women: standardized difference in means 0.36 ± 0.10 ($p < .01$). A meta-regression was performed to assess the effect of PCA duration, which showed a significant correlation between PCA duration and sex effect. The longer the duration of the PCA measurements, the greater the observed sex effect (Fig. 4.2). After 72 h of PCA the sex effect accumulated to a large effect size of 0.8. In contrast, no sex differences were observed in the studies from group B, irrespective of the opioid type used.

MIXED μ/κ-OPIOIDS

A total of 14 useful (clinical and experimental) studies on mixed μ/κ-opioids was identified in which 243 men and 239 women were tested.[25,36-44] An analysis on these studies revealed a significant sex effect with greater analgesia/antinociception in women: standardized difference in means 0.45 ± 0.20 ($p = .02$). A sensitivity analysis on the data revealed the dominance of one study on the results of the aforementioned data analysis. Mogil et al.[43] tested the effect of the mixed μ/κ-opioid pentazocine in persons with a dysfunctional melanocortin 1 receptor (MC1r) gene in an experimental setting. They observed a greater antinociceptive effect in women (standardized difference in means = 1.8 ± 0.6, $p = .008$), while in subjects with a normal functioning MC1r gene no significant sex effect was observed. Removal of the data on subjects with a dysfunctional MC1r gene resulted in an effect size of 0.37 ± 0.19 ($p = .06$). A clear trend is present in the data with greater analgesic efficacy in women. Significance would have been reached if the sample sizes were bigger.

Meta-analysis of experimental studies ($n = 7$, including the one unpublished observation) resulted in the absence of a sex effect with standardized difference in means of −0.04 ± 0.17

Table 4.1   Characteristics of Morphine Studies Used in the Meta-Analysis of Niesters et al.[5]

STUDY	SAMPLE SIZE (M/F)	DRUG	TYPE OF PAIN	OUTCOME
		CLINICAL STUDIES		
Aubrun[6]	2,344/1,933	IV morphine	Postoperative	M > F
Bennett[7]	2/8	PCA morphine	Postoperative	M = F
Bijur[8]	41/50	IV morphine	Acute pain in ED	M = F
Bijur[9]	16/19	IV morphine	Acute pain in ED	M = F
Birnbaum[10]	82/54	IV morphine	Acute pain in ED	M = F
Burns[11]	38/46	PCA morphine	Postoperative	F > M
Cepeda[12]	277/423	IV morphine	Postoperative	M > F
Chang[13]	33/61	IV morphine	Acute pain in ED	M = F
Chang[14]	646/662	PCA morphine	Postoperative	F > M
Chia[15]	854/1,444	PCA morphine	Postoperative	F > M
Dahlström[16]	6/4	PCA morphine	Postoperative	M = F
DeKock[17]	111/89	PCA morphine	Postoperative	F > M
Glasson[19]	44/106	PCA morphine	Postoperative	M = F
Joels[21]	235/246	IV morphine	Postoperative	F > M
Larijani[22]	12/25	IV morphine	Postoperative	M > F
Macintyre[24]	486/453	PCA morphine	Postoperative	F > M
Miller[25]	24/22	IV morphine	Acute pain in ED	M = F
Sidebotham[26]	158/142	PCA morphine	Postoperative	F > M
Tsui[28]	419/372	PCA morphine	Postoperative	F > M
		EXPERIMENTAL STUDIES		
Comer[29]	8/10	IM morphine	Cold pressure test	M = F
Fillingim[30]	39/61	IV morphine	Pressure pain	M = F
Pud[32]	12/9	Oral morphine	Cold pressure test	F > M
Sarton[34]	12/12	IV morphine	Electrical pain	F > M
Zacny[35]	15/15	IV morphine	Cold pressure test	M = F
Zacny*	16/16	IV morphine	Cold pressure test	M = F

ED, emergency department; IM, intramuscular; IV morphine, a single or multiple intravenous morphine administrations; PCA morphine, patient-controlled analgesia with intravenous morphine (outcome of these studies is morphine consumption). * Zacny JP. Gender differences in opioid analgesia in human volunteers: morphine, butorphanol and nalbuphin. 2008, unpublished observation.

(p = .82; this analysis includes the study in subjects with a dysfunctional *MC1r* gene).[41-44] In contrast, the meta-analysis of clinical studies (n = 7) yielded a strong sex effect with a standardized difference in means of 0.84 ± 0.30 (p < .01).[25,36-40] The clinical studies were performed predominantly in patients following oral surgery and were performed by a limited number of research centers (four of seven studies came from one center). Furthermore, some publication bias cannot be excluded (fail-safe, N = 3).

Interpretation of the Opioid Data

While our overall quantitative analyses revealed the existence of a small sex difference in the

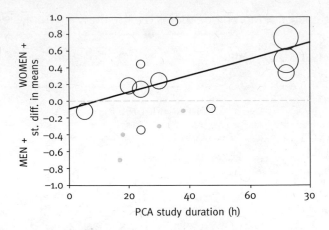

FIGURE 4.2 Meta-regression analysis of patient controlled analgesia (PCA) duration (μ-agonists) versus sex difference effect size (*y*-axis; MEN+ indicates greater analgesic opioid effect in men; WOMEN+ indicates greater opioid analgesic in women). Each of the studies is shown as a circle; the diameter of the circle is proportional to the weight of the study in the analysis. Open circles are morphine PCA studies; gray circles are PCA studies on other μ-opioids.

analgesic efficacy of opioids with a greater effect in women, subanalysis indicated that sex differences are most probably restricted to specific experimental conditions and clinical settings and are limited to specific opioids. Sex differences are most pronounced in clinical studies on morphine PCA, and at present we cannot exclude the existence of sex differences in clinical studies on mixed μ/κ-opioids. This does not mean that we can conclude that sex differences do not exist for other opioids under other conditions than specified here, but the sparse data presently available do not allow any conclusions to be drawn on other opioids in other settings.

With respect to μ-agonists, morphine was the opioid most studied. A small sex effect was observed in experimental studies on morphine, an effect that was dominated by one study. Sarton et al.[34] studied the effect of a 1-h infusion of morphine on transcutaneous electrical pain tolerance and threshold using a population pharmacokinetic/pharmacodynamics (PKPD) study design. This is just one of three studies in our data set that used this approach,[31,33,34] which enables the acquisition of high-quality data allowing (1) the measurement of a sex effect over longer time periods (in this case, 7 h); (2) the assessment of a sex effect due to sex differences in pharmacokinetics, pharmacodynamics, or both; (3) a reliable estimate of the

true opioid potency (rather than of analgesic effect); and (4) a reliable estimate of between- versus within-subject variability. The results of the study are depicted in Figure 4.3A, showing a difference in analgesia during and following the morphine infusion. Peak analgesic effect, while higher in women, is obtained at a later time point than peak analgesia in men. In fact, over the first 60 min, the analgesic effect is greater in men than women. After 60 min this effect is reversed, and at time >240 min no more analgesia is observed in men while analgesia persists in women for times >420 min. The PKPD analysis revealed (1) similar morphine pharmacokinetics in men and women; (2) similar metabolism in men and women with similar concentrations of morphine's metabolites morphine-3-glucuronide and morphine-6-glucuronide; (3) a 80%–100% greater morphine potency in women; and (4) a slower analgesia onset/offset in women by a factor of 2 (half-life for onset of effect = 1.5 h in men versus 3 h in women). To get a better impression of the biphasic nature of the sex difference in morphine-analgesia, we performed a simulation study (see Fig. 4.3B), where we simulated a single morphine infusion at *t* = 0 and observed pain relief for 240 min in men and women using the PKPD data from Sarton et al. The top graph shows the sex orientation with greater analgesic effect in men from

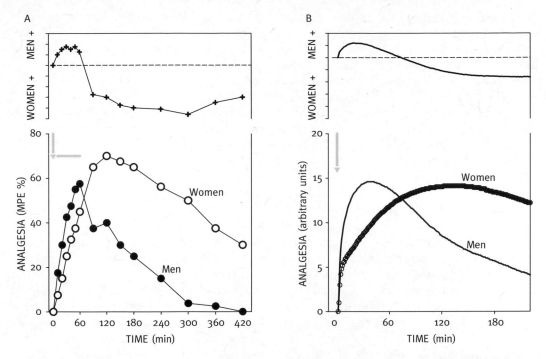

FIGURE 4.3 (*A*) Effect of intravenous morphine (0.1 mg/kg bolus + 0.03 mg/kg per h for 1 h, gray bars) on pain tolerance in 10 men and 10 women as determined from tolerance to a transcutaneous electrical pain stimulus (data are from ref. 34). Initially analgesia is greater but after 60 min women experience greater analgesia. The top graph shows the difference in effect size between men and women. (*B*) Simulation study using PKPD model parameters derived from Sarton et al.[34] A single infusion of 0.1 mg/kg is simulated. Pain responses for men and women are shown together with the difference in effect size (top diagram). MEN+ indicates greater analgesic opioid effect in men; WOMEN+ indicates greater opioid analgesic in women

$t = 0$ to $t = 60$ min (note that this occurs despite greater morphine potency in women), but with greater analgesic effect in women from $t = 60$ min onward. The cause for the biphasic sex effect is the slower onset/offset time for morphine analgesia in women. This may be related to a slower morphine passage across the blood–brain barrier and/or slower opioid receptor kinetics in women. Slower receptor kinetics would result in a slower attachment of morphine to the μ-opioid receptor, but when bound to the receptor it takes longer to get separated again.

The biphasic nature of sex differences in morphine analgesia may well explain the results observed in studies that examine morphine infusions over relatively short periods of time. This is relevant for both experimental and clinical studies on morphine analgesia. For example, Aubrun et al.[6] studied 2,344 men and 1,922 women following abdominal and orthopedic surgery. Morphine doses required to achieve pain relief (a pain score of 3 or less) were assessed with a treatment regimen of 2–3 mg intravenous morphine infusions at 5-min intervals. The sex difference in effect was –0.102 favoring analgesic efficacy in men. Similarly, Cepeda and Carr studied 277 men and 423 women following head/neck, thoracic, abdominal, or orthopedic surgery. Patients received 2.5 mg intravenous morphine at 10-min intervals and the morphine doses until adequate pain relief (pain score 4 or less) was assessed.[12] The sex difference in effect was –0.013, indicating the need for greater morphine doses in women to achieve adequate pain relief in the initial postoperative hours. Studies on patients with acute pain who visited the emergency room and received a single morphine infusion (0.1 mg/kg) observed either no sex difference in morphine analgesia or a greater effect in men (Table 4.1). In contrast, 8 of 11 studies on morphine PCA show that women consume less morphine than men (Fig. 4.2 and Table 4.1). These findings may all be explained by the biphasic nature of sex dependency, with initially a greater morphine analgesic effect in men followed by greater analgesia in women. The duration of the relative period of greater analgesia in men is dependent on the infusion scheme, but it appears to be between 60 and 180 min following the initiation of therapy. Our analyses indicates that sex differences in morphine analgesia (and possibly more general opioid analgesia) are complex and dependent on opioid pharmacokinetics (with possibly sex differences in passage across the blood–brain barrier and receptor kinetics) and opioid pharmacodynamics (a true sex difference in opioid potency). This then suggests that for human data, a meta-analysis on pooled data is not advisable and studies need to be stratified by study design (e.g., for clinical studies Groups A versus B; for experimental studies [long-term] PKPD studies versus [short-term] observational studies). In Group A, PCA studies were collected that were performed for at least 17 h, ample time for the sex effect to develop toward the direction of a greater effect in women. In Group B studies were collected that tested opioid effect for no longer than 4–6 hours, a time span in which either the sex effect is toward greater analgesia in men or no sex differences become apparent. Two PKPD experimental studies on alfentanil and morphine's active metabolite morphine-6-glucuronide showed absence of sex effect in analgesic potency or analgesia onset/offset times.[31,33] These data suggest that sex differences may be opioid dependent and that conclusions drawn from studies on morphine should not be extrapolated to other opioids.

Studies utilizing PCA tend to measure opioid consumption rather than specific measures of opioid efficacy or pain relief. It is possible that opioid consumption per se differs between the sexes and is unrelated to analgesic endpoints (i.e., titration to adequate pain relief). For example, sex differences in the incidence of opioid side effects (such as nausea/vomiting, sedation, dysphoria, light headedness/dizziness, feeling of drug high, etc.) or the fear of opioid use (related to fear of addiction/abuse, respiratory depression, sedation, nausea/vomiting, etc.) may cause women to consume fewer opioids. However, most of the PCA studies do also give pain scores during PCA treatment and either pain scores were not different between men and women, or pain was greater in men. This suggests that opioid consumption in PCA studies reflects titration to pain relief and is not driven (restricted) by non-analgesia-related factors.

The results of the meta-analysis on mixed μ/κ-opioids showed a clear sex difference in clinical studies, especially in studies on third molar extraction or endodontic surgery.[25,36–40] Pain relief was assessed after a single opioid administration for up to 3 h (24 h in one study). In contrast, no sex differences were observed in experimental studies (with the exception of one study performed in persons with a dysfunction MC1r gene), similarly lasting no longer than 1–3 h.[36–41] The discrepancy in these study results cannot simply be explained by sex differences in either pharmacokinetics or pharmacodynamics of the drugs tested. As stated earlier, third molar surgery may possibly result in a peripheral inflammatory/nociceptive response with high sensitivity to κ-opioids restricted to women, and the strong influence of a dysfunctional MC1r gene in an experimental study may indicate that other genetic traits within the sexes may also have a profound influence.

NONOPIOID ANALGESICS

Nonsteroidal Anti-Inflamatory Drugs

Averbuch and Katzper performed a meta-analysis on seven double-blind studies on the efficacy of the nonsteroidal anti-inflammatory drug (NSAID) ibuprofen on post-third-molar extraction dental pain.[45] The studies were submitted electronically to the US Food and Drug Administration. Subjects in the studies were aged 15 years or older and had moderate to severe pain before the initiation of treatment (pain score > 50 mm or a 100 mm visual analog scale). Efficacy endpoints included pain intensity and pain relief during the 6 hours following surgery and time to rescue medication. A total of 195 women and 119 men were included in the analysis. The meta-analysis demonstrated the well-established analgesic effects of ibuprofen, but it failed to indicate sex differences in any of the efficacy parameters ($p = .62$). Analyses of the individual studies indicated a significant sex effect in just two of the studies (analgesic effects observed were greater in men than women in one study and the reverse in the other study). One additional study on ibuprofen (800 mg, oral) was performed in volunteers (10 men/10 women), showing an analgesic effect to electrical transcutaneous pain in men only.[46] This is remarkable as in clinical models ibuprofen is an active analgesic in both sexes. One study on a different NSAID, ketorolac, in healthy volunteers (25 men/25 women), using cold pressor pain tolerance as efficacy parameter, showed no sex differences.[47] In summary, the current data on the efficacy of NSAIDs in men versus women do not permit the conclusion that significant sex differences in analgesic effect exist.

Ketamine

Sigtermans et al.[48] examined possible sex differences of the N-methyl-D-aspartate (NMDA) receptor antagonist ketamine in humans. The authors performed a PKPD modeling study and assessed the effect of a 2-h increasing intravenous (IV) infusion of S-ketamine (the S(+)-enantiomer) in healthy volunteers (10 men/10 women; duration of study was 6 h). The results are shown in Figure 4.4C. An evident difference in response to a heat pain stimulus is observed with a greater analgesic effect in men. However, this difference in therapeutic effect is fully explained by differences in the pharmacokinetics of ketamine between the sexes; women demonstrating lower concentrations of both the parent (ketamine) and active metabolite (norketamine; Fig. 4.4A and 4.4B). Ketamine potency did not differ between men and women (C_{50} 370 ng/ml in the two sexes). In a separate study, sex differences in the side effects of ketamine also were observed with greater side effects (cognitive decline) from racemic ketamine in men relative to women (plasma concentrations were not obtained).[49] The results of Sigtermans et al.[48] suggest that

these later observations may also be related to sex difference in ketamine's pharmacokinetics. The study from Sigtermans et al. exemplifies the need for a PKPD study design to fully understand possible sex difference in analgesic efficacy. However, a clear conclusion on the existence of a sex effect in the analgesic effect of NMDA receptor antagonists cannot be concluded from this one experimental study.

Local Anesthetics

We retrieved five studies from the literature on the effect of local anesthetics in adult humans that allowed a quantitative assessment of an analgesic sex effect of these agents (two experimental studies and three clinical studies):

- In an experimental study on the effect of iontophoretic lidocaine in healthy volunteers (21 women/23 men), men rated the pain induced by a pressure stimulus less painful than women (difference in effect size about 20%).[50]
- Healthy volunteers (20 women/10 men) received a buccal infiltration with lidocaine and epinephrine (1:100,000), and their pain threshold to an electrical stimulus (using an electric pulp tester) was assessed. Pain threshold was higher in men, indicating a better analgesic effect in men.[51]
- In a clinical study on the effectiveness of EMLA cream (a cream consisting of lidocaine and prilocaine) for skin analgesia during transcutaneous endomyocardial biopsy, females had greater pain scores than men (50 men/19 women).[52]
- In 35 men and 35 women undergoing anorectal surgery, the minimum local analgesic concentration of ropivacaine (as determined by Dixon's up-and-down sequential allocation method) for caudal analgesia in patients was 31% greater in women.[53]
- The effect of patient-controlled epidural analgesia was tested in postsurgical patients (1,094 men/659 women). These patients received a mixture of bupivacaine and fentanyl and had similar anesthetic/opioid consumption during the first three postoperative days.[54]

Four of the five studies indicate greater efficacy of local anesthetics in men. However, the data should be interpreted with caution. The number of studies is limited, sample sizes

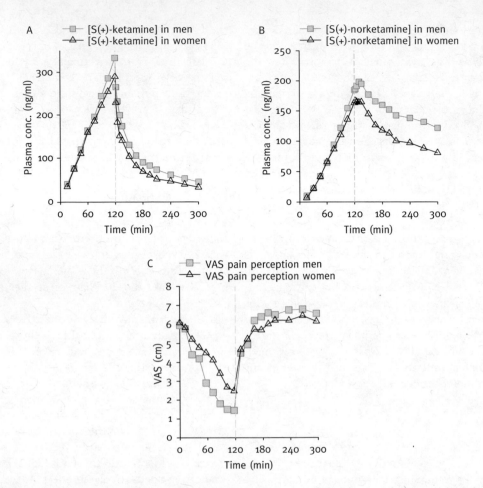

FIGURE 4.4   Effect of a 2-h S-ketamine infusion on plasma concentrations S-ketamine (*A*), plasma S-norketamine concentrations (*B*), and pain intensity in response to a heat pain stimulus on the lower arm (*C*) in 10 men and 10 women (data are from Sigtermans M, Dahan A, Mooren R, et al. S[+]-ketamine effect on experimental pain and cardiac output: a population pharmacokinetic-pharmacodynamic modeling study in healthy volunteers. *Anesthesiology* 2009;111:892–903). The observed sex difference in pain intensity is fully explained by sex differences in S-ketamine and S-norketamine pharmacokinetics. S-ketamine potency did not differ between the sexes. Horizontal lines indicate the end of the S-ketamine infusion (from *t* = 0 to *t* = 2 h).

were small, and in three studies a drug combination was given (EMLA, lidocaine + epinephrine, bupivacaine + fentanyl), making interpretation of data difficult, as we remain uninformed on the contributions and influence of the individual agents used. Also, the design of most of the studies is such that pain is assessed only once, after administration of the anesthetic. Thus, sex differences in basal pain perception could drive the findings. That is, it is possible that the anesthetics work equally well in both sexes, but women have more pain from the procedure.

In conclusion, the evidence for the existence of sex difference in the analgesic effects of local anesthetics remains small, and although four of the five aforementioned studies point toward greater analgesic efficacy from local anesthetics in men, further data are required before definitive conclusions can be drawn.

SUMMARY AND FINAL REMARKS

Evidence regarding the existence of sex differences in the efficacy of analgesics in humans is meager. Although meta-analysis of pooled data from 50 studies showed a slight statistically significant difference favoring analgesic effects of opioids in women, more detailed meta-analysis of the studies that stratified for various μ- and μ/κ-opioid drugs in experimental and clinical settings revealed little evidence for clear differences of effect between the sexes. This systematic review of the literature indicates that the strongest evidence for sex differences exists for clinical studies using mixed μ/κ-opioids and clinical studies PCA with morphine. The latter showed greater morphine analgesic efficacy in women (irrespective of age). The observation from the meta-regression analysis that a linear relationship exists between the duration of PCA and the results from a PKPD modeling study on IV morphine efficacy in healthy volunteers, jointly, indicate that apart from a true pharmacodynamic difference in morphine's behavior, there exists a difference in morphine onset/offset times. This then explains the findings of greater analgesia/antinociception in men in studies testing the short-term effect of intravenous morphine in both experimental and clinical studies compared to the greater analgesia/antinociception observed in women as time progresses.

In addition, an item that remains understudied is the interaction between age and sex differences in opioid effect. Eight studies give data on opioid effect in men versus women at a postmenopausal age (>50 years old).[6,14,15,17,21–23,28] Two of these found the loss of a sex difference at ages >60 years,[6,17] the majority observed the persistence of sex differences, although in all studies opioid doses (consumption or IV dose for adequate pain relief) were significantly smaller in older patients (>60 years).[14,15,21–23,28] No studies addressed the extremes of old age. Taken the fact that the world population is aging with more people aged >80 years than ever (octogenarians are currently increasing at 3.8%/year and 65% of them are female, while 83% of persons >100 years are female),[55] we would encourage further study on the existence of sex differences in analgesic pharmacokinetics and/or pharmacodynamics in older patients (>80 years).

A second item that remains understudied is the possible existence of sex differences in analgesics in chronic pain patients. Only few studies report the effect of sex (often included as covariate in the analysis) on analgesic efficacy in patients taking opioids for chronic pain. Five studies that do report on sex effect on opioids for treatment of cancer and noncancer pain indicate absence of a significant sex difference (in terms of dosage required for adequate pain relief).[56–60] However, interpretation of these data is difficult as pretreatment pain and the development of the underlying disease process may differ between the sexes and consequently may affect the study outcome. Furthermore, since the weights of the patients are not reported, a difference in weight between the sexes may be a confounder that requires attention in further studies. Finally, there is some evidence that hyperalgesia from sustained opioid therapy in chronic pain is sex dependent with greater hyperalgesia in women.[61] If true, sex differences in hyperalgesia may coexist with sex differences in analgesia. This analgesia–hyperalgesia interaction will determine the development of the analgesic pattern and as such is an important area for further research.

REFERENCES

1. Craft RM. Sex differences in opioid analgesia: "from mouse to man." *Clin J Pain* 2003; 19:175–86.
2. Dahan A, Kest B, Waxman AR, Sarton E. Sex-specific responses to opiates: animal and human studies. *Anesth Analg* 2008;107:83–95.
3. Fillimgim RB, King CD, Ribeiro-Dasilva MC, Rahim-Williams B, Riley JL. Sex, gender, and pain: a review of recent clinical and experimental findings. *J Pian* 2009;10:447–85.
4. Mogil JS, Bailey AL. Sex and gender differences in pain and analgesia. *Prog Brain Res* 2010;186:141–57.
5. Niesters M, Dahan A, Kest B, et al. Do sex differences exist in opioid analgesia? A systematic review and meta-analysis of human experimental and clinical studies. *Pain* 2010;151:61–8.
6. Aubrun F, Salvi N, Coriat P, Riou B. Sex- and age-related differences in morphine requirements for postoperative pain relief. *Anesthesiology* 2005;103:156–60. *Anaesthesia* 1985;40:529–32.
7. Bennett R, Batenhorst R, Graves DA, Foster TS, Griffen WO, Wright BD. Variation in

postoperative analgesic requirements in the morbidly obese following gastric bypass surgery. *Pharmacotherapy* 1982;2:50–53.

8. Bijur PE, Esses D, Birnbaum A, Chang AK, Schechter C, Gallagher EJ. Response to morphine in male and female patients: analgesia and adverse events. *Clin J Pain* 2008(a,b,c);24:192–8.

9. Bijur PE, Schechter C, Esses D, Chang AH, Gallagher EJ. Intravenous bolus of ultra-low-dose naloxone added to morphine does not enhance analgesia in emergency department patients. *J Pain* 2006;7:75–81.

10. Birnbaum A, Esses D, Bijur PE, Holden L, Gallagher EJ. Randomized double-blind placebo-controlled trial of two intravenous morphine dosages (0.10 mg/kg and 0.15 mg/kg) in emergency department patients with moderate to severe acute pain. *Ann Emerg Med* 2006;48:164–72.

11. Burns JW, Hodsman NBA, McLintock TTC, Gillies GWA, Kenny GNC, McArdle CS. The influence of patient characteristics on the requirement for postoperative analgesia. *Anaesthesia* 1989;44:2–6.

12. Cepeda MS, Carr DB. Women experience more pain and require more morphine than men to achieve a similar degree of analgesia. *Anesth Analg* 2003;97:1464–8.

13. Chang AK, Bijur PE, Meyer RH, Kenny MK, Solorzano C, Gallagher EJ. Safety and efficacy of hydromorphone as an analgesic alternative to morphine in acute pain: a randomized clinical trial. *Ann Emerg Med* 2003;10:390–2.

14. Chang KY, Tsou MY, Chan KH, Sung CS, Chang WK. Factors affecting patient-controlled analgesia requirements. *J Formos Med Assoc* 2006;105:918–25.

15. Chia YY, Chow LH, Hung CC, Liu K, Ger LP, Wang PN. Gender and pain upon movement are associated with the requirements for postoperative patient-controlled *iv* analgesia: a prospective survey of 2,298 Chinese patients. *Can J Anaesth* 2002;49:249–55.

16. Dahlström B, Tamsen A, Paalzow L, Hartvig P. Patient-controlled analgesic therapy, part IV: Pharmacokinetics and analgesic plasma concentrations of morphine. *Clin Pharmacokinet* 1982;7:266–79.

17. DeKock M, Scholtes JL. Postoperative P.C.A. in abdominal surgery: analysis of 200 consecutive patients. *Acta Anaesth Belg* 1991;42:85–91.

18. Fukuda K, Hayashida M, Ide S, et al. Association between *OPRM1* gene polymorphisms and fentanyl sensitivity in patients undergoing painful cosmetic surgery. *Pain* 2009;147:194–201.

19. Glasson JC, Sawyer WT, Lindley CM, Ginsberg B. Patient-specific factors affecting patient-controlled analgesia dosing. *J Pain Palliat Care Pharmacother* 2002;16:5–21.

20. Gourlay GK, Kowalski SR, Plummer JL, Cousins MJ, Armstrong PJ. Fentanyl blood concentration-analgesic response relationship in the treatment of postoperative pain. *Anesth Analg* 1988;67:329–37.

21. Joels CS, Mostafa G, Matthews BD, et al. Factors affecting intravenous analgesic requirements after colectomy. *J Am Coll Surg* 2003;197:780–5.

22. Larijani GE, Goldberg ME, Gratz I, Warshal DP. Analgesic and hemodynamic effects of a single 7.5-mg intravenous dose of morphine in patients with moderate-to-severe postoperative pain. *Pharmacotherapy* 2004;24:1675–80.

23. Lehmann KA, Gördes B. Postoperative on-demand analgesie mit buprenorphin. *Anaesthesist* 1988;37:65–70.

24. Macintyre PE, Jarvis DA. Age is the best predictor of postoperative morphine requirements. *Pain* 1995;64:357–64.

25. Miller PL, Ernst AA. Sex differences in analgesia: a randomized trial of µ versus κ opioid agonists. *Southern Med J* 2004;97:35–41.

26. Sidebotham D, Dijkhuizen MRJ, Schug SA. The safety and utilization of patient-controlled analgesia. *J Pain Symp Manag* 1997;14:202–9.

27. Tamsen A, Hartvig P, Fagerlund C, Dahlström B. Patient-controlled analgesic therapy, part II: individual analgesic demand and analgesic plasma concentrations of pethidine in postoperative pain. *Clin Pharmacokinet* 1982;7:164–75.

28. Tsui SL, Tong WN, Irwin M, Ng KFJ, Chan WS, Yang J. The efficacy, applicability and side-effects of postoperative intravenous patient-controlled morphine analgesia: an audit in 1223 Chinese patients. *Anaesth Intens Care* 1996;24:658–64.

29. Comer SD, Cooper ZD, Kowalczyk WJ, et al. Evaluation of potential sex differences in the subjective and analgesic effects of morphine in normal, healthy volunteers. *Psychopharmacology* 2010;208:45–55.

30. Fillingim RB, Ness TJ, Glover TL, et al. Morphine responses and experimental pain: Sex differences in side effects and cardiovascular responses but not analgesia. *J Pain* 2005;6:116–24.

31. Olofsen E, Romberg R, Bijl H, et al. Alfentanil and placebo analgesia: no sex differences detected in models of experimental pain. *Anesthesiology* 2005;103:120–29.

32. Pud D, Yarnitsky D, Sprecher E, Rogowski Z, Adler R, Eidenberg E. Can personality traits and gender predict the response to morphine? An experimental cold pain study. *Eur J Pain* 2006;10:103–12.

33. Romberg R, Olofsen E, Sarton E, den Hartigh J, Taschner PEM, Dahan A. Pharmacokinetic-pharmacodynamic modeling of morphine-6-glucuronide-induced analgesia in healthy volunteers. *Anesthesiology* 2004;100:120–33.

34. Sarton E, Olofsen E, Romberg R, et al. Sex differences in morphine analgesia: an experimental study in healthy volunteers. *Anesthesiology* 2000;93:1245–54.

35. Zacny JP. Gender differences in opioid analgesia in human volunteers: cold pressor and mechanical pain. *NIDA Res Mon* 2002;182: 22–3.

36. Gear RW, Miaskowski C, Gordon NC, Paul SM, Heller PH, Levine JD. Kappa-opioids produce significantly greater analgesia in women than in men. *Nat Med* 1996;2:1248–50.

37. Gear RW, Miaskowski C, Gordon NC, Paul SM, Heller PH, Levine JD. The kappa opioid nalbuphine produces gender- and dose-dependent analgesia and antianalgesia in patients with postoperative pain. *Pain* 1999;83:339–45.

38. Gordon NC, Gear RW, Heller PH, Miaskowski PC, Levine JD. Enhancement of morphine analgesia by the $GABA_B$ agonist baclofen. *Neurosci* 1995;69:345–49.

39. Lehmann KA, Tenbuhs B. Patient-controlled analgesia with nalbuphine, a new narcotic agonist-antagonist, for the treatment of postoperative pain. *Eur J Clin Pharmacol* 1986;31:267–76.

40. Ryan JL, Jureidini B, Hodges JS, Baisden M, Swift JQ, Bowles WR. Gender differences in analgesia for endodontic pain. *J Endod* 2008;34:552–6.

41. Fillingim RB, Hastie BA, Ness TJ, Glover TL, Campbell CM, Staud R. Sex-related psychological predictors of baseline pain perception and analgesic responses to pentazocine. *Biol Psychol* 2005;69:97–112.

42. Fillingim RB, Ness TJ, Glover TL, Campbell CM, Price DP, Staud R. Experimental pain models reveal no sex differences in pentazocine analgesia in humans. *Anesthesiology* 2004;100:1263–70.

43. Mogil JS, Wilson SG, Chesler EJ, et al. The melanocortin-1 receptor gene mediates female-specific mechanisms of analgesia in mice and humans. *Proc Natl Acad Sci USA* 2003;100: 4867–72.

44. Zacny JP, Beckman NJ. The effects of cold-water stimulus on butorphanol effects in males and females. *Pharmacol Biochem Behav* 2004;78:653–9.

45. Averbuch M, Katzper M. A search for sex differences in response to analgesia. *Arch Int Med* 2000;160:3424–8.

46. Walker SJ, Camody JJ. Experimental pain in healthy human subjects: gender differences in nociception and in response to ibuprofen. *Anesth Analg* 1998;86:1257–62.

47. Comptom P, Charuvastra VC, Ling W. Effect of keterolac and gender on human cold pressor pain tolerance. *Clin Exp Pharmacol Physiol* 2003;30:759–63.

48. Sigtermans M, Dahan A, Mooren R, et al. S(+)-ketamine effect on experimental pain and cardiac output: a population pharmacokinetic-pharmacodynamic modeling study in healthy volunteers. *Anesthesiology* 2009;111:892–903.

49. Morgan CJA, Perry EB, Cho H-S, Krystal JH, D'Souza DC. Greater vulnerability to the amnesic effects of ketamine in males. *Pyschophramacol* 2006;187:405–14.

50. Robinson ME, Riley JR, Brown FF, Gremillion H. Sex differences in response to cutaneous anesthesia: a double blind randomized study. *Pain* 1998;77:143–9.

51. Tófoli GR, Ramacciato JC, Volpato MC, et al. Anesthetic efficacy and pain induced by dental anesthesia: the influence of gender and menstrual cycle. *Oral Surg Oral Med Oral Pathol Oral Radiol Endod* 2007;103:e34–8.

52. Leloudis DH, Kittleson MM, Felker M, et al. Topical anesthesia with EMLA reduces pain during endomyocardial biopsy: a randomized trial. *J Heart Lung Transplant* 2006;25:1164–6.

53. Li Y, Zhou Y, Chen H, Feng Z. The effect of sex on the minimum local analgesic concentration of ropivacaine for caudal anesthesia in anorectal surgery. *Anesth Analg* 2010;110:1490–3.

54. Chang KY, Dai CY, Ger LP, Fu MJ, et al. Determinants of patient-controlled epidural analgesia requirements: a prospective analysis in 1753 patients. *Clin J Pain* 2006;22:751–6.

55. Department of Economic and Social Affairs, Population Division. World population ageing: 1950–2050. Available at: http://www.un.org/esa/population/publications/worldageing19502050/. (accessed on June 2, 2012).

56. Sittl R, Nuijten M, Nutrup BP. Changes in the prescribed daily doses of transdermal fentanyl and transdermal buprenorphine during treatment of patients with cancer and noncancer pain in Germany: results of a retrospective cohort study. *Clin Ther* 2005;27:1022–31.

57. Likar R, Kayser H, Sittl R. Long-term management of chronic pain with transdermal buprenorphine: a multi-center, open-label, follow-up study in patients from three short-term clinical trials. *Clin Ther* 2006;28:943–52.

58. Kalso E, Simpson KH, Slappendel R, Dejonckheere J, Richarz U. Predicting long-term response to strong opioids in patients with low

back pain: findings from a randomized, controlled trial of transdermal fentanyl and morphine. *BMC Med* 2007;5:39.

59. Peniston JH, Gould E. Oxymorphone extended release for the treatment of chronic low back pain: a retrospective pooled analysis of enriched-enrollment clinical trial data stratified according to age, sex, and prior opioid use. *Clin Ther* 2009;31:347–59.

60. Mercadante S, Casucio A, Pumo S, Fulfaro F. Factors influencing the opioid response in advanced cancer patients with pain followed at home: the effects of age and gender. *Support Care Cancer* 2000;8:123–30.

61. Cohen SP, Christo PJ, Wang S, et al. The effect of opioid dose and treatment duration on the perception of a painful standardized clinical stimulus. *Reg Anes Pain Med* 2008;199–206.

SECTION TWO

BIOPSYCHOSOCIAL FACTORS CONTRIBUTING TO SEX DIFFERENCES

5

SEX-DEPENDENT GENETIC CONTRIBUTIONS TO PAIN AND ANALGESIA

Jeffrey S. Mogil

THE ORIGIN OF SEX DIFFERENCES IN PAIN AND ANALGESIA

The observation of differences in pain or analgesic sensitivity between men and women—inconsistent in effect size but consistent in direction—is sufficiently well accepted by now[1-5] that researchers are starting to move on from simply documenting the phenomenon to attempting to explain it. The default assumption is that gonadal hormones act as modulatory factors affecting pain sensitivity or analgesic potency, and indeed much evidence has been gathered in humans and rodents documenting that estrogen, progesterone, and testosterone levels can affect pain (see ref. 3). That being said, the existing evidence is highly contradictory, as exemplified by the title of a workshop at the 13th World Congress of Pain: "Are estrogens pro-nociceptive or anti-nociceptive?"

There are potential explanations of sex differences other than activational modulation by gonadal hormones. Gonadal hormones may have organizational effects on the development of pain systems, for which some evidence has been amassed in rodents (e.g., ref. 6). There may be direct effects of genetic (rather than hormonal) sex, for example the effects of females possessing two copies of relevant X-linked genes. Using the "four core genotype" mouse model, in which transgenic manipulations were used to dissociate hormonal and genetic sex in four mouse lines (XX female, XY male, XX "male," and XY "female"),[7] Arnold and colleagues have demonstrated significant effects of genetic sex on tail-withdrawal, hot-plate, and formalin sensitivity.[8-9] Sex differences in pain sensitivity might be explained by purely experiential differences between the genders, for example, if childbirth alters the anchoring of pain scale usage,[10] or by sociocultural factors such as gender role expectations.[11]

The final and admittedly most radical possibility, albeit the one I wish to discuss in this chapter, is that pain physiology actually differs between the sexes to the extent that talking about "modulation" by gonadal hormones is misleading. That is, what if pain systems evolved somewhat or even largely separately in males and females, and thus feature different component proteins (and thus genes)? It is not difficult to assume rather different adaptive pressures on the development of pain and especially pain modulation systems between the sexes, which may have experienced cutaneous and visceral pain at greatly differing frequency throughout evolution. An alternate explanation of the existence of *qualitatively* different pain processing between the sexes derives from the observation that pain modulatory circuitry in the central nervous system may have "piggybacked" on top of reproductive circuitry[12]; by this notion the reason for sex differences in pain is simply because there are sex differences in reproduction.

How would one determine whether such qualitative sex differences exist? The observation of "all-or-none" effects of receptor activation or antagonism would provide evidence, as would sex-specific effects of genetic null mutations or sex-specific genetic associations/linkages. Note that the existence of a qualitative sex difference does not preclude the simultaneous observation of a quantitative sex difference, since the operation of sex-specific mechanisms may not have equal "output" in terms of pain levels or analgesic potency or efficacy. Note also that gonadal hormones may still play important organizational and/or activation roles in such qualitative sex differences. In a number of examples to be provided herein, gonadal hormones appear to represent a "switching" mechanism. Over a certain threshold level (levels maintained at all times in normal males and females) the sex-dependent system is enabled; after gonadectomy the same system is disabled, and (in some cases) the organism can switch over to the system normally used by the other sex.

This chapter will endeavor to provide some striking examples of qualitative sex differences in pain and analgesia, with most of the evidence provided by sex/genetic interactions. In addition to supporting the notion that men and women really have "different brains" when it comes to pain, these examples call into question what a "sex difference" (or, for that matter, a "genetic difference") actually is.

STRAIN-DEPENDENT SEX DIFFERENCES AND SEX-DEPENDENT STRAIN DIFFERENCES IN PAIN AND ANALGESIA

To my knowledge, the first specific explicit mention of sex and strain interactions in a pain-related trait was the observation that male Sprague Dawley rats were 25% more sensitive to morphine than females of this strain, whereas Wistar-Furth rats of both sexes were equisensitive.[13] The first systemic study of this interaction was performed by Kest and colleagues.[14] Male and female mice of 11 inbred mouse strains were tested for nociceptive sensitivity on the 49°C tail-withdrawal test, and for intracerebroventricular morphine inhibition of that thermal pain. In this study, as expected, female mice exhibited mean tail-withdrawal latencies almost 0.5 s shorter than those of males, and thus were more sensitive than males overall (see Fig. 5.1). However, this overall difference was driven by large sex differences in just three strains (AKR/J, C3H/HeJ, and C57BL/6J); all others exhibited either no sex differences or sex differences too small to observe with the sample size employed (see Fig. 5.1). The morphine analgesia data were even more interesting. In three strains (AKR/J, C57BL/6J, and SWR/J), significant male>female analgesic sensitivity was observed. In seven strains, no sex differences emerged. In one strain, however, a significant sex difference was observed in the *reverse* direction, such that CBA/J females were >5-fold more sensitive to morphine than CBA/J males.

The finding that sex differences can be observed on some genetic backgrounds but not others has been observed repeatedly, by ourselves in mice and rats,[15–17] by Rady and Fujimoto using mice,[18] and in the laboratory of Mitchell J. Picker using rats.[19–22] Although there is contradictory evidence regarding exactly which genotypes show sex differences, even within-laboratory, the general conclusion that sex differences are dependent on genotype is quite robust. The interaction is not at all limited to thermal nociception, as sex differences in mechanical allodynia following experimental mononeuropathy are observed in Sprague Dawley and Long-Evans but not Holtzman rats.[23,24] Neither is the interaction limited to morphine analgesia, being observed for a number of compounds acting at μ- and κ-opioid receptors,[19–21] as well as for nonopioid analgesics like WIN55,212–2, epibatidine, and indomethacin.[16–17] Of great interest as well, the modulatory effects of estrus cyclicity[15] and gonadectomy[25] in female mice and rats are themselves strain dependent. Finally, there is one direct demonstration that sex and genotype interact in the determination of the

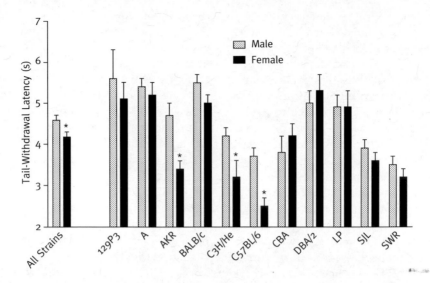

FIGURE 5.1 Sex–genotype interactions in baseline sensitivity to noxious thermal stimuli on the 49°C tail-withdrawal test. Bars represent mean ± SEM latency (s) to withdraw tail from the hot water. *p < .05 compared to males. As can be seen, the overall sex difference (All Strains; left) is accounted for largely by sex differences in three particular strains: AKR, C3H/He, and C57BL/6.

modulatory effect of an environmental manipulation. Maternal separation in infancy produced increased sensitivity to thermal nociception in adult, female Lewis rats, but not female Fischer 344 rats or males of either strain.[26]

If sex differences may or may not be observed in various genotypes, it should also sometimes be the case that strain differences are observed in one sex but not the other. We have in fact noted this on a number of occasions,[14–17] as has the Picker laboratory.[20] For example, in a study by Calderone et al.,[27] electric shock jump latencies were longer in 129/J mice relative to C57BL/6J mice, but only in females; males of these strains did not differ.

STRAIN, SEX, AND THEIR INTERACTION AS SOURCES OF VARIABILITY IN PAIN SENSITIVITY

We performed a study attempting to quantify sources of variability in a very large (>8,000-subject) archival study of baseline sensitivity on the 49°C hot water tail-withdrawal test.[28,29] The data set was comprised of every mouse tested by me or in my laboratory on this test over an 8-year period, and it was subjected to an automated machine-learning technique called classification and regression tree (CART) analysis. CART revealed the relative importance of various factors in explaining the considerable interindividual variability in withdrawal latencies in the data set; the second most important factor overall was genotype, and sex was the sixth most important factor.[28] This heuristic finding led us to perform a fully crossed and balanced study conducted on a single day, in which strain, sex, tester, time, and cage order were systematically varied. We found that strain accounted for 27% of the overall variance, and sex by itself only 0.4% of the variance. However, interactions of sex with other factors (including strain) accounted for almost 10% of the variance.[29]

SEX-SPECIFIC EFFECTS OF NULL MUTATIONS

One of the most prolific molecular genetics approaches to pain biology has been the creation and testing of the transgenic knockout mouse. Taking advantage of homologous recombination (the switching of highly similar segments of DNA during meiosis), one can replace an endogenous gene with a disrupted version and inject the "transgene" into developing mouse blastocysts to eventually produce mice with a null mutation of the targeted gene (see ref. 30). Our *PainGenes Database* (paingeneticslab.ca/4105/06_02_pain_genetics_database.asp) tracks the progress of this technique as applied to pain[31]; as of this writing 369 different knockout mice have been demonstrated to have an altered pain "phenotype" (i.e., more or less sensitive to pain, to inflammatory or neuropathic hypersensitivity, or to an analgesic) compared to their "wild-type" control strain.

Of course, the vast majority of published studies in this domain (like every other domain of pain research) feature the testing of male subjects only or are silent on the issue of sex differences.[32] A few studies have, however, specifically observed sex differences in either the effect of the null mutation on the pain state or observed that sex differences observed in wild-type mice were absent in knockout mice. A compilation of such findings is shown in Table 5.1. As an example, Mitrovic and colleagues[33] observed that the increased sensitivity of female wild-type (C57BL/6J strain) mice compared to males on the radiant heat tail-flick and hot-plate tests was ameliorated in G protein–coupled inwardly rectifying potassium channel 2 (GIRK2) knockout mice, suggesting that GIRK2 might be responsible for the sex difference. A similar pattern was observed for morphine inhibition of thermal pain on these assays: female wild-type mice exhibited less morphine analgesia than male wild types, whereas male and female knockout mice were equisensitive (although

Table 5.1   Sex-Specific Knockout Mouse Phenotypes

GENE	PROTEIN NAME	TYPE	ASSAY	SEX DIFFERENCE	REFERENCE
Avpr1a	Vasopressin-1A receptor	Conv.	Pain, capsaicin analgesia, stress	♂ phenotype only ♂ phenotype only	89
Asic1/2/3	Acid-sensing ion channel 1, 2, 3	DN	Pain, multiple	♂ phenotype only	34
Gabrb3	g-aminobutyric acid (GABA-A) receptor, β_3 subunit	Conv.	Pain, mechanical	♂ phenotype only	92
Gnaz	Guanine nucleotide binding protein, α_z subunit	Conv.	Pain, heat	♀ phenotype only	93
Kcnj6	G-protein-coupled inwardly rectifying potassium channel 2	Conv.	Pain, heat analgesia, multiple	WT: ♂<♀ KO: ♂ = ♀	33,94
Oprk1	κ-opioid receptor	Conv.	Pain, heat	♀ phenotype only	95
Oprm1	μ-Opioid receptor	Conv.	Analgesia, stress	WT: ♂<♀ KO: ♂ = ♀	96
Ptgs2	Prostaglandin-endoperoxide synthase 2 (COX-2)	HET	Pain, inflammatory	♀ phenotype only	97
Trpa1	Transient receptor potential cation channel, A1	Conv.	Pain, cold	♀ phenotype only	98

Conv., conventional null mutant; DN, dominant negative (triple) mutant; HET, heterozygote.

less sensitive than wild types of either sex).[33] A more obvious sex difference was observed by Chanda and colleagues,[34] who reported that the various alterations in pain phenotypes of male dominant-negative mutants lacking all acid-sensing ion channels (ASICs)[35] simply could not be observed in females, in which wild-type and knockout mice were equisensitive on every assay (see Fig. 5.2).

SEX-DEPENDENT GENETIC LINKAGES AND ASSOCIATIONS

Null mutant phenotypes can provide evidence that a particular gene (and the protein it encodes) is required for pain processing, but not that a particular gene plays a role in pain-related variability.[36] For the latter, genetic linkage or genetic association data are required.[37] Because of statistical power limitations imposed by the size of compiled genetic pedigrees, linkage mapping in humans is only useful for the discovery of genes responsible for monogenic traits with high penetrance, for example, congenital insensitivity to pain syndromes[38] or familial hemiplegic migraine syndromes.[39] I am unaware of any pain-relevant human linkage mapping findings with a reported sex difference. In animal models, where very large (and simple) pedigrees can be easily generated, linkage mapping is known as quantitative trait locus (QTL) mapping,[37] and a number of pain-relevant QTL studies (and their successors, haplotype mapping studies) performed in rats and mice have been published.[40–60] Some of these have featured sex-dependent effects, as shown in Table 5.2. All three types of sex-specific linkages[61] have been observed: (1) sex-specific effects (whereby a gene affects a trait only in one sex but not the other), (2) sex-biased effects (a gene affects both sexes but to differing degrees), and (3) sex-antagonistic effects (a gene affects both

A. von Frey Test (mechanical)

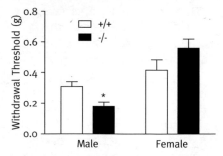

B. Tail-Clip Test (mechanical)

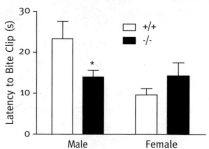

C. Formalin Test (late phase; inflammatory)

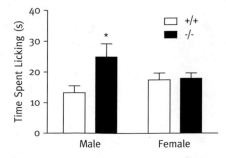

D. Zymosan Test (inflammatory)

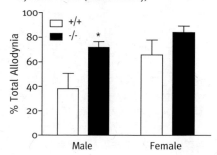

FIGURE 5.2 An example of a sex-dependent phenotype of a null mutant. Data presented here are from wild-type (+/+) and dominant negative triple null mutant (–/–) mice lacking acid-sensing ion channel (ASIC) currents from *Asic1*, *Asic2*, and *Asic3*. Bars represent mean ± SEM in every case. *$p < .05$ compared to +/+ within sex.

Table 5.2 Sex-Specific Genetic Linkages and Associations

GENE	PROTEIN	SPECIES	TRAIT	SEX DIFFERENCE	REFERENCE
Calca	Calcitonin-related polypeptide, α	Mouse	Pain, heat	♂>♀	48
Mc1r	Melanocortin-1 receptor	Mouse, human	Analgesia, κ-opioid	♀ only	46
Oprd1	δ-Opioid receptor	Mouse	Pain, heat	♂>♀	41
		Human	Pain, heat	♂>♀	69
Oprk1	κ-Opioid receptor (presumed)	Mouse	Analgesia, morphine	♀ only	43
Oprm1	μ-Opioid receptor	Human	Pain, heat pain, mechanical	♂ up; ♀ down ♂ only	70

sexes but in opposite directions). An intriguing example is that of Bergeson and colleagues,[43] regarding morphine analgesia in mice. Of the five significant QTLs (genomic regions containing a trait-relevant DNA variant) reported, two were wholly sex-specific. On mouse chromosome 9, at approximately cM from the centromere, a QTL was uncovered with a combined *p*-value of 6 × 10^6 in females; the analogous *p*-value for male data was .19. The gene underlying this QTL has yet to be identified. More intriguing, though, is another female-specific QTL on chromosome 1, at approximately 10 cM (female: *p* = .00002; male: *p* = .3). Nearby on mouse chromosome 1 is the *Oprk1* gene, coding for the κ-opioid receptor. Although it has never been formally proven that the chromosome 1 QTL is actually *Oprk1*, a number of findings in humans and rodents suggest that μ-opioid (the binding site for morphine) and κ-opioid receptors interact positively in females but negatively in males.[62–66] Most recently, work from Alan Gintzler's laboratory has demonstrated that spinal μ- and κ-opioid receptors can form heterodimers in the spinal cord in females but not males.[67] Thus, the genetic status of the κ-opioid receptor gene, *Oprk1*, could be expected to contribute to morphine analgesic magnitude in females but not males, a compelling hypothesis for the female-specific QTL.

Not being limited to pedigrees, genetic association studies are now far more common than linkage mapping studies, and many investigations

of experimental and chronic pain have now been performed using this technique (see ref. 68). I am aware of only three sex-specific genetic association findings of relevance to pain (see also Table 5.2). Using the CART analysis described earlier, the Phe27→Cys variant of the *OPRD1* gene was found to be associated with 49°C heat pain intensity in men but not women.[69] This is intriguing because a sex-biased (male > female) linkage of the mouse *Oprd1* gene to sensitivity on the 54°C hot-plate assay was previously observed.[41] A sex-specific effect of the well-studied A118G (Asn40→Asp) variant of *OPRM1*, the μ-opioid receptor gene, on pressure pain thresholds was observed by Fillingim and colleagues,[70] with inheritance of the minor "G" allele associated with higher thresholds in men but not women. Another group subsequently observed such an association in females, but with another variant (IVS2 + 31G>A) within the *OPRM1* gene (men were not studied). Finally, a sex-specific genetic association of the melanocortin-1 receptor gene, *MC1R*, to pentazocine inhibition of both ischemic and thermal pain was observed.[46] This finding will be discussed later.

Sex-specific genetic linkages and associations have been found repeatedly in other domains,[71] with some arguing that failing to model for sex-specific genetic architecture may hamper the ability of linkage mapping to identify QTLs.[71] Wang and colleagues[72] specifically developed a computational model to do this and detected sex-specific haplotypes within the human *OPRD1* gene (encoding the δ-opioid receptor) relevant to pressure pain thresholds. However, it has been argued that such sub-group comparisons are inherently problematic, and most studies are underpowered to detect interactions with sex.[73]

SEX-SPECIFIC ROLES IN PAIN OF THE N-METHYL-D-ASPARTATE AND MELANOCORTIN-1 RECEPTORS

Genetic studies in mice and humans have led to the discovery of a robust and wide-ranging sex difference in pain processing: the male-specific role of the N-methyl-D-aspartate receptor (NMDAR) and the analogous female-specific role of the melanocortin-1 receptor (MC1R). The story begins with behavior pharmacology experiments performed in the early 1990s.[74] In these studies, a low dose of the NMDAR antagonist, MK-801 (dizocilpine), was found to attenuate forced cold water swim stress-induced analgesia (SSIA), but only in male mice. Female mice displayed SSIA of equivalent magnitude, but it was neither opioid (i.e., reversible by naloxone) or NMDAR mediated.[74]

It appeared that we had uncovered evidence for a wholly female-specific system, and not simply a modulation of a common system, because gonadectomy of female mice reinstated MK-801's effect; that is, gonadectomized female mice were apparently using the "male" NMDAR-based system.[74] Furthermore, estrogen replacement to gonadectomized females restored MK-801 insensitivity, apparently switching mice back to the "female" system. This "switching" hypothesis was confirmed by a number of follow-up studies, including the demonstration that organizational hormonal manipulations could affect SSIA mediation,[75] that the switching could be produced by acute progesterone treatment in addition to chronic estrogen treatment,[76] and that postestropausal female mice reverted to the male system.[77] Independent investigations in the Kavaliers laboratory revealed that the very same sexual dimorphism (i.e., reversible by NMDAR antagonism in males but not females) also characterized SSIA, predator exposure-related analgesia, biting fly–induced analgesia, and κ-opioid analgesia in mice.[78–80]

Using a QTL mapping strategy specifically to shed light on the identity of the female-specific system, we discovered a strong and unambiguously female-specific QTL for SSIA on distal mouse chromosome 8, which we named *Siafq1*.[42] Later work confirmed this region to also be linked, in females only, to U50,488 analgesia.[46] We chose the *Mc1r* gene, encoding the MC1R, to be the most likely candidate in the genomic region, since immunohistochemistry had revealed a dense pocket of MC1Rs in the analgesia-relevant midbrain periaqueductal gray.[81] Genetic and pharmacologic studies in mice were designed to evaluate the candidacy of *Mc1r*. First, we obtained mice with a spontaneous mutation of the *Mc1r* gene, called recessive yellow or "*e/e*" (C57BL/6-*Mc1r^{e/e}*).[82] These mice were not at all deficient in their analgesic response to U50,488 (in fact, the female *e/e* mice displayed slightly higher analgesia), and male mutants showed the expected MK-801 reversal of analgesia. However, MK-801 was also found to reverse U50,488 analgesia in female *e/e* mice (but not female wild-type controls), suggesting that they had "switched" over to using the male system.[46] That is, it appeared as if female *e/e* mutants were using the male system because the female system was not available to them, directly implicating MC1Rs as being part of the female system. To provide convergent evidence, a MC1R-selective peptide antagonist was injected into outbred mice of both sexes. The antagonist had no effect in male mice whatsoever; in female mice, it produced a clear potentiation of U50,488 analgesia and rendered such analgesia newly sensitive to blockade by MK-801.[46] That is, antagonist treatment also induced female mice to switch to the male system.

Thus, convinced that *Mc1r* very likely represented the female-specific QTL for κ-opioid analgesia (and very likely being *Siafq1*), we attempted a translational genetic association study to investigate the impact of genotype at the human *Mc1r* analog, *MC1R*. This gene is well known for its prodigious variability and is known to explain the large majority of cases of red headedness (see ref. 83). We recruited men and women of different hair colors and measured their sensitivity to pain before and after administration of the κ-opioid-acting drug, pentazocine (0.5 mg/kg). Participants were sequenced at *MC1R* to establish their genotype; only inheritance of multiple variants is associated with nonfunctioning MC1Rs and red hair.[84] For both assays, we found that *MC1R* genotype did not affect pentazocine analgesia in men. In women, on the other hand, those with multiple variants (all redheads, although not all redheads had multiple variants) displayed significantly higher pentazocine analgesia[46] (see Fig. 5.3).

Finally, very recent work performed in the laboratory of Ben Kest suggests that this very same sexual dimorphism is involved in the physiology of opioid-induced hyperalgesia, a phenomenon whereby chronic exposure to μ-opioid agonists leads, paradoxically, to increased pain sensitivity (see ref. 85). In mice, continuous infusion of morphine using subcutaneously implanted osmotic pumps leads to robust hyperalgesia on the tail-withdrawal test. This hyperalgesia is sex-specific in its presentation, with males displaying temporary hyperalgesia that resolves after 6 days and females displaying apparently permanent (>12 day-long) hyperalgesia.[86] In both sexes,

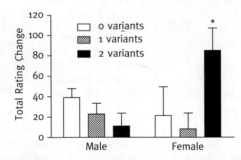

FIGURE 5.3 An example of a sex-dependent genetic association. Men and women were tested for thermal pain sensitivity (10 heat pulses at 52°C) and inhibition of that pain by pentazocine (0.5 mg/kg), and their *MC1R* gene was sequenced. Subjects were stratified by the number of DNA variants encountered, 0 (the "wild-type" sequence), 1 (one variant; functional receptor), or 2 (two variants, nonfunctional receptor). Bars represent mean ± SEM pain ratings (on a 0–100 numerical rating scale), expressed as change from baseline to pentazocine; higher bars indicate more pentazocine analgesia. *p < .05 compared to other genotypes within sex.

naltrexone administration does not block the hyperalgesia (although it does block the initial morphine analgesia), attesting to the nonopioid nature of the hyperalgesia phenomenon. As in the previous studies with SSIA and κ-opioid analgesia, here too NMDAR antagonism (using either MK-801 or the competitive antagonist, LY235959) was successful in reversing morphine hyperalgesia in male and ovariectomized female mice, but not intact female mice or estrogen-replaced ovariectomized female mice.[86] Morphine hyperalgesia was also completely absent in *e/e* mutant female mice, suggesting that MC1Rs were required for this phenomenon in females (although in this case no switching was observed).[87] Just as MK-801 could reverse morphine hyperalgesia in male mice, so could MC1R antagonism using MSG606 reverse the phenomenon in female mice.[87] Finally, just as progesterone injection was shown to be able to activate female-specific κ-opioid analgesia mechanisms in ovariectomized mice, so too can progesterone activate female-specific morphine hyperalgesia mechanisms.[88] I note that although the precise relationship between κ-opioid analgesia and morphine hyperalgesia physiology has yet to be elucidated, the congruence of these two sets of findings could not possibly be coincidental.

A SEX–GENE–STRESS INTERACTION IN PAIN AND ANALGESIA

A remarkable set of recent findings is deserving of mention,[89] if only to provide an example that pain biology may be even more complex than the interactions described thus far. A QTL mapping study of chemical/inflammatory pain using the formalin test yielded two significant QTLs.[90] One of these, on mouse chromosome 9, was for early/acute phase (0–10 min postinjection) nociception, and we have subsequently demonstrated that the responsible gene is *Atp1b3*, encoding the β_3 subunit of the sodium-potassium ATPase (pump).[57] The second QTL, linked to late/tonic (10–60 min postinjection) nociception, was located on distal mouse chromosome 10. A number of years of breeding and testing congenic, recombinant congenic, and subcongenic strains refined the position of the responsible gene to a 3.4 Mb region, and subsequent haplotype mapping refined the position further, to approximately 100 kb.[89] Only two genes are found in this region, *Avpr1a* (encoding the vasopressin-1A receptor; V1AR) and *Ppm1h* (encoding the protein phosphatase 1H). As there was previous tentative evidence that vasopressin may modulate pain, we concluded that *Avpr1a* was likely responsible for the linkage, and we confirmed this hypothesis with strain-dependent gene expression data and a positive knockout phenotype on the formalin test. In fact, we tested the *Avpr1a* knockout mouse on an entire battery of nociceptive assays, and in addition to the formalin test only one assay exhibited a genotype difference: the capsaicin test. This was fortuitous, since the capsaicin test can be performed in humans as well as mice.

Two studies were thus undertaken in humans. First, an *AVPR1A* genetic association study was performed on capsaicin pain data already collected at Johns Hopkins University.[91] Second, we attempted to investigate whether a stable vasopressin analog, desmopressin, would produce inhibition of capsaicin pain in normal volunteers. Both studies appeared to fail. There was no genetic association to capsaicin pain observed to either of two *AVPR1A* variants genotyped, and desmopressin did not produce analgesia. However, further examination of the data sets revealed surprisingly robust interactions with sex and stress levels at the time of testing. We found that, in men experiencing stress at the time of capsaicin administration (presumably *due* to the impending capsaicin administration), pain ratings were in fact significantly associated with inheritance of a single nucleotide polymorphism, rs10877969, near the promoter region of *AVPR1A*. There was no effect in women, nor any effect in male subjects who were stress-free. The same sorts of interactions could also be observed in the desmopressin experiment, such that desmopressin *did* produce significant inhibition of capsaicin pain in stress-free individuals only. The correlation between stress levels and desmopressin efficacy was significant only in male subjects of one genotype at rs10877969.[89]

Newly armed with the knowledge that *AVPR1A* affects pain and vasopressin analgesia in males only and in a stress-dependent manner, we conducted new experiments in the laboratory mouse. These revealed that, in mice too, *Avpr1a* genotype affects formalin and capsaicin pain only in mice not habituated to the testing environment (i.e., experiencing testing-related stress), and that, in mice too, vasopressin only produces analgesia in nonstressed mice (i.e., habituated to the testing environment). Although the *Avpr1a* genotype affects pain levels in female mice too, the interaction between genotype and stress is only seen in males. We went on to demonstrate that V1ARs are crucial for stress-induced analgesia in male but not female mice.[89]

These data are not only a compelling example of mouse-to-human-to-mouse translational research but suggest that both sex differences and genetic effects can be even more complex than previously thought, since they can interact with environmental factors (in this case, acute stress) in addition to each other.

THE TIP OF THE ICEBERG?

The observations described herein are compelling, but their impact depends crucially on the prevalence of such qualitative sex differences. Are they rare examples of limited differences in a neurobiological system largely shared by males and females? Or do they represent the tip of an iceberg in which the neurobiology of pain is largely different in males and females, a fact until now almost completely obscured by the limited investigation into the topic? Obviously, time will tell. Although the sex differences in pain demonstrated in the field so far have no enormous implications for clinical treatment of pain in men and women, the future may bring truly individualized treatment of pain by sex.

REFERENCES

1. Niesters M, Dahan A, Kest B, et al. Do sex differences exist in opioid analgesia? A systematic review and meta-analysis of human experimental and clinical studies. *Pain* 2010;151(1):61–8.
2. Mogil JS, Bailey AL. Sex and gender differences in pain and analgesia. *Prog Brain Res* 2010;186:141–157.

3. Fillingim RB, King CD, Riberio-Dasilva MC, Rahim-Williams B, Riley JL, III. Sex, gender, and pain: a review of recent clinical and experimental findings. *J Pain* 2009;10(5):447–85.

4. Paller CJ, Campbell CM, Edwards RR, Dobs AS. Sex-based differences in pain perception and treatment. *Pain Med* 2009;10(2):289–99.

5. Greenspan JD, Craft RM, LeResche L, et al. Studying sex and gender differences in pain and analgesia: a consensus report. *Pain* 2007; 132(Suppl 1):S26–45.

6. Cicero TJ, Nock B, O'Connor L, Meyer ER. Role of steroids in sex differences in morphine-induced analgesia: activational and organizational effects. *J Pharmacol Exp Ther* 2002;300(2):695–701.

7. Arnold AP, Chen X. What does the "four core genotypes" mouse model tell us about sex differences in the brain and other tissues? *Front Neuroendocrin* 2008;30:1–9.

8. Gioiosa L, Chen X, Watkins R, et al. Sex chromosome complement affects nociception in tests of acute and chronic exposure to morphine in mice. *Horm Behav* 2008;53:124–30.

9. Gioiosa L, Chen X, Watkins R, Umeda EA, Arnold AP. Sex chromosome complement affects nociception and analgesia in newborn mice. *J Pain* 2008;9(10):962–9.

10. Robinson ME, Gagnon CM, Dannecker EA, Brown JL, Jump RL, Price DD. Sex differences in common pain events: expectations and anchors. *J Pain* 2003;4(1):40–5.

11. Robinson ME, Riley JL, III, Myers CD, et al. Gender role expectations of pain: relationship to sex differences in pain. J Pain 2001;2:251–7.

12. Bodnar RJ, Commons K, Pfaff DW. *Central Neural States Relating Sex and Pain*. Baltimore, MD: Johns Hopkins University Press; 2002.

13. Kasson BG, George R. Endocrine influences on the actions of morphine. IV. Effects of sex and strain. *Life Sci* 1984;34:1627–34.

14. Kest B, Wilson SG, Mogil JS. Sex differences in supraspinal morphine analgesia are dependent on genotype. *J Pharmacol Exp Ther* 1999;289(3):1370–5.

15. Mogil JS, Chesler EJ, Wilson SG, Juraska JM, Sternberg WF. Sex differences in thermal nociception and morphine antinociception in rodents depend on genotype. *Neurosci Biobehav Rev* 2000;24:375–89.

16. Wilson SG, Smith SB, Chesler EJ, et al. The heritability of antinociception: common pharmacogenetic mediation of five neurochemically distinct analgesics. *J Pharmacol Exp Ther* 2003;304(2):547–59.

17. Wilson SG, Bryant CD, Lariviere WR, et al. The heritability of antinociception II: pharmacogenetic mediation of three over-the-counter analgesics in mice. *J Pharmacol Exp Ther* 2003;305:755–64.

18. Rady JJ, Fujimoto JM. Analgesic response in offspring of crosses between heroin δ (Swiss Webster) and μ (ICR) responding mice. *Pharmacogenetics* 1997;7:429–33.

19. Terner JM, Barrett AC, Cook CD, Picker MJ. Sex differences in (-)-pentazocine antinociception: comparison to morphine and spiradoline in four rat strains using a thermal nociceptive assay. *Behav Pharmacol* 2003;14:77–85.

20. Cook CD, Barrett AC, Roach EL, Bowman JR, Picker MJ. Sex-related differences in the antinociceptive effects of opioids: importance of rat genotype, nociceptive stimulus intensity, and efficacy at the μ opioid receptor. *Psychopharmacology* 2000;150:430–42.

21. Barrett AC, Cook CD, Terner JM, Roach EL, Syvanthong C, Picker MJ. Sex and rat strain determine sensitivity to κ opioid-induced antinociception. *Psychopharmacology* 2002;160:170–81.

22. Terner JM, Barrett AC, Lomas LM, Negus SS, Picker MJ. Influence of low doses of naltrexone on morphine antinociception and morphine tolerance in male and female rats of four strains. *Pain* 2006;122:90–101.

23. LaCroix-Fralish ML, Mogil JS, Weinstein JN, Rutkowski MD, DeLeo JA. The magnitude of mechanical allodynia in a rodent model of lumbar radiculopathy is dependent on strain and sex. *Spine* 2005;30(16):1821–7.

24. DeLeo JA, Rutkowski MD. Gender differences in rat neuropathic pain sensitivity is dependent on strain. *Neurosci Lett* 2000;282:197–9.

25. Terner JM, Barrett AC, Grossell E, Picker MJ. Influence of gonadectomy on the antinociceptive effects of opioids in male and female rats. *Psychopharmacology* 2002;163:183–93.

26. Stephan M, Helfritz F, Pabst R, von Horsten S. Postnatally induced differences in adult pain sensitivity depend on genetics, gender and specific experiences: reversal of maternal deprivation effects by additional postnatal tactile stimulation or chronic imipramine treatment. *Behav Brain Res* 2002;13:149–58.

27. Calderone BJ, George TP, Zachariou V, Picciotto MR. Gender differences in learned helplessness behavior are influenced by genetic background. *Pharmacol Biochem Behav* 2000;66(4):811–7.

28. Chesler EJ, Wilson SG, Lariviere WR, Rodriguez-Zas SL, Mogil JS. Influences of laboratory environment on behavior. Nat Neurosci 2002;5:1101–2.

29. Chesler EJ, Wilson SG, Lariviere WR, Rodriguez-Zas SL, Mogil JS. Identification and

ranking of genetic and laboratory environment factors influencing a behavioral trait, thermal nociception, via computational analysis of a large data archive. *Neurosci Biobehav Rev* 2002;26:907–23.

30. Mogil JS, Grisel JE. Transgenic studies of pain. *Pain* 1998;77(2):107–28.

31. LaCroix-Fralish ML, Ledoux JB, Mogil JS. The Pain Genes Database: an interactive web browser of pain-related transgenic knockout studies. *Pain* 2007;131(1–2):3.e1–e4.

32. Mogil JS, Chanda ML. The case for the inclusion of female subjects in basic science studies of pain. *Pain* 2005;117(1–2):1–5.

33. Mitrovic I, Margeta-Mitrovic M, Bader S, Stoffel M, Jan LY, Basbaum AI. Contribution of GIRK2-mediated postsynaptic signaling to opiate and α2-adrenergic analgesia and analgesic sex differences. *Proc Natl Acad Sci USA* 2003;100(1):271–6.

34. Chanda ML, Mogil JS. Sex differences in the effects of amiloride on formalin test nociception in mice. *Am J Physiol Regul Integr Comp Physiol* 2005;291(2):R335–42.

35. Mogil JS, Breese NM, Witty M-F, et al. Transgenic expression of a dominant-negative ASIC3 subunit leads to increased sensitivity to mechanical and inflammatory stimuli. *J Neurosci* 2005;25(43):9893–901.

36. Mogil JS, McCarson KE. Finding pain genes: bottom-up and top-down approaches. *J Pain* 2000;1(Suppl 1):66–80.

37. Lander ES, Schork NJ. Genetic dissection of complex traits. *Science* 1994;265:2037–48.

38. Verpoorten N, De Jonghe P, Timmerman V. Disease mechanisms in hereditary sensory and autonomic neuropathies. *Neurobiol Dis* 2006;21:247–55.

39. Ferrari MD, van den Maagdenberg AMJM, Frants RR, Goadsby PJ. Migraine as a cerebral ionopathy with impaired central sensory processing. In: Waxman SG, ed. *Molecular Neurology*. New York: Elsevier; 2007: 439–61.

40. Belknap JK, Mogil JS, Helms ML, et al. Localization to chromosome 10 of a locus influencing morphine analgesia in crosses derived from C57BL/6 and DBA/2 mouse strains. *Life Sci* 1995;57:PL117–24.

41. Mogil JS, Richards SP, O'Toole LA, Helms ML, Mitchell SR, Belknap JK. Genetic sensitivity to hot-plate nociception in DBA/2J and C57BL/6J inbred mouse strains: possible sex-specific mediation by δ2-opioid receptors. *Pain* 1997;70(2–3):267–77.

42. Mogil JS, Richards SP, O'Toole LA, et al. Identification of a sex-specific quantitative trait locus mediating nonopioid stress-induced analgesia in female mice. *J Neurosci* 1997; 17(20):7995–8002.

43. Bergeson SE, Helms ML, O'Toole LA, et al. Quantitative trait loci influencing morphine antinociception in four mapping populations. *Mamm Genome* 2001;12:546–53.

44. Seltzer Z, Wu T, Max MB, Diehl SR. Mapping a gene for neuropathic pain-related behavior following peripheral neurectomy in the mouse. *Pain* 2001;93:101–6.

45. Furuse T, Miura Y, Yagasaki K, Shiroishi T, Koide T. Identification of QTLs for differential capsaicin sensitivity between mouse strains KJR and C57BL/6. *Pain* 2003;105:169–75.

46. Mogil JS, Wilson SG, Chesler EJ, et al. The melanocortin-1 receptor gene mediates female-specific mechanisms of analgesia in mice and humans. *Proc Natl Acad Sci USA* 2003;100(8): 4867–72.

47. Devor M, Gilad A, Arbilly M, et al. *pain1*: a neuropathic pain QTL on mouse chromosome 15 in a C3HxC58 backcross. *Pain* 2005;116:289–93.

48. Mogil JS, Meirmeister F, Seifert F, et al. Variable sensitivity to noxious heat is mediated by differential expression of the CGRP gene. *Proc Natl Acad Sci USA* 2005;102:12938–43.

49. Liang D-Y, Liao G, Lighthall GK, Peltz G, Clark DJ. Genetic variants of the P-glycoprotein gene *Abcb1b* modulate opioid-induced hyperalgesia, tolerance and dependence. *Pharmacogenet Genom* 2006;16:825–35.

50. Liang D-Y, Liao G, Wang J, et al. A genetic analysis of opioid-induced hyperalgesia in mice. *Anesthesiology* 2006;104:1054–62.

51. Mogil JS, Ritchie J, Sotocinal SG, et al. Screening for pain phenotypes: analysis of three congenic mouse strains on a battery of nine nociceptive assays. *Pain* 2006;126(1–2):24–34.

52. Devor M, Gilad A, Arbilly M, et al. Sex-specific variability and a "cage effect" independently mask a neuropathic pain quantitative trait locus detected in a whole genome scan. *Eur J Neurosci* 2007;26:681–8.

53. Dominguez CA, Lidman O, Hao JX, et al. Genetic analysis of neuropathic pain-like behavior following peripheral nerve injury suggests a role of the major histocompatibility complex in development of allodynia. *Pain* 2008;136(3):313–9.

54. Nissenbaum J, Shpigler H, Pisante A, et al. *pain2*: neuropathic pain QTL identified on rat chromosome 2. *Pain* 2008;135:92–7.

55. Smith SB, Marker CL, Perry C, et al. Quantitative trait locus and computational mapping identifies *Kcnj9* (GIRK3) as a candidate gene

affecting analgesia from multiple drug classes. *Pharmacogenet Genom* 2008;18:231–41.

56. Kest B, Smith SB, Schorscher-Petcu A, et al. *Gnao1* (Gαo protein) is a likely genetic contributor to variation in physical dependence on opioids in mice. *Neuroscience* 2009;162:1255–64.

57. LaCroix-Fralish ML, Mo G, Smith SB, et al. The β3 subunit of the Na+,K+-ATPase affects pain sensitivity. *Pain* 2009;144:294–302.

58. Fortin A, Diez E, Ritchie J, et al. Positional cloning of a quantitative trait locus contributing to pain sensitivity: possible mediation by *Tyrp1* (tyrosinase-related protein 1). *Genes Brain Behav* 2010;9:856–67.

59. Nissenbaum J, Devor M, Seltzer Z, et al. Susceptibility to chronic pain following nerve injury is genetically affected by *CACNG2*. *Genome Res* 2010;20:1180–90.

60. Nair HK, Hain H, Quock RM, et al. Genomic loci and candidate genes underlying inflammatory nociception. *Pain* 2011;152:599–606.

61. Anholt RR, Mackay TFC. Quantitative genetic analyses of complex behaviours in *Drosophila*. *Nature Rev Genet* 2004;5:838–49.

62. Gear RW, Gordon NC, Heller PH, Paul SM, Miaskowski C, Levine JD. Gender difference in analgesic response to the kappa-opioid pentazocine. *Neurosci Lett* 1996;205:207–9.

63. Gear RW, Miaskowski C, Gordon NC, Paul SM, Heller PH, Levine JD. Kappa-opioids produce significantly greater analgesia in women than in men. *Nat Med* 1996;2(11):1248–50.

64. Gear RW, Miaskowski C, Gordon NC, Paul SM, Heller PH, Levine JD. The kappa opioid nalbuphine produces gender- and dose-dependent analgesia and antianalgesia in patients with postoperative pain. *Pain* 1999;83:339–45.

65. Tershner SA, Mitchell JM, Fields HL. Brainstem pain modulating circuitry is sexually dimorphic with respect to mu and kappa opioid receptor function. *Pain* 2000;85:153–9.

66. Liu N-J, von Gizycki H, Gintzler AR. Sexually dimorphic recruitment of spinal opioid analgesic pathways by the spinal application of morphine. *J Pharmacol Exp Ther* 2007;322:654–60.

67. Chakrabarti S, Liu N-J, Gintzler AR. Formation of μ-/κ-opioid receptor heterodimer is sex-dependent and mediates female-specific opioid analgesia. *Proc Natl Acad Sci USA* 2010; 107(46):20115–9.

68. LaCroix-Fralish ML, Mogil JS. Progress in genetic studies of pain and analgesia. *Annu Rev Pharmacol Toxicol* 2009;49:97–121.

69. Kim H, Neubert JK, San Miguel A, et al. Genetic influence on variability in human acute experimental pain sensitivity associated with gender, ethnicity and psychological temperament. *Pain* 2004;109(3):488–96.

70. Fillingim RB, Kaplan L, Staud R, et al. The A118G single nucleotide polymorphism of the μ-opioid receptor gene (OPRM1) is associated with pressure pain sensitivity in humans. *J Pain* 2005;6:159–67.

71. Weiss LA, Pan L, Abney M, Ober C. The sex-specific genetic architecture of quantitative traits in humans. *Nature Genet* 2006;38(2):218–22.

72. Wang C, Cheng Y, Liu T, et al. A computational model for sex-specific genetic architecture of complex traits in humans: implications for mapping pain sensitivity. *Mol Pain* 2008;4:13.

73. Patsopoulos NA, Tatsioni A, Ioannidis JP. Claims of sex differences: an empirical assessment in genetic associations. *JAMA* 2007; 298(8):880–93.

74. Mogil JS, Sternberg WF, Kest B, Marek P, Liebeskind JC. Sex differences in the antagonism of swim stress-induced analgesia: effects of gonadectomy and estrogen replacement. *Pain* 1993;53:17–25.

75. Sternberg WF, Mogil JS, Kest B, et al. Neonatal testosterone exposure influences neurochemistry of swim stress-induced analgesia in adult mice. *Pain* 1996;63:321–6.

76. Sternberg WF, Chesler EJ, Wilson SG, Mogil JS. Acute progesterone can recruit sex-specific neurochemical mechanisms mediating swim stress-induced and kappa-opioid analgesia in mice. *Horm Behav* 2004;46(4):467–73.

77. Sternberg WF, Ritchie J, Mogil JS. Qualitative sex differences in κ-opioid analgesia in mice are dependent on age. *Neurosci Lett* 2004;363:178–81.

78. Kavaliers M, Choleris E. Sex differences in *N*-methyl-D-aspartate involvement in κ opioid and non-opioid predator-induced analgesia in mice. *Brain Res* 1997;768:30–6.

79. Kavaliers M, Colwell DD, Choleris E. Sex differences in opioid and *N*-methyl-D-aspartate mediated non-opioid biting fly exposure induced analgesia in deer mice. *Pain* 1998;77(2):163–77.

80. Kavaliers M, Galea LAM. Sex differences in the expression and antagonism of swim stress-induced analgesia in deer mice vary with the breeding season. *Pain* 1995;63:327–34.

81. Xia Y, Wikberg JES, Chhajlani V. Expression of melanocortin 1 receptor in periaqueductal gray matter. *Neuroreport* 1995;6:2193–6.

82. Cone RD, Lu D, Koppula S, et al. The melanocortin receptors: agonists, antagonists, and the hormonal control of pigmentation. *Rec Prog Horm Res* 1996;51:287–317.

83. Rees JL, Birch-Machin M, Flanagan N, Healy E, Phillips S, Todd C. Genetic studies of the human melanocortin-1 receptor. *Ann NY Acad Sci* 1999;885:134–42.

84. Scott MC, Wakamatsu K, Ito S, et al. Human *melanocortin 1 receptor* variants, receptor function and melanocyte response to UV radiation. *J Cell Sci* 2002;115:2349–55.

85. Angst MS, Clark JD. Opioid-induced hyperalgesia: a qualitative systematic review. *Anesthesiology* 2006;104(3):570–87.

86. Juni A, Klein G, Kowalczyk B, Ragnauth A, Kest B. Sex differences in hyperalgesia during morphine infusion: effect of gonadectomy and estrogen treatment. *Neuropharmacology* 2008;54: 1264–70.

87. Juni A, Cai M, Stankova M, et al. Sex-specific mediation of opioid-induced hyperalgesia by the melanocortin-1 receptor. *Anesthesiology* 2010; 112:181–8.

88. Waxman AR, Juni A, Kowalczyk W, Arout C, Sternberg WF, Kest B. Progesterone rapidly recruits female-typical opioid-induced hyperalgesic mechanisms. *Physiol Behav* 2010; 101:759–63.

89. Mogil JS, Sorge RE, LaCroix-Fralish ML, et al. Pain sensitivity and vasopressin analgesia are mediated by a gene-sex-environment interaction. *Nat Neurosci* 2011;14:1569–1573.

90. Wilson SG, Chesler EJ, Hain HS, et al. Identification of quantitative trait loci for chemical/inflammatory nociception in mice. *Pain* 2002;96(3):385–91.

91. Campbell CM, Edwards RR, Carmona C, et al. Polymorphisms in the GTP cyclohydrolase gene (*GCH1*) are associated with ratings of capsaicin pain. *Pain* 2009;141:114–8.

92. DeLorey TM, Sahbaie P, Hashemi E, Li W-W, Salehi A, Clark DJ. Somatosensory and sensorimotor consequences associated with the heterozygous disruption of the autism candidate gene, Gabrb3. *Behav Brain Res* 2011;216:36–45.

93. Leck KJ, Bartlett SE, Smith MT, et al. Deletion of guanine nucleotide binding protein αz subunit in mice induces a gene dose dependent tolerance to morphine. *Neuropharmacology* 2004;46:836–46.

94. Marker CL, Stoffel M, Wickman K. Spinal G-protein-gated K+ channels formed by GIRK1 and GIRK2 subunits modulate thermal nociception and contribute to morphine analgesia. *J Neurosci* 2004;24(11):2806–12.

95. Martin M, Matifas A, Maldonado R, Kieffer BL. Acute antinociceptive responses in single and combinatorial opioid receptor knockout mice: distinct mu, delta and kappa tones. *Eur J Neurosci* 2003;17:701–8.

96. Contet C, Gaveriaux-Ruff C, Matifas A, Caradec C, Champy M-F, Kieffer BL. Dissociation of analgesic and hormonal responses to forced swim stress using opioid receptor knockout mice. *Neuropsychopharmacology* 2006;31:1733–44.

97. Ballou LR, Botting RM, Goorha S, Zhang J, Vane JR. Nociception in cyclooxygenase isozyme-deficient mice. *Proc Natl Acad Sci USA* 2000;97(18):10272–6.

98. Kwan KY, Allchorne AJ, Vollrath MA, et al. TRPA1 contributes to cold, mechanical and chemical nociception but is not essential for hair-cell transduction. *Neuron* 2006;50:277–89.

6

ROLE OF SEX HORMONES IN PAIN AND ANALGESIA

Rebecca Craft

INTRODUCTION

In the past few decades, research on the influence of sex hormones on pain has increased dramatically. A PubMed search conducted in May 2011 using the terms "estradiol and pain" yielded approximately 1,200 articles, with over 70% of those articles published since 1990 (see Fig. 6.1). Research on sex hormone modulation of the analgesic effects of drugs, although still comparatively sparse, is also on a rising trajectory (Fig. 6.1).

The broad focus of this chapter is on the effects of the primary sex hormones—estradiol, progesterone, and testosterone—on pain and analgesia. Sexual differentiation of sensitivity to pain and analgesia can be attributed in part to both organizational and activational effects of sex hormones. Organizational effects refer to sex hormone effects that result in permanent structural and functional differentiation of biological substrates that is typically due to testosterone exposure early in life (in mammals, beginning before birth). Activational effects of sex hormones are those that promote male or female characteristics in adulthood (at puberty and thereafter, primarily via testosterone and estradiol); these effects are considered impermanent, as they may change according to the hormone state of the individual. Because hormone manipulations are

difficult to conduct in very young animals (and unethical to conduct in very young humans), we have relatively little information on organizational sex hormone effects on pain and analgesia. Thus, this chapter will focus primarily on the activational effects of sex hormones. Even this is a very large topic, so the primary emphasis will be on sex hormone modulation of analgesia. First, what is the evidence from animal and human studies that sex hormones modulate analgesia produced by opioids, cannabinoids, nonsteroidal anti-inflammatory drugs (NSAIDs), and alpha-2 adrenergic drugs? Second, what pharmacokinetic and pharmacodynamic mechanisms may explain the modulatory effects of sex hormones on analgesia?

It should be noted that pregnancy-induced analgesia is not addressed in this chapter; interested readers are encouraged to peruse the work of Dr. Alan Gintzler, who has uncovered many mechanisms underlying the dramatic changes in pain sensitivity resulting from pregnancy-induced elevations in estradiol and progesterone.[1,2]

SEX HORMONE MODULATION OF PAIN

The greater prevalence of many types of chronic pain in women than in men[3,4] strongly

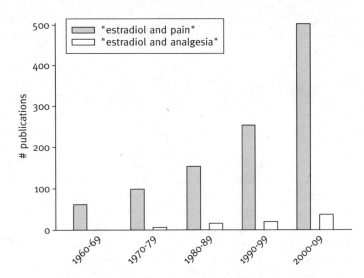

FIGURE 6.1   Results of a PubMed search conducted on May 29, 2011. The terms "estradiol" and "pain" were entered, yielding 1,161 citations; 83 citations dating from 2010–2011 (and 1 from 1959) are not included on the plot. The terms "estradiol" and "analgesia" then were entered, yielding 87 citations; 6 citations dating from 2010–2011 are not included on the plot.

implicates sex hormones as pain modulators. Although there is some evidence for fluctuations in pain across the menstrual cycle in women, the fluctuations observed in normally cycling women in laboratory pain studies are far from robust.[5,6] Sex hormone modulation of acute pain is also only inconsistently reported.[7,8] The most abundant evidence at present for sex hormone effects on pain is estradiol modulation of chronic pain. However, even for this single hormone, generalizations such as "estradiol worsens pain" or "estradiol alleviates pain" simply cannot be made: estrogens have extremely diverse effects on many different systems of the body, such that their effects on pain depend on the extent to which a particular type of chronic pain involves particular systems of the body (e.g., cardiovascular vs. immune).[8] Additionally, *changes* in estradiol level rather than simply the presence or absence of estradiol can strongly influence pain. For example, the decline in estradiol such as occurs after ovulation, at the end of the luteal phase, or upon termination of estradiol supplementation or replacement can precipitate migraine in women.[9] Estradiol-related migraine is believed to be caused by direct effects of estradiol on vasodilation as well as estradiol modulation of sensitivity to various vasoactive agents (e.g.,

CGRP, ACh).[10] In contrast to estradiol effects on migraine, which may primarily involve the cardiovascular system, estradiol effects on chronic pain such as in temporomandibular disorder likely reflect the composite effects of estradiol on immune, skeletal, and nervous systems. For example, estradiol can increase immune responses (thereby increasing inflammation and worsening pain), promote bone deposition (thereby protecting against pain caused by joint degeneration), and increase firing of sensory afferents in the temporomandibular joint area (thereby worsening pain).[8] Although it can be difficult to predict the balance among all these estradiol effects in terms of overall pain levels in women at any given point in time, the predominant outcome appears to be a worsening of pain. In fact, recent reports suggest that women with particular estrogen receptor polymorphisms are at higher risk for a number of chronic pain disorders.[11] Finally, given the increasing evidence for ovarian hormone modulation of mood and cognition,[12–14] there is potential for indirect effects of ovarian hormones on pain perception via hormone effects on emotional and cognitive processing. This latter question remains largely unaddressed, but studies demonstrating that administration of sex hormones directly into limbic areas such as the amygdala can modulate pain responses in animals[15–16] suggest that it merits further consideration.

SEX HORMONE MODULATION OF ANALGESIA

Opioids

Sex differences in opioid analgesia have been reported in a number of animal and human studies over the past two decades. In a recent review of studies conducted in humans, Niesters and colleagues[17] concluded that the prototypical mu opioid agonist morphine is a more effective analgesic in women than in men, based on experimental pain studies and clinical studies involving the use of patient-controlled analgesia (also see Chapter 4, this volume). Although data on other mu opioid agonists as well as mixed mu-kappa opioid agonists are less convincing, mu-kappa opioid analgesia against clinical pain also appears to be greater in women than in men.[17] In contrast, a majority of animal (particularly rat) studies on sex differences in opioid antinociception demonstrate greater potency and sometimes greater efficacy of mu and mu-kappa opioid agonists in *males*.[18–22] As for selective kappa opioid agonists, which have only been studied in animals, sex differences are mixed; however, greater antinociceptive potency and/or efficacy in females than in males is reported with greater frequency than for mu opioid agonists.[23]

It should be noted that nearly all sex difference studies in rodents have examined opioid antinociception only acutely. Because male rats in particular may develop morphine tolerance more readily than females, after some days of morphine treatment, *females* may show greater antinociceptive potency than males.[24–26] As noted by Niesters and colleagues,[17] in human studies sex differences tend to be greater with more prolonged opioid treatment; thus, the very short time period over which opioid antinociception is typically examined in animal studies may contribute to the apparent species difference in the direction of sex differences observed. This hypothesis could be tested in animal experiments by assessing opioid antinociceptive potency over a matter of weeks rather than on a single day. Furthermore, using an analgesic self-administration paradigm in rodents that are in chronic pain[27] would better approximate the patient-controlled analgesia studies that have been used to compare opioid analgesic potency/efficacy in humans. Whether the long-standing discrepancy between human and animal studies can be resolved by using more comparable methodological approaches to assessing analgesic effectiveness remains to be seen.

When observed, sex differences in opioid analgesia have been shown to be sex hormone dependent. Organizational sex hormone effects—which can only be investigated experimentally in animal studies—appear to be responsible for sexual differentiation of mu opioid antinociceptive potency. Specifically, sex differences in the acute antinociceptive potency of morphine can be eliminated by early neonatal castration of male rats or neonatal testosterone treatment of females.[28–31] Once rodents are adults, estradiol (and rarely testosterone and progesterone) has been shown to modulate mu opioid antinociceptive sensitivity.[7] Regarding activational effects, female rats of various strains show fluctuating sensitivity to mu opioid agonist-induced antinociception across the estrous cycle,[32–33] typically with lowest sensitivity during vaginal estrus, which occurs approximately 1 day after peak ovarian hormone levels and roughly corresponds to ovulation and the period of sexual receptivity in the rat. Numerous studies support the hypothesis that estradiol is the ovarian hormone responsible for estrous stage–related fluctuations in mu opioid agonist sensitivity. When administered "chronically"—typically, a single high-dose injection with a 48-hour interval before testing, or via Silastic implant—estradiol generally decreases antinociceptive sensitivity to morphine in ovariectomized female rats.[32,34,35] However, when administered acutely (single injection with ≤24 hour-interval before testing), estradiol may increase opioid antinociception. For example, estradiol significantly increased morphine antinociceptive potency when assessed 4–24 hours later, but it decreased morphine antinociceptive potency when assessed 48 hours after estradiol administration.[36] These time-dependent changes likely reflect the fluctuations observed in gonadally intact females across the estrous cycle, as their estradiol levels wax and wane.

As for kappa opioid agonist-induced antinociception, only a few studies have examined sex hormone modulation, primarily in adult animals. For example, Mokha and colleagues recently reported that intrathecal U50,488 was antinociceptive only in proestrous (peak or rising estradiol and progesterone) female rats, not in diestrous (low estradiol and progesterone) females or in males; the greater effect in proestrous females can be attributed to estradiol, as ovariectomy abolished U50,488 sensitivity and estradiol treatment dose dependently reinstated it.[37] Several other studies, though not all, also report fluctuating kappa opioid antinociception across the estrous cycle[38] or enhanced kappa opioid agonist-induced antinociception when ovariectomized females are treated with estradiol, including studies in rhesus monkeys.[39,40] Thus, estradiol may have opposing effects on mu versus kappa opioid agonist-induced antinociception—attenuating mu opioid antinociception while enhancing kappa opioid antinociception (when opioid antinociception is examined 48 hours after hormone treatment). Opposing effects of estradiol on mu versus kappa sensitivity may contribute to the sometimes conflicting results obtained when examining sex differences in, and sex hormone modulation of, antinociception produced by mixed-action, mu-kappa opioids.

Very few investigators have examined progesterone's effects on opioid antinociception thus far (except in models of pregnancy, where progesterone in combination with estradiol exerts profound effects on endogenous opioid function.[1] We have found that s.c. progesterone alone rarely alters opioid antinociceptive potency in ovariectomized female rats, nor does it typically alter estradiol's effect.[32,41] In contrast, intrathecal (but not i.m.) progesterone given to intact female rats enhanced sufentanil-induced antinociception.[42] Finally, although acute systemic progesterone has not been found to alter the potency of U50,488-induced antinociception per se, it does alter the *mechanism* by which U50,488 produces antinociception in ovariectomized female mice (i.e., from NMDA-sensitive, male-like antinociception to NMDA-insensitive antinociception seen in intact females).[43]

To date, only one study has been conducted in humans to examine menstrual cycle–related changes in sensitivity to the analgesic effects of opioids. In a laboratory study, normally cycling women showed greater morphine analgesia against ischemic (but not heat or pressure) pain when they were in the follicular phase compared to the luteal phase.[44] This cycle-related difference was not observed for pentazocine, and no cycle effects were observed in women taking oral contraceptives.[44] Given that changes in opioid analgesic sensitivity in female rats tend to be observed around the time of ovulation, it will be important in future human studies to include an ovulatory phase test (no small challenge in terms of scheduling women participants). Additionally, the possible acute modulatory effects of estradiol and progesterone on opioid analgesic sensitivity have not been examined yet in humans; an experimental design similar to that used by Zubieta and colleagues[45] in which women are treated acutely with estradiol during the early follicular phase (when endogenous ovarian hormones are low) would be informative. In that study, exogenous estradiol was found to modulate brain mu opioid receptor occupancy and women's pain perception, suggesting that estradiol's effects on opioid sensitivity observed in female rodents may generalize to women.

Cannabinoids

There is tremendous interest in the analgesic potential of cannabinoids. During the past 15 years, 16 US states plus Washington, D.C. and Canada have legalized marijuana use for medical purposes; chronic pain is commonly listed among the conditions for which marijuana can be used. A number of controlled studies demonstrate the utility of cannabinoids as analgesics against postoperative pain,[46] neuropathic pain,[47–49] and experimental pain (intradermal capsaicin-induced, radiant heat).[50–52] Sex differences in cannabinoid analgesia have not yet been investigated in humans; however, several rodent studies suggest that cannabinoids such as Δ^9-tetrahydrocannabinol (THC), 11-OH-THC, and CP55,940 are more potent—and in a few cases, more efficacious—in producing antinociception in females than in males.[53–56]

THC-induced antinociception also appears to be sex hormone dependent. First, gonadally intact, cycling female rats showed significantly greater sensitivity to THC-induced antinociception in late proestrus or estrus than in diestrus, when THC was administered systemically[57] or intracerebroventricularly.[58] Chronic estradiol exposure via Silastic capsule implant enhanced THC-induced antinociception in ovariectomized female rats,[57] suggesting that the enhanced THC sensitivity observed in late proestrous females is due to estradiol. However, acute injection of estradiol in ovariectomized mice *attenuated* the antinociceptive effect of WIN55,212–2.[59] These apparently discrepant results may simply reflect the time-dependent effects of estradiol. We are currently using a more sophisticated hormone replacement regimen that better models the rat estrous cycle, to provide a clearer picture of cyclic ovarian hormone modulation of cannabinoid antinociception.

As for other sex hormones, testosterone did not significantly alter THC-induced antinociception in castrated male rats, in the only study that has examined this hormone.[57] Progesterone also has been examined in a single study, and it did not significantly alter antinociception produced by the cannabinoid WIN55,212-2.[59] The combination of estradiol and progesterone has not yet been examined. Thus far, ovarian hormone modulation of mu opioid and cannabinoid antinociception in adult females appears to occur in a compensatory manner: when females' sensitivity to mu opioids is falling (proestrus to estrus), their sensitivity to cannabinoids is rising.

Nonsteroidal Anti-Inflammatory Drugs

A few studies have been conducted to examine sex differences in analgesia produced by NSAIDs (see Chapter 4 for a summary of the human data). Although animal studies are typically utilized to more comprehensively compare analgesic potency and efficacy, a PubMed search ("NSAID and sex differences and pain") revealed no studies of sex differences in NSAID-induced antinociception in animals. However, a recent study examined the modulation of NSAID-induced antinociception by estradiol in ovariectomized female rats. Both estradiol and a COX-2 inhibitor (NS398) given alone reduced intraplantar carrageenan-induced thermal hyperalgesia; when coadministered, their effects were generally additive with the exception that estradiol appeared to prolong the effects of the COX-2 inhibitor.[60] Estradiol did not significantly alter the effects of a COX-1 inhibitor in this assay, and estradiol enhancement of NS398-induced anti-hyperalgesia did not appear to be related to prostaglandin levels.[60] In conclusion, the existing literature provides little evidence for either sex differences in, or sex hormone modulation of, NSAID-induced analgesia; however, this research topic has received very little attention to date. Given the extremely widespread use of NSAID analgesics clinically, more comprehensive sex comparisons and gonadal hormone manipulation studies are needed.

Alpha-2 Adrenergic Agonists

Alpha-2 adrenergic agonists like clonidine and dexmedetomidine are used clinically as adjunctive anesthetics and analgesics for postoperative pain.[61,62] Several rodent studies demonstrate significantly greater clonidine-induced antinociception in males compared to females.[63–65] Furthermore, sex hormones may dramatically modulate clonidine-induced antinociception in adult rats. In adult males, castration abolishes, and testosterone (but not estradiol) replacement reinstates clonidine-induced antinociception.[63,66,67] In cycling females, male-like sensitivity to clonidine-induced antinociception is evident in proestrous females, whereas those in diestrous, and ovariectomized, estradiol-treated females are considerably less sensitive to clonidine.[65,66] Sex comparisons of alpha-2 adrenergic analgesia have not yet been conducted in humans. However, sex differences in local vascular responses have been observed using a highly selective alpha-2 adrenergic agonist, azepexole,[68] suggesting that the sex differences in alpha-2 adrenergic analgesia observed in animal studies should be examined in humans.

Mechanisms of Sex Hormone Modulation of Analgesia: Pharmacokinetics

Theoretically, sex hormones could influence an organism's response to analgesic (and other) drugs via pharmacokinetic and pharmacodynamic mechanisms. Regarding pharmacokinetic mechanisms, many studies have demonstrated sex differences and/or sex hormone effects on the distribution, metabolism, and excretion of therapeutic drugs. For example, the CYP3A family of cytochrome P450 enzymes—which are involved in the metabolism of over 50% of drugs, including some opioids and cannabinoids—has approximately 50% more activity in women than in men; furthermore, membrane transport of some drugs is greater in men than in women, and estrogens and androgens can modulate the expression of various cytochrome P450 enzymes.[69-75] The current consensus, however, is that only for a few drugs are these sex differences and hormone effects of substantial clinical importance. In addition, sex differences in pharmacokinetics for a given drug are not always the same in humans and rats. For the most widely used analgesic drugs such as opioids and NSAIDs, there is limited evidence for sex differences in one or more pharmacokinetic parameters in humans. In the only human study in which both analgesic action and pharmacokinetics of morphine were compared in men versus women, i.v. morphine was more potent in women yet had a slower onset and offset; peak plasma concentrations of morphine and its two metabolites did not differ between the sexes.[76] The authors conclude that although morphine is initially more effective in men, this is simply due to the slower onset in women, and over a longer period of time, greater analgesic potency of morphine in women is likely due to pharmacodynamic rather than pharmacokinetic factors.

Several studies have found no significant differences in plasma levels of morphine in female versus male rodents despite greater morphine antinociceptive potency in males.[77-79] However, two studies report greater morphine levels in the *brains* of males compared to females,[77-80] and one study reports substantially lower morphine-3-glucuronide levels in males compared to females—both of which could contribute to greater morphine-induced antinociception in males compared to females.[79] Central pharmacodynamic explanations cannot be ruled out, however, because microinjection of mu opioid agonists into the cerebral ventricles or into pain-related brain areas such as the periaqueductal gray (PAG) still leads to greater antinociception in males compared to females.[81-86, 111] Thus, based on current evidence, it can be concluded that sex differences in, and sex hormone modulation of, pharmacokinetic factors contributes to but does not fully explain sex differences in opioid analgesia in either rats or humans.

As for cannabinoids, a recent study reported significantly higher AUC and C_{max} (and shorter T_{max}) in women than in men for THC and 11-OH-THC, the major active metabolite of THC.[87] A single rodent study has examined the relationship between sex differences in THC-induced antinociception and THC pharmacokinetics. Although plasma and brain levels of THC itself did not differ between female and male rats, females showed more 11-OH-THC and other metabolites in brain; furthermore, blocking cytP450 metabolism of THC completely eliminated sex differences in THC-induced antinociception.[88] Sex differences in, and sex hormone modulation of, cytochrome P450 enzymes that metabolize THC are known to exist in rodents and monkeys.[89,90] Thus, peripheral pharmacokinetic factors clearly contribute to male-female differences in cannabinoid antinociception in the rat. Still, pharmacodynamic explanations cannot be ruled out, given that significant sex differences in THC-induced antinociception were observed after THC was administered directly into the brain.[58]

As for NSAIDs, a single study reported that after treatment with weight-adjusted dose(s) of aspirin, peak plasma levels of salicylic acid—the major active metabolite of aspirin—were significantly higher in women than in men; these sex differences could be attributed to slower absorption and faster elimination in men compared to women.[91] Because there are no published studies comparing the analgesic effects of aspirin in males versus females of any species, it is unclear whether sex differences in the pharmacokinetics of aspirin result in sex differences in its analgesic effects. However, aspirin–triggered 15-epi-lipoxin A_4, an endogenous autacoid with anti-inflammatory properties, showed age-related increases in women but decreases in men given a low dose of aspirin.[92] This sex difference in an anti-inflammatory property of aspirin may contribute to sex differences in the therapeutic utility of aspirin for various chronic inflammatory diseases.

Mechanisms of Sex Hormone Modulation of Analgesia: Pharmacodynamics

As noted earlier, one of the first indicators that central pharmacodynamic mechanisms could also be important in mediating sex differences in, and sex hormone modulation of, antinociception was the fact that group differences persisted even when opioids and cannabinoids were microinjected directly into the brain. A key sexually differentiated brain area that contributes to sex differences in opioid, and perhaps other drug-induced analgesia, is the descending pain modulatory pathway. Through a series of elegant studies conducted over the past few years, Murphy and colleagues demonstrated that morphine attenuates persistent pain-induced Fos expression in the PAG of male but not female rats, and that morphine activates significantly more PAG neurons that project to the rostral ventromedial medulla in males than in females.[93] Within the PAG, sexually differentiated mu opioid antinociception can be attributed to GABAergic control of output neurons rather than the output neurons themselves, since direct activation of output neurons resulted in equivalent antinociception in female and male rats.[86] When rats are exposed to an acute noxious stimulus, pain-related cells in the rostral ventromedial medulla fire less in estradiol-treated female rats than in no-hormone controls, which may reflect estradiol's effect upstream in the PAG.[94] Using an irreversible, mu opioid receptor–selective antagonist to reduce the number of available receptors in the PAG resulted in a greater reduction in morphine antinociceptive potency in females compared to males, suggesting that females have a lower receptor reserve than do males.[95] Indeed, PAG mu opioid receptor expression is lowest in proestrous and estrous females, and these groups show significantly lower morphine antinociceptive potency than diestrous females and males.[85] Although yet to be demonstrated in PAG neurons, estradiol can uncouple hypothalamic mu

opioid receptors from their G proteins [96] as well as induce internalization of mu opioid receptors.[97] All of these pharmacodynamic mechanisms could contribute to reduced mu opioid antinociception in females, particularly during the period following peak estradiol levels.

Opioids are potent analgesics when administered intrathecally, and they may act peripherally as well; thus, sex differences in spinal and peripheral sensitivity to opioids could also contribute to sex differences in analgesia when opioids are administered systemically. Although no sex differences in antinociception have been reported after intrathecal morphine administration in the rat,[98,99] a peripherally restricted opioid agonist was more potent in males than in females against visceral pain[98] and arthritis pain.[100] Additionally, despite equivalent potency between males and females, i.t. morphine-induced antinociception required *kappa opioid receptor activation* only in proestrous females,[99] which was later discovered to result from ovarian hormone-induced spinal mu-kappa opioid receptor heterodimerization.[101] Thus, there appear to be multiple pharmacodynamic mechanisms underlying sex differences in opioid antinociception, at least in the rat.

To date, there is little information available regarding pharmacodynamic mechanisms underlying differential antinociception produced by nonopioid analgesics in males versus females or in females in different estrous stages. Cannabinoid antinociception after site-specific drug administration has been compared in only one study: i.c.v. THC produced significantly greater antinociception in females in late proestrus compared to those in estrus and males.[58] Sex, estrous cycle, and estradiol treatment have been reported to alter brain CB1 receptor density[102–105] and endocannabinoid production[106] in some brain areas; the extent to which these cellular mechanisms relate to cannabinoid antinociception remains to be discovered. It should be noted that at least in some cases, estradiol-induced changes in receptor density do not correlate with estradiol modulation of antinociception (e.g., alpha-2 adrenergic receptors).[66] However, an early finding of greater peripheral cannabinoid receptor density in women compared to men (on leukocytes)[107] suggests that sex differences in the analgesic effects of cannabinoids on chronic pain are worth investigating in humans.

One additional pharmacodynamic mechanism merits mention in relation to sex differences in—and possibly sex hormone modulation of—pain and analgesia. This mechanism involves a particular type of ion channel—the G protein–activated, inwardly rectifying potassium type 2 (GIRK2) channel. GIRK2 channels mediate the postsynaptic inhibition of neural firing caused by opioids and some other analgesics; thus, their activity is central to pain control.[108] In 2003, two independent laboratories reported that when GIRK2 channels were eliminated via gene knockout, pain responses to some noxious stimuli and antinociception produced by various drugs and stress were significantly altered in mice—in a sex-dependent manner in some cases.[64,109] For example, GIRK2 knockout decreased thermal nociceptive latencies in males but not females, and decreased morphine- and clonidine-induced antinociception more in males than females, eliminating the sex differences in antinociception.[64] GIRK2 gene expression in spinal cord and brain is already somewhat greater in male than in female rats at 1 week of age, and in adults, GIRK2 gene expression may be modulated by sex hormones in both females and males.[110] Thus, it is possible that sex hormone modulation of expression of this single type of potassium channel—which is known to mediate the analgesic effects of multiple drugs—contributes to sex hormone modulation of analgesia produced by opioids, alpha-2 adrenergic agonists, and other analgesics.

CONCLUSION

The exploration of sex hormone modulation of pain and analgesia is still in its infancy. Early data indicate that sex hormones can modulate both pharmacokinetic and pharmacodynamic factors that contribute to sex differences in analgesia produced by opioids and other analgesics. Estradiol, in particular, modulates female rats' sensitivity to nociceptive stimuli and to antinociception produced by opioids (mu and kappa), cannabinoids, and alpha-2 adrenergic drugs; two studies suggest that

ovarian hormones also may modulate opioid analgesia in humans. Future sex comparison and especially hormone manipulation studies in humans, as well as animal studies that better reflect the human clinical conditions in which analgesics are widely used—and the long duration for which they are used—will be crucial for determining to what extent sex differences in, and sex hormone modulation of, pain and analgesia really matter.

REFERENCES

1. Dawson-Basoa ME, Gintzler AR. Estrogen and progesterone activate spinal kappa-opiate receptor analgesic mechanisms. *Pain* 1996;64:169–77.
2. Gintzler AR, Schnell SA, Gupta DS, Liu N-J, Wessendorf MW. Relationship of spinal dynorphin neurons to δ-opioid receptors and estrogen receptor α: anatomical basis for ovarian sex steroid opioid antinociception. *J Pharmacol Exp Ther* 2008;326:725–31.
3. Unruh AM. Gender variations in clinical pain experience. *Pain* 1996;65:123–67.
4. Johannes CB, Le TK, Zhou X, Johnston JA, Dworkin RH. The prevalence of chronic pain in United States adults: results of an internet-based survey. *J Pain* 2010;11:1230–9.
5. Riley JL, Robinson ME, Wise EA, Price DD. A meta-analytic review of pain perception across the menstrual cycle. *Pain* 1999;81:225–35.
6. Sherman JJ, LeResche L. Does experimental pain response vary across the menstrual cycle? A methodological review. *Am J Physiol Regul Integr Comp Physiol* 2006;291:R245–56.
7. Craft RM, Mogil JS, Aloisi AM. Sex differences in pain and analgesia: the role of gonadal hormones. *Eur J Pain* 2004;8:397–411.
8. Craft RM. Modulation of pain by estrogens. *Pain* 2007;132:S3–12.
9. Brandes JL. The influence of estrogen on migraine. A systematic review. *JAMA* 2006;15:1824–30.
10. Gupta S, Mehrotra S, Villalón C, et al. Effects of female sex hormones on responses to CGRP, acetylcholine, and 5-HT in rat isolated arteries. *Headache* 2007;47:564–75.
11. Ribeiro-Dasilva MC, Line SRP, Godoy dos Santos MCL, Arthuri MT, Hou W, Fillingim RB. Estrogen receptor-α polymorphisms and predisposition to TMJ disorder. *J Pain* 2009;10:527–33.
12. LaCreuse A. Effects of ovarian hormones on cognitive function in nonhuman primates. *Neuroscience* 2006;138:859–67.

13. McEwen BS. Stress, sex, and neural adaptation to a changing environment: mechanisms of neuronal remodeling. *Ann NY Acad Sci* 2010;1204: E38–59.

14. Jacobs E, D'Esposito M. Estrogen shapes dopamine-dependent cognitive processes: implications for women's health. *J Neurosci* 2011;31: 5286–93.

15. Frye CA, Walf AA. Estrogen and/or progesterone administered systemically or to the amygdala can have anxiety-, fear-, and pain-reducing effects in ovariectomized rats. *Behav Neurosci* 2004;118:306–13.

16. Myers B, Schulkin J, Greenwood-Van Meerveld B. Sex steroids localized to the amygdala increase pain responses to visceral stimulation in rats. *J Pain* 2011;12:486–94.

17. Niesters M, Dahan A, Kest B, et al. Do sex differences exist in opioid analgesia? A systematic review and meta-analysis of human experimental and clinical studies. *Pain* 2010;151:61–8.

18. Craft RM. Sex differences in opioid analgesia: "from mouse to man." *Clin J Pain* 2003;19:175–86.

19. Craft RM. Sex differences in analgesic, reinforcing, discriminative and motoric effects of opioids. *Exp Clin Psychopharmacol* 2008;16:376–85.

20. Fillingim RB, Gear RW. Sex differences in opioid analgesia: clinical and experimental findings. *Eur J Pain* 2004;8:413–25.

21. Dahan A, Kest B, Waxman A, Sarton E. Sex-specific responses to opiates: animal and human studies. *Anesth Analg* 2008;107:83–95.

22. Bodnar RJ, Kest B. Sex differences in opioid analgesia, hyperalgesia, tolerance and withdrawal: central mechanisms of action and roles of gonadal hormones. *Horm Behav* 2010;58:72–81.

23. Rasakham K, Liu-Chen L-Y. Sex differences in kappa opioid pharmacology. *Life Sci* 2011;88: 2–16.

24. Craft RM, Stratmann JA, Bartok RE, Walpole TI, King SJ. Sex differences in development of morphine tolerance and dependence in the rat. *Psychopharmacology* 1999;143:1–7.

25. Mousavi Z, Shafaghi B, Kobarfard F, Jorjani M. Sex differences and role of gonadal hormones on glutamate level in the nucleus accumbens in morphine tolerant rats: a microdialysis study. *Eur J Pharmacol* 2007;554:145–9.

26. Loyd DR, Morgan MM, Murphy AZ. Sexually dimorphic activation of the periaqueductal gray—rostral ventromedial medullary circuit during the development of tolerance to morphine in the rat. *Eur J Neurosci* 2008;27:1517–24.

27. Martin TJ, Kim SA, Buechler NL, Porreca F, Eisenach JC. Opioid self-administration in the nerve-injured rat. *Anesthesiology* 2007; 106:312–22.

28. Cicero TJ, Nock B, O'Connor L, Meyer ER. Role of steroids in sex differences in morphine-induced analgesia: activational and organizational effects. *J Pharmacol Exp Ther* 2002;300:695–701.

29. Krzanowska EK, Ogawa S, Pfaff DW, Bodnar RJ. Reversal of sex differences in morphine analgesia elicited from the ventrolateral periaqueductal gray in rats by neonatal hormone manipulations. *Brain Res* 2002;929:1–9.

30. Borzan J, Fuchs PN. Organizational and activational effects of testosterone on carageenan-induced inflammatory pain and morphine analgesia. *Neuroscience* 2006;143:885–93.

31. Craft RM, Ulibarri C. Sexual differentiation of rat reproductive vs. opioid antinociceptive systems. *Gender Med* 2009;6:209–24.

32. Stoffel EC, Ulibarri CM, Craft RM. Gonadal steroid hormone modulation of nociception, morphine antinociception and reproductive indices in male and female rats. *Pain* 2003;103: 285–302.

33. Terner JM, Lomas LM, Picker MJ. Influence of estrous cycle and gonadal hormone depletion on nociception and opioid antinociception in female rats of four strains. *J Pain* 2005;6:372–83.

34. Sandner A, Eisenach JC. Estrogen reduces efficacy of μ- but not κ-opioid agonist inhibition in response to uterine cervical distension. *Anesthesiology* 2002;96:375–80.

35. Ji Y, Murphy AZ, Traub RJ. Estrogen modulation of morphine analgesia of visceral pain in female rats is supraspinally and peripherally mediated. *J Pain* 2007;8:494–502.

36. Craft RM, Ulibarri C, Leitl MD, Sumner JE. Dose- and time-dependent estradiol modulation of morphine antinociception in adult female rats. *Eur J Pain* 2008;12:472–9.

37. Lawson KP, Nag S, Thompson AD, Mokha SS. Sex-specificity and estrogen-dependence of kappa opioid receptor-mediated antinociception and antihyperalgesia. *Pain* 2010;151:806–15.

38. Clemente JT, Parada CA, Veiga MCA, Gear RW, Tambeli CH. Sexual dimorphism in the antinociceptio mediated by kappa opioid receptors in the rat temporomandibular joint. *Neurosci Lett* 2004;372:250–5.

39. Negus SS, Mello NK. Opioid antinociception in ovariectomized monkeys: Comparison with antinociception in males and effects of estradiol replacement. *J Pharmacol Exp Ther* 1999;290:1132–40.

40. Negus SS, Mello NK. Effects of gonadal steroid hormone treatments on opioid

antinociception in ovariectomized rhesus monkeys. *Psychopharmacology* 2002;159:275–83.

41. Stoffel EC, Ulibarri CM, Folk JE, Rice KC, Craft RM. Gonadal hormone modulation of mu, kappa, and delta opioid antinociception in male and female rats. *J Pain* 2005;6:261–74.

42. Jayaram A, Carp H. Progesterone-mediated potentiation of spinal sufentanil in rats. *Obstet Anesth* 1993;76:745–50.

43. Sternberg WF, Chesler EJ, Wilson SG, Mogil JS. Acute progesterone can recruit sex-specific neurochemical mechanisms mediating swim stress-induced and kappa-opioid analgesia in mice. *Horm Behav* 2004;46:467–73.

44. Ribeiro-Dasilva MC, Shinal RM, Glover T, et al. Evaluation of menstrual cycle effects on morphine and pentazocine analgesia. *Pain* 2011;152:614–22.

45. Smith YR, Stohler CS, Nichols TE, Bueller JA, Koeppe RA, Zubieta J-K. Pronociceptive and antinociceptive effects of estradiol through endogenous opioid neurotransmission in women. *J Neurosci* 2006;26:5777–85.

46. Holdcroft A, Maze M, Doré C, Tebbs S, Thompson S. A multicenter dose-escalation study of the analgesic and adverse effects of an oral cannabis extract (Cannador) for postoperative pain management. *Anesthesiology* 2006;104:1040–6.

47. Karst M, Salim K, Burstein S, Conrad I, Hoy L, Schneider U. Analgesic effects of the synthetic cannabinoid CT-3 on chronic neuropathic pain. *JAMA* 2003;290:1757–62.

48. Nurmikko TJ, Serpell MG, Hoggart B, Toomey PJ, Morlion BJ, Haines D. Sativex successfully treats neuropathic pain characterized by allodynia: a randomized, double-blind, placebo-controlled clinical trial. *Pain* 2007;133:210–20.

49. Ellis RJ, Toperoff W, Vaida F, et al. Smoked medicinal cannabis for neuropathic pain in HIV: a randomized, crossover clinical trial. *Neuropsychopharmacology* 2009;34:672–80.

50. Wallace M, Schulteis G, Atkinson JH, et al. Dose-dependent effects of smoked cannabis on capsaicin-induced pain and hyperalgesia in healthy volunteers. *Anesthesiology* 2007;107:785–96.

51. Greenwald MK, Stitzer ML. Antinociceptive, subjective and behavioral effects of smoked marijuana in humans. *Drug Alc Depend* 2000;59:261–75.

52. Naef M, Curaotolo M, Petersen-Felix S, Arendt-Nielsen L, Zbinden A, Brenneisen R. The analgesic effects of oral delta-9-tetrahydrocannabinol (THC), morphine and a THC-morphine combination in healthy subjects

under experimental pain conditions. *Pain* 2003;105:79–88.

53. Tseng AH, Craft RM. Sex differences in antinociceptive and motoric effects of cannabinoids. *Eur J Pharmacol* 2001;430:41–7.

54. Romero EM, Fernandez B, Sagredo O, et al. Antinociceptive, behavioural and neuroendocrine effects of CP55,940 in young rats. *Devel Brain Res* 2002;136:85–92.

55. Wiley JL, O'Connell MM, Tokarz ME, Wright MJ. Pharmacological effects of acute and repeated administration of Δ^9-tetrahydrocannabinol in adolescent and adult rats. *J Pharmacol Exp Ther* 2007;320:1097–05.

56. Wiley JL, Evans RL. To breed or not to breed? Empirical evaluation of drug effects in adolescent rats. *Int J Dev Neurosci* 2009;27:9–20.

57. Craft RM, Leitl MD. Gonadal hormone modulation of the behavioral effects of Δ^9-tetrahydrocannabinol in male and female rats. *Eur J Pharmacol* 2008;578:37–42.

58. Wakley AA, Craft RM. Antinociception and sedation following intracerebroventricular administration of Δ^9-tetrahydrocannabinol in female vs. male rats. *Behav Brain Res* 2011;216:200–6.

59. Kalbasi Anaraki D, Sianati S, Sadeghi M, et al. Modulation by female sex hormones of the cannabinoid-induced catalepsy and analgesia in ovariectomized mice. *Eur J Pharmacol* 2008;586:189–96.

60. Hunter KA, Barr GA, Shivers K-Y, et al. Interactions of estradiol and NSAIDS on carrageenan-induced hyperalgesia. *Brain Res* 2011;1382:181–8.

61. Cormack JR, Orme RM, Costello TG. The role of α2-agonists in neurosurgery. *J Clin Neurosci* 2005;12:375–8.

62. Chan AK, Cheung CW, Chong YK. Alpha-2 agonists in acute pain management. *Expert Opin Pharmacother* 2010;11:2849–68.

63. Kiefel JM, Bodnar RJ. Roles of gender and gonadectomy in pilocarpine and clonidine analgesia in rats. *Pharmacol Biochem Behav* 1992;41:153–8.

64. Mitrovic I, Margeta-Mitrovic M, Bader S, Stoffel M, Jan LY, Basbaum AI. Contribution of GIRK2-mediated postsynaptic signaling to opiate and α_2-adrenergic analgesia and analgesic sex differences. *Proc Natl Acad Sci USA* 2003;100:271–6.

65. Nag S, Mokha SS. Activation of alpha$_2$-adrenoceptors in the trigeminal region produces sex-specific modulation of nociception in the rat. *Neuroscience* 2006;142:1255–62.

66. Thompson AD, Angelotti T, Nag S, Mokha SS. Sex-specific modulation of spinal nociception

by α_2-adrenoceptors: differential regulation by estrogen and testosterone. *Neuroscience* 2008;153:1268–77.

67. Nag S, Mokha SS. Testosterone is essential for α_2-adrenoceptor-induced antinociception in the trigeminal region of the male rat. *Neurosci Lett* 2009;467:48–52.

68. King D, Etzel JP, Chopra S, et al. Human response to α2-adrenergic agonist stimulation studied in an isolated vascular bed in vivo: biphasic influence of dose, age, gender, and receptor genotype. *Clin Pharmacol Ther* 2005;77:388–403.

69. Meibohm B, Beierle I, Derendorf H. How important are gender differences in pharmacokinetics? *Clin Pharmacokinet* 2002;41:329–42.

70. Anakk S, Ku CY, Vore M, Strobel HW. Insights in gender bias: rat cytochrome P450 3A9. *J Pharmacol Exp Ther* 2003;305:703–9.

71. Morris ME, Lee H-J, Predko LM. Gender differences in the membrane transport of endogenous and exogenous compounds. i 2003;55:229–40.

72. Gandhi M, Aweeka F, Greenblatt RM, Blaschke TF. Sex differences in pharmacokinetics and pharmacodynamics. *Annu Rev Pharmacol Toxicol* 2004;44:499–523.

73. Zhang H, Cui, D, Wang B, et al. Pharmacokinetic drug interactions involving 17α-ethinylestradiol. *Clin Pharmacokinet* 2007;46:133–57.

74. Chang S-Y, Chen C, Yang Z, Rodrigues D. Further assessment of 17α-ethinyl estradiol as an inhibitor of different human cytochrome P450 forms in vitro. *Drug Metab Dispos* 2009;37:1667–75.

75. Monostory K, Pascussi J-M, Kobori L, Dvorak Z. Hormonal regulation of CYP1A expression. *Drug Metab Rev* 2009;41:547–72.

76. Sarton E, Olofsen E, Romberg R, et al. Sex differences in morphine analgesia. *Anesthesiology* 2000;93:1245–54.

77. Craft RM, Kalivas PW, Stratmann JA. Sex differences in discriminative stimulus effects of morphine in the rat. *Behav Pharmacol* 1996;7:764–78.

78. Cicero TJ, Nock B, Meyer ER. Sex-related differences in morphine's antinociceptive activity: relationship to serum and brain morphine concentrations. *J Pharmacol Exp Ther* 1997;282:939–44.

79. Baker L, Ratka A. Sex-specific differences in levels of morphine, morphine-3-glucuronide, and morphine antinociception in rats. *Pain* 2002;95:65–74.

80. Candido J, Lutfy K, Billings B, et al. Effect of adrenal and sex hormones on opioid analgesia and opioid receptor regulation. *Pharmacol Biochem Behav* 1992;42:685–92.

81. Kepler KL, Kest B, Kiefel JM, Cooper ML, Bodnar RJ. Roles of gender, gonadectomy and estrous phase in the analgesic effects of intracerebroventricular morphine in rats. *Pharmacol Biochem Behav* 1989;34:119–27.

82. Boyer JS, Morgan MM, Craft RM. Microinjection of morphine into the rostral ventromedial medulla produces greater antinociception in male compared to female rats. *Brain Res* 1998;796:315–8.

83. Kest B, Wilson SG, Mogil JS. Sex differences in supraspinal morphine analgesia are dependent on genotype. *J Pharmacol Exp Ther* 1999;289:1370–75.

84. Tershner SA, Mitchell JM, Fields HL. Brainstem pain modulating circuitry is sexually dimorphic with respect to mu and kappa opioid receptor function. *Pain* 2000;85:153–9.

85. Loyd DR, Wang X, Murphy AZ. Sex differences in μ-opioid receptor expression in the rat midbrain periaqueductal gray are essential for eliciting sex differences in morphine analgesia. *J Neurosci* 2008;28:14007–17.

86. Bobeck EN, McNeal AL, Morgan MM. Drug dependent sex-differences in periaqueductal gray mediated antinociception in the rat. *Pain* 2009;147:210–6.

87. Nadulski T, Pragst F, Weinberg G, et al. Randomized, double-blind, placebo-controlled study about the effects of cannabidiol (CBD) on the pharmacokinetics of Δ^9-tetrahydrocannabinol (THC) after oral application of THC verses standardized cannabis extract. *Ther Drug Monit* 2005;27:799–810.

88. Tseng AH, Harding JW, Craft RM. Pharmacokinetic factors in sex differences in Δ^9-tetrahydrocannabinol-induced behavioral effects in rats. *Behav Brain Res* 2004;154(1):77–83.

89. Narimatsu S, Watanabe K, Yamamoto I, Yoshimura H. Sex differences in the oxidative metabolism of Δ^9-tetrahydrocannabinol in the rat. *Biochem Pharmacol* 1991;41:1187–94.

90. Funahashi T, Tanaka Y, Yamaori S, et al. Stimulatory effects of testosterone and progesterone on the NADH- and NADPH-dependent oxidation of 7β-hydroxy-Δ^8-tetrahydrocannabinol to 7-oxo-Δ^8-tetrahydrocannabinol in monkey liver microsomes. *Drug Metab Pharmakinet* 2005;20:358–67.

91. Trnavská Z, Trnavsky K. Sex differences in the pharmacokinetics of salicylates. *Eur J Clin Pharmacol* 198325:679–82.

92. Chiang N, Hurwitz S, Ridker PM, Serhan CN. Aspirin has a gender-dependent impact on anti-inflammatory 15-epi-lipoxin A_4 formation. *Arterioscler Thromb Vasc Biol* 2006;26:e14–7.

93. Loyd DR, Murphy AZ. The role of the peri-aqueductal gray in the modulation of pain in males and females: are the anatomy and physiology really that different? *Neural Plast* 2009;2009:462879. Epub.

94. Craft RM, Morgan MM, Lane DA. Oestradiol dampens reflex-related activity of on- and off-cells in the rostral ventromedial medulla of female rats. *Neuroscience* 2004;125:1061–8.

95. Bernal SA, Morgan MM, Craft RM. PAG mu opioid receptor activation underlies sex differences in morphine antinociception. *Behav Brain Res* 2007;177:126–33.

96. Kelly MJ, Lagrange AH, Wagner EJ, Rønnekleiv OK. Rapid effects of estrogen to modulate G protein-coupled receptors via activation of protein kinase A and protein kinase C pathways. *Steroids* 1999;64:64–75.

97. Micevych PE, Rissman EF, Gustafsson JA, Sinchak K. Estrogen receptor-alpha is required for estrogen-induced mu-opioid receptor internalization. *J Neurosci Res* 2003;71:802–10.

98. Ji Y, Murphy AZ, Traub RJ. Sex differences in morphine-induced analgesia of visceral pain are supraspinally and peripherally mediated. *Am J Physiol Regul Integr Comp Physiol* 2006;29:R307–14.

99. Liu N-J, von Gizycki H, Gintzler AR. Sexually dimorphic recruitment of spinal opioid analgesic pathways by the spinal application of morphine. *J Pharmacol Exp Ther* 2007;322:654–60.

100. Cook CD, Nickerson MD. Nociceptive sensitivity and opioid antinociception and antihyperalgesia in Freund's adjuvant-induced arthritic male and female rats. *J Pharmacol Exp Ther* 2005;313:449–59.

101. Chakrabarti S, Liu N-J, Gintzler AR. Formation of μ-/κ-opioid receptor heterodimer is sex-dependent and mediates female-specific opioid analgesia. *Proc Natl Acad Sci USA* 2010;107:20115–9.

102. Bonnin A, Fernandez-Ruiz JJ, Martin M, Rodriguez de Fonseca R, Hernandez ML, Ramos JA. Delta-9-tetrahydrocannabinol affects mesolimbic dopaminergic activity in the female rat brain: interactions with estrogens. *J Neural Transm [GenSect]* 1993;92:81–95.

103. Rodriguez de Fonseca F, Cebeira M, Ramos JA, Martin M, Fernandez-Ruiz JJ. Cannabinoid receptors in rat brain areas: sexual differences fluctuations during estrous cycle and changes after gonadectomy and sex steroid replacement. *Life Sci* 1994;54:159–70.

104. Gonzalez S, Bisogno T, Wenger T, et al. Sex steroid influence on cannabinoid CB1 receptor mRNA and endocannabinoid levels in the anterior pituitary gland. *Biochem Biophys Res Comm* 2000;270:260–6.

105. Riebe CJ, Hill MN, Lee TT, Hillard CJ, Gorzalka BB. Estrogenic regulation of limbic cannabinoid receptor binding. *Psychoneuroendocrinology* 2010;35:1265–9.

106. Bradshaw HB, Rimmerman N, Krey JF, Walker JM. Sex and hormonal cycle differences in rat brain levels of pain-related cannabimimetic lipid mediators. *Am J Physiol Regul Integr Comp Physiol* 2006;291:R349–58.

107. Onaivi ES, Chaudhuri G, Abaci AS, et al. Expression of cannabinoid receptors and their gene transcripts in human blood cells. *Prog Neuropsychopharmacol Biol Psychiatry* 1999;23:1063–77.

108. Lüscher C, Slesinger PA. Emerging roles for G protein-gated inwardly rectifying potassium (GIRK) channels in health and disease. *Nat Rev Neurosci* 2010;11:301–15.

109. Blednov YA, Stoffel M, Alva H, Harris RA. A pervasive mechanism for analgesia: activation of GIRK2 channels. *Proc Natl Acad Sci USA* 2003;100:277–82.

110. Ahangar N, Kazemi B, Jorjani M. Effects of gonadal steroid hormones on $GIRK_2$ gene transcription in the rat central nervous system. *Neurosci Lett* 2008;431:201–5.

111. Krzanowska EK, Bodnar RJ. Morphine antinociception elicited from the ventrolateral periaqueductal gray is sensitive to sex and gonadectomy differences in rats. *Brain Res* 1999;821:224–30.

7

ROLE OF PSYCHOSOCIAL FACTORS AND PSYCHOLOGICAL INTERVENTIONS

Edmund Keogh

INTRODUCTION

Pain involves more than just sensory processes; it includes emotional, cognitive, and social factors. Furthermore, the treatment of pain, especially in its chronic state, is often delivered with reference to how a person thinks, feels, and behaves, as well as the environment (e.g., family) in which one finds oneself. Consideration of the psychosocial factors that influence the perception and experience of pain and pain-related behaviors is, therefore, very relevant to those interested in differences between men and women. This chapter will provide an overview of the role that psychosocial factors have in understanding why there may be sex differences (and similarities) in pain, and it will consider whether there are differences in how men and women respond to psychological interventions for pain. The chapter will highlight current gaps in our knowledge base, as well as consider possible directions for future research.

COGNITIVE FACTORS (THOUGHTS, BELIEFS, AND EXPECTATIONS)

Cognition refers to a wide range of processes, encompassing the type of thoughts we have and the style of thought processing, through to careful consideration of the cognitive architecture involved (e.g., attention, memory). When considering sex differences in pain, research has tended to focus on two thought processes: pain-related catastrophizing and gender-role expectations.

Catastrophizing

Catastrophizing is a cognitive style associated with excessive rumination and worry about pain, as well as exaggeration of the negative consequences of painful events.[1] It is related to increased pain and disability, and it is an important predictor of outcome. It also seems as if females are more likely to engage in pain-related catastrophizing, in both healthy and patient groups.[1-4] For example, Keefe et al.[2] found that within a group of adult chronic pain patients, females reported higher levels of pain-related catastrophizing than males. Similarly, Keogh and Eccleston[3] report a study on adolescents attending a chronic pain clinic, and they found that females report more catastrophic thoughts than males. While some studies fail to find such group differences,[5,6] the general pattern suggests a fairly reliable difference between the sexes.

This negative style of thinking may also help explain some of the differences in male and female pain experiences.[2,3,7-11] For example,

Sullivan et al.[11] examined whether levels of catastrophizing affect responses to a cold pressor task. They not only found sex differences in experimental pain but that levels of catastrophizing mediated this relationship. In other words, the reason why females reported higher levels of experimental pain seemed to be due to their higher tendency to engage in catastrophic thinking. Mediation effects have been reported in chronic pain as well. For example, Keefe et al.[2] also found that sex differences in pain were mediated by pain-related catastrophizing in a group of chronic pain patients with osteoarthritis. A similar pattern has been found in children, with suggestions that catastrophizing might explain why there are sex differences in intervention responses.[3,8] Together, these studies certainly suggest that pain-related catastrophizing is an important cognitive variable, which may help explain why there are sex differences in pain.

Gender-Role Expectations

Social factors play an important role in shaping our behaviors, which includes belief systems about femininity and masculinity. Such gender-related beliefs about pain are thought to partly explain the differences between men and women.[12] Research has focused on understanding the nature of these beliefs, as well as establishing what influence they may have on pain experiences.[5,13–19] For example, Robinson et al.[17] found that both men and women view males as being less willing to report pain, whereas females are viewed as more sensitive. In a second study, Robinson et al.[15] found that the worst conceivable pain for men relates to injury, whereas for women it is childbirth or menstrual pain. Gender-role beliefs also exist for pain-related behaviors. Keogh and Denford[5] found that the typical woman is viewed as being more likely to engage in catastrophizing, distraction, and praying as coping strategies, whereas the typical man is viewed as being more likely to ignore pain sensations.

These studies confirm that we hold certain beliefs and expectations about pain, which depend on the perceived gender of the person. Importantly, such gender-role beliefs may also help explain why there are sex differences in pain and pain behavior. For example, gender-role beliefs have been found to explain differences in experimental pain responses between men and women.[20–22] Using a thermal heat stimulus to induce pain, Wise et al.[21] found that sex differences in pain responses were explained by gender-role beliefs. A similar finding was reported by Robinson et al.[20] using a temporal summation methodology. However, other studies have reported that sex differences remained significant even after controlling for gender roles.[22,23] Interestingly, the possible influence of gender expectations extends to how we perceive pain in others.[18,20] In one study, using video clips of people engaging in a cold pressor pain task, Robinson and Wise[18] found that observers rated the video clips of males as having less pain than the female clips. They also found that female observers reported greater pain in the clips than male observers, and that these observer sex differences were explained by their gender-role expectations. Thus, not only do gender beliefs influence how people behave when in pain but such expectations also influence how we view others. This suggests that social-cognitive factors play a role in shaping how we think about pain, as well as partly explain why men and women differ in their pain experiences.

Positive Thinking

Alongside catastrophizing and gender-role beliefs, there are a wide range of other cognitive factors that may be potentially important within the context of sex differences in pain. However, these alternatives have not yet been explored in sufficient detail to be able to draw any definite conclusions, but nevertheless they hint toward areas for future investigation. For example, there have been developments within the field of positive cognitions and beliefs, including constructs such as self-efficacy, resilience, and optimism.[24] Self-efficacy relates to the beliefs one has in being able to achieve goals, and it has been shown in at least one study that it might help explain sex differences in pain.[25,26] Psychological resilience refers to a more general ability to maintain psychological well-being despite aversive life events. Again there are only a few studies that have examined for sex differences, but there are suggestions that women may benefit more from positive thinking in the context of pain.[27–29] For example, Keogh et al.[29] found that an acceptance approach to coping resulted in less pain in women compared to men, whereas Ong et al.[27] found that positive thinking was more of a benefit to women in terms of pain-related catastrophizing. Given the general emergence of positive psychology as a distinct and established area of research, it is likely that we will see further examples where these constructs are applied to pain. This, in turn, may reveal cognitive styles of thinking that may selectively serve as protective factors for men and women.

SEX DIFFERENCES IN PAIN-RELATED EMOTIONS AND EMOTIONAL RESPONSES

Given the importance that emotional factors have in the perception and experience of pain, some have considered whether they help explain sex differences. The main emotions to be considered are anxiety and depression, which is unsurprising given the general focus on these emotions in mainstream psychology, as well as the fact that women generally report higher levels of both emotions when compared to men.[30,31]

Anxiety

Some have found evidence that women report higher levels of pain-related anxiety than men.[32–35] However, this difference is not consistently found.[36,37] For example, when Edwards et al.[36] examined 215 patients referred for multidisciplinary pain treatment, no significant differences were found between men and women on a pain anxiety measure. One reason for this discrepancy could be due to variability between studies (e.g., acute vs. chronic conditions), as well as issues associated with how anxiety constructs are measured.[38] However, there are also inconsistencies within studies.[33,39,40] For example, McCracken and Keogh[33] did not find sex differences in anxiety sensitivity within a sample of chronic pain patients, but they did find a sex difference in pain-related anxiety.

In a study of 83 children with acute postsurgical pain, Pagé et al.[39] found that sex differences in general anxiety and anxiety sensitivity, but not for pain-related anxiety or depression.

There have also been attempts to consider whether the relationship between anxiety and pain is similar in men and women.[36,37,41–45] Edwards et al.[36] found that within chronic pain patients, males who were high in anxiety reported higher pain severity and interference than those low in anxiety; this was not found within females. These investigators later reported that pre-treatment anxiety was a significant predictor of responses to pain treatment for males but not females.[44] Similarly, in a large sample of 1,709 individuals with whiplash, Elklit and Jones[41] found a stronger relationship between anxiety and disability in men than women. A similar relationship has also been found in healthy groups, within an experimental pain-induction study using capsaicin.[45] Therefore, it seems that men show a stronger relationship between anxiety and pain-related outcomes, that is, anxiety seems to have more of an effect on men than women.

While it is tempting to draw such conclusions, there are examples where this relationship has not been found,[46,47] as well as examples where the opposite pattern is reported. Anxiety sensitivity, which is related to the fear of bodily sensations, is one such case, in that it seems to show a stronger relationship with pain in women.[48,49] For example, Keogh and Birkby[48] found that healthy females who are high in anxiety sensitivity tend to report more experimental pain than low-anxiety counterparts. Similarly, in some acute pain settings, anxiety sensitivity is more strongly related to the pain reports of female patients than males.[49] However, even here there are inconsistencies,[33,50] and the number of studies conducted are few in number.

Depression

A second emotion considered in the context of sex differences in pain is depression. Evidence suggests a higher comorbidity between pain and depression in women,[51,52] and some studies with chronic pain patients find females report more depression than men.[8,36,53] For example, Keogh et al.[8] found that females (mean = 17) had higher Beck Depression Inventory (BDI) scores than males (mean = 13). However, others have reported mixed findings or failed to find sex differences.[46,54–58] Interestingly, in a comprehensive investigation of 481 patients with chronic pain who completed the BDI-2 scale, Harris and D'Eon[58] only found a few sex differences on the items. Furthermore, they failed to find sex differences in the factor structure or item loadings, or in the subscale and total scores. Together, this suggests that there are mixed findings when it comes to sex differences in depression within the context of pain.

Like anxiety, some studies have directly examined for sex differences in the relationship between depression and pain. In contrast to anxiety, some studies suggest that depression may be more strongly related to pain in women when compared to men.[46,53,55,57] For example, Keogh et al.[46] found that depression was more strongly related to pain-related disability in women. In a second study, Hirsch et al.[59] found that negative mood mediates the relationship between pain and disability in women. However, there are also inconsistencies.[54,60] For example, Edwards et al.[36] failed to find any interaction between gender and depression on pain severity, interference, or general activity, and Wasan et al.[54] found a stronger relationship between self-reported depression and pain in men compared to women.

Thus, it seems unclear whether there are sex differences in the relationship between depression and pain. When they are found, it seems as if depression may be more strongly related to pain in women. This confusion is not helped by the fact that there are only a few published studies to draw on. Once this position changes, we should have a better idea as to the extent to which role emotions such as depression play in understanding why there are sex differences in pain.

BEHAVIORAL FACTORS

Pain behaviors usually refer to a range of different activities that men and women engage in when they are in pain. This section will consider whether there are sex differences in health and pain-seeking behaviors, as well as differences in the use of pain coping strategies.

Pain-Related Coping Behaviors

Pain-related coping refers to strategies people engage in when trying to deal with pain. One approach has been to examine what health care support people seek out when they are in pain. Studies into health-seeking behavior and health care utilization suggest that there are sex differences, with women being more likely to seek support when compared to men.[61,62] Women are also more likely to make use of pain services, and they are more actively involved in using both over-the-counter and prescription analgesics.[63–66] Biases in health-seeking behaviors are not limited to obtaining services from health professionals, in that there also seem to be sex differences in the general use of social support systems. Indeed, in both adult and adolescent samples, females have been found to report a greater likelihood of using social support systems compared to males.[3,6,67,68] Reasons why these differences in health-seeking behavior exist are multifaceted, and they may reflect the fact that women are less likely to avoid health problems and are socialized to engage in health care systems more than men.[12]

Pain-related coping incorporates a wide range of different strategies, not just support seeking. A review by Unruh[6] suggested that there may be sex differences in the range of pain coping strategies, with women engaging in a wider range of strategies than men. Specific usage has also been examined.[68–70] For example, in a community-based survey of 309 people, Unruh et al.[68] found that as well as using more social support, women also reported a greater use of problem solving, positive self-statements, and palliative behaviors than men. Grossi et al.[70] report a study on 446 patients with chronic musculoskeletal pain and found females scored higher on catastrophizing, diverting attention, praying/hoping, behavioral activity, and pain behaviors, but no differences on ability to control pain, ignoring, or reinterpreting sensations scales. Interestingly, when they controlled for other group differences (e.g., work, distress, pain), most of these sex differences in coping were no longer significant; the exception was a complex interaction between gender and post-traumatic responses on catastrophizing. Two studies on children suggest that as well as girls reporting using a greater use of social support, boys more frequently engage in distraction-type strategies for pain.[3,67]

Thus, it seems that females may be more likely to engage in a wider range of health-seeking behaviors, especially those that involve seeking help from others. There are inconsistencies, however,[5,36,60,71] and even if there are differences in the pain coping strategies used, this does not necessarily mean that they are equally effective, and they may to some extent depend on context.[72]

Nonverbal Pain Behaviors

When a person is in pain, he or she exhibits a range of behaviors that function to inform others that he or she is in pain and requires help. These cues are often nonverbal and include facial expressions, vocalizations, and posture/movements. Being able to effectively recognize pain is extremely important in order to ensure it is correctly managed, and it highlights the fact that pain behaviors are not only expressed (or encoded) by an individual but need to be detected or recognized (decoded) by an observer. Given that there are known sex differences in both emotional expression and nonverbal communication,[73] this has led some to consider whether there are sex differences in the encoding and decoding of pain cues in nonverbal domains.

Within the domain of facial expressions, some have found encoding differences in the cues used to express pain.[74,75] For example, Prkachin and Solomon[75] examined nonverbal facial expresions to a range of motion exercise in a group of adults with chronic shoulder pain. They found that men showed more pain than women. However, there generally seem to be more studies that fail to find significant differences in facial expression cues of pain than actually find them.[76–78] In terms of the recognition or decoding on facial expressions of pain, there seems to be more consistent evidence for possible sex differences.[77,79–81] For example, Hill and Craig[80] found that females were more accurate in recognizing pain cues, whereas Prkachin et al.[81] found that females were more sensitive to facial displays of pain than males. Together this would suggest that there may not

be differences in the facial encoding of pain, but that there may be sex differences in the decoding of pain-related facial expressions.

While studies have considered facial expressions of pain, this has not been extensively examined within vocal or body expression domains. Indeed, there are limited examples of sex differences in the encoding and decoding of vocal and body-related cues within pain, and so few conclusions can really be made at present. However, this is an emerging area that highlights that pain behaviors are interpreted by observers, and that sex-related factors may be important.

EFFECT OF SOCIAL CONTEXT AND INTERPERSONAL INTERACTIONS

The previous section highlights that pain does not occur in isolation, and in fact it is very much seen as a social behavior that is shared between individuals.[12,82] The potential for pain and pain behaviors to be influenced by the social interactions between males and females has also been directly considered. Given that pain behaviors are thought to be influenced and shaped by the wider context in which people find themselves, this section will consider how social-contextual factors impact on pain and pain-related behaviors in men and women.

Effect of Gender Context on Pain Reports

Some have considered the way the sex of an observer may impact on the pain responses of a participant. These usually take the form of laboratory-based experimental pain studies in which both the experimenter's sex and the participant's sex are considered.[83,84] In a now classic study, Levine and Desimone[84] conducted a cold pressor study and found that when the experimenter was female, males reported less pain than when the experimenter was male. Another approach has been to consider interactions between patient and family members.[85,86] For example, some studies have examined parental responses and how these may affect how a child responds to pain. In adult studies, investigations have focused on the patient and his or her spouse, looking for ways in which pain behaviors may be reinforced.[87,88] For example, Smith et al.[88] asked chronic pain patients to engage in a set of everyday tasks. Importantly, the behaviors of the patients' spouse were also examined to see whether the sex of the spouse was important. Here they found that husbands were less likely to engage in facilitative behaviors compared to wives. These studies suggest that pain does not occur in a vacuum but can be influenced by the presence of others, which in turn may depend on the sex of those involved.

Effect of Gender Context on Health Carer Behavior

The gender context has also been considered in terms of those observing and treating people in pain. Indeed, there is evidence to suggest that the type of pain medication received by patients may be linked to whether they are male or female.[89-90] For example, Michael et al.[91] report a study on the pre-hospital emergency treatment received by individuals with an injury, and they found that females were less likely to receive analgesia than males. In another study, Lord et al.[90] found that when analgesia was administered, women were less likely to receive morphine than men. Similar biases have been reported within hospital settings.[92-95] While it may seem as though gender-related biases exist in the administration of pain medication, a recent review by LeResche[96] concluded that such biases have been inconsistently reported in clinical studies. For example, studies often fail to consider the dose of analgesics administered, sex differences in weight, and/or adequately assess levels of pain. This unfortunately limits the conclusions we can draw at present.

The possibility that such treatment biases are due to how observers interpret a person's pain have, however, been explored in experimental studies.[79,97-101] Using pain vignettes, Bernardes and Lima[98] found that when the character was female, pain was viewed as less severe and credible than if the character was male. In a series of studies making use of virtual patients,[79,99,100] varying the sex of the patients led to differences in the estimates of pain and treatment needs made by observers. For example, Hirsch et al.[79] found that when the virtual patients was female, observers rated them as being in greater pain, less able to cope, and in greater need of medical help. These studies suggest that a health carer's interpretation of patients' pain behaviors may to some extent depend on whether the patient is male or female.

SEX DIFFERENCES IN PSYCHOLOGICAL INTERVENTIONS AND TREATMENTS

This chapter has demonstrated that there is good evidence that psychosocial factors play an important role in understanding why there are sex differences in pain, with a suggestion that there may be treatment-related effects. Given that pain interventions, especially those focused on chronic pain management, take a multidisciplinary approach, it is possible that there are important sex-related differences in treatment responses. This section will consider the evidence that there are sex differences in interventions and treatments for pain that involve a psychological component.

Sex Differences in Pain Intervention Responses

One way to determine whether there are sex differences in treatment responses has been to manipulate the coping instructions given to participants to see whether this has an effect on pain outcomes. Most of these studies employ experimental pain induction paradigms, where it is relatively easy to vary coping instructions given to healthy participants.[3,5,29,50,68,102-104] A number of these studies have compared simple distraction-type instructions with those that involve some form of focus on the pain. For example, using the cold pressor task, Keogh et al.[103] found that men seem to benefit from focusing on the sensory component of pain, whereas women did not. Women have also been found to find emotion-based coping less useful[104] and perhaps benefit more from acceptance-based coping strategies.[102] Of course, these are experimental studies in healthy groups, and so far there have been few examples where different coping strategies are compared within chronic pain samples in terms of whether they are associated with sex-specific differences in chronic pain outcome.

A second method can be seen in studies that examine the effects of expectation, including the role of placebo analgesia.[105-109] Some have found that placebo effects may be stronger in males than females. For example, Aslaksen et al.[105] report a study in which males showed greater placebo analgesia (pain unpleasantness report) to thermal heat when compared to females. Also, there is also at least one study that suggests that there may be sex differences in nocebo effects as well.[106] However, it should be noted that there are only a few examples, which limits any definite conclusion. Even so, given that there may be sex differences in analgesic efficacy[110] (also see Chapter 4, this volume), this would seem a useful line of research for the future.

Sex Differences in Nonpharmacological Treatment Responses

A few studies have examined for possible sex differences in responses to nonpharmacological interventions for chronic pain. Most have looked at treatment responses to some form of multimodal intervention in adult chronic pain sufferers.[8,111-117] Some have found that females benefit more from these treatment interventions than males.[113,115] For example, Jensen et al.[115] report a study on patients with chronic spinal pain in which treatment-outcome responses to physical therapy, cognitive-behavioral therapy, and a combination were compared to a waiting list control. Improvements in quality of life outcomes at 18 months post treatment were related to the cognitive-behavioral conditions, but only in females. Similarly, Hampel et al.[113] found that females showed better mental health outcomes compared to males, following treatment (although this difference was not found for other outcomes).

Others report contradictory findings, suggesting that males may show better responses to treatment.[8,116] For example, McGeary et al.[116] reported a large study on 1,827 patients with a chronic spinal condition who entered a multimodal treatment program and were followed up after 1 year. In this study men seemed to show better outcomes on a range of measures, including disability and depression. However, some have reported fairly limited or no between-sex

differences following treatment,[114,117] whereas others find mixed results that depend on the outcome measures being considered.[112] For example, Edwards et al.[112] found that a multidisciplinary treatment program resulted in lower pain severity in men, and lower pain interference and greater activity levels in women. Two studies have shown that cognitive-emotional factors may play a role in some of these sex differences.[8,111] For example, Burns et al.[111] found that anger expressions may moderate sex differences in treatment outcomes, whereas Keogh et al.[8] implicated pain-related catastrophizing as a mediator in explaining treatment differences between males and females.

Although most of these treatment outcome studies have examined responses within adult samples, there are also a few examples that have examined for sex differences in adolescents with chronic pain.[118,119] For example, Hechler et al.[119] examined responses to multimodal treatment in both child and adolescent groups. Although both sexes showed improvements following the intervention, females were found to report higher pain intensity scores at 3 and 12 months after treatment, and they had a higher school absence rate at 12 months. Females were also more likely to continue using analgesics following treatment. Interestingly, no sex differences were found in changes associated with disability or coping. In a second study, Hechler et al.[118] examined for sex differences in treatment-related changes in coping strategies within a group of adolescents with chronic pain. They found that while both sexes decreased in their use of social support, this was stronger in boys compared to girls. When related to changes in pain intensity, a decrease in social support use was related to lower pain in girls, but not boys. No such effects were found for disability.

Despite the limited number of studies that have looked for sex differences in response to multidisciplinary pain treatments, it seems that both adult and child groups do show differences. However, the actual direction and/or pattern of results is confusing, and more studies are required to help clarify this position. It is somewhat disappointing to report that despite there being a number of pharmacological studies, there are few studies that have focused on sex differences in treatment effect associated with nonpharmacological interventions. Future research needs to be more systematic in looking for, and reporting sex differences in, all forms of treatment-outcome investigation.

CONCLUSIONS AND FUTURE DIRECTIONS

This chapter has considered some of the psychosocial factors that have been examined within the context of sex differences in pain. The focus has been to consider differences in what men and women think (cognition), feel (emotion), and do (behavior) when in pain, and whether these differences help understand some of the variation between the sexes. What becomes apparent is that there are indeed a number of interesting differences that emerge. For example, there seem to be general sex differences in health-seeking behaviors and coping strategies. There is good evidence that pain-related catastrophizing may play an important role, as well as suggestions that anxiety may be differentially related to pain, depending on whether the person is male or female. Interestingly, some of the more convincing evidence stems from studies that consider the impact of people's beliefs and expectations have about typical "male" and "female" pain behaviors. This is particularly pertinent when one pairs this with findings that pain behaviors, as well as treatment, may be affected by observer behaviors. Indeed, what seems to be emerging from the literature is that pain does not occur in isolation and that we really need to start considering the way in which the pain behaviors of males and females are shaped and managed. Relevant to this are the recent advances in paediatric pain research, where it has not only been shown that parents play an important role in shaping pain behaviors, but that there may also be sex differences in how children and adolescences respond to pain.

Despite two decades of research, there are still relatively few studies that considered whether there are sex differences in nonpharmacological pain interventions. A few studies suggest that men and women might differ in the efficacy of some psychologically based interventions, but on the whole, relatively few studies have actively considered and designed interventions taking sex differences into consideration. It therefore comes as no surprise to discover that there have been relatively few studies that have considered sex differences in the development of psychological treatment interventions. Fortunately, these unanswered questions pave the way for future research into the psychosocial influences that may help explain the nature and extent of sex differences in pain. In time, this position will hopefully change, and by increasing our knowledge about the psychosocial processes involved, this may manifest into specific recommendations as to how best manage pain in a sex-specific way.

REFERENCES

1. Sullivan MJL, Bishop SR, Pivik J. The pain catastrophizing scale: development and validation. *Psychol Assessment* 1995;7(4):524–32.
2. Keefe FJ, Lefebvre JC, Egert JR, Affleck G, Sullivan MJ, Caldwell DS. The relationship of gender to pain, pain behavior, and disability in osteoarthritis patients: the role of catastrophizing. *Pain* 2000;87(3):325–34.
3. Keogh E, Eccleston C. Sex differences in adolescent chronic pain and pain-related coping. *Pain* 2006;123(3):275–84.
4. Osman A, Barrios FX, Gutierrez PM, Kopper BA, Merrifield T, Grittmann L. The pain catastrophizing scale: further psychometric evaluation with adult samples. *J Behav Med* 2000;23(4):351–65.
5. Keogh E, Denford S. Sex differences in perceptions of pain coping strategy usage. *Eur J Pain* 2009;13(6):629–34.
6. Unruh AM. Gender variations in clinical pain experience. *Pain* 1996;65(2–3):123–67.
7. Edwards RR, Haythornthwaite JA, Sullivan MJ, Fillingim RB. Catastrophizing as a mediator of sex differences in pain: differential effects for daily pain versus laboratory-induced pain. *Pain* 2004;111(3):335–41.
8. Keogh E, McCracken LM, Eccleston C. Do men and women differ in their response to interdisciplinary chronic pain management? *Pain* 2005;114(1–2):37–46.
9. Khan RS, Ahmed K, Blakeway E, et al. Catastrophizing: a predictive factor for postoperative pain. *Am J Surg* 2011;201(1):122–31.
10. Sullivan MJL, Thorn B, Haythornthwaite JA, et al. Theoretical perspectives on the relation

between catastrophizing and pain. *Clin J Pain* 2001;17(1):52–64.

11. Sullivan MJL, Tripp DA, Santor D. Gender differences in pain and pain behavior: the role of catastrophizing. *Cognit Ther Res* 2000;24(1):121–34.

12. Bernardes SF, Keogh E, Lima ML. Bridging the gap between pain and gender research: a selective literature review. *Eur J Pain* 2008;12(4):427–40.

13. Myers CD, Tsao JCI, Glover DA, Kim SC, Turk N, Zeltzer LK. Sex, gender, and age: contributions to laboratory pain responding in children and adolescents. *J Pain* 2006;7(8):556–64.

14. Pool GJ, Schwegler AF, Theodore BR, Fuchs PN. Role of gender norms and group identification on hypothetical and experimental pain tolerance. *Pain* 2007;129(1–2):122–9.

15. Robinson ME, Gagnon CM, Dannecker EA, Brown JL, Jump RL, Price DD. Sex differences in common pain events: expectations and anchors. *J Pain* 2003;4(1):40–5.

16. Robinson ME, Gagnon CM, Riley JL, Price DD. Altering gender role expectations: effects on pain tolerance, pain threshold, and pain ratings. *J Pain* 2003;4(5):284–8.

17. Robinson ME, Riley JL, Myers CD, et al. Gender role expectations of pain: relationship to sex differences in pain. *J Pain* 2001;2(5):251–7.

18. Robinson ME, Wise EA. Gender bias in the observation of experimental pain. *Pain* 2003;104(1–2):259–64.

19. Fowler SL, Rasinski HM, Geers AL, Helfer SG, France CR. Concept priming and pain: an experimental approach to understanding gender roles in sex-related pain differences. *J Behav Med* 2011;34(2):139–47.

20. Robinson ME, Wise EA, Gagnon C, Fillingim RB, Price DD. Influences of gender role and anxiety on sex differences in temporal summation of pain. *J Pain* 2004;5(2):77–82.

21. Wise EA, Price DD, Myers CD, Heft MW, Robinson ME. Gender role expectations of pain: relationship to experimental pain perception. *Pain* 2002;96(3):335–42.

22. Myers CD, Robinson ME, Riley JL, Sheffield D. Sex, gender, and blood pressure: contributions to experimental pain report. *Psychosom Med* 2001; 63(4):545–50.

23. Otto MW, Dougher MJ. Sex-differences and personality-factors in responsivity to pain. *Percept Motor Skill* 1985;61(2):383–90.

24. Stewart DE, Yuen T. A systematic review of resilience in the physically ill. *Psychosomatics* 2011;52(3):199–209.

25. Jackson T, Iezzi T, Gunderson J, Nagasaka T, Fritch A. Gender differences in pain perception: the mediating role of self-efficacy beliefs. *Sex Roles* 2002;47(11–12):561–8.

26. Strong J, Ashton R, Chant D. The measurement of attitudes towards and beliefs about pain. *Pain* 1992;48(2):227–36.

27. Ong AD, Zautra AJ, Reid MC. Psychological resilience predicts decreases in pain catastrophizing through positive emotions. *Psychol Aging* 2010;25(3):516–23.

28. Mcrae K, Ochsner KN, Mauss IB, Gabrieli JJD, Gross JJ. Gender differences in emotion regulation: an fMRI study of cognitive reappraisal. *Group Processes Intergroup Relations* 2008;11(2):143–162.

29. Keogh E, Bond FW, Hanmer R, Tilston J. Comparing acceptance- and control-based coping instructions on the cold-pressor pain experiences of healthy men and women. *Eur J Pain* 2005;9(5):591–8.

30. McLean CP, Anderson ER. Brave men and timid women? A review of the gender differences in fear and anxiety. *Clin Psychol Rev* 2009;29(6):496–505.

31. Ustun TB. Cross-national epidemiology of depression and gender. *J Gend Specif Med* 2000;3(2):54–8.

32. Heft MW, Meng X, Bradley MM, Lang PJ. Gender differences in reported dental fear and fear of dental pain. *Community Dent Oral Epidemiol* 2007;35(6):421–8.

33. McCracken LM, Keogh E. Acceptance, mindfulness, and values-based action may counteract fear and avoidance of emotions in chronic pain: an analysis of anxiety sensitivity. *J Pain* 2009;10(4):408–15.

34. Tashani OA, Alabas OA, Johnson MI. Cold pressor pain responses in healthy Libyans: effect of sex/gender, anxiety, and body size. *Gend Med* 2010;7(4):309–19.

35. Carleton RN, Abrams MP, Asmundson GJ, Antony MM, McCabe RE. Pain-related anxiety and anxiety sensitivity across anxiety and depressive disorders. *J Anxiety Disord* 2009;23(6):791–8.

36. Edwards RR, Augustson EM, Fillingim RB. Sex-specific effects of pain-related anxiety on adjustment to chronic pain. *Clin J Pain* 2000;16(1):46–53.

37. McCracken LM, Houle T. Sex-specific and general roles of pain-related anxiety in adjustment to chronic pain: a reply to Edwards et al. *Clin J Pain* 2000;16(3):275–6.

38. Mounce C, Keogh E, Eccleston C. A principal components analysis of negative affect-related constructs relevant to pain: evidence for a three component structure. *J Pain* 2010;11(8):710–7.

39. Page MG, Campbell F, Isaac L, Stinson J, Martin-Pichora AL, Katz J. Reliability and validity of the Child Pain Anxiety Symptoms Scale (CPASS) in a clinical sample of children and adolescents with acute postsurgical pain. *Pain* 2011;152(9):1958–65.

40. Keogh E, Book K, Thomas J, Giddins G, Eccleston C. Predicting pain and disability in patients with hand fractures: comparing pain anxiety, anxiety sensitivity and pain catastrophizing. *Eur J Pain* 2010;14(4):446–51.

41. Elklit A, Jones A. The association between anxiety and chronic pain after whiplash injury: gender-specific effects. *Clin J Pain* 2006;22(5):487–90.

42. Jones A, Zachariae R, Arendt-Nielsen L. Dispositional anxiety and the experience of pain: gender-specific effects. *Eur J Pain* 2003;7(5):387–95.

43. Logan DE, Rose JB. Gender differences in post-operative pain and patient controlled analgesia use among adolescent surgical patients. *Pain* 2004;109(3):481–7.

44. Edwards RR, Augustson E, Fillingim RB. Differential relationships between anxiety and treatment-associated pain reduction among male and female chronic pain patients. *Clin J Pain* 2003;19(4):208–16.

45. Frot M, Feine JS, Bushnell MC. Sex differences in pain perception and anxiety. A psychophysical study with topical capsaicin. *Pain* 2004;108(3):230–36.

46. Keogh E, McCracken LM, Eccleston C. Gender moderates the association between depression and disability in chronic pain patients. *Eur J Pain* 2006;10(5):413–22.

47. Lautenbacher S, Rollman GB. Sex differences in responsiveness to painful and non-painful stimuli are dependent upon the stimulation method. *Pain* 1993;53(3):255–64.

48. Keogh E, Birkby J. The effect of anxiety sensitivity and gender on the experience of pain. *Cogn Emot* 1999;13(6):813–29.

49. Keogh E, Hamid R, Hamid S, Ellery D. Investigating the effect of anxiety sensitivity, gender and negative interpretative bias on the perception of chest pain. *Pain* 2004;111(1–2):209–17.

50. Thompson T, Keogh E, French CC. Sensory focusing versus distraction and pain: moderating effects of anxiety sensitivity in males and females. *J Pain* 2011;12(8):849–58.

51. Bingefors K, Isacson D. Epidemiology, co-morbidity, and impact on health-related quality of life of self-reported headache and musculoskeletal pain: a gender perspective. *Eur J Pain* 2004;8(5):435–50.

52. Tsang A, Von Korff M, Lee S, et al. Common chronic pain conditions in developed and developing countries: gender and age differences and comorbidity with depression-anxiety disorders. *J Pain* 2008;9(10):883–91.

53. Bolton JE. Psychological distress and disability in back pain patients: evidence of sex differences. *J Psychosom Res* 1994;38(8):849–58.

54. Wasan AD, Anderson NK, Giddon DB. Differences in pain, psychological symptoms, and gender distribution among patients with left- vs right-sided chronic spinal pain. *Pain Med* 2010;11(9):1373–80.

55. Haley WE, Turner JA, Romano JM. Depression in chronic pain patients: relation to pain, activity, and sex differences. *Pain* 1985;23(4):337–43.

56. Haythornthwaite JA, Sieber WJ, Kerns RD. Depression and the chronic pain experience. *Pain* 1991;46(2):177–84.

57. Novy DM, Nelson DV, Averill PM, Berry LA. Gender differences in the expression of depressive symptoms among chronic pain patients. *Clin J Pain* 1996;12(1):23–9.

58. Harris CA, D'Eon JL. Psychometric properties of the Beck Depression Inventory—second edition (BDI-II) in individuals with chronic pain. *Pain* 2008;137(3):609–22.

59. Hirsh AT, Waxenberg LB, Atchison JW, Gremillion HA, Robinson ME. Evidence for sex differences in the relationships of pain, mood, and disability. *J Pain* 2006;7(8):592–601.

60. Kaczynski KJ, Claar RL, Logan DE. Testing gender as a moderator of associations between psychosocial variables and functional disability in children and adolescents with chronic pain. *J Pediatr Psychol* 2009;34(7):738–48.

61. Green CA, Pope CR. Gender, psychosocial factors and the use of medical services: a longitudinal analysis. *Soc Sci Med* 1999;48(10):1363–72.

62. Weir R, Browne G, Tunks E, Gafni A, Roberts J. Gender differences in psychosocial adjustment to chronic pain and expenditures for health care services used. *Clin J Pain* 1996;12(4):277–90.

63. Antonov KI, Isacson DG. Prescription and nonprescription analgesic use in Sweden. *Ann Pharmacother* 1998;32(4):485–94.

64. Isacson D, Bingefors K. Epidemiology of analgesic use: a gender perspective. *Eur J Anaesthesiol* 2002;19:5–15.

65. Paulose-Ram R, Hirsch R, Dillon C, Losonczy K, Cooper M, Ostchega Y. Prescription and non-prescription analgesic use among the US adult population: results from the third

National Health and Nutrition Examination Survey (NHANES III). *Pharmacoepidemiol Drug Saf* 2003;12(4):315–26.

66. Wu LT, Pilowsky DJ, Patkar AA. Non-prescribed use of pain relievers among adolescents in the United States. *Drug Alcohol Depend* 2008; 94(1–3):1–11.

67. Lynch AM, Kashikar-Zuck S, Goldschneider KR, Jones BA. Sex and age differences in coping styles among children with chronic pain. *J Pain Symptom Manage* 2007;33(2):208–16.

68. Unruh AM, Ritchie J, Merskey H. Does gender affect appraisal of pain and pain coping strategies? *Clin J Pain* 1999;15(1):31–40.

69. Christensen U, Schmidt L, Hougaard CO, Kriegbaum M, Holstein BE. Socioeconomic position and variations in coping strategies in musculoskeletal pain: a cross-sectional study of 1,287 40- and 50-year-old men and women. *J Rehabil Med* 2006;38(5):316–21.

70. Grossi G, Soares JJF, Lundberg U. Gender differences in coping with musculoskeletal pain. *Int J Behav Med* 2000;7(4):305–21.

71. Hermann C, Hohmeister J, Zohsel K, Ebinger F, Flor H. The assessment of pain coping and pain-related cognitions in children and adolescents: current methods and further development. *J Pain* 2007;8(10):802–13.

72. Tamres LK, Janicki D, Helgeson VS. Sex differences in coping behavior: a meta-analytic review and an examination of relative coping. *Pers Soc Psychol Rev* 2002;6(1):2–30.

73. Vigil JM. A socio-relational framework of sex differences in the expression of emotion. *Behav Brain Sci* 2009;32(5):375–90; discussion 391–428.

74. Guinsburg R, de Araujo Peres C, Branco de Almeida MF, et al. Differences in pain expression between male and female newborn infants. *Pain* 2000;85(1–2):127–33.

75. Prkachin KM, Solomon PE. The structure, reliability and validity of pain expression: evidence from patients with shoulder pain. *Pain* 2009;139(2):267–74.

76. Kunz M, Gruber A, Lautenbacher S. Sex differences in facial encoding of pain. *J Pain* 2006;7(12):915–28.

77. Simon D, Craig KD, Gosselin F, Belin P, Rainville P. Recognition and discrimination of prototypical dynamic expressions of pain and emotions. *Pain* 2008;135(1–2):55–64.

78. Vervoort T, Goubert L, Crombez G. The relationship between high catastrophizing children's facial display of pain and parental judgment of their child's pain. *Pain* 2009;142(1–2):142–8.

79. Hirsh AT, Alqudah AF, Stutts LA, Robinson ME. Virtual human technology: capturing sex, race, and age influences in individual pain decision policies. *Pain* 2008;140(1):231–8.

80. Hill ML, Craig KD. Detecting deception in facial expressions of pain: accuracy and training. *Clin J Pain* 2004;20(6):415–22.

81. Prkachin KM, Mass H, Mercer SR. Effects of exposure on perception of pain expression. *Pain* 2004;111(1–2):8–12.

82. Craig KD. The social communication model of pain. *Canadian Psychology* 2009;50(1):22–32.

83. Kallai I, Barke A, Voss U. The effects of experimenter characteristics on pain reports in women and men. *Pain* 2004;112(1–2):142–7.

84. Levine FM, Desimone LL. The effects of experimenter gender on pain report in male and female subjects. *Pain* 1991;44(1):69–72.

85. Evans S, Tsao JC, Lu Q, et al. Sex differences in the relationship between maternal negative life events and children's laboratory pain responsivity. *J Dev Behav Pediatr* 2009;30(4):279–88.

86. Keefe FJ, Crisson J, Urban BJ, Williams DA. Analyzing chronic low back pain: the relative contribution of pain coping strategies. *Pain* 1990;40(3):293–301.

87. Romano JM, Jensen MP, Turner JA, Good AB, Hops H. Chronic pain patient-partner interactions: further support for a behavioral model of chronic pain. *Behav Ther* 2000;31(3):415–50.

88. Smith SJ, Keefe FJ, Caldwell DS, Romano J, Baucom D. Gender differences in patient-spouse interactions: a sequential analysis of behavioral interactions in patients having osteoarthritic knee pain. *Pain* 2004;112(1–2):183–7.

89. Cicero TJ, Aylward SC, Meyer ER. Gender differences in the intravenous self-administration of mu opiate agonists. *Pharmacol Biochem Behav* 2003;74(3):541–9.

90. Lord B, Cui J, Kelly AM. The impact of patient sex on paramedic pain management in the prehospital setting. *Am J Emerg Med* 2009; 27(5):525–9.

91. Michael GE, Sporer KA, Youngblood GM. Women are less likely than men to receive prehospital analgesia for isolated extremity injuries. *Am J Emerg Med* 2007;25(8):901–6.

92. Calderone KL. The influence of gender on the frequency of pain and sedative medication administered to postoperative patients. *Sex Roles* 1990;23(11–12):713–25.

93. Chen EH, Shofer FS, Dean AJ, et al. Gender disparity in analgesic treatment of emergency department patients with acute abdominal pain. *Acad Emerg Med* 2008;15(5):414–8.

94. Roger VL, Farkouh ME, Weston SA, et al. Sex differences in evaluation and outcome of unstable angina. *JAMA* 2000;283(5):646–52.

95. Zegre-Hemsey J, Sommargren CE, Drew BJ. Initial ECG acquisition within 10 minutes of arrival at the emergency department in persons with chest pain: time and gender differences. *J Emerg Nurs* 2011;37(1):109–12.

96. Leresche L. Defining gender disparities in pain management. *Clin Orthop Relat Res* 2011; 469(7):1871–7.

97. Bernardes SF, Lima ML. Being less of a man or less of a woman: perceptions of chronic pain patients' gender identities. *Eur J Pain* 2010;14(2):194–9.

98. Bernardes SF, Lima ML. On the contextual nature of sex-related biases in pain judgments: the effects of pain duration, patient's distress and judge's sex. *Eur J Pain* 2011;15(9):950–7.

99. Wandner LD, Stutts LA, Alqudah AF, et al. Virtual human technology: patient demographics and healthcare training factors in pain observation and treatment recommendations. *J Pain Res* 2010;3:241–7.

100. Alqudah AF, Hirsh AT, Stutts LA, Scipio CD, Robinson ME. Sex and race differences in rating others' pain, pain-related negative mood, pain coping, and recommending medical help. *J Cyber Ther Rehabil* 2010;3(1):63–70.

101. Weisse CS, Sorum PC, Sanders KN, Syat BL. Do gender and race affect decisions about pain management? *J Gen Intern Med* 2001;16(4):211–7.

102. Keogh E, Barlow C, Mounce C, Bond FW. Assessing the relationship between cold pressor pain responses and dimensions of the anxiety sensitivity profile in healthy men and women. *Cogn Behav Ther* 2006;35(4):198–206.

103. Keogh E, Hatton K, Ellery D. Avoidance versus focused attention and the perception of pain: differential effects for men and women. *Pain* 2000;85(1–2):225–30.

104. Keogh E, Herdenfeldt M. Gender, coping and the perception of pain. *Pain* 2002;97(3):195–201.

105. Aslaksen PM, Bystad M, Vambheim SM, Flaten MA. Gender differences in placebo analgesia: event-related potentials and emotional modulation. *Psychosom Med* 2011;73(2):193–9.

106. Klosterhalfen S, Kellermann S, Braun S, et al. Gender and the nocebo response following conditioning and expectancy. *J Psychosom Res* 2009;66(4):323–8.

107. Compton P, Charuvastra VC, Ling W. Effect of oral ketorolac and gender on human cold pressor pain tolerance. *Clin Exp Pharmacol Physiol* 2003;30(10):759–63.

108. Gear RW, Miaskowski C, Gordon NC, Paul SM, Heller PH, Levine JD. The kappa opioid nalbuphine produces gender- and dose-dependent analgesia and antianalgesia in patients with postoperative pain. *Pain* 1999;83(2):339–45.

109. Aslaksen PM, Flaten MA. The roles of physiological and subjective stress in the effectiveness of a placebo on experimentally induced pain. *Psychosom Med* 2008;70(7):811–8.

110. Niesters M, Dahan A, Kest B, et al. Do sex differences exist in opioid analgesia? A systematic review and meta-analysis of human experimental and clinical studies. *Pain* 2010;151(1):61–8.

111. Burns JW, Johnson BJ, Devine J, Mahoney N, Pawl R. Anger management style and the prediction of treatment outcome among male and female chronic pain patients. *Behav Res Ther* 1998;36(11):1051–62.

112. Edwards RR, Doleys DM, Lowery D, Fillingim RB. Pain tolerance as a predictor of outcome following multidisciplinary treatment for chronic pain: differential effects as a function of sex. *Pain* 2003;106(3):419–26.

113. Hampel P, Graef T, Krohn-Grimberghe B, Tlach L. Effects of gender and cognitive-behavioral management of depressive symptoms on rehabilitation outcome among inpatient orthopedic patients with chronic low back pain: a 1 year longitudinal study. *Eur Spine J* 2009;18(12):1867–80.

114. Hooten WM, Townsend CO, Bruce BK, Shi Y, Warner DO. Sex differences in characteristics of smokers with chronic pain undergoing multidisciplinary pain rehabilitation. *Pain Med* 2009;10(8):1416–25.

115. Jensen IB, Bergstrom G, Ljungquist T, Bodin L, Nygren AL. A randomized controlled component analysis of a behavioral medicine rehabilitation program for chronic spinal pain: are the effects dependent on gender? *Pain* 2001;91(1–2):65–78.

116. McGeary DD, Mayer TG, Gatchel RJ, Anagnostis C, Proctor TJ. Gender-related differences in treatment outcomes for patients with musculoskeletal disorders. *Spine J* 2003;3(3):197–203.

117. Hooten WM, Townsend CO, Decker PA. Gender differences among patients with fibromyalgia undergoing multidisciplinary pain rehabilitation. *Pain Med* 2007;8(8):624–32.

118. Hechler T, Kosfelder J, Vocks S, et al. Changes in pain-related coping strategies and their importance for treatment outcome following multimodal inpatient treatment: does sex matter? *J Pain* 2010;11(5):472–83.

119. Hechler T, Blankenburg M, Dobe M, Kosfelder J, Hubner B, Zernikow B. Effectiveness of a multimodal inpatient treatment for pediatric chronic pain: a comparison between children and adolescents. *Eur J Pain* 2010;14(1):97, e91–9.

SECTION THREE

FEMALE-SPECIFIC PAIN

8

CURRENT MANAGEMENT OF
LABOR PAIN

Cynthia A. Wong

INTRODUCTION

Childbirth pain is arguably the most severe pain most women will endure in their lifetimes. James Young Simpson pioneered the modern era of childbirth analgesia in 1847 when he administered ether, and later chloroform, to women in childbirth. Early in the 20th century *Dämmerschlaf*, or "twilight sleep," was introduced, and the use of single-shot spinal, lumbar, and caudal epidural, paravertebral, and pudendal nerve blocks for obstetric analgesia were described. Well over half a century ago the first published report of continuous caudal analgesia for childbirth launched the use of continuous neuraxial (spinal and epidural) analgesia for labor and delivery analgesia. Current management of childbirth analgesia includes an array of regional nerve blocks, systemic analgesic, and nonpharmacologic techniques. Pharmacologic and nonpharmacologic techniques can be used together or alone. This chapter will summarize the physiology of childbirth pain, labor, and delivery analgesic techniques, and it will briefly describe the effects of labor analgesia on the mother and infant.

PATHOPHYSIOLOGY OF CHILDBIRTH PAIN

The pain and suffering associated with labor and vaginal delivery vary widely among parturients.

Unfortunately, few if any validated tools exist to measure the prevalence, intensity, and quality of labor pain. Melzack et al. used the McGill Pain Questionnaire to measure pain during labor and delivery (Fig. 8.1).[1] Pain scores for childbirth were higher than those associated with cancer pain, phantom limb pain, and postherpetic neuralgia, and higher in nulliparous than parous women.

During the first stage of labor (start of labor until complete cervical dilation) pain signals predominantly originate from dilation (tissue distension, stretching, and tearing) of the cervix and the lower uterine segment. As the fetus descends in the birth canal during the late first stage and second stage of labor (complete cervical dilation until delivery), stretching and tearing of fascia and subcutaneous tissues, and pressure on the skeletal muscles of the perineum, are additional sources of pain.

First-stage labor pain from the cervix and lower uterine segment are transmitted via visceral afferent nerve fibers that accompany sympathetic nerve fibers and enter the spinal cord at the tenth, eleventh, and twelfth thoracic and first lumbar spinal segments (Fig. 8.2). These visceral C-fibers terminate in the ipsilateral dorsal and ventral horns of the spinal cord in a loose network of synapses, as well as crossing the midline to the contralateral side. Second-stage

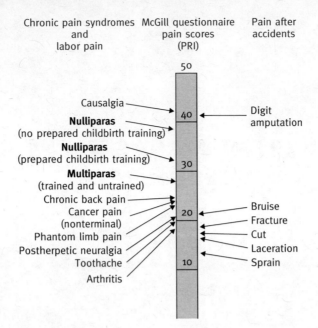

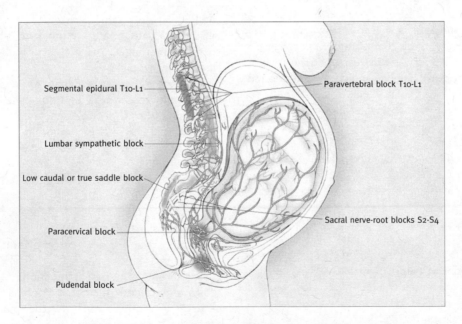

FIGURE 8.1 Comparison of pain scores using the McGill Pain Questionnaire obtained from women during labor and from patients in general hospital clinics and an emergency department. The pain rating index (PRI) represents the sum of the rank values for all words chosen from 20 sets of pain descriptions. (Used with permission from Melzack R. The myth of painless childbirth [The John J. Bonica Lecture]. *Pain* 1984;19[4]:321–337.)

FIGURE 8.2 Transmission of labor pain. Labor pain has a visceral component and a somatic component. Noxious impulses from the uterus and cervix follow afferent sensory-nerve fibers that accompany sympathetic nerves, traveling through the paracervical region and the pelvic and hypogastric plexus to enter the lumbar sympathetic chain and the dorsal horn of the spinal cord through the white rami communicantes of the T10, T11, T12, and L1 spinal nerves. Noxious impulses from the vagina and perineum travel via the pudendal nerve to enter the spinal cord at S2 to S4. (Used with permission from Eltzschig HK, Lieberman ES, Camann WR. Regional anesthesia and analgesia for labor and delivery. *N Eng J Med* 2003; 348[4]:319–332.)

labor pain from the somatic sensory impulses from the vagina and perineum are transmitted via the pudendal nerves to the second, third, and fourth sacral spinal segments, and they terminate in the ipsilateral superficial laminae of the dorsal horn. There is minimal rostrocaudal fiber extension. Thus, the pain of the first stage of pain tends to be diffuse in nature, and it is often referred to the dermatomes supplied by the same spinal cord segments that receive input from the uterus and cervix (T10 to L1). Additionally, during the late first stage and second stage of labor, pressure on one or more roots of the lumbosacral plexus may result in aching, burning, or cramping discomfort in the thigh, legs, and lower back. Abnormal fetal position (e.g., occiput posterior) may worsen this type of pain.

The current treatment of labor pain is based on our knowledge of the anatomic and physiologic basis of childbirth pain. Thus, bilateral paracervical plexus or lumbar sympathetic blockade blocks the visceral pain of the first stage of labor (Fig. 8.2). Bilateral pudendal nerve blockade blocks sacral somatic pain caused by descent of the fetus in the birth canal. By blocking both the low thoracic and sacral dermatomes, neuraxial blockade (spinal or epidural) is the only technique that provides complete analgesia for the first and second stages of labor.

The severity and duration of labor pain and suffering may be influenced by a number of psychological and physical factors. Psychological factors include fear, apprehension, and anxiety.[2] Education, motivation, and cultural factors influence the affective and behavioral dimensions of pain, although they probably minimally affect actual pain sensation. For example, women who had predelivery psychoprophylaxis training manifested little or no pain behavior during childbirth, although after delivery most of them indicated the process had been quite painful.[3]

Physical factors that affect labor pain include maternal age and parity, the condition of the cervix at the onset of labor, and the size and position of the fetus relative to the size and shape of the birth canal. The parous cervix is generally more dilated and effaced at the onset of labor and therefore less sensitive than the nulliparous cervix. Older nulliparas usually experience longer and more painful labors than younger nulliparas.[1] The intensity of uterine contractions tends to be greater in nulliparous than parous women early in labor; the reverse is true as labor advances. Dystocia from a large baby, contracted pelvis, or abnormal presentation or position is often associated with greater pain.

NONPHARMACOLOGIC METHODS OF LABOR ANALGESIA

Nonpharmacologic techniques to mitigate the pain and suffering of childbirth are often touted as alternative therapies to pharmacologic analgesia, but these techniques should also be considered complementary to pharmacologic analgesia. Most of these interventions have not been subject to rigorous scientific study; therefore, conclusions about their efficacy are not possible.[4-8]

Antenatal *childbirth education* is widely practiced. Studies investigating the role of childbirth education in influencing outcomes such as use of analgesia, duration of labor, mode of delivery, and incidence of non-reassuring fetal status are of mediocre quality and the results are inconsistent. For example, observational studies have found that participation in childbirth education classes is associated with a decreased, increased, and no change in the rate of neuraxial analgesia.

Emotional support during childbirth is often provided by the parturient's partner or friend(s). Evidence is inconsistent as to whether this type of support affects childbirth pain. Controlled trials and several systematic analyses have concluded that women who receive continuous labor support (nonmedical support by a trained person, e.g., a doula) have shorter labors, fewer operative deliveries, fewer analgesic interventions, and greater satisfaction.[9]

Intradermal water injection is one of the few nonpharmacologic techniques that have been rigorously studied. Randomized controlled trials have consistently found that the technique effectively reduces severe back pain during labor, although the rate of use of other analgesic modalities was not different in the treatment compared to control group.[4,10] Small volumes of sterile water (0.05 to 0.1 mL) are injected at four sites on the lower back using an insulin or tuberculin syringe. There are no known maternal or fetal side effects. The mechanism of analgesia is unclear.

Hydrotherapy is the immersion of the parturient in warm water deep enough to cover the abdomen. Systematic reviews of randomized controlled trials have concluded that hydrotherapy is associated with less pain and use of other analgesia modalities, without adverse effect on the duration of labor, mode of operative delivery, or neonatal outcome.[11,12]

Self-hypnosis requires the prenatal training of the mother, and sometimes her partner, by a trained hypnotherapist. A meta-analysis of five randomized controlled trials of self-hypnosis concluded that the use of pharmacologic analgesia methods was decreased in the hypnosis compared to controlled group.[13] Data were inconclusive or limited regarding progress of labor and neonatal outcomes.

Acupuncture is a component of traditional Chinese medicine. Although a number of randomized controlled trials have compared acupuncture and acupressure to placebo or sham procedures, systematic reviews have concluded that a high risk of bias exists in most studies.[14,15] Meta-analyses of these trials have concluded that women randomized to acupuncture had modestly lower pain scores and lower use of epidural and systemic opioid analgesia than women randomized to control groups.

Transcutaneous electrical nerve stimulation (TENS) is the application of low-intensity, high-frequency electrical impulses via surface electrodes applied to the lower back. The buzzing, electrical current sensation caused by the TENS unit may reduce the parturient's awareness of labor pain. Results of studies are inconsistent, but in general, labor pain does not appear to be lessened nor is the use of other analgesic modalities.[8] However, TENS use appears safe for both the mother and the fetus.

INHALATION ANALGESIA

Current methods of systemic labor analgesia are systemic opioid analgesia and inhalation analgesia. Inhalation analgesia for labor and vaginal delivery is unusual in the United States, but it is more common in other countries. Currently, the only inhaled anesthetic agent in common use is nitrous oxide. It is available in the United Kingdom as Entonox®, a mixture of 50% nitrous oxide and 50% oxygen. A disadvantage of its use is that special scavenging equipment is necessary to ensure the safe administration of the drug without contamination of the environment. Environmental contamination results in exposure of health care workers and contributes to the greenhouse effect.[16]

Use of *nitrous oxide* for labor analgesia is controversial[17]; studies are conflicting as to whether the drug actually provides benefit, and well-conducted studies are lacking. At best, analgesia is incomplete. The most recent review in 2002[18] summarized the results of 11 randomized controlled trials; only one was published after 1996. This review concluded that current published work does not provide clear objective evidence of analgesic efficacy of nitrous oxide.

The intermittent use of nitrous oxide has been traditionally thought to be safe for the mother and fetus/neonate. Maternal drowsiness may occur in up to 24% of women and is dose dependent.[18] The risk of maternal hypoxemia may be increased by concomitant use of nitrous oxide and systemic opioids.[19] Well-conducted toxicity studies are lacking.

SYSTEMIC OPIOID ANALGESIA

Systemic opioid analgesia is widely used throughout the world, although its use for labor analgesia lacks rigorous scientific study. Existing data suggest that opioids provide little significant analgesia.[20-22] There is a high incidence of dose-related maternal and fetal side effects. Historically, meperidine has been the most commonly used systemic opioid. However, in the past decade, because of concerns of lack of efficacy and presence of side effects, there has been a move away from its use for the treatment of other pain conditions.[23,24] Meperidine also has adverse effects on the neonate[21]; thus, other opioid agonists and agonist-antagonists are increasingly used for labor analgesia (Table 8.1). Unfortunately, there are few studies comparing opioids for labor analgesia, and there is little evidence that one opioid is better than another.[21, 22] Maternal side effects include sedation, nausea, vomiting, dysphoria, delayed gastric emptying, and respiratory depression. All opioids cross the placenta. In utero opioid exposure results in a slower fetal heart rate and decreased beat-to-beat variability.[25] The opioid dose and timing of administration influence the risk of neonatal respiratory depression. The active metabolite of meperidine, normeperidine, has a half-life of 60 hours in neonates.[26]

Patient-controlled intravenous opioid analgesia (PCIA) may have advantages compared to nurse- or midwife-administered opioid analgesia, including superior analgesia with smaller drug doses, lower incidence of maternal and fetal side effects, patient control of analgesia, and increased patient satisfaction. Meperidine, nalbuphine, fentanyl, and more recently, remifentanil, have been used for PCIA (Table 8.2). Several randomized controlled trials of remifentanil PCIA compared to epidural analgesia found more effective analgesia with epidural analgesia.[27,28] Maternal sedation and oxygen desaturation were more common in

Table 8.1 Drugs for Systemic Opioid Labor Analgesia

DRUG	DOSE RANGE
Meperidine[a]	25–50 mg IV
	50–100 mg IM
Morphine	2–5 mg IV
	5–10 mg IM
Hydromorphone	1 mg IV or IM
Fentanyl	25–50 µg IV
	100 µg IM
Nalbuphine	10–20 mg IV or IM
Butorphanol	1–2 mg IV or IM
Tramadol	50–100 mg IV or IM

[a]Meperidine is less preferred than other opioids because of its adverse neonatal effects due to accumulation of meperidine and the active metabolite, normeperidine; a single dose only is advised.[21]

IM, intramuscular; IV, intravenous.

Table 8.2 Patient-Controlled Intravenous Analgesia Regimens

DRUG	PATIENT-CONTROLLED BOLUS DOSE	LOCKOUT INTERVAL (MIN)
Meperidine	10–15 mg	8–20
Fentanyl	10–25 µg	5–12
Remifentanil (bolus only)	0.4–0.5 µg/kg	2–3
Remifentanil (bolus plus background infusion)	Infusion rate: 0.05 µg/kg/min Bolus dose 0.25 µg/kg	2–3

the remifentanil PCIA groups, although neonatal outcome did not differ in these small studies.[27,28]

Compared to other opioids, remifentanil may have theoretical advantages for PCIA because of its short latency (time to peak effect after IV administration is 60 to 90 seconds).[29] Additionally, because of its rapid metabolism by plasma esterases, it may be safer for the mother and neonate. Systematic review and meta-analysis suggest that pain scores after 1 hour are lower with remifentanil compared to meperidine.[30] Data were insufficient to assess side effect profiles.

NEURAXIAL ANALGESIA

Neuraxial labor analgesia is the most complete and effective method of pain relief during childbirth. It is the only method that provides complete analgesia without maternal or fetal sedation. The use of neuraxial analgesia for childbirth has increased dramatically in the United States over the past 40 years.[31] In the most recent US survey performed in 2001, over 60% of women in large hospitals received neuraxial analgesia during labor.[31] The United Kingdom National Health Service Maternity Statistics of 2005–2006 reported that one-third of parturients chose neuraxial analgesia during childbirth.[32]

Continuous lumbar epidural analgesia and combined spinal-epidural (CSE) analgesia are the most common techniques. The duration of labor is unpredictable; therefore, techniques utilizing neuraxial catheters offer the most flexibility. Continuous spinal analgesia provides excellent labor analgesia,[33] but it is currently an uncommon technique because it requires dural puncture with a large-bore needle. Small "microcatheters" have not been commercially available in the United States, and large catheters are associated with an unacceptably high risk of postdural puncture (spinal) headache.

Contraindications to neuraxial analgesia include patient refusal, coagulopathy, infection at the puncture site, and lack of experienced anesthesia providers. Relative contraindications include hemorrhage or other causes of hypovolemia, untreated systemic infection, preload-dependent cardiac disease, and lumbar spine pathology.

Lumbar epidural analgesia has been the mainstay of neuraxial labor analgesia for many years. Typically, an epidural catheter is threaded into the lumbar epidural space via a mid- to low-lumbar interspace. In case of need for intrapartum cesarean delivery, the ability to quickly convert from epidural *analgesia* to epidural *anesthesia* is a major benefit of epidural labor analgesia.

Randomized studies consistently demonstrate that pain scores are lower and patients are more satisfied with epidural analgesia compared to other nonneuraxial analgesic techniques.[34] Complete labor analgesia requires blockade of low thoracic and sacral spinal cord segments. Injection of anesthetic agents into the lumbar epidural space allows spread of the anesthetic solution both cephalad and caudad.

Combined spinal-epidural analgesia has become increasingly popular in the past decade. After advancing the epidural needle into the epidural space, a long spinal needle is passed through the epidural needle, which functions as an introducer. Drug(s) are injected into the intrathecal space, the spinal needle is removed, and a catheter is threaded into the epidural space. Onset of analgesia is significantly faster with CSE compared to epidural analgesia (2 to 5 min vs. 15 to 20 min).[35] In early labor, complete analgesia can be obtained with the intrathecal injection of lipid-soluble opioids such as fentanyl or sufentanil, without local anesthetics. This technique avoids the motor blockade associated with neuraxial local anesthetics, and it decreases the risk of hypotension. The spinal opioid dose is significantly less than that required for systemic or epidural administration and does not result in maternal or neonatal sedation. This technique is ideal for parturients who wish to ambulate. The addition of local anesthetic to a lipid-soluble opioid results in sacral analgesia within several minutes. Because sacral analgesia is necessary in the late first stage and second stage of labor, the rapid onset of sacral analgesia seen with the CSE technique is a distinct advantage for women in whom analgesia is initiated late in labor and who require sacral analgesia for adequate pain relief.

There are several disadvantages of CSE analgesia. Dural puncture is required, albeit with a small-gauge needle. However, the risk of postdural (spinal) headache is not greater with CSE compared to epidural analgesia.[35] The incidence of pruritus is higher with intrathecal versus epidural opioids.[35] After the initiation of CSE analgesia it will be unclear for 1 to 2 hours whether the epidural catheter is properly sited in the epidural space, as the initial analgesia is provided with the spinal component of the technique. Therefore, CSE analgesia may not be the technique of choice if a functioning epidural catheter is critical to the safe care of the patient (e.g., high likelihood of urgent cesarean delivery or an anticipated difficult airway during general anesthesia).

DRUGS FOR NEURAXIAL LABOR ANALGESIA

The ideal analgesic drug or drug combination for neuraxial labor analgesia would provide rapid onset of effective analgesia with minimal motor blockade, minimal risk of maternal toxicity, and negligible effect on uterine activity and uteroplacental perfusion. Placental transfer would be limited, as well as direct or indirect effects on the fetus and neonate. Finally, the ideal drug would have a long duration of action. Unfortunately, the perfect drug(s) does not currently exist, but the combination of a long-acting amide local anesthetic with a lipid-soluble opioid allows this goal to be approached.

Traditionally, neuraxial local anesthetics, in particular bupivacaine, were administered to block both the visceral and somatic pain of labor. The discovery in 1976 of opiate receptors in the dorsal horn of the spinal cord launched a new era in neuraxial labor analgesia.[36] Neuraxial opioid administration results in opioid binding to these spinal cord receptors with minimal systemic opioid side effects. Neuraxial local anesthetics and opioids appear to act synergistically to provide neuraxial analgesia.[37]

Contemporary neuraxial labor analgesia most often incorporates low doses of a long-acting local anesthetic with a lipid-soluble opioid, both for the initiation and maintenance of analgesia. The combination of a local anesthetic with a lipid-soluble opioid allows the use of lower doses of each drug, thus minimizing undesirable side effects, including motor blockade from high doses of local anesthetic or sedation from high doses of epidural opioid. The addition of a lipid-soluble opioid to local anesthetics shortens latency.[38]

Bupivacaine has been the time-honored workhorse of epidural and spinal analgesia for many years (Table 8.3). It is most often used in combination with fentanyl or sufentanil to induce epidural and CSE analgesia. Placental transfer is minimal because the drug is highly protein bound; duration of analgesia is approximately 2 hours after a bolus dose. Ropivacaine and levobupivacaine are amide local anesthetics with similar characteristics to bupivacaine, and they are also commonly used for neuraxial labor analgesia. Compared to an equipotent sensory dose of bupivacaine, ropivacaine may be associated with less motor blockade[39]; however, this characteristic may not be clinically relevant when low doses of bupivacaine are used.[40]

The lipid-soluble opioids fentanyl and sufentanil are usually combined with a local anesthetic for the initiation of spinal and epidural analgesia. Doses commonly used for initiation and maintenance of neuraxial analgesia have been shown to be safe for both the mother and neonate.[41] Neuraxial morphine is not normally used for labor analgesia because of its long latency. Additionally, its long duration of action results in bothersome side effects (pruritus, nausea, and vomiting) long after delivery.

Adjuvants for neuraxial labor analgesia include epinephrine and clonidine. Both drugs

Table 8.3 Drugs for Neuraxial Labor Analgesia

| | INITIATION OF ANALGESIA | | MAINTENANCE OF ANALGESIA[c] |
	EPIDURAL ANALGESIA[a]	SPINAL ANALGESIA	EPIDURAL ANALGESIA
Local Anesthetics[b]			
Bupivacaine	0.625–1.25 mg/mL	1.25–2.5 mg	0.625–1.0 mg/mL
Ropivacaine	0.8–2.0 mg/mL	2.5–4.5 mg	0. 8–2.0 mg/mL
Levobupivacaine	0.625–1.25 mg/mL	2.5–4.5 mg	
Opioids[b]			
Sufentanil	5–10 µg	1.5–5 µg	0.2–0.33 µg/mL
Fentanyl	50–100 µg	15–25 µg	1.5–3 µg/mL

[a]The volume required to initiate epidural labor analgesia is 5 to 15 mL of local anesthetic solution injected into the lumbar epidural space.

[b]The local anesthetic dose/concentration and the fentanyl or sufentanil dose are reduced if the drugs are combined, or if a local anesthetic-containing epidural test dose is administered before the initiation dose.

[c]Continuous infusions usually consist of a local anesthetic combined with an opioid, administered at a rate of 6 to 15 mL/h into the lumbar epidural space.

contribute to analgesia by binding to spinal cord α_2-adrenergic receptors. Additionally, epinephrine decreases the uptake of local anesthetics and opioids from the epidural space secondary to vasoconstriction.

MAINTENANCE OF NEURAXIAL LABOR ANALGESIA

Epidural labor analgesia may be maintained until after delivery with intermittent bolus injection, continuous epidural infusion, or patient-controlled epidural analgesia. A dilute solution of bupivacaine or ropivacaine combined with fentanyl or sufentanil is commonly used (Table 8.1). Continuous epidural infusions compared to intermittent bolus injections have the advantage of fewer "top-up" injections and increased patient satisfaction. The disadvantage of infusions is higher total drug dose compared to intermittent injections.[42]

Patient-controlled epidural analgesia (PCEA) allows patient-titrated bolus injections with or without a background infusion. PCEA compared to continuous infusion analgesia results in greater patient satisfaction and a lower average hourly dose of bupivacaine (and therefore less motor block) and less need for physician intervention.[43,44] The protocols for PCEA vary widely. At one extreme, most of the hourly dose is administered via a background infusion; the parturient treats breakthrough pain by supplementing the infusion with self-administered boluses. At the other extreme, the entire dose is self-administered via intermittent boluses; there is no background infusion. A recent review suggests that administration of approximately one-third of the hourly dose via a continuous infusion may minimize the incidence of breakthrough pain while optimizing individual patient titration and drug dose.[44]

Many women like to move around during labor. They dislike being confined to bed and prefer to walk to the toilet or sit in a chair at the bedside. The term "walking" epidural analgesia was first coined to describe CSE opioid analgesia because motor function was maintained and the ability to walk was not impaired. However, the term can be applied to any neuraxial analgesic technique that allows safe ambulation. This can be achieved with the use of pure opioid, or low-dose local anesthetic-opioids techniques, and maintenance techniques that favor intermittent bolus dose administration over continuous infusion. Ambulation per se has not been shown to positively or negatively affect the progress or outcome of labor; however, dense motor blockade may adversely affect the spontaneous vaginal delivery rate (*vide infra*). Thus, the goal of the anesthesia provider should be to minimize motor blockade, regardless of whether the patient wishes to ambulate.

SIDE EFFECTS OF NEURAXIAL LABOR ANALGESIA

Common side effects of neuraxial labor analgesia include hypotension and pruritus; fetal bradycardia and maternal hyperthermia are less common side effects. Neuraxial labor analgesia is not associated with an increased risk of nausea and vomiting, although both are common during labor. Hypotension is the result of local anesthetic blockade of the sympathetic nervous system, leading to vasodilation, increased venous capacitance, decreased preload, and decreased cardiac output. Because uterine blood flow is not autoregulated, a decrease in maternal blood pressure results in a decrease in uteroplacental perfusion. Therefore, maternal blood pressure and fetal heart rate are monitored at frequent intervals. Hypotension should be treated with small bolus doses of intravenous vasopressor, such as ephedrine or phenylephrine, and repositioning the mother in the lateral position in order to avoid aortocaval compression.

Pruritus is more common after intrathecal than epidural or systemic opioid administration. The incidence and severity are dose related.[45,46] The cause is unknown; it is not histamine related and is readily treated with μ-opioid receptor antagonists or agonist-antagonists. Epidural labor analgesia is associated with maternal fever in a subset of women.[47] The mechanism is unknown, although evidence suggests an inflammatory mechanism may play a role. The clinical implications of this elevation in temperature are unclear.

Fetal bradycardia, not associated with maternal hypotension, sometimes occurs within 15 to 45 minutes after initiation of epidural or CSE analgesia. The mechanism is unclear; however, it is hypothesized that an increase in uterine tone, and a subsequent decrease in uteroplacental perfusion, is responsible for the bradycardia.[48] The initiation of analgesia is associated with an acute decrease in maternal plasma epinephrine levels.[49] Because epinephrine is a tocolytic, the rapid decline in plasma levels may contribute to an increase in uterine tone. The bradycardia usually resolves with conservative therapy, including discontinuing exogenous oxytocin and the administration of an intravenous fluid bolus. The cesarean delivery rate is not higher in women with neuraxial analgesia-associated fetal bradycardia.[50-52]

Observational studies suggest that women who receive epidural labor analgesia have a higher risk of intrapartum and postpartum urinary retention compared to women who receive other forms of analgesia or no analgesia.[53] It is unclear whether this finding reflects a cause-and-effect relationship or patient selection bias; however, differences among groups appear to resolve by postpartum day one.[53]

COMPLICATIONS OF NEURAXIAL ANALGESIA

Complications of neuraxial labor analgesia include breakthrough pain and unintentional dural puncture with an epidural needle. Rare complications include infection (epidural abscess, meningitis), high- or total spinal anesthesia, direct trauma to nerve tissue, and unintentional intravascular injection of local anesthetics, resulting in local anesthetic systemic toxicity. Although 30% to 50% of women complain of back pain after delivery, randomized controlled trials have failed to show a significant relationship between epidural analgesia and long-term backache. [54,55] The incidence of unintentional dural puncture in obstetric patients is approximately 1.5%.[56] Fifty to sixty percent of these patients will suffer from a postdural puncture headache.

EFFECTS OF ANALGESIA ON THE PROGRESS AND OUTCOME OF LABOR

Whether neuraxial labor analgesia affects the progress of labor and mode of delivery is controversial. No randomized trials have compared neuraxial or systemic opioid analgesia to no analgesia. For ethical reasons, these trials are unlikely to ever be completed. Therefore, the effect of any type of analgesia, be it neuraxial or systemic, on the outcome of labor is not known.

Although early investigators noted that neuraxial analgesia appeared to be an effective treatment for dysfunctional labor,[57-59] observational studies consistently identified an association between neuraxial analgesia, prolonged labor, and operative delivery. In contrast, randomized controlled trials comparing neuraxial labor analgesia to systemic opioid analgesia have found no difference in the rate of cesarean delivery between groups.[34,60] Observational data suggest that women with more pain during labor (and thus more likely to request analgesia) have a higher risk of cesarean delivery.[61-63] This association may explain the observed association between neuraxial analgesia and operative delivery. Fetal macrosomia, malposition, and dysfunctional labor may cause more painful labor and are associated with a higher rate of cesarean delivery.

Similarly, observational studies have found an association between the initiation of neuraxial analgesia in early (latent phase) labor and increased rate of cesarean delivery. Randomized controlled trials, however, have uniformly demonstrated that early labor neuraxial compared to systemic opioid analgesia does not adversely affect the progress and outcome of labor, and may actually result in faster labor.[64,65]

In contrast to its lack of effect on the rate of cesarean delivery, neuraxial analgesia may increase the risk of instrumental vaginal delivery. Randomized controlled trials comparing neuraxial to systemic opioid analgesia have assessed the risk of instrumental vaginal delivery as a secondary outcome. Systematic review of these trials has concluded that the rate of instrumental forceps delivery may be increased.[34,60] However, several limitations of the trial designs may limit general conclusions. First, the treatment (neuraxial) group in many of the trials received epidural analgesia with bupivacaine 2.5 mg/mL, a higher dose than the current norm. In several randomized controlled trials comparing neuraxial techniques to each other, women randomized to receive epidural analgesia with bupivacaine 2.5 mg/mL had a higher rate of instrumental vaginal delivery than women randomized to receive low-dose bupivacaine-opioid (≤ bupivacaine 1 mg/mL) techniques.[66,67] Thus, the goal of the anesthesia provider should be to provide analgesia with low-concentration local anesthetic-opioid mixtures in order to decrease the risk of instrumental vaginal delivery.

FETAL AND NEONATAL EFFECTS OF NEURAXIAL ANALGESIA

Neuraxial analgesia may affect the fetus directly, indirectly, or both. Scientifically rigorous studies are lacking, and many studies are dated. The neonatal depressant effects of drugs administered to the mother in the intrapartum period are usually assessed with neurobehavioral testing.[68] Unfortunately, these tests lack specificity and are quite subjective. However, evidence for a direct adverse effect of low-dose local anesthetic/opioid neuraxial analgesia is lacking. Compared to epidural bupivacaine analgesia, systemic meperidine analgesia is associated with a greater loss of FHR variability and fewer FHR accelerations,[25] and a higher incidence of neonatal respiratory depression.[69]

The indirect fetal effects of epidural and intrathecal analgesia may be more significant than the direct effects. Fetal bradycardia after initiation of neuraxial analgesia was discussed previously. Maternal hypotension may cause a decrease in uteroplacental perfusion and fetal oxygenation. Neuraxial opioid administration may cause maternal respiratory depression, especially when coadministered with systemic opioids or other central nervous system depressants. Obviously, if the mother has severe respiratory depression and hypoxemia, fetal hypoxemia and hypoxia will follow.

OTHER REGIONAL ANALGESIC TECHNIQUES

Neuraxial analgesia is the most effective and flexible analgesic technique for labor and delivery; however, some parturients may have contraindications to neuraxial analgesia, or they may not want it. Other nerve blocks provide acceptable, albeit less flexible, analgesia (Table 8.4).

Afferent nerves from the uterus and cervix can be blocked with the deposition of local anesthetic around the *paracervical* (Frankenhäuser's) ganglia. Bilateral block provides analgesia for the first stage of labor, before fetal descent, without somatic sensory or motor block. However, somatic pain caused by distension of the pelvic floor, vagina, or perineum is not relieved and analgesia is not continuous. Fetal bradycardia is the most common fetal complication; the etiology is unknown. Serious maternal complications are uncommon. Unintentional direct fetal scalp injection is more likely to occur when the block is performed in the presence of advanced cervical dilation (>8 cm).

Table 8.4   Regional and Nerve Blocks for Labor Analgesia

REGIONAL AND NERVE BLOCK	ANALGESIA	STAGE LABOR
Cervical plexus block	Uterus and cervix	First
Lumbar sympathetic block	Uterus and cervix	First
Pudendal block	Vagina and perineum	Second
Epidural block[a]	Uterus and cervix/vagina and perineum	First and second
Spinal block[b]	Uterus and cervix/vagina and perineum	First and second

[a]Usually maintained with an epidural catheter. Labor analgesia can be converted to surgical anesthesia for cesarean delivery by the injection of concentrated local anesthetic solutions.

[b]Usually performed as a component of a combined-spinal epidural technique.

Similar to a paracervical block, *paravertebral lumbar sympathetic blockade* interferes with transmission of visceral afferent nerve impulses from the uterus and cervix and provides analgesia for the first stage of labor. The technique is technically more difficult to learn and perform, requires bilateral injection, and is not continuous. However, it provides first-stage analgesia without any motor block, is associated with less fetal bradycardia than a paracervical block, and may be useful for patients with previous back surgery.

The pudendal nerve innervates the vaginal, vulva, and perineum. *Bilateral pudendal nerve block* provides anesthesia for spontaneous vaginal and low- or outlet-forceps delivery, but not mid-forceps delivery or exploration of the upper vagina, cervix, or uterine cavity. The pudendal nerve can be blocked via the transperineal or transvaginal route. Most obstetricians in the United States employ the transvaginal route. Maternal and fetal complications of pudendal nerve block are unusual. Fetal complications include fetal trauma and direct fetal injection of local anesthetic.

Perineal infiltration of local anesthetic is often performed immediately before or after delivery to provide anesthesia for an episiotomy or repair. Perineal infiltration provides no motor relaxation. Complications included direct injection of local anesthetic into the fetal scalp, resulting in neonatal local anesthetic toxicity.

CONCLUSION

Childbirth pain is one of the most painful experiences women will endure in their lifetimes. Labor and delivery pain can be treated most effectively, safely for the mother and baby, with neuraxial (spinal or epidural) analgesia. However, this mode of analgesia is labor intensive and expensive, and it is not an option for many women in developing countries. Systemic opioid analgesia is widely used in many settings, but it has not been well studied and is not effective for many women. More sophisticated methods of delivering systemic opioids, such as patient-controlled techniques, and newer drugs, such as remifentanil, offer promise of improved analgesia. Nonpharmacologic techniques may mitigate labor pain and suffering, but they have also not been well studied. Further study is required to identify low-cost, effective methods and drugs for labor analgesia.

REFERENCES

1. Melzack R. The myth of painless childbirth (the John J. Bonica lecture). *Pain* 1984;19(4):321–37.
2. Lang AJ, Sorrell JT, Rodgers CS, Lebeck MM. Anxiety sensitivity as a predictor of labor pain. *Eur J Pain* 2006;10(3):263–70.
3. Bonica JJ. *Principles and Practice of Obstetric Analgesia and Anesthesia*. Philadelphia, PA: FA Davis; 1969.
4. Simkin P, Bolding A. Update on nonpharmacologic approaches to relieve labor pain and prevent suffering. *J Midwifery Womens Health* 2004;49(6): 489–504.
5. Field T. Pregnancy and labor alternative therapy research. *Altern Ther Health Med* 2008;14(5): 28–34.
6. Tournaire M, Theau-Yonneau A. Complementary and alternative approaches to pain relief during labor. *Evid Based Complement Alternat Med* 2007;4(4):409–17.
7. Smith CA, Collins CT, Crowther CA. Aromatherapy for pain management in labour. *Cochrane Database Syst Rev* 2011;(7):CD009215.
8. Dowswell T, Bedwell C, Lavender T, Neilson JP. Transcutaneous electrical nerve stimulation (TENS) for pain relief in labour. *Cochrane Database Syst Rev* 2009;(2):CD007214.
9. Hodnett ED, Gates S, Hofmeyr GJ, Sakala C, Weston J. Continuous support for women during childbirth. *Cochrane Database Syst Rev* 2011;(2): CD003766.
10. Hutton EK, Kasperink M, Rutten M, Reitsma A, Wainman B. Sterile water injection for labour pain: a systematic review and meta-analysis of randomised controlled trials. *BJOG* 2009;116(9): 1158–66.
11. Simkin PP, O'Hara M. Nonpharmacologic relief of pain during labor: systematic reviews of five methods. *Am J Obstet Gynecol* 2002;186 (5 Suppl):S131–59.
12. Cluett ER, Nikodem VC, McCandlish RE, Burns EE. Immersion in water in pregnancy, labour and birth. *Cochrane Database Syst Rev* 2004;(2):CD000111.
13. Smith CA, Collins CT, Cyna AM, Crowther CA. Complementary and alternative therapies for pain management in labour. *Cochrane Database Syst Rev* 2006;(4):CD003521.

14. Smith CA, Collins CT, Crowther CA, Levett KM. Acupuncture or acupressure for pain management in labour. *Cochrane Database Syst Rev* 2011;(7): CD009232.

15. Cho SH, Lee H, Ernst E. Acupuncture for pain relief in labour: a systematic review and meta-analysis. *BJOG*;117(8):907–20.

16. Yentis S. The use of Entonox® for labour pain should be abandoned. *Int J Obstet Anesth* 2001;10(1): 25–7.

17. American College of Nurse-Midwives. Nitrous oxide for labor analgesia. *J Midwifery Womens Health*;55(3):292–6.

18. Rosen MA. Nitrous oxide for relief of labor pain: a systematic review. *Am J Obstet Gynecol* 2002;186(5 Suppl):S110–26.

19. Lucas DN, Siemaszko O, Yentis SM. Maternal hypoxaemia associated with the use of Entonox in labour. *Int J Obstet Anesth* 2000;9(4):270–2.

20. Nelson KE, Eisenach JC. Intravenous butorphanol, meperidine, and their combination relieve pain and distress in women in labor. *Anesthesiology* 2005;102(5):1008–13.

21. Anderson D. A review of systemic opioids commonly used for labor pain relief. *J Midwifery Womens Health* 2011;56(3):222–39.

22. Ullman R, Smith LA, Burns E, Mori R, Dowswell T. Parenteral opioids for maternal pain relief in labour. *Cochrane Database Syst Rev* 2010;(9):CD007396.

23. Latta KS, Ginsberg B, Barkin RL. Meperidine: a critical review. *Am J Ther* 2002;9(1):53–68.

24. Gordon DB, Jones HD, Goshman LM, Foley DK, Bland SE. A quality improvement approach to reducing use of meperidine. *Jt Comm J Qual Improv* 2000;26(12):686–99.

25. Hill JB, Alexander JM, Sharma SK, McIntire DD, Leveno KJ. A comparison of the effects of epidural and meperidine analgesia during labor on fetal heart rate. *Obstet Gynecol* 2003;102(2):333–7.

26. Caldwell J, Wakile LA, Notarianni LJ, et al. Maternal and neonatal disposition of pethidine in childbirth—a study using quantitative gas chromatography-mass spectrometry. *Life Sci* 1978;22(7):589–96.

27. Douma MR, Middeldorp JM, Verwey RA, Dahan A, Stienstra R. A randomised comparison of intravenous remifentanil patient-controlled analgesia with epidural ropivacaine/sufentanil during labour. *Int J Obstet Anesth* 2011;20(2):118–23.

28. Volmanen P, Sarvela J, Akural EI, Raudaskoski T, Korttila K, Alahuhta S. Intravenous remifentanil vs. epidural levobupivacaine with fentanyl for pain relief in early labour: a randomised, controlled, double-blinded study. *Acta Anaesthesiol Scand* 2008;52(2):249–55.

29. Hinova A, Fernando R. Systemic remifentanil for labor analgesia. *Anesth Analg* 2009;109(6): 1925–9.

30. Leong WL, Sng BL, Sia AT. A comparison between remifentanil and meperidine for labor analgesia: a systematic review. *Anesth Analg* 2011; 113(4):818–25.

31. Bucklin BA, Hawkins JL, Anderson JR, Ullrich FA. Obstetric anesthesia workforce survey: twenty-year update. *Anesthesiology* 2005;103(3):645–53.

32. Richardson A, Mmata C. *National Health Service Maternity Statistics 2005–2006*. The Information Centre; 2007

33. Arkoosh VA, Palmer CM, Yun EM, et al. A randomized, double-masked, multicenter comparison of the safety of continuous intrathecal labor analgesia using a 28-gauge catheter versus continuous epidural labor analgesia. *Anesthesiology* 2008;108(2):286–98.

34. Anim-Somuah M, Smyth R, Howell C. Epidural versus non-epidural or no analgesia in labour. *Cochrane Database Syst Rev* 2005;(4):CD000331.

35. Simmons SW, Cyna AM, Dennis AT, Hughes D. Combined spinal-epidural versus epidural analgesia in labour. *Cochrane Database Syst Rev* 2007;(3):CD003401.

36. Pert CB, Kuhar MJ, Snyder SH. Opiate receptor: autoradiographic localization in rat brain. *Proc Natl Acad Sci USA* 1976;73(10):3729–33.

37. Polley LS, Columb MO, Wagner DS, Naughton NN. Dose-dependent reduction of the minimum local analgesic concentration of bupivacaine by sufentanil for epidural analgesia in labor. *Anesthesiology* 1998;89(3):626–32.

38. Justins DM, Francis D, Houlton PG, Reynolds F. A controlled trial of extradural fentanyl in labour. *Br J Anaesth* 1982;54(4):409–14.

39. Beilin Y, Guinn NR, Bernstein HH, Zahn J, Hossain S, Bodian CA. Local anesthetics and mode of delivery: bupivacaine versus ropivacaine versus levobupivacaine. *Anesth Analg* 2007;105(3):756–63.

40. Beilin Y, Halpern S. Focused review: ropivacaine versus bupivacaine for epidural labor analgesia. *Anesth Analg* 2010;111(2):482–7.

41. Bader AM, Fragneto R, Terui K, Arthur GR, Loferski B, Datta S. Maternal and neonatal fentanyl and bupivacaine concentrations after epidural infusion during labor. *Anesth Analg* 1995;81(4):829–32.

42. Hicks JA, Jenkins JG, Newton MC, Findley IL. Continuous epidural infusion of 0.075% bupivacaine for pain relief in labour. *Anaesthesia* 1988;43(4):289–92.

43. van der Vyver M, Halpern S, Joseph G. Patient-controlled epidural analgesia versus

continuous infusion for labour analgesia: a meta-analysis. *Br J Anaesth* 2002;89(3):459–65.

44. Halpern SH, Carvalho B. Patient-controlled epidural analgesia for labor. *Anesth Analg* 2009; 108(3):921–8.

45. Wong CA, Scavone BM, Loffredi M, Wang WY, Peaceman AM, Ganchiff JN. The dose-response of intrathecal sufentanil added to bupivacaine for labor analgesia. *Anesthesiology* 2000;92(6):1553–8.

46. Herman NL, Choi KC, Affleck PJ, et al. Analgesia, pruritus, and ventilation exhibit a dose-response relationship in parturients receiving intrathecal fentanyl during labor. *Anesth Analg* 1999;89(2):378–83.

47. Segal S. Labor epidural analgesia and maternal fever. *Anesth Analg* 2010;111(6):1467–75.

48. Clarke VT, Smiley RM, Finster M. Uterine hyperactivity after intrathecal injection of fentanyl for analgesia during labor: a cause of fetal bradycardia? *Anesthesiology* 1994;81(4):1083.

49. Shnider SM, Abboud TK, Artal R, Henriksen EH, Stefani SJ, Levinson G. Maternal catecholamines decrease during labor after lumbar epidural anesthesia. *Am J Obstet Gynecol* 1983;147(1):13–5.

50. Albright GA, Forster RM. Does combined spinal-epidural analgesia with subarachnoid sufentanil increase the incidence of emergency cesarean delivery? *Reg Anesth* 1997;22(5):400–5.

51. Mardirosoff C, Dumont L, Boulvain M, Tramer MR. Fetal bradycardia due to intrathecal opioids for labour analgesia: a systematic review. *Br J Obstet Gynaecol* 2002;109(3):274–81.

52. Van de Velde M, Teunkens A, Hanssens M, Vandermeersch E, Verhaeghe J. Intrathecal sufentanil and fetal heart rate abnormalities: a double-blind, double placebo-controlled trial comparing two forms of combined spinal epidural analgesia with epidural analgesia in labor. *Anesth Analg* 2004;98(4):1153–9.

53. Weiniger CF, Wand S, Nadjari M, et al. Post-void residual volume in labor: a prospective study comparing parturients with and without epidural analgesia. *Acta Anaesthesiol Scand* 2006;50(10):1297–303.

54. Loughnan BA, Carli F, Romney M, Dore CJ, Gordon H. Epidural analgesia and backache: a randomized controlled comparison with intramuscular meperidine for analgesia during labour. *Br J Anaesth* 2002;89(3):466–72.

55. Howell CJ, Kidd C, Roberts W, et al. A randomised controlled trial of epidural compared with non-epidural analgesia in labour. *BJOG* 2001;108(1):27–33.

56. Choi PT, Galinski SE, Takeuchi L, Lucas S, Tamayo C, Jadad AR. PDPH is a common complication of neuraxial blockade in parturients: a meta-analysis of obstetrical studies. *Can J Anaesth* 2003;50(5):460–9.

57. Climie CR. The place of continuous lumbar epidural analgesia in the management of abnormally prolonged labour. *Med J Aust* 1964;2:447–50.

58. Moir DD, Willocks J. Management of incoordinate uterine action under continuous epidural analgesia. *Br Med J* 1967;3(5562):396–400.

59. Reich AM. Paravertebral lumbar sympathetic block in labor: a report on 500 deliveries by a fractional procedure producing continuous conduction anesthesia. *Am J Obstet Gynecol* 1951;61(6):1263–76.

60. Sharma SK, McIntire DD, Wiley J, Leveno KJ. Labor analgesia and cesarean delivery: an individual patient meta-analysis of nulliparous women. *Anesthesiology* 2004;100(1):142–8.

61. Alexander JM, Sharma SK, McIntire DD, Wiley J, Leveno KJ. Intensity of labor pain and cesarean delivery. *Anesth Analg* 2001;92(6):1524–8.

62. Hess PE, Pratt SD, Soni AK, Sarna MC, Oriol NE. An association between severe labor pain and cesarean delivery. *Anesth Analg* 2000;90(4):881–6.

63. Panni MK, Segal S. Local anesthetic requirements are greater in dystocia than in normal labor. *Anesthesiology* 2003;98(4):957–63.

64. Wong CA, Scavone BM, Peaceman AM, et al. The risk of cesarean delivery with neuraxial analgesia given early versus late in labor. *N Engl J Med* 2005;352(7):655–65.

65. Wang F, Shen X, Guo X, Peng Y, Gu X. Epidural analgesia in the latent phase of labor and the risk of cesarean delivery: a five-year randomized controlled trial. *Anesthesiology* 2009;111(4):871–80.

66. Comparative Obstetric Mobile Epidural Trial Study Group UK. Effect of low-dose mobile versus traditional epidural techniques on mode of delivery: a randomised controlled trial. *Lancet* 2001;358(9275):19–23.

67. Nageotte MP, Larson D, Rumney PJ, Sidhu M, Hollenbach K. Epidural analgesia compared with combined spinal-epidural analgesia during labor in nulliparous women. *N Eng J Med* 1997;337(24):1715–9.

68. Camann W, Brazelton TB. Use and abuse of neonatal neurobehavioral testing. *Anesthesiology* 2000;92(1):3–5.

69. Ramin SM, Gambling DR, Lucas MJ, Sharma SK, Sidawi JE, Leveno KJ. Randomized trial of epidural versus intravenous analgesia during labor. *Obstet Gynecol* 1995;86(5):783–9.

9

PAIN IN PREGNANCY

Maryam Jowza, Geeta Nagpal, Christopher M. Viscomi, and James P. Rathmell

INTRODUCTION

The appearance of musculoskeletal pain during the course of normal pregnancy is almost universal. In some cases, the pain can be severe, and it can limit almost any activity. Many women enter pregnancy with preexisting painful disorders, and management of ongoing pain and painful exacerbations can be challenging. This chapter will review the clinical characteristics, diagnosis, and approach to management of some of the more common painful conditions that occur during the course of pregnancy.

PREGNANCY-RELATED LOW BACK PAIN

Pregnancy-related low back pain is characterized as pain occurring in the lumbosacral region (Fig. 9.1). Fifty percent of women will experience low back pain during their pregnancies, and this is commonly looked upon as a normal part of pregnancy.[1] In one-third of pregnant women, back pain is severe and compromises normal everyday activity.[2] The pain is similar to the low back pain women experience in the nonpregnant state and is often described as dull and aching in nature. There can be a limitation in range of motion of the lumbar spine, and pain is often exacerbated by both forward flexion and palpation of the erector spinae muscles.[3]

The onset of low back pain occurs most commonly around the 18th week of pregnancy, with the peak intensity between the 24th and 36th weeks.[3] However, pregnancy-related low back pain can start as early as the first trimester or as late as several weeks postpartum. Sixteen percent of women with pregnancy-related low back pain report persistent pain 6 years later; pregnancy is a well-recognized risk factor for the development of persistent low back pain.[4]

The etiology of pregnancy-related low back pain is likely multifactorial. The lumbar lordosis, to balance the anterior weight of the womb, becomes markedly accentuated during pregnancy and may represent a mechanical cause for the pain.[5] Endocrine changes during pregnancy may also play a role in the development of back pain. Relaxin, a polypeptide secreted by the corpus luteum, softens the ligaments around the pelvic joints and cervix, allowing accommodation of the developing fetus and facilitating vaginal delivery. This laxity may cause pain by allowing an exaggerated range of motion.[6]

Evaluation of the pregnant patient with low back pain must begin with a thorough history and physical examination. The aim is to exclude other causes of pain that are obstetric complications. Preterm labor, placental abruption,

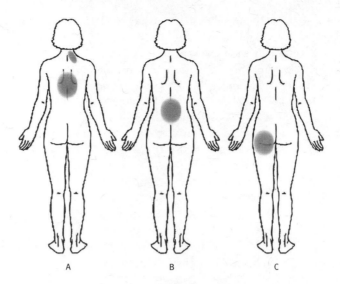

FIGURE 9.1 Three types of pain were reported by a group of 855 women studied between 12 menstrual weeks of pregnancy and delivery. Forty-nine percent of women reported back pain at some point during pregnancy: (A) high back pain by 10%; (B) low back pain by 40%; (C) sacroiliac pain by 50%. (Adapted with permission from reference Ostgaard HC, Andersson GBJ, Karlsson K. Prevalence of back pain in pregnancy. *Spine* 1991;16:549–52.)

degeneration of uterine fibroids, round ligament pain, and chorioamnionitis can all present with low back pain. Urologic disorders, including hydonephrosis, pyelonephrosis, and renal calculi, may also present with low back discomfort. A history of trauma, cancer, drug abuse, neurologic symptoms, and fever should initiate a workup for serious causes of pain. With signs of focal infection and tenderness over the spinous processes, a diagnosis of osteomyelitis may be suggested. Positive straight leg raise (typical low back pain with radiation to the ipsilateral lower extremity on flexion of the leg at the hip with the knee held in full extension) is consistent with herniated nucleus pulposus; subluxation of the sacroiliac joint typically produces pain limited to the lumbosacral junction when performing the same maneuver. The presence of neurologic signs, including loss of bowel or bladder function, sensory or motor deficit, or loss of deep tendon reflexes, may suggest cauda equina syndrome or lumbar nerve root compression.[3] The appearance of symptoms arising from compression of the cauda equina is rare and most often stems from a large central disc herniation; lateral disc herniations are far more common and may cause neurologic signs and symptoms arising from involvement of a single spinal nerve.

Although radicular symptoms often accompany low back pain during pregnancy, herniated nucleus pulposus has an incidence of only 1:10,000 pregnancies.[7] Magnetic resonance imaging of the lumbar spine in pregnant patients with or without back pain demonstrates the same prevalence of lumbar disc herniation as nonpregnant asymptomatic patients.[3] Imaging studies also reveal that pregnant women do not have an increased prevalence of lumbar disc abnormalities.[8] Direct pressure of the fetus on the lumbosacral nerves or lumbar plexus has been postulated as a more common cause of radicular symptoms than disc herniation.

The diagnosis of pregnancy-related low back pain is largely based solely on clinical criteria. As discussed subsequently in this chapter in the section on pelvic girdle pain, X-ray imaging techniques such as computed tomography scans are not ideal in pregnancy. However, pregnancy is not an absolute contraindication to radiographic evaluation. No detectable growth or mental abnormalities have been associated with fetal exposure to less than 10 rads—the dose received during a typical three-view spinal series typically does not exceed 1.5 rads.[9] Nonetheless, plain radiographs seldom contribute vital information—primarily when fracture, dislocation, and destructive lesions of the bone are suspected. MRI is thought to be safe throughout pregnancy, although there are no studies with long-term follow-up. Therefore, its use should be reserved for those patients where there is strong suspicion of abnormality.[3]

Electrodiagnostic studies (collectively referred to as electromyography and nerve conduction studies [EMG/NCV]) serve as good screening tests in the patient with new onset of low back pain accompanied by sensory or motor symptoms. When the clinical presentation is confusing, EMG/NCV can aid in differentiating peripheral nerve lesions, polyneuropathies, and plexopathies from single radiculopathies. However, false-negative EMG/NCV results are common, especially in the case of a herniated nucleus pulposus causing compression of a single nerve root.[10]

There are some studies that suggest that the risk of low back pain during pregnancy can be reduced by physical exercise and fitness prior to pregnancy.[11] However, there is a paucity of studies dealing specifically with prevention of low back pain during pregnancy after conception.

Treatment of pregnancy-related low back pain begins with patient education about the common causes of back pain during pregnancy. Back care classes are commonly available and focus on anatomy, ergonomics, correct posture, and relaxation techniques.[3] If the pain remains poorly controlled, referral to a physical therapist for instruction in body mechanics and low back exercises may be beneficial. In a recent Cochrane review of the treatment of low back pain, pregnancy-specific exercise programs, physiotherapy, and acupuncture added to usual prenatal care appeared to reduce back pain more than usual prenatal care.[12] When compared to physiotherapy, acupuncture may be more effective. Participation in water gymnastics programs also reduced the number of back pain–related work absences.[12]

PELVIC GIRDLE PAIN

Pelvic girdle pain (PGP) is a clinical syndrome occurring during pregnancy that is distinct from pregnancy-related low back pain. Women with PGP report pain extending from the posterior iliac crest and gluteal fold over the anterior and posterior elements of the bony pelvis. The same or similar syndromes have carried other names, including symphasis pubis dysfunction, pelvic joint insufficiency, pelvic girdle relaxation, and posterior pelvic pain. Pain is often described as stabbing, sometimes burning, in the region of the sacroiliac joints and can extend anteriorly to region of pubic symphasis. Radiation of pain to the groin, perineum, and posterior thigh in a nondermatomal pattern is common. The location of pain can change during the course of pregnancy.

The onset of PGP occurs from the first trimester to 1 month postpartum, though onset of symptoms during the third trimester is most common. In most patients, symptoms subside by 6 months postpartum. The actual incidence is difficult to establish, given the wide array of symptoms and absence of specific diagnostic criteria. The reported incidence of PGP ranges from 16% to 25%.[13,14]

The etiology of PGP remains unclear, but it is likely multifactorial with mechanical, hormonal, and genetic influences. Mechanical factors relate to separation of the pubic symphysis during pregnancy. Hormonal changes include elevated levels of progesterone and relaxin. Genetic influence is likely based on the increased prevalence of PGP among first-degree relatives.[13]

Diagnosis of PGP is largely based on clinical criteria. The aim of the history and physical is to exclude other causes of pain and "red flag" conditions such as inflammatory, infectious, or neoplastic causes. Many women with PGP have tenderness to deep palpation of the suprapubic and sacroiliac region along the course of the long posterior sacroiliac and sacrotuberous ligaments. The pubic symphysis itself is often tender. Because there is no specific diagnostic test for PGP, Leadbetter developed a scoring system based on five discrete symptoms to aid in screening pregnant women.[15] The symptoms thought to be associated with PGP include pubic bone pain on walking, turning over in bed, climbing stairs, standing on one leg, and previous damage to back or pelvis. Each of the previous symptoms earns one point, and a score of 2 or more is considered diagnostic for PGP (Table 9.1).

Radiographic evaluation is rarely undertaken during pregnancy for fear of causing adverse

Table 9.1   Clinical Scoring System for Establishing a Diagnosis of Symphysis Pubis Dysfunction (Pelvic Girdle Pain) during Pregnancy

- Pubic bone pain on walking
- Pubic bone pain on turning over in bed
- Pubic bone pain on climbing stairs
- Pubic bone pain on standing on one leg
- Previous damage to back or pelvis

Note: Using a score of 1 for each of the following symptoms, a score of 2 and above is considered diagnostic of symphysis pubis dysfunction.[15]

effects on the developing fetus, and it is generally used in postpartum women. Investigations include anterior-posterior (AP) inlet and outer pelvic films to quantify the degree of symphaseal separation. Cortical sclerosis and spurring can also be identified on X-ray. Subtle symphasis separation can be detected with single-limb or flamingo stances. On the AP view, a step off of more than 2 mm (or 7 mm on flamingo views) denotes pelvic instability by some authors. The severity of pain, however, does not correlate with the degree of separation.

Magnetic resonance imaging can safely be used during pregnancy. It offers enhanced soft tissue visualization and can aid in the differential diagnosis. Some authors have also made use of transvaginal and transperineal ultrasound to visualize the pubic symphysis. It is unclear which among these diagnostic approaches is best, and it is also unclear that imaging offers any further information to guide clinical management beyond that offered by history and physical examination alone.

Guided local anesthetic injection into the sacroiliac joint or the pubic symphysis can have diagnostic and therapeutic value. As most clinicians wish to limit exposure to ionizing radiation during pregnancy, ultrasound can be used effectively to guide needle placement adjacent to the sacroiliac joint. Relief after an intra-articular injection is indicative only of intra-articular pathology. Extra-articular pathologies contributing to pelvic girdle pain such as strain of the superficial long sacroiliac joint ligament are unlikely to improve after an intra-articular injection.

There are a limited number of high-quality studies on the management of PGP during pregnancy. Treatment options during pregnancy are also limited by potential hazard to the fetus. After delivery, the majority of women do improve within a few months. Nonpharmacologic treatment modalities used during pregnancy include physical therapy with pelvic tilt exercises, rotational manipulation of the sacroiliac joint, water gymnastics, transcutaneous electrical stimulation (TENS), and acupuncture.[12] With use of TENS during pregnancy, there is theoretical concern about inadvertent induction of labor through use of certain acupuncture points as well as fetal cardiac conduction disturbances with passage of current through the fetal heart. Limited data suggest that TENS is safe during pregnancy. A recent Cochrane review on use of TENS for treatment of pain during labor found no deleterious effects on the mother or the fetus.[16] Given the theoretical concerns, some experts recommend keeping the current density low and avoiding certain acupuncture points when TENS is used during pregnancy.[17]

Migraine Headache during Pregnancy and Lactation

Clinicians are often confronted with the occurrence of headache during pregnancy as recurring headaches happen most commonly during the childbearing years. Migraine headaches are among the most common type of headache in women during pregnancy and can be a disabling. The prevalence of migraine among women is greater than in men, and this is thought in part due to the influence of female sex hormones. Migraine headaches vary with the female reproductive events that include menarche, menstruation, oral contraceptives, pregnancy, and menopause.[18] Eighty percent of female migraineurs report the onset of migraine headaches between the ages of 10 and 39 years, suggesting that sex hormones do play a significant role in the pathogenesis.[19] They typically improve in the first trimester of pregnancy, when there is a sudden and sustained increase in estrodiol levels. In fact, 50%–80% of patients who suffer from migraines experience a significant reduction in frequency or total cessation of migraine attacks during pregnancy. However, women with headaches persisting into the second trimester are less likely to improve thereafter.

Migraine headaches rarely begin during pregnancy (<3%) and if they do, they typically begin during the first trimester. New headaches or significant changes in headache symptoms or activity during pregnancy require evaluation to differentiate between benign and pathologic causes of headache. One report of nine women presenting with migraine-like headaches during pregnancy found that four were severely thrombocytopenic, two met criteria for preeclampsia, and one had a threatened abortion.[20] The literature is replete with reports of intracranial pathology that mimicked migraines during pregnancy, including strokes, pseudotumor cerebri, tumors, aneurysms, arteriovenous malformations, and cerebral venous thrombosis.[21] Metabolic causes of headache during pregnancy include illicit drug use (most notably, cocaine),[22] anti-phospholipid antibody syndrome, and choriocarcinoma.[23]

Pregnancy outcomes, including preterm labor, low birth weights, or congenital abnormalities, do not seem to be impacted by the occurrence of migraine headaches during pregnancy. However, a number of studies have shown an association between the history of the migraine and an increased risk of preeclampsia during pregnancy. A prospective study of 485 patients with migraines prior to pregnancy revealed a 10-fold increased incidence of preeclampsia compared with the general population.[24]

Patients who present with their first severe headache during pregnancy should be promptly and thoroughly evaluated. Only when secondary causes of headache in pregnancy, including head trauma, cerebral venous thrombosis, pre-eclampsia, subarachnoid hemmorhage, ischemic stroke, vasculitis, or dehydration, have been ruled out should pregnant women be diagnosed with a primary headache. The first step is a detailed history and neurologic examination. Focal neurologic abnormalities, papilledema, and seizures in the setting of headache warrant further investigation. Suggested diagnostic tests for new onset headache during pregnancy include urinalysis, blood chemistries, hematologic studies, liver function tests, and coagulation studies. Brain imaging is also an important component of the workup. Magnetic resonance imaging without gadolinium is safe throughout pregnancy and should be the imaging modality of choice. In the patient who presents with sudden onset of the "worst headache of my life," a subarachnoid hemorrhage should be ruled out.[21] In these patients computed tomography (CT) of the brain is the preferred imaging modality. If CT of the brain is negative for hemorrhage, a lumbar puncture should be performed, and the spinal fluid evaluated for subarachnoid blood and infectious causes of headache. Use of CT during pregnancy increases the subsequent risk of childhood cancer in the fetus. The decision to proceed with CT imaging during pregnancy is complex; basic guidelines and a framework for decision making are widely available.[25] Progressively worsening headaches in the setting of sudden weight gain should suggest preeclampsia or pseudotumor cerebri. Elevated blood pressure and proteinuria points toward preeclampsia; visual disturbances, hyperreflexia, and elevated serum uric acid can also be found in patients with preeclampsia.

Postpartum headache is common and occurs in 30%–40% of all women.[20,22] Most occur in the first week after delivery, and about 50% of those who experience relief of their migraine during pregnancy have recurrence a short time after delivery. This phenomenon may be secondary to the rapid ovarian withdrawal of progesterone and estradiol. Lactation can inhibit ovulatory cycles during the peurperium and is characterized by increased levels of prolactin and low levels of estradiol. In bottle-feeding women, the hormonal cycle is rapidly restored, which may contribute to it being a main risk factor for postnatal recurrence of migraine.[26]

For pregnant women with a history of migraines prior to pregnancy and a normal neurological examination, the therapeutic challenge is to achieve control of the headaches while minimizing risk to the fetus. Nonpharmacologic techniques, including relaxation, biofeedback, and elimination of certain foods, often suffice for treatment. Marcus et al.[27] demonstrated significant reduction in headache, which continued throughout pregnancy and at the 1-year follow-up, using a combination of relaxation training, thermal biofeedback, and physical therapy exercises. The next section discusses some of the frequently used pharmacologic agents used for treatment of migraine headaches and their use during pregnancy.

ACETAMINOPHEN

If pharmacologic therapy appears warranted, acetaminophen (Pregnancy Category B) is safe and effective.[28] Acetaminophen has no known teratogenic properties, does not inhibit prostaglandin synthesis or platelet function, and is hepatotoxic only in extreme overdose.[29] Acetaminophen does enter breast milk, although maximal neonatal ingestion would be less than 2% of a maternal dose.[30] Acetaminophen is considered compatible with breastfeeding.[31] A drawback to acetaminophen is the potential for medication overuse and rebound headache, which could develop into daily chronic headaches.

CAFFEINE

Caffeine is a methylxanthine often used in combination analgesics for the management of vascular headaches. It is readily absorbed from the gastrointestinal tract and crosses the placenta such that concentrations in the fetus are similar to maternal plasma levels.[32] While older studies suggest that caffeine use during pregnancy may lead to spontaneous abortion, intrauterine growth restriction, low birth weight, and prematurity, more recent studies do not.[33] Although the data are not strongly compelling against caffeine use in pregnancy, most obstetricians recommend that pregnant women limit caffeine intake to less than 300 mg per day. To date, there is no evidence for birth defects related to caffeine.[34] Caffeine use is also associated with certain cardiovascular changes. Ingestion of modest doses of caffeine (100 mg/m^2, a dose similar to that found in 2 cups of brewed coffee) in caffeine-naïve subjects produces increased maternal heart rate and mean arterial pressure, increased peak aortic flow velocities, and decrease in fetal heart rate.[35] The modest decrease in fetal heart rate and increased frequency of fetal heart rate accelerations may confound interpretation of fetal heart tracings. There are reports of fetal arrhythmias secondary to excessive maternal caffeine ingestion. The rhythm disturbances include supraventricular tachyarrhythmias, atrial flutter, and premature atrial contractions.[36]

Moderate ingestion of caffeine during lactation (up to 2 cups of coffee per day) does not appear to affect the infant. Breast milk usually contains less than 1% of the maternal dose of caffeine, with peak breast milk levels appearing 1 hour after maternal ingestion. Excessive caffeine use may cause increased wakefulness and irritability in the infant.[37]

SUMATRIPTAN

Sumatriptan is a selective serotonin agonist that has achieved widespread use because of its efficacy in the treatment of migraine headaches. Sumatriptan is advantageous in the treatment of migraine headache in pregnancy because it does not share uterine contractile properties with ergotamine. It, along with all other triptans, is considered to be Pregnancy Category C by the Food and Drug Administration (FDA). In January, 1996, Glaxo-Wellcome established a registry to prospectively evaluate the risk of sumatriptan use during pregnancy.[38] The accumulated evidence from sumatriptan's pregnancy registry and other studies suggest that this drug is a safe therapeutic option for the treatment of migraine attacks in pregnant women. To date, the evidence for safety of other triptans during pregnancy is also reassuring, though more studies are needed.[39,40,41]

A minimal amount of sumatriptan is excreted into breast milk, and it is considered safe to use while breastfeeding. The use of sumatriptan during lactation has not been well studied. One study of a single 6 mg subcutaneous sumatriptan administration to lactating women found total breast milk sumatriptan to be only 0.24% of the maternal dose. Since sumatriptan is poorly absorbed from the infant gastrointestinal tract, only 14% of the drug ingested by the fetus would be bioavailable. Even this minor exposure could be largely avoided by expressing and discarding all milk for 8 hours after injection.[42]

NONSTEROIDAL ANTI-INFLAMMATORY DRUGS

Ibuprofen and naproxen are the most commonly used nonsteroidal anti-inflammatory drugs (NSAIDs) for abortive management of migraines; however, they are FDA Pregnancy Category C prior to 30 weeks and Category D in the third trimester. Like acetaminophen, NSAIDs are safe in the postpartum period with breastfeeding. The short-term use of mild opioid analgesics like hydrocodone, alone or in combination with acetaminophen, also appears to carry little risk (Table 9.2). Use of opioids during pregnancy is discussed in detail elsewhere in this text. When oral analgesics prove ineffective, hospital admission and administration of parenteral opioids may be required.

MIGRAINE PROPHYLAXIS

A history of three to four incapacitating headaches per month warrants consideration of prophylactic therapy.[28] If the frequency of the headache or headaches is less than three to four per month, but they are severe and unmanageable with acute therapies, prophylactic therapy should be considered to prevent maternal dehydration, which could cause fetal distress. Some of the commonly used medications for migraine prophylaxis will be discussed.

ANTICONVULSANTS

A number of anticonvulsant medications are used for migraine prophylaxis as well as chronic pain conditions. Most data regarding the fetal risk in women taking anticonvulsants are derived from the treatment of epilepsy. Although epilepsy itself is not associated with increased risk of congenital malformations, some theoretical risk may exist. Despite this, data from anticonvulsant use in epileptic women are used to assess risk of the same medications when used for pain conditions. Recently, the American Academy of Neurology and American Epilepsy Society subcommittee undertook a systematic review of the evidence for teratogenic potential and perinatal outcomes among pregnant women on antiepileptic medication.[43,44] The review found that valproic

Table 9.2   Oral Analgesics for Treating Pain during Pregnancy

DRUG	EQUIANALGESIC ORAL DOSE (MG)	HOW SUPPLIED	FDA RISK CATEGORY
Acetaminophen	—	325-, 500-, 625-mg tabs; 500-mg/15-mL elixir	B
Codeine	60	15-, 30-, 60-mg tabs; 15-mg/5-mL elixir	C[a]
Acetaminophen with codeine	—	300–15, 300–30, 300–60 mg tabs; 120–12/5 mL elixir	C[a]
Hydrocodone	60	[b]	B[a]
Acetaminophen with hydrocodone	—	500–2.5, 500–5, 500–7.5, 660–10 mg tabs; 500–7.5/15 mL elixir	C[a]
Oxycodone	10	5-mg tabs; 5-mg/5-mL elixir	B[a]
Acetaminophen with oxycodone	—	325–5, 500–5 mg tabs; 325–5/5 mL elixir	C[a]
Morphine	10	15-, 30-mg tabs; 10-, 20-mg/5-mL elixir	B[a]
Hydromorphone	2	2-, 4-, 8-mg tabs; 5-mg/5-mL elixir	B[a]

Note:. There is wide variability in the duration of analgesic action from patient to patient. All of the oral agents listed are generally started with dosing every 4–6 h; the dosing interval can then be adjusted as needed to maintain adequate analgesia.

[a]All opioid analgesics are FDA Risk Category D if used for prolonged periods or in large doses near term.

[b]There is no oral formulation of hydrocodone alone available in the United States.

acid exposure, especially in the first trimester, contributes to neural tube defects, facial cleft, and possibly hypospadias. The review also found that neonates of women taking anticonvulsants were also more likely to be small for gestational age and have lower Apgar scores. Treatment with valproic acid is more likely to be associated with a major congenital malformation than treatment with carbamazepine or lamotrigine. There is a possible dose relationship for development of congenital malformations for valproic acid during the first trimester. Though not consistent throughout all of the studies, valproic acid dose of greater than 1,000 mg daily may be associated with greatest risk of malformations.

In the same review, carbamazepine was associated with increased risk of cleft palate, but this was not confirmed by another study focusing specifically on carbamazepine using the EUROCAT (European Surveillance of Congenital Anomalies) database. Though this study did not find an association between carbamazepine and clefts, it did find an association with spina bifida.

First-trimester topiramate therapy has been associated with a higher risk of major malformations with cleft lip being the most commonly cited malformation.[45] Its use has also been linked with low birth weight.[46] The studies on topiramate, however, are limited.

Gabapentin is an anticonvulsant that is being used for treatment of neuropathic pain syndromes. Very little and conflicting information exists about the safety of gabapentin in pregnant women. In their prescribing information, the manufacturer reports a series of nine women who received gabapentin during their pregnancy.[47] Four women elected pregnancy termination, four had normal outcomes, and one neonate had pyloric stenosis and an inguinal hernia.

In a pilot study on use of gabapentin for treatment of hyperemesis gravidum two of the seven treated women gave birth to babies with congenital defects. In these two cases, gabapentin was started at 8 and 9 weeks gestation. One defect was a tethered cord, which occurred in a woman who had undergone in vitro fertilization for conception, and the other defect was hydronephrosis.[48] The link between gabapentin and the defects is unclear.

The results of the Gabapentin Registry Study do not show an increased risk for adverse maternal and fetal events. However, because of the small number of patients, there are insufficient data to counsel patients regarding the fetal risk of gabapentin use during pregnancy.[49]

β-BLOCKERS

Propranolol and other β-blockers are utilized in the chronic prophylaxis against migraine and nonmigraine vascular headaches. Most studies on β-blocker use during pregnancy involve women being treated for hypertension as opposed to migraine prophylaxis, and hypertension itself may increase the risk for small gestational age newborns.[50] A 2009 Cochrane review looking at β-blocker use for mild to moderate hypertension during pregnancy found that the effect of β-blockers on perinatal outcome is unclear.[51] Fetal effects that are noted with maternal use of propranolol and other β-blockers include decreased weight, potentially due to a modest decrease in maternal cardiac output, with consequent diminished placental perfusion.[52] Patients should be aware that fetal toxicity can result in complications, including intrauterine growth restriction, hypoglycemia, bradycardia ,and respiratory depression.[53] Longer acting agents should lead to less fluctuation in both maternal and fetal blood concentrations, and perhaps less fluctuation in the drug effects on fetal heart rate. The FDA rates all β-blockers as Category C with the exception of atenolol, which is rated as Category D.

In the lactating mother, propranolol doses of up to 240 mg/day appear to have minimal neonatal effects. The average neonatal exposure at this maternal dose is less than 1% of the therapeutic dose.[53] Atenolol is concentrated in breast milk, but it still results in subtherapeutic levels in the infant.[54]

ANTIDEPRESSANTS

While antidepressants are effective for prophylactic therapy in nonpregnant patients, the most commonly utilized medications of this class are FDA Category C or D. Imipramine and nortriptyline are FDA Category D, while amitryptyline and desipramine are rated as

Category C.[21] The selective serotonin receptor inhibitors are Category B or C and can be used with caution, especially if there is comorbid depression. There are very limited data, leading most physicians to avoid these medications. Withdrawal syndromes have been reported in neonates born to mothers using nortriptyline, imipramine, and desipramine with symptoms including irritability, colic, tachypnea, and urinary retention.[55] Amitriptyline, nortriptyline, and desipramine are all excreted into human milk. Pharmacokinetic modeling suggests that infants are exposed to about 1% of the maternal dose.[56] In a critical review of the literature regarding use of antidepressants during breastfeeding, Wisner et al. concluded that amitriptyline, nortriptyline, desipramine, clomipramine, and sertraline were not found in quantifiable amounts in nurslings and that no adverse effects were reported. The authors recommend use of these agents as the antidepressants of choice for breastfeeding women.

Duloxetine (a selective serotonin reuptake inhibitor) is representative of a new class of drug that combines inhibition of serotonin and norepinephrine reuptake. Duloxetine is efficacious for both depression and neuropathic pain, and it may have particular efficacy in diabetic neuropathy. Duloxetine is FDA pregnancy Category C, indicating potential risk and benefit. Neonates born to mothers receiving selective serotonin reuptake inhibitor or serotonin–norepinephrine reuptake inhibitors drugs may have a withdrawal reaction as discussed earlier. Although the relative risks and benefits of breastfeeding when a woman is receiving duloxetine have not been fully evaluated, the manufacturer advises against breastfeeding.

CALCIUM CHANNEL BLOCKERS

Limited anecdotal experience with calcium channel blockers (verapamil, nifedipine, and diltiazem are all FDA Category C) or mini-dose aspirin (80 mg/day) suggests they may be effective prophylactic agents during pregnancy.[21]

PAIN IN THE PREGNANT PATIENT WITH SICKLE CELL DISEASE

Sickle cell disease is an inherited multisystem disorder. The presence of abnormal hemoglobin within red blood cells leads to the cardinal features of the disease: chronic hemolytic anemia and recurrent painful episodes. Vaso-occlusive crisis is the most common maternal complication noted in parturients with sickle cell hemoglobinopathies.[57] Vaso-occlusive crises follow a characteristic pattern of recurrent sudden attacks of pain, usually involving the abdomen, chest, vertebrae, and extremities. Painful episodes occurred at some time during the course of 50% of pregnancies.

Most crises during pregnancy are vaso-occlusive and are often precipitated by urinary tract infection, preeclampsia/eclampsia, thrombophlebitis, or pneumonia. Clinically, the individual will describe pain in the bones or joints but may also perceive the soft tissues as being affected. Visceral pain is also common and may be related to events in the liver or spleen. Painful episodes can be variable in severity and duration with most episodes lasting from 3–5 days.[58]

Because laboratory evaluation is nonspecific, diagnosis of vaso-occlusive crisis begins with excluding other causes for the painful episode, particularly occult infection.

Management of vaso-occlusive crisis during pregnancy is primarily supportive and symptomatic. A 2009 Cochrane review of intervention for treating a sickle cell crisis during pregnancy attempted to assess effectiveness and safety of commonly used treatment regimens, including red cell transfusion, oxygen therapy, intravenous hydration, analgesic drugs, and steroids; there are no randomized clinical trials on this topic, in part because pregnant women tend to be excluded from clinical trials.[59] Most clinicians begin management of a vaso-occlusive crisis with aggressive hydration to increase intravascular volume and decrease blood viscosity.[60] Supplemental oxygen is provided to patients with hypoxemia. Partial exchange transfusions to reduce polymerized hemoglobin S remain an integral part of the management of sickle cell disease[61]; prophylactic transfusion may reduce the incidence of severe complications during pregnancy.[62]

Education about how pregnancy interacts with sickle cell disease can help to reduce depression or anxiety, often decreasing the pain that the patient is experiencing. Biofeedback has been shown to reduce the pain of sickle cell crises and the number of days that analgesics were taken.[63] Physical therapy techniques (exercise, splinting, local application of heat) can also be helpful.[64] TENS may be helpful when pain is isolated to a limited region.[65] The severity of pain dictates the pharmacologic approach to managing sickle cell pain. Although nonopioid analgesics may suffice, oral or parenteral opioids are often required. Acetaminophen remains the nonopioid analgesic of choice during pregnancy. While NSAIDs can be useful adjuncts, particularly for controlling bone pain, they should be used cautiously during pregnancy. Oral analgesic combinations containing acetaminophen and hydrocodone or another weak-to-moderate potency opioid can be added for more severe pain.

For the hospitalized patient with severe sickle cell pain, potent opioid analgesics administered intravenously may be necessary to adequately control pain (Table 9.3). Morphine sulfate is well tolerated and effective for control of severe sickle cell pain[66]; fentanyl and hydromorphone provide reasonable alternatives in patients who cannot tolerate morphine. Administration of morphine via a patient-controlled analgesia (PCA) device allows the patient a sense of control over his or her illness. Weisman and Schecter[67] point out that significantly higher doses of opioids may be necessary for the control of vaso-occlusive crisis pain as compared to postoperative pain. One management approach is to aggressively treat individuals with severe sickle cell pain with potent opioids administered via PCA, most often using morphine. As the pain of vaso-occlusive crisis begins to resolve, patients can be transitioned to a long-acting oral opioid, such as sustained-release morphine. This approach allows earlier ambulation and hospital discharge. All opioids are then tapered over the following 7–10 days.

The use of regional anesthesia has not been formally studied in sickle cell disease. There are case reports describing epidural analgesia for treatment of a sickle cell crisis during pregnancy in parturients with pain localized to the trunk or lower extremities.[68,69] This technique offers the theoretic advantage of increased microvascular blood flow while providing pain relief without opioids.

SUMMARY

Pain is a common symptom during pregnancy and lactation. Most painful conditions are benign and self-limited. A clear explanation about these common disorders is all that is needed to reassure most patients. Many are easily managed using nonpharmacologic approaches. Disorders associated with chronic, recurrent pain can also manifest during the course of pregnancy and lactation, and we have chosen to discuss two of the more common and challenging among them: migraine headache and sickle cell pain crises. Knowing the typical manifestations and time course will allow the clinician to remain vigilant for other serious causes of pain and to guide effective treatment.

Table 9.3   Analgesics for Moderate to Severe Pain during Pregnancy

DRUG	EQUIANALGESIC PARENTERAL DOSE	EQUIANALGESIC ORAL DOSE
Fentanyl	100 µg	—
Hydro-morphone	1.5 mg	7.5 mg
Morphine	10 mg	30–60 mg
Meperidine	75 mg	300 mg

Note. There is wide variability in the duration of analgesic action from patient to patient. All of the parenteral agents listed are generally started with dosing every 3–4 h and the oral agents every 4–6 h. The dosing interval can then be adjusted as needed to maintain adequate analgesia.

REFERENCES

1. Ostgaard HC, Andersson GBJ, Karlsson K. Prevalence of back pain in pregnancy. *Spine* 1991;16:549–52.
2. Mogren I, Pohjanen A. Low back pain and pelvic pain during pregnancy prevelance and risk factors. *Spine* 2005;30:983–91.
3. Vermani E, Mittal R, Weeks A. Pelvic girdle pain and low back pain in pregnancy: a review. *Pain Practice* 2010;10:60–71.
4. Gutke A, Ostgaard HC, Oberg B. Predicting persistent pregnancy related low back pain. *Spine* 2008;33:386–393.

5. MacEvilly M, Buggy D. Back pain and pregnancy: a review. *Pain* 1996;64:405–14.
6. Daly JM, Frame PS, Rapoza PA. Sacroiliac subluxation: a common, treatable cause of low-back pain in pregnancy. *Fam Practice Res J* 1991;11:149–59.
7. LaBan MM, Perrin JCS, Latimer FR. Pregnancy and the herniated lumbar disc. *Arch Phys Med Rehabil* 1983;64:319–21.
8. Weinreb JC, Wolbarsht LB, Cohen JM, Brown CE, Maravilla KR. Prevalence of lumbosacral intervertebral disc abnormalities in MR images of pregnant and asymptomatic non pregnant women. *Radiology* 1989;170:125–8.
9. Schwartz RB. Neurodiagnostic imaging of the pregnant patient. In: Devinsky O, Feldmann E, Mainline B, eds. *Neurological Complications of Pregnancy*. New York: 1994; Raven Press: 243–8.
10. Wilbourn AJ, Aminoff MJ. Electrodiagnosis. In: Rothman RH, Simeone FA, eds. *The Spine*. Philadelphia, PA: 1992; WB Saunders: 163–71.
11. Ostgaard HC, Zetherstrom G, Roos-Hansson E, Svanberg B. Reduction of back and posterior pelvic pain in pregnancy. *Spine* 1994;19:894–900.
12. Pennick V, Young G. Inerventions for preventing and treating pelvic and back pain in pregnancy. *Cochrane Database Syst Rev* 2007;(2):CD001139.
13. Kanakaris NK, Roberts CS, Giannoudis PV. Pregnancy-related pelvic girdle pain: an update. *BMC Med* 2011;15:15.
14. Albert HB, Godskesen M, Korsholm L, Westergaard JG. Incidence of four syndromes of pregnancy related pelvic joint pain. *Spine* 2002;27:2831–4.
15. Leadbetter R, Mawer D, Lindow S. The development of a scoring system for symphysis pubis dysfunction. *J Obstet Gynaecol* 2006;26:20–3.
16. Dowswell T, Bedwell C, Lavender T, Neilson JP. Transcutaneous electrical nerve stimulation (TENS) for pain relief in labour. *Cochrane Database Syst Rev* 2009;(2):CD007214.
17. Coldron, Y, Crothers E, Haslam J, Notcutt W, Sidney D, Thomas R. Tim Watson ACPWH guidance on the safe use of transcutaneous electrical nerve stimulation for musculoskeletal pain during pregnancy. 2007. Available at: http://www.oaa-anaes.ac.uk/assets/_managed/editor/File/PDF/info_for_mothers/TENS%20Statement%20JUNE%2007%20ACPWH%20Final.pdf. (accessed on December 25, 2011).
18. Kvisvik EV, Stovner LJ, Helde G, Bovim G, Linde M. Headache and migraine during pregnancy and puerperium: the MIGRA-study. *J Headache Pain* 2011;12:443–51.
19. Menon R, Bushnell, C. Headache and pregnancy. *Neurologist* 2008; 14:108–19.
20. Chanceller MD, Wroe SJ. Migraine occurring for the first time during pregnancy. *Headache* 1990;30:224–7.
21. Hainline B. Neurological complications of pregnancy: headache. *Neurol Clin* 1994;12:443–60.
22. Levine SR, Brust JC, Futrell N, et al. Cerebrovascular complications of the use of the "crack" form of alkaloidal cocaine. *N Engl J Med* 1990;323:699–704.
23. Donaldson JO. Thrombophillic coagulopathies and pregnancy associated cerebrovascular disease. *Current Obstet Gynaecol* a991;1:186–92.
24. Chen TC, Leviton A. Headache recurrence in pregnant women with migraine. *Headache* 1994;34: 107–10.
25. Coakley F, Gould R, Laros Jr, RK, Thiet M. Guidelines for the use of CT and MRI during pregnancy and lactation. Available at: http://www.radiology.ucsf.edu/patient-care/patient-safety/ct-mri-pregnancy#summary. (accessed on December 25, 2011).
26. Nappi RE, Albani F, Sances G, Terreno E, Brambilla E, Polatti F. Headaches during pregnancy. *Curr Pain Headache Rep* 2011;15:289–94.
27. Marcus DA, Scharff L, Turk D. Nonpharmacological management of headaches during pregnancy. *Psychosom Med* 1995;57:527–35.
28. Silverstein SD. Headaches and women: treatment of the pregnant and lactating migraineur. *Headache* 1993;33:533–40.
29. Paracetamol. *IARC Monogr Eval Carcinog Risks Hum* 1990;50:307–32.
30. Notorianni LJ, Oldham HG. Passage of paracetamol into human milk. *Br J Clin Pharmacol* 1987;24:63–7.
31. American Academy of Pediatrics Committee on Drugs. The transfer of drugs and other chemicals into human milk. *Pediatrics* 2001;108:776–89.
32. Kuczkowski KM. Caffeine in pregnancy. *Arch Gynecol Obstet* 2009;280:695–8.
33. Brent RL, Christian MS, Diener RM. Evaluation of the reproductive and developmental risks of caffeine. *Birth Defects Res B Dev Reprod Toxicol* 2011;92:152–87.
34. Browne ML, Hoyt AT, Feldkamp ML, et al. Maternal caffeine intake and risk of selected birth defects in the National Birth Defects Prevention Study. *Birth Defects Res A Clin Mol Teratol* 2011;91:93–101.
35. Miller RC, Watson WJ, Hackney AC, Seeds JW. Acute maternal and fetal cardiovascular effects of caffeine ingestion. *Am J Perinatol* 1994;11:132–6.

36. Hadeed A, Siegel S. Newborn cardiac arrhythmias associated with maternal caffeine use during pregnancy. *Clinical Pediatrics* 1993;32:45–7.

37. Findlay JW, DeAngelis RL, Kearney MF, Welch RM, Findlay JM. Analgesic drugs in breast milk and plasma. *Clinical Pharmacol Ther* 1981;29:625–33.

38. Personal communication, June 1997, Robbin Eldridge, Senior Pregnancy Registry Monitor, Worldwide Epidemiology, Glaxo Wellcome, Five Moore Drive, Research Triangle Park, NC 27009.

39. Cunnington, M. The safety of sumatriptan and naratriptan in pregnancy: what have we learned? *Headache* 2009;49:1414–22.

40. Hilaire M. Treatment of migraine headaches with sumatriptan in pregnancy. *Ann Pharmachother* 2004;38:1726–9.

41. Lucas S. Medication use in the treatment of migraine during pregnancy and lactation. *Curr Pain Headache Rep* 2009;13:329–98.

42. Wojnar-Horton RE, Hackett LP, Yapp P, Dusci LJ, Paech M, Ilett KF. Distribution and excretion of sumatriptan in human milk. *Br J Clin Pharmacol* 1996;41:217–21.

43. Harden CL, Hopp J, Ting TY, et al. Practice parameter update: management issues for women with epilepsy—focus on pregnancy (an evidence-based review): obstetrical complications and change in seizure frequency: report of the Quality Standards Subcommittee and Therapeutics and Technology Assessment Subcommittee of the American Academy of Neurology and American Epilepsy Society. *Neurology* 2009;73:126–32.

44. Harden CL, Meador KJ, Pennell PB, et al. Practice parameter update: management issues for women with epilepsy—focus on pregnancy (an evidence-based review): teratogenesis and perinatal outcomes: report of the Quality Standards Subcommittee and Therapeutics and Technology Assessment Subcommittee of the American Academy of Neurology and American Epilepsy Society. *Neurology* 2009;73:133–41.

45. Hunt S, Russell A, Smithson WH, et al. Topiramate in pregnancy: preliminary experience from the UK Epilepsy and Pregnancy Register. *Neurology* 2008;71:272–6.

46. Herndandez-Diaz S, Mittendorf R, Holmes LB. Comparative safety of topiramate during pregnancy [abstract]. *Birth Defects Research (Part A)* 2010;88:408.

47. Gabapentin prescribing information. Park-Davis, a division of Pfizer, Inc. 2011. Available at: http://labeling.pfizer.com/ShowLabeling.aspx?id=630. (accessed on December 25, 2011).

48. Guttuso T Jr, Robinson LK, Amankwah KS. Gabapentin use in hyperemesis gravidarum: a pilot study. *Early Hum Dev* 2010;86:65–6.

49. Montouris G. Gabapentin exposure in human pregnancy: results from the Gabapentin Pregnancy Registry. *Epilepsy Behav* 2003;4:310–17.

50. Nakhai-Pour HR, Rey E, Bérard A. Antihypertensive medication use during pregnancy and the risk of major congenital malformations or small-for-gestational-age newborns. *Birth Defects Res B Dev Reprod Toxicol* 2010;89:147–54.

51. Magee LA, Duley L. Oral beta-blockers for mild to moderate hypertension during pregnancy. *Cochrane Database Syst Rev* 2003;(3):CD002863.

52. Pruyn SC, Phelan JP, Buchanan GC. Long term propranolol therapy in pregnancy: maternal and fetal outcome. *Am J Obstet Gynecol* 1979;135:485–9.

53. Bauer JH, Pape B, Zajicek J, Groshong T. Propranolol in human plasma and breast milk. *Am J Cardiol* 1979;63:860–2.

54. White WB, Andreoli JW, Wong SH, Cohn RD. Atenolol in human plasma and breast milk. *Obstet Gynecol* 1984;63:42–4.

55. American Academy of Pediatrics. Use of psychoactive medication during pregnancy and possible effects on the fetus and newborn. Committee on Drugs. *Pediatrics* 2000;105:880–7.

56. Wisner KL, Perel JM, Findling RL. Antidepressant treatment during breast-feeding. *Am J Psychiatr* 1996;153:1132–7.

57. Powars DR, Sandhu M, Niland-Weiss J, Johnson C, Bruce S, Manning PR. Pregnancy in sickle cell disease. *Obstet Gynecol* 1986;67:217–28.

58. Shapiro B, Dinges DF, Orne ED. Recording of crisis pain in sickle cell disease. *Adv Pain Res Ther* 1990;15:313–21.

59. Martí-Carvajal AJ, Peña-Martí GE, Comunián-Carrasco G, Martí-Peña AJ. Interventions for treating painful sickle cell crisis during pregnancy. *Cochrane Database Syst Rev* 2009;(1):CD006786.

60. Martin JN, Martin RW, Morrison JC. Acute management of sickle cell disease in pregnancy. *Clin Perinatol* 1986;13:853–68.

61. Wayne AS, Kevy SV, Nathan DG. Transfusion management of sickle cell disease. *Blood* 1993;81:1109–23.

62. Howard RJ, Tuck SM, Pearson TC. Pregnancy in sickle cell disease in the UK: results of a multicentre survey of the effect of prophylactic blood transfusion on maternal and fetal outcome. *Br J Obstet Gynaecol* 1995;102:947–51.

63. Cozzi L, Tyron WW, Sedlaceck K. The effectiveness of biofeedback assisted relaxation in modifying sickle cell crisis. *Biofeedback Self Regul* 1987;12:51–61.

64. Alcorn R, Bowser B, Henley EJ, Holloway V. Fluidotherapy and exercise in the management of sickle cell anemia. *Phys Ther* 1984;64:1520–2.

65. Wang WC, George SL, Wilimas JA. Transcutaneous nerve stimulation treatment of sickle cell pain. *Acta Haematol* 1988;80:99–102.

66. Chamberlain G. Medical problems in pregnancy II. *BMJ* 1991;302:1327–30.

67. Weisman SJ, Schechter NL. Sickle cell anemia: pain management. In: Sinatra RS, Hord AH, Ginsberg B, Preble LM, eds. *Acute Pain: Mechanisms and Management*. St. Louis, MO: Mosby Year Book; 1992: 508–16.

68. Finer P, Blair J, Rowe P. Epidural analgesia in the management of labor pain and sickle cell crisis: a case report. *Anesthesiology* 1988;68:799–800.

69. Winder AD, Johnson S, Murphey J, Ehsanipoor RM. Epidural analgesia for treatment of sickle cell crisis during pregnancy. *Obstet Gynecol* 2011;118:495–7.

10

THE OPIOID-TOLERANT PREGNANT PATIENT

Nilda E. Salaman and May L. Chin

INTRODUCTION

Chronic pain is a burgeoning health issue. Pain relief as a fundamental human right continues to be addressed by international organizations such as the World Health Organization (WHO), the International Association for the Study of Pain (IASP), and the European Federation of IASP Chapters (EFIC).[1–3] In the United States, the Institute of Medicine recently published a "blueprint" for enhancing access, and quality of pain relief, through improved patient care, education, and research.[4] Opioid analgesics are commonly prescribed for pain; this use has increased significantly as health care providers recognize the need to provide adequate pain relief, particularly in patients with chronic pain. The widespread use of opioids has led to increased challenges in treating these patients, many of whom may present with opioid tolerance, dependency, and addiction.[5]

The pregnant patient presents a unique situation that encompasses the dynamic changes of pregnancy and the presence of a developing fetus. The goal in such a patient is balancing the mother's need for adequate pain control without incurring harm or adverse drug exposure to the fetus or neonate. Unrelieved pain in the pregnant patient, as well as the presence of opiates in maternal blood, adversely affects

the fetus and neonate.[6–8] Hence, pregnancy in a woman presents an added challenge in pain management.

The opioid-tolerant pregnant patient includes those who are on opioid analgesics for chronic pain and/or those who use opioids and other drugs illicitly. Many of these patients are seen in the acute, subacute, or chronic care settings, where practitioners are often unable or unwilling to adequately address their pain issues. In this chapter we will address: (a) pain management in an opioid-tolerant patient who is pregnant; and (b) considerations for fetal well-being when treating such a patient. The terms *addiction*, *opioid tolerance*, *opioid dependence*, *physical dependence*, and *withdrawal syndrome* are defined in Appendix A.

INCIDENCE OF PREGNANT WOMEN WHO MAY BE OPIOID TOLERANT

It is reported that 3% to 16% of the general population has an addiction disorder.[9] There is scant information available on the incidence of pregnant women who may be opioid tolerant. The available information is gathered from observational studies on women with addiction to illicit drugs and who are on methadone maintenance programs. Between 2002 and 2004, an estimated 6% of pregnant women used nonmedical prescription drugs and more than two-thirds of these women also took pain relievers, such as oxycodone.[10] The 2009–2010 US National Survey on Drug Use and Health reported that 4.4% of pregnant women aged 15 to 44 years used illicit drugs.[11] This number was significantly lower compared to that of non-pregnant women in the same age group who used illicit drugs (10.9%).

The United Kingdom Advisory Council on the Misuse of Drugs reported that approximately 6,000 babies, or 1% of all deliveries, are born to mothers who abuse drugs each year.[12] The European Monitoring Centre for Drugs and Drug Addiction reported as many as 30,000 pregnant women using opioids annually.[13] Nonetheless, the true prevalence of drug use in pregnant women is unclear, although it appears to be less widespread than use of nicotine (16.3%) or alcohol (10.3%).[14]

CHANGES IN PREGNANCY THAT AFFECT PAIN PERCEPTION AND DRUG DISPOSITION

Anatomic and physiological changes during pregnancy are largely attributed to the hormonal effects, namely those of estrogen and progesterone. Estrogen levels increase dramatically in the first trimester and then plateau during the second and third trimesters.[15] The relationship between estrogen and pain is complex.[16] Estrogen acts as a pain-modulating messenger, in which a rise in estrogen levels may result in pain reduction.[17] But findings also suggest that estrogen may be counterproductive to pain relief and may contribute to increased pain.[16] Other neurohumoral changes may alter or

reduce pain perception. For instance, reduced anesthetic requirements during pregnancy are associated with elevated progesterone levels in the cerebrospinal fluid,[18–20] and low levels of substance P (a neuropeptide associated central hyperexcitability and increased sensitivity to pain) typically occur during pregnancy.[21] Perhaps these changes help prepare the pregnant patient for the painful process of labor.

Pharmacokinetic and pharmacodynamic changes during pregnancy affect the absorption, metabolism and sensitivity to drugs (Table 10.1). By the fifth week of gestation, pregnant women experience a 50% increase in cardiac output, reflecting a 25% increase each in stroke volume and heart rate. Elevated intravascular volume contributes to an increase in renal plasma flow and an increase in glomerular filtration rate. The increase in renal elimination influences drug disposition and therefore the dosing of medications.

Blood flow to the dermis is increased three- to four-fold at term pregnancy, contributing to an increase in skin temperature. This change may influence the transdermal absorption of drugs such as clonidine, fentanyl, and lidocaine. Pulmonary changes include increased minute ventilation and increased tidal volume, which may increase the absorption of inhaled substances.

Drug absorption from the gastrointestinal tract may be enhanced by decreased motility and prolonged intestinal transit time.[22] Decreased gut motility, including delay in gastric emptying during labor, may be exacerbated by opioid analgesics. The increase in mean plasma volume and body fat may prolong drug half-lives due to an increase in the volume of

Table 10.1   Physiologic Changes during Pregnancy[15]

Increased cardiac output 50%: stroke volume, 25%; heart rate, 25%

Increased renal plasma flow 75%, GFR, renal elimination

Increased blood flow to various organs (uterus, dermis, kidneys)

Increased minute ventilation, tidal volume; **decreased** residual lung volume

Decreased gastrointestinal transit time; **delayed** gastric emptying during labor

Increased hepatic blood flow, bile excretion; **altered** enzyme induction

Increased extracellular fluid, total body water, total body weight, body fat composition

Decreased albumin concentration, protein binding

---

distribution, and the decrease in protein binding and hepatic biotransformation may lead to higher free drug concentrations.[15]

MATERNAL-PLACENTAL-FETAL DRUG TRANSFER

Pain management in the pregnant patient is complicated by the combined effects of analgesics on the uterine vascular resistance, the placental perfusion, and the direct teratogenic effects of the drugs. The placental transfer of drugs from mother to fetus depends on multiple factors, such as the molecular weight of the drug, the degree of ionization, protein binding, lipid solubility, metabolism, and excretion, as well as maternal pharmacokinetics and hemodynamics.[15] Uncharged, unionized molecules with high lipid solubility and drugs with low protein binding cross the placenta more readily than hydrophilic ionized drugs. With the exception of heparin and insulin, most drugs cross the placenta, including opioid analgesics. The presence of opioids may lead to tolerance in the fetus and the risk of withdrawal symptoms in the neonate.

Fetal development may be adversely affected at any time during gestation. The most vulnerable period in this process is during organogenesis, which occurs between 3 and 8 weeks or 35 to 70 days after the last menstrual period.[23] Direct drug teratogenicity may result in death or produce structural abnormalities, growth retardation, or functional deficiencies. The timing of exposure to the drug is an important consideration, although drug dosage and duration of therapy are also significant. Potential risks from drug exposure include major malformations (first-trimester exposure), low birth weight, neonatal toxicity (third-trimester exposure), postnatal drug dependence, and long-term neurobehavioral effects. In general, drugs account for only a small proportion of the grossly observed fetal abnormalities.[23]

FETAL EFFECTS FROM OPIOID, NONOPIOID, AND ILLICIT DRUGS

Substance abuse (e.g., heroin, cocaine) during pregnancy is associated with increased rates of meconium staining, precipitous delivery, abruptio placenta, premature delivery, intrauterine growth retardation, and neonatal neurobehavioral problems.[24] Opiates appear to be relatively safe when taken for a short period of time. The Collaborative Perinatal Project reported no increased evidence of teratogenicity in 448 mothers exposed to morphine at various stages of pregnancy. In addition, no congenital anomalies were observed with hydrocodone, meperidine, methadone, or oxycodone use during pregnancy.[25] It is unclear, however, what the "safe" time frame is, since there are no studies assessing the effects of long-term opiate therapy in the pregnant human.

Several countries have developed risk classification systems on drug safety during pregnancy. In 1979, the US Food and Drug Administration (FDA) established five categories that classified drugs based on the risks they pose to pregnant women and their fetuses. This system is similar to classification systems in other countries such as Sweden[26] and Australia.[27]

The FDA classification, A, B, C, D, or X (Table 10.2), provides a guide to the relative safety of drugs prescribed to pregnant women.[28,29] The drugs in Categories A and B are generally considered appropriate for use during pregnancy. Category C drugs should be used with caution, drugs in Category D should be avoided, and those in Category X are contraindicated.

In the management of chronic pain, nonopioid drugs are often implemented in a multimodal approach to optimize pain relief and to reduce the use of opioid analgesics. Many of the pharmacologic adjuvants prescribed for pain management fall into Category C or D. A large number of drugs in the United States fall into Category C, in which risk cannot be ruled out since no well-controlled human or animal studies exist.[30] Unfortunately, no single system exists to give the health care provider a clear directive for prescribing drugs to a pregnant patient. This has contributed to angst and uncertainty in choosing an appropriate "risk-reduced" therapy for an expectant mother.

EVALUATION OF THE OPIOID-TOLERANT PREGNANT PATIENT

Because pain is influenced by anatomic, physiologic, and psychosocial factors, adequate

Table 10.2 FDA Classification of Pregnancy Risk Category Drugs Used in Pain Management[28,29]

PREGNANCY RISK CATEGORY	CLASSIFICATION CRITERIA	MEDICATIONS
Category A	Adequate and well-controlled studies in women fail to demonstrate a risk to the fetus in the first trimester of pregnancy. Evidence of risk in the later trimesters of pregnancy is lacking. The possibility of fetal harm appears unlikely.	Prenatal vitamins
Category B	Animal studies have not demonstrated a fetal risk or animal studies indicate a fetal risk not confirmed in well-controlled human studies.	Acetaminophen, Butorphanol, Nalbuphine, Caffeine, Fentanyl, Hydrocodone, Methadone, Meperidine, Morphine, Oxycodone, Oxymorphone, Ibuprofen, Naproxen, Indomethacin[a], Metoprolol, Paroxetine, Fluoxetine, Prednisolone, Prednisone, Ketamine
Category C	Animal studies indicate adverse effects on the fetus, but there are no well-controlled studies in humans or animals.	Aspirin[a], Ketorolac, Celecoxib, Codeine, Gabapentin, Pregabalin, Lidocaine, Mexiletene, Nifedipine, Propranolol, Sumatriptan, Buprenorphine, Gadopentate dimeglumine (contrast)
Category D	There is positive evidence of human fetal risk; however, the benefits from use in certain situations in pregnant women may surpass the potential fetal risks.	Amitriptyline, Imipramine, Diazepam, Phenobarbital, Phenytoin, Valproic acid, Topiramate
Category X	There is positive evidence of fetal risk based on animal and human studies. The risks surpass the potential benefits of use in women who are pregnant and should not be used during pregnancy.	Ergotamine

[a] Full-dose aspirin and nonsteroidal anti-inflammatory drug therapy should be avoided during the third trimester.

treatment necessitates a thorough evaluation. The assessment and management of a pregnant opioid-tolerant patient is best achieved through a collaborative approach that includes the obstetrical team, the pain specialist, and the nursing staff. The initial assessment should include a detailed history of the presenting pain symptom, the current pain management approach, including analgesics tried (opioid and nonopioid), past treatment modalities, comorbid diagnoses (depression/anxiety), and psychosocial history. A focused physical examination and review of diagnostic tests may help to further evaluate the cause of pain and determine the best course of action for both the patient and the fetus.

Clinicians need to determine the underlying pathology for pain regardless of whether the patient is opioid tolerant or has a history of substance abuse. For example, the progression or persistence of a severe headache in a pregnant patient with a history of migraine headaches may signal other treatable and/or life-threatening causes such as preeclampsia, subarachnoid hemorrhage, or intracranial tumor. A team approach may avoid confusion and misunderstanding when decisions and recommendations are coordinated among the different health care providers.

The treatment goals for the opioid-tolerant pregnant patient include decreased pain, improved function, and minimized withdrawal. The patient with a substance abuse disorder may present with significant psychosocial and health-related issues. For instance, the patient's need to sustain the addiction may predispose her to infections, poor prenatal care, and trouble with the law. These patients may also present with comorbid diseases such as cellulitis (from intravenous drug use), end organ damage, hepatitis C, human immunodeficiency virus (HIV), trauma, and malnutrition. In addition, they may also experience behavioral and social problems that frequently exacerbate pain.[31] These patients should not be treated "in a vacuum" if successful therapy is the goal. They require additional services that help reduce the risk of withdrawal and relapse, and the option of drug rehabilitation.

The gestation of the fetus and the estimated time of delivery of the neonate are important considerations in a pain management plan. If further diagnostic studies are to be considered, clinicians should factor in the vulnerable period for central nervous system teratogenesis, which occurs between 10 and 17 weeks of gestation. Nonurgent X-rays and fluoroscopic procedures should be avoided if at all possible during this time. That said, emergent or urgent X-rays are not contraindicated. The American College of Obstetricians and Gynecologists (ACOG) states that "Women should be counseled that X-ray exposure from a single diagnostic procedure does not result in harmful fetal effects. Specifically, exposure to less than 5 rad

[50 mGy] has not been associated with an increase in fetal anomalies or pregnancy loss."[32]

Magnetic resonance imaging (MRI) is considered relatively safe during pregnancy.[33] In comparison, the computed tomography (CT) scan is associated with higher levels of radiation exposure and should be avoided unless the risk-benefit ratio favors its use. In general, the use of contrast material, such as gadolinium-based contrast material, should be avoided during pregnancy.[33] The reason is that after intravenous administration, contrast materials may cross the placental barrier and enter the fetal bloodstream. The contrast material then appears in the fetal bladder and is excreted via urine into the amniotic fluid, where it is subsequently swallowed by the fetus.[34]

OPTIONS FOR PAIN MANAGEMENT

The options for pain management in the opioid-tolerant pregnant patient are based largely on recommendations from retrospective studies, case reports, and expert opinions. The general consensus from these studies suggests maintaining the patient's preexisting opioid requirement with addition of other opioid analgesics as necessary. If feasible, a multimodal approach should be considered. Other possible medications and modalities include anti-inflammatory analgesics, acetaminophen, adjuvant analgesics, use of local anesthetics in regional techniques, and physical therapeutic interventions.[35] Nonpharmacologic modalities should be advocated and encouraged whenever possible and appropriate.

The plan for pain management should take into account the patient's pregnancy stage, in other words, whether the patient is antepartum, in active labor, or postpartum. If the patient is antepartum and not in active labor, clinicians should attempt to stabilize the patient's level of pain and employ services that will help improve function, reduce pain and minimize withdrawal or relapse. If the patient is in active labor, pain management is directed toward maintaining analgesia or anesthesia for labor with expectant vaginal delivery, with or without instrumentation, or surgical delivery by cesarean section. Methods for pain control during labor, including use of systemic opioid analgesics and neuraxial analgesia, will be covered in Chapter 8.

Methadone

Methadone may be a reasonable pain management option in an opioid-tolerant pregnant patient. This drug was first introduced in the 1960s by Nyswander and approved by the FDA for the treatment of heroin addiction.[36,37] Methadone is classified pregnancy Category B drug (Table 10.2). It is a long-acting synthetic opioid analgesic that binds to mu, delta, and kappa receptors. Methadone has a mu-receptor affinity similar to that of morphine but may be more efficacious with repeated dosing.[38] Methadone inhibits the reuptake of monoamines serotonin and norepinephrine. It is anti-hyperalgesic with moderate antagonism of N-methyl-D-aspartate (NMDA) receptor.[39] Activation of the NMDA receptor leads to central sensitization; therefore, blocking this receptor may help prevent the development of tolerance.[40] Methadone is well absorbed from the gastric mucosa and has a high bioavailability of 75%, although this may vary depending on the pharmacokinetics and pharmacodynamics of each individual.

The pregnant patient with opioid tolerance may benefit from methadone therapy if the opioid dose has escalated without adequate pain relief or if opioid side effects limit a dose increase. Instituting methadone with or without short-acting opioids for breakthrough pain may be of some benefit to these patients. Practitioners should exercise caution when converting from a high-dose opioid analgesic regimen to methadone since the equianalgesic conversion ratio is not straightforward. This dose ratio may vary depending on the daily opioid dose the patient is on prior to converting to methadone. For instance, the conversion ratio for a patient on an oral daily dose of morphine ranging from 300 mg to 600 mg is generally 10:1 (morphine to methadone).

Among the Western nations, oral methadone is the preferred maintenance pharmacotherapy for the pregnant heroin user.[41] In the United States, guidelines for administration of methadone were developed in the 1970s and methadone maintenance therapy is considered the standard of care for pregnant women dependent on opioids.[42,43] The goal is to achieve a methadone dose sufficient to prevent symptoms of withdrawal while, at the same time, reducing or eliminating drug craving. Studies of heroin-addicted pregnant women under methadone maintenance therapy report that they benefit from better medical and prenatal care. In addition, they report less maternal illicit drug use at delivery, decreased neonatal abstinence symptoms, and decreased length of hospital stay.[44,45] In fact, stable methadone therapy may reduce the stress on the fetus and prevent withdrawals that may otherwise recur due to an inconsistent presence of illicit drugs or opiates in the mother. Methadone maintenance therapy has been associated with improved perinatal outcomes by reducing the risk of preeclampsia, and improving birthweight and head circumference.[46]

Pregnant patients stabilized on methadone before pregnancy should remain on methadone with dose adjustments at term because methadone metabolism and elimination are increased in pregnancy, and patients may require more than one daily dose to maintain stable blood levels during the third trimester.[47,48] The American Academy of Pediatrics considers prescribed methadone compatible with breastfeeding.[49]

RISKS WITH METHADONE USE

The preterm birth rate among opiate-addicted women treated with methadone (29.1%) is nearly three times the national average for singleton pregnancies (11.1%).[50] The risk of neonatal abstinence syndrome (NAS) is one of the drawbacks of maternal methadone therapy or chronic opiate use in the pregnant woman. Infants born to mothers maintained on methadone are physically dependent on opioids and are at risk for withdrawal symptoms. The half-life of methadone is greater than 24 hours, and acute withdrawal may occur within the first 48 hours after birth and for as long as 7 to 14 days thereafter. Drug accumulation secondary to a long half-life is a potential risk and may lead to sedation, respiratory depression, respiratory arrest, and even death.

Methadone may prolong the rate-corrected QT interval (QTc), resulting in torsades de pointes and sudden cardiac death. Women have a slightly longer QTc interval compared to men and are at greater risk for arrhythmias.[51] Doses greater than 100 mg/day have been associated with prolonged QTc, but this may reverse when the dose is decreased. Even so, sudden cardiac death has been reported with doses as low as 20 mg/day. Clinical guidelines for cardiac safety with methadone treatment advocate risk/benefit discussions, routine electrocardiogram monitoring, patient-specific risk stratification, and increased provider awareness.[52]

Buprenorphine

Buprenorphine has been prescribed since the 1970s for treating moderate to severe pain. It is a semisynthetic agonist-antagonist, acting as partial agonist at the mu receptor and antagonist at the kappa receptor. The effect of buprenorphine at other receptors (delta, nociceptin) has not been fully elucidated, but the known actions at both mu and kappa receptors render the drug useful as an analgesic for maintenance therapy in patients with a history of drug abuse.[53] In the United States, sublingual buprenorphine is prescribed for the treatment of opioid addiction.[54] The parenteral and transdermal formulations are prescribed for the relief of moderate to severe pain.

Buprenorphine has a long duration of action (6 to 8 hours). It has an active metabolite, norbuprenorphine. The analgesic and respiratory depressant effect of 0.3 mg parenteral buprenorphine is equivalent to 10 mg parenteral morphine.[53] At higher doses, a "ceiling effect" is reached with respect to analgesia and respiratory depression. Compared to methadone, buprenorphine has a lower risk for overdose and is associated with less physical dependence and withdrawal effects.

Since buprenorphine is an agonist-antagonist, it may precipitate withdrawal symptoms when administered to individuals on high doses of opioids.[55] This limits the use of this drug for the treatment of acute pain in such patients. Conversely, patients on long-term buprenorphine therapy may require higher doses of an opioid agonist for treatment of acute pain. The following options may be considered for such patients: (a) increase the dose of the buprenorphine; (b) use short-acting analgesics with the baseline maintenance dose of buprenorphine; or (c) replace the buprenorphine with a pure opioid agonist, for example. parenteral fentanyl or morphine.[56,57]

Buprenorphine is classified as a pregnancy Category C drug (Table 10.2). The dose of buprenorphine during the third trimester of pregnancy may need to be adjusted because of increased drug metabolism and elimination. Current information on buprenorphine use for opioid-dependent/tolerant pregnant individuals is limited. Some studies suggest that it is efficacious and reportedly safe for the mother and neonate due to decreased risk of NAS and may therefore serve as an alternative to methadone.[58]

The Maternal Opioid Treatment: Human Experimental Research (MOTHER), a prospective, international study of 131 opioid-dependent mothers and their newborns, reported similar maternal and fetal outcomes from methadone and buprenorphine treatment. The study also reported that newborns in the buprenorphine group were associated with less severe NAS symptoms and required less medication and hospitalization.[59]

Buprenorphine crosses the placenta and is excreted in breast milk. Given the poor oral bioavailability of this drug, infant exposure through breast milk may be minimal with little impact on the NAS scoring. The Center for Substance Abuse Treatment panel states that mothers prescribed buprenorphine may breastfeed unless other contraindications exist.[60]

Ketamine

Ketamine, an N-methyl-D-aspartate (NMDA) antagonist, is an anesthetic drug with "dissociative" properties. It is an FDA approved drug for many decades, but over time its use in the operating room has been surpassed by newer anesthetic drugs. The interest in ketamine was rekindled with the discovery of the role of NMDA receptors in central sensitization, hyperalgesia, and persistent pain.[61]

Multiple case reports indicate a reduction of neuropathic pain and opioid-resistant pain with ketamine.[62] This drug may be given in the perioperative setting as an adjunct to decrease opioid use. Ketamine in subanesthetic doses has been shown to reduce morphine requirements in the first 24 hours after surgery.[63] Hence, ketamine may be considered a useful adjuvant in the management of postcesarean pain in opioid-tolerant patients who do not have the benefit of epidural or intrathecal analgesia.

Potential adverse effects of NMDA antagonists include hallucinations, lightheadedness, dizziness, fatigue, headache, out-of-body sensation, nightmares, and sensory changes. Ketamine has oxytocic properties, resulting in uterine hypertonus at parenteral doses greater than 1.5 to 2.2 mg/kg. It may also be associated with neonatal depression, increased neonatal muscle tone, and elevated maternal blood pressure. However, subanesthetic doses (0.2–1.0 mg/kg IV) have not been associated with these complications.[64] The elimination half-life of ketamine is approximately 2 hours, and the drug is undetectable in the mother's plasma approximately 11 hours after a dose.[64] It is unlikely that the infant will be exposed to significant amounts of ketamine if breast fed after this length of time.

Nonopioid Analgesics

Commonly prescribed nonopioid analgesics include acetaminophen, salicylates, nonsteroidal anti-inflammatory drugs (NSAIDs), antiepileptic drugs, antidepressants, and alpha 2 agonists (clonidine).

Acetaminophen is a pregnancy Category B drug. It is available in oral and intravenous form and can be used at all stages of pregnancy. Acetaminophen is a nonsalicylate similar to aspirin in analgesic potency. Health care providers should exercise caution when treating patients with underlying liver disease since overdosage may lead to fatal hepatotoxicity. The FDA requested pharmaceutical companies to decrease the dose of acetaminophen from 500 mg to 325 mg in combination drugs[65] in an attempt to maintain a lower daily dose of acetaminophen (preferably below 3 grams).

Aspirin (acetylsalicylic acid) is a common analgesic and antipyretic. The usual analgesic adult dose is 325 mg to 650 mg, given once every 4 to 6 hours. Aspirin is a pregnancy Category C drug. The recommended dose during pregnancy is limited to 50 mg/day. Aspirin inhibits platelet function and may contribute to an increased risk of maternal and fetal bleeding. Aspirin has been associated with an increased risk of gastroschisis, intracranial hemorrhage of the premature infant, and premature closure of the ductus arteriosus in utero.[66] Full-dose aspirin and nonsteroidal anti-inflammatory drug therapy should be avoided during the third trimester of pregnancy because of the association of maternal hemorrhage, decreased amniotic fluid volume, and prolonged pregnancy and labor.[66]

Nonsteroidal anti-inflammatory drugs (NSAIDs) are useful adjuncts in the treatment of pain. They have anti-inflammatory and analgesic properties. NSAIDs are classified as Category C prior to 30 weeks and Category D in the third trimester. COX-1 and COX-2 isoenzymes are expressed in the endothelial cell and smooth muscles of the ductus arteriosus and renal tissue. Potential risks with third-trimester exposure include premature closure of the ductus arteriosus, fetal pulmonary hypertension, impaired renal function, and oligohydramnios.[67,68] Constriction of the ductus arteriosus may reverse 24 to 48 hours after withdrawal of the medication.

Anticonvulsant drugs and antidepressants are useful adjuvants in the management of neuropathic pain. Gabapentin and pregabalin are commonly prescribed. They act on the alpha 2 delta subunit of the presynaptic calcium channels. In general, they are safe for long-term use, with good tolerability. The potential adverse side effects of these drugs, as with the older anticonvulsants (carbamazepine and phenytoin), include sedation, dizziness, and impaired mental function, each of which may limit clinical use.

Human birth defects have been reported with topiramate, zonisamide, and gabapentin.[69] Gabapentin has been assigned to pregnancy Category C. Animal studies have reported evidence of fetotoxicity involving delayed ossification in several bones of the skull, vertebrae, forelimbs, and hind limbs. A recent population-based cohort study in Denmark involving 837,795 live-born infants compared the prevalence of major birth defects in those exposed to newer antiepileptic drugs during the first trimester (n = 1,532) to those with no exposure. The study found that exposure in the first trimester to gabapentin ($n = 59$) and exposure to four other antiepileptic drugs (lamotrigine, oxcarbazepine, topiramate, levetiracetam) was not associated with an increased risk of major birth defects.[70] Since these drugs have yet to be extensively studied in the pregnant patient, practitioners should exercise caution when determining the risks and benefits of prescribing adjuvant analgesics in pregnant women.

There is little information on anticonvulsant drugs and breast feeding. One study noted extensive passage of gabapentin into breast milk, but the serum levels of the drug were found to be low in the neonates. Moreover, the breastfed neonates did not exhibit adverse effects consistent with the use of gabapentin.[71]

Selective serotonin reuptake inhibitors and the tricyclic antidepressants, amitriptyline and imipramine, but not doxepin, are thought to be compatible with breastfeeding.[72] The use of antidepressants in the pregnant patient is discussed in Chapter 9 .

NONPHARMACOLOGIC MANAGEMENT

Nonpharmacologic techniques encourage the pregnant patient to take an active role in the management of her pain. These may be useful regardless of whether she is in active labor.

These techniques address the physical sensations of pain and help alleviate pain by promoting self-confidence and coping skills, and by enhancing the psychoemotional and spiritual components of care.[73]

The physical application of hot or cold therapy to the affected area is easy and may be effective in minimizing escalating doses of pharmacologic therapy and their potential side effects.[74] The use of complementary and alternative therapies (massage, relaxation response, biofeedback, meditation) may also provide benefit in terms of reducing pain (Table 10.3).[75] Although few of these techniques have been adequately studied, they are associated with little or no side effects, and they are relatively low cost, which may render them useful as adjunctive treatment in patients with opioid tolerance.

Continuous labor support for women in active labor appears to be highly associated with maternal satisfaction. In randomized controlled trials in North America, continuous labor support by trained laypersons or "doulas" reduced pain (measured indirectly by noting reduced pain medication requirements) and increased maternal satisfaction.[75]

NEONATAL ABSTINENCE SYNDROME

One of the challenges in managing pain in the pregnant opioid-tolerant mother is avoiding

Table 10.3   Nonpharmacologic Methods to Relieve Pain[75]

- Acupuncture and acupressure
- Hypnosis
- Application of heat and cold
- Touch and massage
- Relaxation and breathing
- Transcutaneous electrical nerve stimulation
- Maternal movement and positioning
- Aromatherapy
- Music and audio-analgesia
- Childbirth education
- Continuous labor support
- Baths in labor
- Intradermal water blocks

development of NAS. The manifestations of NAS depend on various factors—the type of maternal drugs, the infant's metabolism and excretion of the active compounds, and the infant's last intrauterine drug exposure.

NAS involves multiple organ systems, namely, the central nervous system, gastrointestinal, autonomic, and respiratory systems. The syndrome is characterized by signs and symptoms consistent with autonomic hyperactivity. The baby may exhibit significant yawning, sneezing, tachypnea, fever, and cerebral irritability such as tremors, increased tone, poor feeding (uncoordinated suck and regurgitation), and, in severe cases, seizures.[76] The signs and symptoms of NAS are nonspecific and can mimic sepsis or other neurologic or gastrointestinal problems. The incidence of NAS is approximately 30% to 90% of mothers on methadone maintenance therapy.[77] The syndrome often manifests in the hours or days following birth, but the onset may be delayed for several days, depending on the half-life of the specific opioid. For instance, with morphine the onset may be 6 to 36 hours, and for methadone, 24 to 72 hours.[78] Other drugs with longer half-lives, such as buprenorphine or sedative-hypnotics, such as benzodiazepines, and barbiturates, may precipitate withdrawal symptoms much later.

In addition to withdrawal symptoms, other opioid effects include low birth weight, intrauterine growth retardation and prematurity, increased weight loss during the early neonatal period, and increased length of hospital stay.[58,79,80] Interestingly, the dose of the opioid (methadone, buprenorphine, slow-release morphine) does not appear to correlate with the incidence of withdrawal or NAS in neonates,[81] although this may be subject to debate. Reports indicate that while up to 90% of newborns exposed to opioids during fetal life display some symptoms of NAS, approximately 50% to 75% will require treatment.[77,82,83]

MANAGEMENT OF NEONATAL ABSTINENCE SYNDROME

Supportive treatment is recommended for NAS. Pharmacologic therapy is instituted when supportive therapy fails to relieve the neonates' symptoms. The opioid antagonist naloxone should be avoided because of risk of inducing sudden withdrawal symptoms, including seizures. Therapy is focused on treating withdrawal symptoms from opioids and other drugs, and being aware that the neonate may have been exposed to multiple drugs if the mother has a history of substance abuse. The use of buprenorphine to treat NAS has become more commonplace as increasing numbers of opioid-tolerant mothers are treated for dependence with buprenorphine. One randomized open label study using sublingual buprenorphine to treat NAS showed a reduction in treatment time and length of stay in comparison to standard opiate therapy.[84] The combined use of opioid and phenobarbital in the management of NAS has been shown to decrease the length of time in severe withdrawal and to decrease the length of hospitalization.[85]

Management of NAS includes frequent monitoring in a newborn nursery unit with experienced personnel or intensive care unit, depending on the severity of symptoms. The Neonatal Abstinence Scoring System score is used to help guide assessment-based therapy. A widely used scoring system is the Finnegan scale, which assesses 21 of the most common signs of neonatal drug withdrawal syndrome. The score provides an objective measure of the severity of the newborns' symptoms and is utilized to monitor the neonates' progress after pharmacotherapy.[79]

BREASTFEEDING

Generally speaking, breastfeeding is encouraged since breast milk confers nutritional and immunologic benefits to the infant. Breastfeeding is not contraindicated in the parturient on opioid maintenance. However, it is contraindicated in the presence of maternal HIV infection since HIV type I can be transmitted through breast milk. This may be controversial in developing countries since breast milk may be the only source of nutrition for the infant.[86]

Breastfeeding promotes mother and child bonding and can potentially decrease the severity of NAS.[87] Most drugs are excreted into the breast milk by passive diffusion. The transfer of drugs into breast milk is governed by the same pharmacodynamic and pharmacokinetic principles that influence transplacental passage of drugs.[87] The drug concentration in breast milk is directly proportional to the corresponding concentration in maternal plasma. The neonatal dose of most medications obtained through breastfeeding is approximately 1% to 2% of the maternal dose; however, most drugs ingested via breast milk rarely reach therapeutic levels in the infant.

The recommendation for pain management in lactating mothers suggests prescribing the lowest effective maternal dose of the drug and timing the breastfeeding before the drug attains peak concentration in the breast milk. Breast milk is produced during and immediately following nursing. To minimize the transfer of medications to the infant, the mother should time her medication intake to achieve the longest interval between drug intake and breast feedings. Opiates, most NSAIDs, local anesthetics, and some of the newer anticonvulsant agents used as adjuvant analgesics appear to be compatible with breastfeeding. More information on medications and lactation may be accessed at: Drugs and Lactation Database (LactMed) at http://toxnet.nlm.nih.gov/cgi-bin/sis/htmlgen?LACT.

SUMMARY

There is a dearth of information in the literature to guide health care providers on how to best manage pain in a pregnant opioid-tolerant patient. General guidelines for evaluating and managing such a patient may be extrapolated, in part, from the recommendations for opioid-tolerant patients who are not pregnant. The pregnant patient is subject to physiological changes that affect pain perception and drug disposition. The challenge lies in providing adequate pain relief in the mother and, at the same time, minimizing exposure of teratogens and drugs to the fetus and neonate. Clinicians should attempt to incorporate a multidisciplinary approach that involves the obstetrician, pain specialist, nursing staff, and other supportive providers (social and psychosocial services). A multimodal approach to therapy, which includes nonpharmacologic as well as appropriate nonopioid adjuvants, should be considered whenever possible.

The patient in active labor may benefit from the early institution of neuraxial analgesia. Supplementation with baseline opioids is often necessary to prevent maternal and fetal withdrawal during the peripartum period, even in the presence of a functioning neuraxial anesthetic. Patients who cannot or do not wish to receive neuraxial analgesia or anesthesia may be managed with opioids and nonpharmacologic modalities. The opioid-tolerant patient often reports higher pain scores and increased sensitivity to painful stimuli and may require larger than expected doses of opioids compared to the opioid-naive patient.[88,89] Consequently, monitoring for respiratory depression and sedation should be available and instituted when indicated. There is an inherent risk of neonatal abstinence syndrome in the presence of opiates and adjuvant analgesics use by the mother. This risk should be anticipated and followed by appropriate care of the neonate.

The opioid-tolerant patient will benefit from continuity of care after delivery and discharge from the medical facility. The patients should resume follow-up with their outpatient programs (e.g., methadone or buprenorphine maintenance program) and with the physician who is responsible for maintaining their chronic pain therapy. However, it is not uncommon for opioid-tolerant patients to experience barriers or difficulty with access to consistent chronic pain relief and/or maintenance programs, and this may complicate their long-term care.

Evidence-based treatment options for the opioid-tolerant pregnant patient are limited, and further research on the opioid-tolerant pregnant patient is needed to help guide practitioners in providing appropriate and optimum care for the mother and developing fetus or newborn.

APPENDIX A

Addiction is a primary, chronic disease of the brain characterized by the compulsive pursuit of reward or relief by substance use despite physical, psychological, or social harm. The American Society of Addiction Medicine published a policy statement on the definition of addiction, available at http://www.asam.org/advocacy/find-a-policy-statement/

view-policy-statement/public-policy-statements/2011/12/15/the-definition-of-addiction.

Opioid dependence is a chronic substance use disorder characterized by a persistent pattern of behavior leading to its continued use.[90]

Opioid tolerance is defined as a state of adaptation that occurs when repeated exposure to a drug diminishes its antinociceptive effect such that a higher dose of the drug is needed to maintain this pharmacologic effect. Opioid tolerance is a predictable pharmacologic adaptation characterized by a rightward shift in the dose–response curve (Fig. 10.1).[91] The other characteristics involve tolerance to the euphoric, sedative, respiratory depressive, and nausea effects from opioids, but not to constipation.[92,93]

Physical dependence is a state of adaptation manifested by a withdrawal syndrome specific to a drug class.[94]

Withdrawal syndrome may occur from (1) an abrupt cessation of an opioid, (2) a decreasing blood level of the drug, or (3) a rapid dose reduction and/or administration of an antagonist agent. Signs and symptoms include yawning, lacrimation, perspiration, mydriasis, tremor, restlessness, myalgias, piloerection, anorexia, nausea, vomiting, abdominal cramps, and diarrhea. The patient may also present with fever, hyperventilation, and hypertension. Other associated symptoms include sleep disturbance, poor concentration, and irritability, all of which may persist even after the acute withdrawal symptoms have subsided.[95]

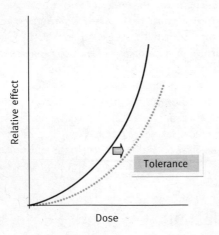

Figure 10.1 Shifts in a dose–response curve with tolerance.[91] There is a shift of the curve to the right, doses higher than initial doses are required to achieve the same effects. (Modified from O'Brien Charles P. Drug addiction. In: Brunton LL, Chabner BA, Knollmann BC, eds. *Goodman & Gilman's The Pharmacological Basis of Therapeutics* 12th ed. New York: McGraw-Hill; 2011)

REFERENCES

1. World Health Organization. *Cancer Pain Relief*. Geneva: World Health Organization; 1986.
2. Brennan F, Carr DB, Cousins M. Pain management: a fundamental human right. *Anesth Analg* 2007;105(1):205–21.
3. Cousins MJ, Lynch ME. The Declaration Montreal: access to pain management is a fundamental human right. *Pain* 2011;152(12):2673–4.
4. *Relieving Pain in America, a Blueprint for Transforming Prevention, Care, Education, and Eesearch*. Washington, DC: Institute of Medicine, The National Academies Press; 2011.
5. Eriksen J, Sjogren P, Bruera E, Ekholm O, Rasmussen NK. Critical issues on opioids in chronic non-cancer pain: an epidemiological study. *Pain* 2006;125(1–2):172–9.
6. Hawkins J. Epidural analgesia for labor and delivery. *New Engl J Med* 2010;362:1503–10.
7. Desmond MM, Wilson GS. Neonatal abstinence syndrome: recognition and diagnosis. *Addict Dis* 1975;2:113–21.
8. Finnegan, L. Kaltenbach, K. Neonatal abstinence syndrome. In: Hoekelman R, Friedman S, Nelson N, Seidel H, ed. *Primary Pediatric Care*. St Louis, MO: Mosby-Year Book; 1992: 1367–78.
9. Jamison R, Ross E, Michna E, Chen L, Holcomb C, Wasan A. Substance misuse treatment for high-risk chronic pain patients on opioid therapy. *Pain* 2010;150(3):390–400.
10. Substance Abuse and Mental Health Services Administration. *Results from the 2009 National Survey on Drug Use and Health: Vol. 1. Summary of National Findings* (Office of Applied Studies, NSDUH Series H-38A, HHS Publication No. SMA 10–4856 Findings). Rockville, MD: Substance Abuse and Mental Health Services Administration.
11. Substance Abuse and Mental Health Services Administration. *Results from the 2010 National Survey on Drug Use and Health: Summary of National Findings* (NSDUH Series H-41, HHS Publication No. SMA 11–4658). Rockville, MD: Substance Abuse and Mental Health Services Administration; 2010.

12. European Monitoring Centre for Drugs and Drug Addiction. Statistical bulletin 2008. Lisbon, Portugal: EMCDDA; 2008.

13. Gyarmathy VA, Giraudon I, Hedrich D, Montanari L, Guarita B, Wiessing L. Drug use and pregnancy–challenges for public health. *Euro Surveill* 2009;14(9):pii=19142.

14. Substance Abuse and Mental Health Services Administration. *Results from the 2008 National Survey on Drug Use and Health: National Findings* (Office of Applied Studies, NSDUH Series H-36, HHS Publication No. SMA 09-4434). Rockville, MD: Substance Abuse and Mental Health Services Administration; 2009.

15. Gaiser R. Physiologic changes of pregnancy. In: Chestnut DH, Polley LS, Tsen LC, Wong CA, eds. *Chestnut's Obstetric Anesthesia, Principles and Practice*. 4th ed. Philadelphia, PA: Mosby, Elsevier; 2009:15–36.

16. Craft RM. Modulation of pain by estrogens. *Pain* 2007;132:S3–12

17. Ji Y, Murphy AZ, Traub RJ. Estrogen modulation of morphine analgesia of visceral pain in female rats is supraspinally and peripherally mediated. *J Pain* 2007;8(6):494–502.

18. Datta S, Hurley RJ, Naulty JS, et al. Plasma and cerebrospinal fluid progesterone concentrations in pregnant and nonpregnant women. *Anesth Analg* 1986;65(9):950–4.

19. Iwasaki H, Collins JG, Saito Y, Kerman-Hinds A. Naloxone-sensitive, pregnancy-induced changes in behavioral responses to colorectal distention: pregnancy-induced analgesia to visceral stimulation. *Anesthesiology* 1991;74(5):927–33.

20. Levinson, GM, Shnider, SM. Anesthesia for surgery during pregnancy. In: Hughes SC, Levinson G, Rosen MA, eds. *Shnider and Levinson's Anesthesia for Obstetrics*. 4th ed. Philadelphia, PA: Lippincott Williams & Wilkins; 2002: 249–266.

21. Dalby PL, Ramanathan S, Rudy TE, et al. Plasma and saliva substance P levels: the effects of acute pain in pregnant and non-pregnant women. *Pain* 1997;69(3):263–7.

22. Parry E, Shields R, Turnbull AC. Transit time in the small intestine in pregnancy. *J Obstet Gynaecol Br Commonw* 1970;77:900–1.

23. Cunningham FG, Leveno KJ, Bloom SL, Hauth JC, Rouse DJ, Spong CY. Teratology and medications that affect the fetus. Available at: http://www.accessmedicine.com/content.aspx?aID=6022358. [accessed on June 7, 2012].

24. McElhatton PR. Pregnancy (2) general principles of drug use in pregnancy. *Pharm J* 2003; 270:232–4.

25. Heinonen OP, Slone D, Shapiro S. *Birth Defects and Drugs in Pregnancy: Maternal Drug Exposure and Congenital Malformations*. Littleton, MA: Publishing Sciences Group; 1977.

26. Sannerstedt R, Lundborg P, Danielsson BR, et al. Drugs during pregnancy: an issue of risk classification and information to prescribers. *Drug Saf* 1996;14(2):69–77.

27. Australian Drug Evaluation Committee, Medicines in Pregnancy Working Party. Prescribing medicines in pregnancy. Available at:ttp://www.tga.gov.au/hp/medicines-pregnancy-categorisation.htm. Accessed June 25, 2012.

28. Food and Drug Administration. Content and format of labeling for human prescription drug and biological products; requirements for pregnancy and lactation labeling. *Federal Register* 2008;73:30831–68.

29. Rathmell JP, Viscomi CM, Ashburn MA. Management of nonobstetric pain during pregnancy and lactation. *Anesth Analg* 1997;85(5): 1074–87.

30. Food and Drug Administration. Labeling requirements for prescription drugs and/or insulin. Available at: http://web.archive.org/web/20080326194429/http://www.fda.gov/cder/pediatric/21cfr20157.htm. [accessed on March 19, 2011].

31. Jones HE, O'Grady K, Dahne J, et al. Management of acute postpartum pain in patients maintained on methadone or buprenorphine during pregnancy. *Am J Drug Alcohol Abuse* 2009; 35(3):151–6.

32. ACOG Committee on Obstetric Practice. Guidelines for diagnostic imaging during pregnancy. *Obstet Gynecol* 2004;104:647–51.

33. McCollough CH, Schueler BA, Atwell TD, et al. Radiation exposure and pregnancy: when should we be concerned? *Radiographics* 2007; 27(4):909–17; discussion 917–918.

34. Dean PB. Fetal uptake of an intravascular radiologic contrast medium. *Rofo* 1977;127(3):267–70.

35. Mehta V, Langford RM. Acute pain management for opioid dependent patients. *Anaesthesia* 2006;61:269–76.

36. Dole VP, Nyswander M A. Medical treatment for diacetylmorphine (heroin) addiction. A clinical trial with methadone hydrochloride. *JAMA* 1965;193:646.

37. Medications development for the treatment of pregnant addicts and their infants. [National Institutes of Drug Abuse, Monograph 149]. Available at: http://archives.drugabuse.gov/pdf/monographs/download149.html. [accessed on March 9, 2011].

38. Davis MP, Walsh D. Methadone for relief of cancer pain: a review of pharmacokinetics, pharmacodynamics, drug interactions and protocols of administration. *Support Care Cancer* 2001;9:73–83.

39. Chung KS. Methadone. In: Sinatra RS, Jahr JS, Watkins-Pitchford JM, eds. *The Essence of Analgesia and Analgesics*. New York: Cambridge University Press; 2011: 127–131.

40. Hewitt DJ. The use of NMDA-receptor antagonists in the treatment of chronic pain. *Clin J Pain* 2000;16(2 Suppl):S73–9.

41. Henry-Edwards S, Gowing L, White J, et al. Clinical guidelines and procedures for the use of methadone in the maintenance treatment of opioid dependence. Commonwealth of Australia (2003), Available at http://www.health.vic.au/dpu/downloads/guidelines-methadone pdf. Accessed on June 27, 2012.

42. Substance Abuse and Mental Health Services Administration. Pregnant substance abusing women. Treatment Improvement Protocol (TIP) Series 2. Available to:http://www.ncbi.nlm.nih.gov/books/bv.fcgi?rid=hstat5.section.22556; DHHS Publication No.(SMA) 95–3056.html

43. NIH Consensus Development Project. Effective medical treatment of opiate addiction. Available at: http://consensus.nih.gov/1997/1998TreatOpiateAddiction108html.htm. [accessed on March 9, 2011].

44. Fischer G. Treatment of opioid dependence in pregnant women. *Addiction* 2000;95:1141–4.

45. Burns, L, Mattick, RP, Lim, K, Wallace, C. Methadone in pregnancy: treatment retention and neonatal outcomes. *Addiction* 2007;102:264.

46. Kandall SR, Doberczak TM, Jantunen M, et al. The methadone maintained pregnancy. *Clin Perinatol* 1999;26:173–83.

47. Wolff K, Boys A, Rostami-Hodjegan A, et al. Changes to methadone clearance during pregnancy. *Eur J Clin Pharmacol* 2005;11:765–8.

48. Almario CV, Seligman NS, Dysart KC, et al. Risk factors for preterm birth among opiate-addicted gravid women in a methadone treatment program. *Am J Obstet Gynecol* 2009;201:326.e1–6

49. American Academy of Pediatrics Committee on Drugs. Transfer of drugs and other chemicals in human milk. *Pediatrics* 2001;108:776–89

50. Martin J.A, Hamilton BE, Sutton PD, et al. Births: final data for 2006. *Natl Vital Stat Rep* 2009;57:1–102.

51. Ebert SN, Liu XK, Woosley RL. Female gender as a risk factor for drug induced cardiac arrhythmias: evaluation of clinical and experimental evidence. *J Womens Health* 1998;7:547–57.

52. Krantz MJ, Martin J, Stimmel B, Mehta D, Haigney MC. QTc interval screening in methadone treatment. *Ann Intern Med* 2009;150(6):387–95.

53. Vadivelu N, Anwar M. Buprenorphine in postoperative pain management. *Anesthesiol Clin* 2010;28:601–9.

54. Drugs.com. Buprenorphine hydrochloride. Available at:http://www.drugs.com/monograph/buprenorphine-hydrochloride.html. [accessed on June 7, 2012].

55. Clark NC, Lintzeris N, Muhleisen PJ. Severe opiate withdrawal in a heroin user precipitated by a massive buprenorphine dose. *Med J Aust* 2002;176:166–7.

56. Gevirtz C, Frost EA, Bryson EO. Perioperative implications of buprenorphine maintenance treatment for opioid addiction. *Int Anesthesiol Clin* 2011;49(1):147–55.

57. Alford DP, Compton P, Samet JH. Acute pain management for patients receiving maintenance methadone or buprenorphine therapy. *Ann Intern Med* 2006;144(2):127–34.

58. Jones HE, Martin PR, Heil SH, et al. Treatment of opioid-dependent pregnant women: clinical and research issues. *J Subst Abuse Treat* 2008;35(3):245–59.

59. Jones HE, Kaltenbach K, Heil SH, et al. Neonatal abstinence syndrome after methadone or buprenorphine exposure. *N Engl J Med* 2010;363(24):2320–31.

60. US Department of Health and Human Services. Clinical guidelines for the use of buprenorphine in the treatment of opioid addiction. A treatment improvement protocol: TIP 40. Available at: http://buprenorphine.samhsa.gov/Bup_Guidelines.pdf. [accessed on October 17, 2010].

61. Bennett GJ. Update on the neurophysiology of pain transmission and modulation: focus on the NMDA-receptor. *J Pain Symptom Manage* 2000;19(Suppl 1):S2–6.

62. Hocking G, Cousins MJ. Ketamine in chronic pain management: an evidence-based review. *Anesth Analg* 2003;97:1730–9.

63. Bell RF, Dahl JB, Moore RA, Kalso E. Perioperative ketamine for acute postoperative pain. *Cochrane Database Syst Rev* 2006;(1):CD004603.

64. Briggs GG, Freeman RK, Yaffe SJ. *Drugs in Pregnancy and Lactation: A Reference Guide to Fetal and Neonatal Risk*. 8th ed. Philadelphia, PA: Lippincott Williams & Wilkins; 2008.

65. FDA Drug Safety Comunication. Prescription acetaminophen products to be limited to 325mg per dosage unit boxed warning will highlight potential for severe liver failure. Available at: http://

www.fda.gov/Drugs/DrugSafety/ucm239821. htm. Accessed on June 27, 2012.

66. James AH, Brancazio LR, Price T. Aspirin and reproductive outcomes. *Obstet Gynecol Surv* 2008;63(1):49–57.

67. Koren G, Florescu A, Costei AM, Boskovic R, Moretti ME. Nonsteroidal antiinflammatory drugs during third trimester and the risk of premature closure of the ductus arteriosus: a meta-analysis. *Ann Pharmacother* 2006;40(5): 824–9.

68. Makol A, Wright K, Amin S. Rheumatoid arthritis and pregnancy: safety considerations in pharmacological management. *Drugs* 2011;71(15):1973–87.

69. Pennell, PB. Antiepileptic drugs during pregnancy: what is known and which AEDs seem to be safest? *Epilepsia* 2008;49(Suppl 9):43–55.

70. Molgaard-Nielsen D, Hviid A. Newer-generation antiepileptic drugs and the risk of major birth defects. *JAMA* 2011;305(19): 1996–2002.

71. Ohman I, Vitols S, Tomson T. Pharmacokinetics of gabapentin during delivery, in the neonatal period, and lactation: does a fetal accumulation occur during pregnancy? *Epilepsia* 2005;46:1621–4.

72. Eberhard-Gran M, Eskild A, Opjordsmoen S. Use of psychotropic medications in treating mood disorders during lactation: practical recommendations. *CNS Drugs* 2006;20(3):187–98.

73. Levin JB, Janata JW. Psychological interventions. In: Waldman SD, ed. *Pain Management*. Vol. 2. Philadelphia, PA: Saunders Elsevier; 2007: 1003–9.

74. Waldman SD, Waldman KA, Waldman HJ. Therapeutic heat and cold in the management of pain. In: Waldman SD, ed. *Pain Management*. Vol. 2. Philadelphia, PA: Saunders Elsevier; 2007: 1033–42.

75. Simkin PT, Bolding PT. Update on nonpharmacologic approaches to relieve labor pain and prevent suffering. *J Midwifery Womens Health* 2004;49(6):489–504.

76. Finnegan L. Influence of maternal drug dependence on the newborn. In: Kacew S, Lock S, eds. *Toxicologic and Pharmacologic Principles in Pediatrics*. New York: Hemisphere; 1988: 183–98.

77. Fischer G, Ortner R, Rohrmeister K, et al. Methadone versus buprenorphine in pregnant addicts: a double-blind, double-dummy comparison study. *Addiction* 2006;101(2):275–81.

78. Jansson LM, Velez M, Harrow C. The opioid-exposed newborn: assessment and pharmacologic management. *Opioid Manag* 2009;5(1):47–55.

79. Finnegan L. Neonatal abstinence syndrome: assessment and pharmacotherapy. In: Rubaltelli FF, Granti B, eds. *Neonatal Therapy: An Update*. New York: Elsevier Science; 1986: 122–46.

80. Doberczak T, Kandall S, Wilets I. Neonatal opiate abstinence syndrome in term and preterm infants. *J Pediatrics* 1991;118:933–7.

81. Rosen T, Pippenger C. Pharmacologic observations on the neonatal withdrawal syndrome. *J Pediatrics* 1976;88:1044–8.

82. Johnson K, Gerada C, Greenough A. Treatment of neonatal abstinence syndrome. *Arch Dis Child Fetal Neonatal* Ed 2003;88:1 F2–F5.

83. Winklbaur B, Kopf N, Ebner N, Jung E, Thau K, Fischer G. Treating pregnant women dependent on opioids is not the same as treating pregnancy and opioid dependence: a knowledge synthesis for better treatment for women and neonates. *Addiction* 2008;103(9):1429–40.

84. Kraft WK, Gibson E, Dysart K, Damle VS, Larusso JL, Greenspan JS. Sublingual buprenorphine for treatment of neonatal abstinence syndrome: a randomized trial. *Pediatrics* 2008;122(3): e601–7.

85. Coyle MG, Ferguson A, Lagasse L, et al. Diluted tincture of opium (DTO) and phenobarbital versus DTO alone for neonatal opiate withdrawal in term infants. *J Pediatr* 2002;140(5):561–4.

86. World Health Organization. *HIV and Infant Feeding: Guidelines for Healthcare Management and Supervisors*. Geneva, Switzerland: WHO; 1998.

87. American Academy of Pediatrics Committee on Drugs. Transfer of drugs and other chemicals in human milk. *Pediatrics* 2001;108:776–89.

88. Compton P, Charuvastra VC, Kintaudi K, Ling W. Pain responses in methadone-maintained opioid abusers. *J Pain Symptom Manage* 2000;20:237–45.

89. Meyer M, Wagner K, Benvenuto A, Plante D, Howard D. Intrapartum and postpartum analgesia for women maintained on methadone during pregnancy. *Obstet Gynecol* 2007;110:261–6.

90. Luscher C. Drugs of abuse. In: Katzung BG, Masters SB, Trevor AJ, eds. *Basic and Clinical Pharmacology*. 12th ed. New York: McGraw-Hill; 2012: 565–580.

91. O'Brien CP. Drug addiction. In: Brunton LL, Chabner BA, Knollmann BC, eds. *Goodman and Gilman's The Pharmacological Basis of Therapeutics*. 12th ed. Available at: http://www.accessmedicine.com/content.aspx?aID=16666364. [accessed on June 7, 2012].

92. Gutstein HB, Akil H. Opioid analgesics. In: Brunton LL, Parker K, Lazo J, Buxton I,

Blumenthal D, eds. *Goodman and Gilman's The Pharmacological Basis of Therapeutics.* 11th ed. New York: McGraw-Hill; 2006: 547–90.

93. Mitra S, Sinatra RS. Acute pain management in patients with opioid dependence and substance abuse. In: Sinatra RS, deLeon-Cassasola OA, Ginsberg B, Viscusi ER, eds. *Acute Pain Management.* New York: Cambridge University Press; 2009; 564–80.

94. American Psychiatric Association. *Diagnostic and Statistical Manual of Mental Disorders.* 4th ed, text revision. Washington, DC: American Psychiatric Association; 2000.

95. Vukmir RB. Drug seeking behavior. *Am J Drug Alcohol Abuse* 2004;30:551–75.

11

CHRONIC PELVIC PAIN:

DYSMENORRHEA AND ENDOMETRIOSIS

Amy Stenson and Andrea J. Rapkin

INTRODUCTION

Chronic pelvic pain (CPP) affects up to 20% of reproductive aged women.[1] Endometriosis is the most common reproductive system diagnosis in women who undergo investigation for CPP. Endometriosis is a chronic disease that is difficult to completely eradicate. Over the course of the reproductive years, women with endometriosis will often require several pharmacological and/or surgical treatments. This chapter will focus on the clinical diagnosis and management of endometriosis, including evidence and specific recommendations for each therapeutic option. Since menstrual pain is the most prevalent symptom of endometriosis, we will also briefly discuss primary dysmenorrhea and other causes of secondary dysmenorrhea. As is the case with most chronic pain disorders, the degree of anatomic pathology in women with endometriosis often fails to explain the severity of the pain and associated symptoms. Recent research suggests that endometriosis can alter neural processing, fostering the development and maintenance of chronic pain.[2] This chapter will also summarize relevant research studies highlighting the interactions of the reproductive, immunological, and central nervous systems (CNS) in this disorder.

DYSMENORRHEA

Dysmenorrhea is a common pain symptom affecting up to 60% of women in the reproductive age group.[3] Menstrual pain in the absence of pelvic pathology is defined as primary dysmenorrhea. Primary dysmenorrhea generally begins with the inception of ovulatory cycles, 1–2 years after menarche, and may persist throughout the reproductive life span. Secondary dysmenorrhea, painful menses associated with underlying pathology, often develops later in the reproductive years. Secondary dysmenorrhea can occur with either ovulatory or anovulatory cycles.[4,5]

PRIMARY DYSMENORRHEA

Progesterone levels decrease in the late luteal phase, triggering the release of lytic enzymes and phospholipids from the secretory endometrium, with the subsequent generation of arachidonic acid and activation of the cyclooxygenase (COX) pathway. Primary dysmenorrhea results from upregulated COX enzyme activity and an increase in prostanoids, leading to higher uterine tone and increased amplitude of uterine contractions.[6] Uterine hypercontractility, decreased uterine blood flow, production of other algesic agents secondary to hypoxia, and increased peripheral nerve hypersensitivity all contribute to the pain.[6,7]

SIGNS AND SYMPTOMS

Symptoms of primary dysmenorrhea are suprapubic cramping accompanied by lower back pain and/or pain that radiates down the anterior thighs, diarrhea, nausea, vomiting, and rarely syncope. The pain is colicky in nature, similar to labor pain, and is often alleviated by movement, counterpressure, heat, or lower abdominal massage. Pain begins a few hours before or just after the beginning of menstrual flow and lasts for 48–72 hours. Signs include suprapubic tenderness with no upper abdominal tenderness or rebound.

DIAGNOSIS

The diagnosis of primary dysmenorrhea depends on confirming the cyclic nature of the pain and excluding pelvic pathology by clinical exam and ancillary laboratory studies. Pelvic infection, such as endometritis or pelvic inflammatory disease, should be ruled out if pain is acute, recent in onset, or associated with risks for or signs of infection. Sexual activity, lack of condom use, fever, peritoneal signs, bilateral adnexal or cervical motion tenderness, or mucopurulent cervical discharge should prompt further testing. Gonorrhea and Chlamydia nucleic acid amplification tests, complete blood count, erythrocyte sedimentation rate, and pregnancy testing may be indicated. The pelvic exam is normal in cases of primary dysmenorrhea. However, tenderness may be noted with the bimanual exam during menses, although severe pain with palpation or cervical motion is absent. The exam should focus on uterine and adnexal size, shape, mobility, and tenderness, as well as the contour of the uterosacral ligaments and rectovaginal septum. Pelvic ultrasound is helpful to confirm normal anatomy, particularly if symptoms persist despite first-line treatment. Laparoscopy is not generally indicated.

MANAGEMENT

The mainstay of therapy for primary dysmenorrhea is the class of drugs known as the prostaglandin synthase inhibitors or non-steroidal anti-inflammatory agents (NSAIDs).[8] Treatment should be initiated 1–3 days prior to the onset of menses or at the first onset of symptoms (mild pain or bleeding) and continued every 6–8 hours for the first 2–3 days of menses. Patients will typically respond within the first cycle. If the initial regimen is not successful, the dosage may be optimized or another type of NSAID tried. The medication is generally well tolerated and side effects are mild (dyspepsia, nausea, diarrhea, fatigue). Contraindications to treatment include gastrointestinal ulcers and hypersensitivity to aspirin.

Another effective treatment for primary dysmenorrhea is hormonal therapy, which is preferable for patients who also desire contraception. Options include the combined estrogen and progesterone oral contraceptive pill (OC), vaginal ring, transdermal patch, progestin-only pill, progestin depo injection or implant, or levonorgesterol-releasing intrauterine device. Hormonal contraception has been shown to be more effective than placebo and results in less absence from work and school.[9] For those using OCs who continue to have bothersome symptom with menses, it is recommended that OCs be given continuously without a pill-free interval or as an extended cycle with a menstrual bleed every 3 months or so.[10] The hormonal contraception creates an endocrine milieu similar to the early proliferative phase of the menstrual cycle when prostaglandin levels are lowest; inhibits ovulation and decreases endometrial proliferation, ultimately resulting in diminished uterine cramping.

Complementary and alternative therapy has been shown to reduce the severity of symptoms, and there is evidence for heat, acupuncture, and transcutaneous electrical nerve stimulation.[11-13] There is currently insufficient evidence to support any particular herbal or vitamin regimen for treatment of dysmenorrhea.

For patients with refractory severe primary dysmenorrhea, an opioid may be added for 2–3 days per month after a thorough physical and psychological evaluation have been conducted to exclude other disease processes. Prior to initiating opioids, when NSAIDs and hormonal contraceptives have failed, consideration should be given to diagnostic laparoscopy to rule out endometriosis or other treatable pathology. Rarely, for women who have contraindications or inability to tolerate hormonal approaches, uterine nerve ablation, presacral neurectomy, or hysterectomy may be necessary to adequately address severe primary dysmenorrhea.[14]

SECONDARY DYSMENORRHEA

Secondary dysmenorrhea is defined as cyclic menstrual pain that is associated with underlying pelvic pathology. Pain frequently begins days or up to 1–2 weeks prior to the onset of menses and continues through the end of bleeding. The differential diagnosis of secondary dysmenorrhea, in order of frequency, includes endometriosis, adenomyosis, nonhormonal intrauterine devices, endometritis, congenital abnormalities of the reproductive system, cervical stenosis, and possibly pelvic congestion syndrome. The diagnosis of secondary dysmenorrhea depends on confirmation of pelvic pathology, which will usually require imaging or laparoscopy. With pain occurring throughout the cycle, the linkage of pain with the premenstrual and menstrual phases may require daily charting of bleeding and pain. NSAIDs and hormonal therapy are less effective for secondary dysmenorrhea, and management generally relies on treatment of the underlying pathology.

ADENOMYOSIS

Adenomyosis is defined as the presence of endometrial stroma and glands within the myometrium, whereas endometriosis is characterized by ectopic endometrium located outside of the uterine cavity. Adenomyosis typically occurs in women over 40 years of age but can be found as early as the late 20s. Risk factors include increasing parity, early menarche, and short menstrual cycles.[15–17] The symptoms of adenomyosis begin up to 2 weeks before the onset of and through the cessation of menses and can include heavy or prolonged menstrual bleeding, dysmenorrhea, and deep dyspareunia.

The diagnosis is made clinically. On physical exam, the uterus is globular, mildly enlarged, tender, and mobile. Although transvaginal ultrasound and pelvic magnetic resonance imaging may suggest the diagnosis, scans are accurate in less than 30% of the cases.[18] Adenomyosis is a histological diagnosis that can only be made definitively if the patient undergoes hysterectomy. Adenomyosis and endometriosis often coexist; the underlying disease processes and treatment strategies are similar, although patients with adenomyosis are more likely to benefit from hysterectomy or uterine artery embolization.[16,19]

ENDOMETRIOSIS

Endometriosis is defined as the presence of endometrial glands and stroma in extrauterine sites. The implants are typically found in the dependent portions of the pelvis, including uterine serosa, ovaries, and pelvic peritoneum; in the large bowel; and in 14% of the cases, the appendix. Rarely the lungs or other distant sites can be affected. Estrogen-dependent in nature, endometriosis affects women of reproductive age and becomes inactive after menopause, unless hormonal therapy is used.[20–23] Dysmenorrhea, deep dyspareunia, dyschezia, abnormal uterine bleeding, and subfertility are the hallmark symptoms. However, moderate to severe debilitating chronic pain can occur. Some women are asymptomatic with endometriosis discovered at the time of infertility investigation or surgery for a pelvic mass. Endometriosis is associated with significant social and physical debility, increased medical costs, high rates of emergency department visits, and substantial time lost from work.[24,25]

The prevalence of endometriosis in the general population is not known but has been reported for certain subgroups. In women undergoing a benign gynecologic surgery, endometriosis has been observed in only 1%–7% of women, while for women undergoing diagnostic laparoscopy for chronic pelvic pain, endometriosis is found in 12%–32% of patients.[26,27] In adolescents who come to surgical exploration for the evaluation of severe refractory chronic pelvic pain, the prevalence of endometriosis may be as high as 50%.[28] Risk factors for chronic pain associated with endometriosis include nulliparity, early menarche, late menopause, short menstrual cycles, prolonged menses, Müllerian anomalies, and low body mass index.[22, 29,30]

PATHOGENESIS

The definitive pathogenesis of endometriosis has not been established; however, there are several predominant hypotheses.[31] The "implantation" theory proposes that endometrial cells are shed during menstruation and transported retrograde through the fallopian tubes into the peritoneal cavity, where they implant on pelvic structures. This theory is supported by the observation that the incidence of endometriosis is increased with partial obstruction of the menstrual flow (such as transverse vaginal septum or other uterine Müllerian anomalies),[32] though rates of retrograde menstruation are similar in women with and without endometriosis. The "direct transplantation theory" poses that endometrial cells are disseminated throughout the body through blood vessels or the lymphatic system. The third theory suggests that the peritoneal cavity contains undifferentiated cells that undergo "coelomic metaplasia" and become endometrial tissue. Development of endometriosis is also related to additional factors such as immune system functioning, genetic predisposition, and CNS input, which will be discussed later. There is significant variation in the appearance, location, and extent of endometriotic lesions.

ENDOMETRIOTIC LESIONS

Grossly, lesions are divided into three categories: superficial peritoneal, deeply infiltrating (DIE), and ovarian (cystic) endometriosis, called endometriomas.[33–35] Laparoscopy allows for biopsy of lesions for histological confirmation.[36] A visual survey without biopsy is accepted as the standard for diagnosis but may lead to misclassification of lesions because it does not accurately assess the depth of lesions. Histological diagnosis of disease is important because minimal or mild disease seen on survey is frequently not confirmed by biopsy,[37,38] and superficial peritoneal lesions frequently have an atypical appearance and may be confused with scarring or other pelvic pathology.[39]

SPECTRUM OF PAIN

A causal relationship between specific endometriotic lesions and pain has not been definitively established. The location and burden of lesions often have little or no relation to the magnitude or location of pain that a woman experiences.[40–42] Women with minimal lesions and low-stage disease based on the American Society of Reproductive Medicine (ASRM) criteria may experience severe pain, while others with extensive endometriosis and large ovarian endometriotic cysts (endometriomata) may be asymptomatic. Any of the three lesion types can be associated with CPP.[43] The presence of an endometrioma is not correlated with the severity of dysmenorrhea.[44] However, endometriomas may suggest the presence of more severe DIE in the cul de sac.[45] DIE of the rectovaginal septum or vagina has been more consistently associated with severe pain, dyspareunia, and gastrointestinal symptoms; in particular, dyschezia.[43,46] Local inflammation is part of the tissue response to endometriosis and generally leads to the formation of adhesions.[47,48] The relationship between adhesions, pain, and endometriosis is also not well understood,[37,47,49,50] as many women with severe adhesions have no pain and adhesiolysis is not invariably associated with diminution of pain.[51]

Since lesion size and location do not correlate well with symptom severity and location of pain, explaining the genesis of pain has proved challenging. The range of pain symptoms encompassed by endometriosis also typically extends beyond the reproductive tract; muscular pain, urinary urgency, urinary frequency, bladder pain, dyschezia, irritable bowel–like symptoms, and chronic noncyclical abdominal-pelvic pain are common. There is a great degree of variability in the nature and severity of pain among individuals. Chronologically, the initiation of the pain syndrome generally begins with cyclic pain (dysmenorrhea), which can progress over time to include prolonged cyclic pain and chronic acyclic pelvic pain and dysfunctional activity and pain in other pelvic visceral and somatic structures that share innervations with the reproductive tract.[52] The constellation of pain symptoms, chronicity, and association with other chronic pain syndromes reflects the variable activity of the lesions, the involvement of the immune system, and characteristics of the upregulated and sensitized CNS[52] (see later discussion).

CLINICAL ASSESSMENT

Endometriosis is suspected clinically based on a history of severe dysmenorrhea and cyclic pelvic pain. Particular attention should be paid to the timing, location, and symptoms associated with the pain. The pain begins up to 2 weeks prior to menses and may be sharp or pressure-like in nature. It is often localized to the midline of the lower abdomen with radiation to the back. Associated symptoms include dyparenunia (deep thrust), dyschezia, urinary frequency or urgency, bloating, and rarely hematochezia or hematuria. A history of infertility or subfertility is common. Another important aspect of the history is the responsiveness of the pain to prior treatment modalities, particularly hormonal therapy.

The physical exam may elicit focal tenderness of the uterus, rectovaginal septum, or uterosacral ligaments. The bimanual exam may identify uterosacral nodularity, a fixed retroverted uterus, or laterally deviated cervix resulting from fibrosis from endometriosis. Fullness of the adnexa on bimanual exam suggests an ovarian endometrioma.

A definitive diagnosis can only be made surgically. However, ultrasound may help identify endometriotic cysts, which can generally be distinguished from other types of adnexal masses and are homogenous, hemorrhagic appearing cysts persisting over a few menstrual cycles. CA-125 can be elevated, but this marker and others that have been described are nonspecific and generally not helpful.[53]

Direct visualization by laparoscopy or laparotomy establishes the diagnosis of endometriosis. Lesions vary widely in appearance. Early lesions may appear as active red flame, colorless vesicles, or reddish petechial lesions, while long-standing lesions frequently have a brown-black powder burn, fibrotic appearance. Common lesion sites include the posterior cul de sac, uterosacral ligaments, adnexae, and pelvic peritoneum. Suspicious lesions should be biopsied to confirm diagnosis histologically.

Endometriosis is staged using the ASRM classification system based on lesion size, depth, location, and associated adhesions observed during surgery. It is limited by an inability to correlate pain with physical findings and falls short of being able to predict patient outcomes such as pain or infertility.[54] Pain in endometriosis is usually classified as dysmenorrhea, dyspareunia, or CPP and absent, mild, moderate, or severe in intensity. This system fails to capture the specific pain characteristics of each patient and hampers the ability to assess individual outcomes.[55,56] A detailed, individualized history is needed, as well as a physical exam that includes the mapping of pain by attempting to reproduce the pain during a single-digit pelvic exam of vagina and pelvic floor muscles, in addition to examimation of the urinary bladder, cervix, paracervical region, cardinal and broad ligaments, uterus, ovaries, uterosacral ligaments, and rectum.

It is important to exclude or treat other comorbid conditions or "pain generators" that may be contributing to or causing pain. Subacute pelvic infection and disorders of the genitourinary, gastrointestinal, myofascial, and neurologic systems should be excluded.[24,57] In particular, other pain conditions such as irritable bowel syndrome, gastroesophageal reflux disease, painful bladder/interstitial cystitis, myofascial pain, low back pain, fibromyalgia, migraines, and other headache disorders must be considered. Chronic fatigue syndrome and mood or anxiety disorders, including depression, generalized anxiety and panic disorder, and posttraumatic stress syndrome, may play a significant role in negatively impacting the quality of life for individuals with endometriosis.[58] All of these factors should be considered when planning therapy for patients, and a multidisciplinary approach is generally optimal.

MECHANISMS OF PAIN IN ENDOMETRIOSIS

While surgical destruction of lesions leads to pain relief in some patients, suggesting that the lesions themselves play a role in the generation of pain, the mechanisms by which they cause pain are unclear.[37] Pain frequently returns with or without evidence of lesions,[59] and severity of pain is not correlated with extent of lesion severity.[36] Furthermore, patients with minimal or mild disease are more likely to experience a recurrence of symptoms soon after treatment.[60] CNS remodeling is likely to play a role in the pain symptoms of these patients. There are a few hypotheses regarding how endometriosis lesions engage the nervous system and produce pain. The following types of translational and clinical evidence will be discussed: de novo innervation of implants, infiltration or compression of existing pelvic nerve fibers, production of algesic substances, and hormonal modulation.

INNERVATIONS

Endometriosis requires vacularization of lesions to survive, and these blood vessels are innervated with sensory and sympathetic fibers.[61,62] When angiogenesis occurs, the nerves supplying the vessels may "sprout" and invade endometriotic lesions under the influence of such chemicals as vascular endothelial growth factor (VEGF) and nerve growth factor (NGF).[63-65] This direct sensory and sympathetic innervation of ectopic endometriotic lesions has been shown both in rat models and in lesions from women.[52,66] In a rodent model of endometriosis (ENDO), pieces of uterine horn sutured to the bowel mesentery simulate endometriotic growths, develop hormonal sensitivity, and produce pain behavior.[66] Histologically, the lesions vascularize and develop a nerve supply (neuroangiogenesis), demonstrating immunohistological staining consistent with both sensory and autonomic functions. In the rat ENDO model, pain symptoms manifest as estrous cycle–dependent pain behavior, vaginal hyperalgesia, increased abdominal muscle activity,[67] and increased bladder irritability as manifested by lower urinary micturition threshold.[68] As in women, the severity of pain behavior in the ENDO rats does not correlate with the volume of the endometriotic growths.[69] When the ectopic lesions develop a nerve supply, there is increased communication between the endometriotic growths and the dorsal root neurons and other regions of the CNS.[52,70] This access to the CNS has been suggested to underlie the increased pain perception as well as the viscero-visceral and viscero-somatic sensitization and the viscero-muscular reflex changes seen in ENDO rats and women with endometriosis.

Histological studies of implants in women are analogous to the rat ENDO findings.[52]

Women with higher chronic pelvic pain, dysmenorrhea, and dyspareunia scores exhibited endometriotic lesions with a higher mean percentage or density of nerve fibers[71] and also a greater degree of intraneurial infiltration by endometriosis.[72] DIE lesions (the lesions associated with the highest correlation with pain symptoms) have denser sympathetic and parasympathetic innervations than peritoneal or ovarian implants.[73-75] Increased nerve fiber density has also been documented in DIE implants in ovarian endometriomas and of the bowel.[73,76,77] DIE vaginal endometriotic nodules also have greater nerve density than the surrounding vaginal tissue.[78] Mast cells may also contribute to the hyperalgesia and pain in endometriosis. Increased numbers of activated and degranulated mast cells were intimately associated with nerves in the most painful DIE lesions.[79] However, although more research is needed, it appears that in less deeply infiltrating implants the direct correlation between nerves and pain may not be substantiated: pain has not been correlated with nerve fiber density in adhesions, peritoneum, or endometriomas.[80,81]

Pain can also be augmented by compression or infiltration of existing nerves near or within lesions. This can contribute to pain when deeply infiltrating lesions invade highly innervated structures like the uterosacral ligaments.[82,83]

There are also nerve fibers, particularly sensory C fibers in the uterine endometrium and myometrium in women with endometriosis, which are absent or rare in women without endometriosis.[84,85] It has been suggested that detection of nerve fibers in the endometrium via deep biopsy could be a useful diagnostic tool with sensitivity (98%) and specificity (83%) similar to laparoscopy.[86]

CENTRAL NERVOUS SYSTEM FACTORS

Central sensitization is defined as "an increase in the excitability of neurons so that normal input elicits an exaggerated response."[87] This may be an important mechanism underlying pain hypersensitivity in endometriosis. Central neural processing initiated with peripheral sensitization may become independently maintained and, thus, central sensitization occurs in a similar manner to the formation of other memories.[88,89] The pain becomes independent of the original stimulus and therapies directed at the periphery are less likely to alleviate pain.[2]

In the rat ENDO model, afferent fibers from the mesenteric implants in the rat enter the spinal cord well above the region of the cord that receives input from the vagina and lower pelvis (e.g., bladder, vagina, the lower abdominal wall muscles), suggesting altered intersegmental and CNS modulation of sensory information. The vaginal hyperalgesia in the ENDO rats is increased when the mesenteric ENDO cysts are resected surgically but only incompletely removed.[90] Hypothetically, the surgery may exacerbate the noxious stimulus to the afferent fibers in the ENDO and thereby upregulate CNS neurotransmission. Furthermore, the CNS effects in the setting of endometriosis are not solely under the influence of estradiol.[90]

Evidence for central sensitization in women with endometriosis was established by Bajaj et al. Injection of hypertonic saline into muscles of the hand produced increased pain intensity, pain area, and hypersensitivity to pressure stimulation of the hand compared to control women.[91] The CNS mechanisms underlying the genesis and maintenance of pain in women and in the animal models are an area of active research.

VISCERO-VISCERAL CROSS-SENSITIZATION

The incidence of other pelvic pain syndromes in women with endometriosis is high, suggesting mechanisms of "cross-talk" between organ systems contribute to the pain.[68,92] It is thought that most cross-talk occurs at the spinal cord level.[2] In rodents, for example, inflammation of the uterus directly affects the colon, leading to increased pERK and substance P in the dorsal root ganglia.[93] Inflammation of either the bladder or colon cross-sensitizes the other organ, possibly via a mast cell–mediated process and afferent C fibers.[94]

ALGESIC SUBSTANCES

Algesic agents increase neural activation. Relevant inflammatory mediators for endometriosis-related pain include prostaglandins, cytokines, and various peptides such as NGF, transforming growth factor beta-1 (TGFβ-1), and tumor necrosis factor alpha (TNF-α). It has been suggested that pro-inflammatory factors are released into the peritoneal fluid, where they may elicit pain by activation of sensory nerve fibers.[31] Angiogenic factors such as VEGF, insulin-like growth factor, interleukins (IL-6 and IL-8), and TGF-β have also been identified in pelvic peritoneal fluid and are thought to play a role in the development of increased vasculature around endometriotic implants and, as noted earlier, novel innervations.[95] DIE endometriotic lesions are associated with both increased microvascular density and increased angiogenic growth factor expression.[96] The process of neuroangiogenesis, which involves the recruitment and development of nerves and vasculature in ectopic endometriotic implants, may have important implications for novel targeted therapy.[95]

Pro-inflammatory cytokine production is associated with chronic pain states in both animals and humans.[97,98] It has been demonstrated that administration of inflammatory cytokines in animal models results in illness, increased sensitivity to stimuli and hyperalgesia; and that administration of IL-1 receptor antagonist or TNF-α antagonist will reverse the pain.[99,100] In endometriosis these same cytokines are found in peritoneal fluid.[97] Unfortunately, TNF-α inhibitors have not been found to be effective for pain in women with endometriosis.[101]

NGF increases neuronal growth and may act on nerves to produce pain by increasing the sensitivity and excitability of receptors.[102] In deep adenomyotic nodules, NGF concentrations have been correlated with pain and hyperalgesia.[70] Transforming growth factor beta-1 (TGFβ-1) has been implicated in modulating the pain of dysmenorrhea, and high levels of TGFβ-1 have been found in DIE lesions.[103]

In the rat ENDO model, the degree of vaginal hyperalgesia is directly correlated with levels of NGF and VEGF in the lesions.[104] Sympathetic and sensory fibers respond to NGF [105] and convey hormonally modifiable information bidirectionally. Further support for the neurovascular connection lies in the strong association between sympathetic nerve fibers and blood vessels in endometiotic lesions infiltrating the uterosacral ligaments.[106] These findings suggest that endometriosis is a "neurovascular condition" similar to a headache, a concept that has also been suggested clinically.[104]

C-fibers are found in ectopic endometriotic growths in the rat model and in women.[66,71,73,107] Normally silent, they respond to noxious events by conveying sensory information to the CNS and by releasing algesic substances such as Substance P, CGRP, tackykinins, somatostatin, nitric oxide, and other factors into the peritoneal environment.[108,109] This efferent process may lead to increased local vascular permeability and inflammation, termed "neurogenic inflammation."[110,111] The nerves may become sensitized and continue to exhibit electrical activity even after the original stimulus resolves.[112]

NEUROENDOCRINE AND OTHER HORMONAL FACTORS

The hypothalamic-pituitary-adrenal (HPA) axis is activated in animal models during tonic and phasic pain, which is a stressful event.[113] HPA activation results in increases in glucocorticoid secretion, loss of monoaminergic tone, and ultimately an increase in pain.[114] Prolonged activation of the HPA axis results in dysregulation, increased hormone production, and resistance to glucocorticoids, which, in turn, leads to an increased cytokine production. This process may contribute to peripheral and/or central sensitization. Similar to fibromyalgia and other inflammatory diseases in endometriosis, a dysfunctional HPA, axis is likely to contribute to the development of a chronic pain state.[2,115,116] Therapies that reduce estradiol and/or alter progesterone levels are often successful in alleviating pain for women with endometriosis, suggesting that these two hormones play an important role in the generation and/or maintenance of endometriosis pain.[117,118] The mechanisms underlying how hormones modulate pain are not well understood. Females suffer from more medically unexplained pain conditions and autoimmune disorders than do males. Additionally, pain disorders are often more severe in the premenstrual phase of the cycle. Estrogen and progesterone have myriad effects within the CNS.[2] Estradiol has been shown to influence peripheral sensory and sympathetic neurons as well as modulate central neuronal activity in pain states.[119-121] One example is how neurons in the thalamus process information related to the reproductive tract. In a rat model, estradiol was associated with increased thalamic response thresholds for cervical and vaginal stimulation.[122] This may help explain why hormonal therapy that lowers estradiol levels is sometimes effective for relief of pain even in the absence of visible endometriosis lesions or in women with bladder pain syndrome or irritable bowel syndrome.

In a rat ENDO model, the degree of vaginal hyperalgesia is affected by the phases of the ovarian estrous cycle with parallel histological changes in endometriosis lesions.[123] The ENDO rats have greater degrees of vaginal hyperalgesia and abdominal wall muscle activity in the presence of high levels of estradiol. Even in those rats whose ENDO cysts are completely removed and pain thus eliminated, the hyperalgesia returns when estradiol levels are increased.[90,123] These findings suggest that estradiol modulation of the pain response may occur at the level of the CNS rather than at the level of the lesion. A "memory" of CNS changes induced by growths may be created and later "recalled" by increased levels of estradiol.[2]

REPRODUCTIVE ORGANS' CONTRIBUTION TO PAIN

Uterine Endometrium and Myometrium

Normal menstrual endometrium contains cytokines, chemokines, leukocytes, VEGF, metalloproteinases, and prostaglandins. Alteration of these factors (cytokines, chemokines, etc.) may contribute to the process of nerve sprouting and sensitization.[124-126] These factors are produced in response to ovarian steroids and may be altered by hormonal treatment.[127] In endometriosis, there are subtle shifts in the endometrium that favor production of cytokines, prostaglandins, metalloproteinases, and estrogen. These factors are amplified when the endometrium attaches to mesothelial cells.[128] Women with endometriosis are often relatively "progesterone resistant," a finding that may be of key importance in development of endometriosis and pain and may be reversed with use of high-dose progestins.[129] As noted, nerve fibers in the endometrium of women with endometriosis have been observed, although how this finding will be used clinically has not yet been determined.[85,86,130,131] Hormonal modulation of the nerve growth in endometrium is an area of active research.

The theory of retrograde menstruation is the most widely accepted theory for how endometriosis develops; however, a more detailed explanation of the genetic, histological, inflammatory, or autoimmune risk factors has not been forthcoming. Uterine prostaglandins are found in higher concentrations in women with dysmenorrhea and may contribute to inflammation and sensitization if not treated.[132] Heavier menses is reported in women with endometriosis, and outflow obstruction of menses is a risk factor for the development of endometriosis and pain.[133,134] With removal of the obstruction, lesions and pain often resolve. The uterine endometrium appears to play a key role in the genesis of endometriosis. However, much work remains to be done to better understand its contribution to pain and how this can be modulated.

Increased nerve growth in the myometrium of women with pain compared with normal healthy women has been documented.[104] Contractions of the uterus are present throughout the menstrual cycle.[135] In normal women these contractions start in the fundus and propagate to the cervix during menses. These contractions are inhibited in women on oral contraceptives.[136,137] Prostaglandins may play a role in regulating myometrial contractions since use of PGE-2 and PGF-2α increases contractions and NSAIDs blunt contractions. It is believed that women with endometriosis have hyperkinetic or dyskinetic contraction patterns that hinder menstrual emptying. The pressure and frequency of contractions is higher and may lead to an increase in retrograde menses and deposition of debris and factors that could lead to nerve sprouting, inflammation, and sensitization in endometriosis.[2,138,139]

OVARIES AND PERITONEAL FLUID

The ovarian cycle is complex, regulated by the hypothalamic-pituitary ovarian axis and leading to events that may increase cytokines and inflammation.[140,141] Women with endometriosis generally have regular monthly menstrual cycles. Ovarian follicles have been shown to have 100-fold higher levels of hormones than plasma and, when ovulation occurs, hormones and cytokines are released into the abdominal/pelvic cavity.[142,143] This process is likely to contribute to pain through their actions on neurons. Oral contraceptives significantly diminish the release of hormones and fluid volume from the ovaries.[144]

The peritoneal fluid arises from vascular leakage and follicular fluid release and contains macrophages, cytokines, and interleukins.[98] In the setting of endometriosis, inflammation activates macrophages, which release cytokines, growth factors, and angiogenic factors that may contribute to nerve sprouting and sensitization.[98,145] Progestins in vitro have been shown to decrease macrophage production of cytokines, decrease angiogenesis, and increase natural killer cell activity, which may partially explain their effectiveness in vivo.[146,147]

MANAGEMENT OF ENDOMETRIOSIS AND ENDOMETRIOSIS-RELATED PAIN

First-line treatment of women with suspected endometriosis or adenomyosis is based on clinical, nonsurgical diagnosis. Surgery is reserved for women who are infertile, have an adnexal mass, or have failed initial medical management. Surgery is costly, invasive, and should be preformed by highly experienced laparoscopic surgeons. Medical management is recommended by an expert consensus panel, due to the low cost, excellent response rate, and low risk of this line of treatment. However, no studies have directly compared medical versus surgical therapy for the initial management of endometriosis. Primary medical management consists of a trial of at least one NSAID, followed by or with the addition of combined or progestin-only hormonal contraceptives for decidualization of implants and menstrual cycle control. There is a paucity of comparative data regarding the optimal therapy to target the symptoms of endometriosis.

ANALGESICS

Analgesic drugs (including NSAIDs and opioids) are commonly used to alleviate pain in women with endometriosis and are considered an important part of first-line therapy. However, there is a lack of conclusive evidence of their effectiveness in treating this disorder.[148] Attention should be directed to insure the optimal dosage and timing of administration for each NSAID and trying different regimens. Further research is warranted to determine the most effective regimens and to delineate the role of each type of NSAID in endometriosis-related pain relief.[2]

Opioids should be used cautiously in patients with chronic pain from endometriosis and only considered as a last resort when other treatment modalities have proved ineffective. Randomized clinical trial data supporting the use of opioids for endometriosis-related pain is lacking. In general, one should avoid daily opioids and place the main thrust of medical management on hormonal therapy. Hormonal therapy has the potential to reverse or decrease the progression of endometriosis and is generally well tolerated, especially if intrauterine progestins are included in the armamentarium. For those women with contraindications to hormonal therapy and NSAIDS, or in whom NSAIDS are ineffective, opioids are very reasonable for cyclic menstrual pain episodes and infrequent intermenstrual pain flares. However, for those women with severe, daily pain, uncontrolled with hormonal approaches and NSAIDS (or if these are contraindicated), surgery should be considered. Laparoscopic surgery can be very effective for 5 years or more, but up to 20% of women may not have prolonged relief with conservative surgery and this percentage increases over time. Repeated yearly or biannual laparoscopies are not indicated. Alternatively, surgery may no longer reveal evidence of endometriosis. In these cases, multidisciplinary therapy, including cognitive-behavioral pain management, is recommended, even if opioids are ultimately required. All pain generators should be explored once again before settling on chronic use of opioids (e.g., neuropathy, abdominal wall and pelvic floor myofascial abnormalities, bladder or gastrointestinal etiologies, and psychosocial issues, including depression or drug seeking).

If a physician deems that opioids are necessary, clear documentation of prior treatment failures and patient counseling is warranted. Opioids should be provided on a scheduled basis. A written narcotic contract should be created after the mutual decision is made to embark on provision of chronic opioid therapy. The contract should outline the following agreements: to allow the clinic access to prior treatment records, to obtain opioid medications from only one provider, to agree to frequent and consistent follow-up visits, to avoid illicit drugs and alcohol, and to agree to intermittent drug testing and psychological evaluation if needed; early refills and replacements of prescriptions are not allowed. The patient should be frequently reevaluated to assess the adequacy of pain relief, level of functioning, and quality of life.[149,150]

HORMONAL MODULATION: OVERVIEW

Endometriosis is an estrogen-dependent disease state, and the mainstay of hormonal therapy focuses on suppressing ovarian functioning, thereby lowering estrogen levels to those within the therapeutic window.[36] Equally effective options for management include combined estrogen-progestin OCs, depo or oral medroxyprogesterone acetate (MPA), other progestins such as gestrinone or norethindrone acetate, androgen derivatives such as danazol, and gonadotropin- releasing hormone (GnRH) agonists.[151–153] (See Table 11.1.) It has been shown that lesions are still present during hormonal treatment[154] but considered quiescent and perhaps neurologically inactive. When estrogen levels return to normal once ovulation and menstruation are restored, the pain often returns within a variable period of time.

ESTROGEN-PROGESTIN COMBINED CONTRACEPTIVES

Combined estrogen-progestin regimens suppress ovulation, thin the endometrium, promote decidualization, and lead to atrophy of endometriotic implants.[155] OCs have been

Table 11.1 Pharmacologic Options for Management of Endometriosis

CLASS	DRUG NAME	DOSAGE	DISADVANTAGES
Analgesics	Ibuprofen	400–800 mg PO tid to qid	Contraindicated for women with gastrointestinal issues, bleeding disorders, renal disease
	Naproxen sodium	500–550 mg bid	
	Mefemamic acid	500 mg x 1, then 250 mg q 6 hr PO	
Combined estrogen-progestin	Oral contraceptive pills	One pill taken daily May be taken cyclically or continuously	Spotting or breakthrough bleeding (esp. extended or continuous use)
	Transdermal patch	Apply to skin weekly x 3 weeks	Side effects: weight gain, nausea, breast tenderness a Increased risk of VTE
	Transvaginal ring	Placed vaginally monthly for 3 weeks	
Progestins	MPA	10 mg PO tid (max. dose 100 mg q day)	Side effects: nausea, breast tenderness, fluid retention, weight gain, depression, spotting/irregular bleeding
	MPA depot injection	150 mg IM q 2 weeks until amenorrhea then 150 mg q 3 months	
	Norethindrone acetate	5 mg q day (max dose 15 mg q day)	Loss of bone mineral density (MPA-depot)
	Levonorgestrel-releasing IUD	Replace every 5 years	Increased cramping (IUD)
	Etonorgestrel subdermal implant (Implanon)	Replace every 3 years	
Danazol	Oral	150–200 mg tid	Severe side effects (oral): weight gain, hirsuitism, decreased breast size, oily skin, acne, muscle cramps, hot flashes, mood changes, depression
	Vaginal	100–200 mg qd	
			May decrease HDL
Aromatase inhibitors	Anastrozle	1 mg PO q day	Bone loss
	Letrozole	2.5 mg PO q day	Cause multifollicular cyst development
			Must be prescribed with OCP or GnRH agonist to suppress ovulation
GnRH agonist	Nafarelin acetate (nasal)	200 mcg bid	Severe side effects: hot flushes, mood changes, vaginal dryness, sleep disturbance, headaches.
	Leuprolide acetate (IM)	3.75 mg q month 11.25 mg q 3 months	
	Goserelin acetate (Sub-Q)	3.6 mg SubQ q 28 days	Accelerates bone loss

(continued)

Table 11.1   (*Continued*)

CLASS	DRUG NAME	DOSAGE	DISADVANTAGES
Add-back therapy	Norethindrone acetate	5 mg PO q day	Recommended first line for preservation of bone density and relief of vasomotor sx
	Estrogen plus medroxyprogesterone acetate	0.625 mg/5 mg PO q day	Use for women who do not tolerate norethindrone add-back therapy

HDL, high-density lipoprotein; IUD, intrauterine device; MPA, medroxyprogesterone acetate; OCP, oral contraceptive pills; VTE, venous thromboembolism.

shown to be effective for pain reduction of moderate to severe dysmenorrhea due to endometriosis in a double-blind placebo-controlled trial.[156] This study also demonstrated a reduction in the volume of ovarian endometriomas for women given the OCs. For women who desire contraception, combined estrogen-progestin regimens are an excellent option. They have the advantage of long-term safety and relatively few side effects such that they may be taken indefinitely during the reproductive years. These regimens are highly effective when taken either cyclically (21/7 or 24/4 on/off regimens) or in an extended regimen without cessation of active pills. They can be administered orally, vaginally (contraceptive ring), or percutaneously (contraceptive patch), depending on tolerability and patient preference. There is no evidence that continuous OC use is superior to cyclic (21/7) or tricyclic (menstrual period once in 3 months) therapy for relieving the noncyclic pain of endometriosis.[157] The patient response is highly individual. If a patient does not respond to a cyclic regimen, then switching to a continuous regimen may be effective. A 3- to 6-month trial of therapy is recommended before switching to another treatment modality. Side effects are generally mild but can include nausea/vomiting, bloating, irregular bleeding, headache, moodiness, and breast tenderness. When given continuously, these regimens are more likely to result in breakthrough bleeding or spotting, which may not be tolerable for some patients. However, over 6 months or so, a continuous regimen generally leads to amenorrhea. Other uncommon adverse events include venous thrombosis and embolism, cardiovascular disease, stroke, headaches, and increased risk for cervical cancer. However, OC use decreases the risk of ovarian cancer, endometrial cancer, and colon cancer, and it does not appear to affect the incidence of breast cancer, although data are conflicting.[158] These events are rare but should be considered in patients with a personal or family history. Absolute contraindications to the use of OCs include previous thromboembolic event or stroke, a history of an estrogen-dependent tumor, active liver disease, pregnancy, undiagnosed abnormal uterine bleeding, hypertriglyceridemia, and heavy smoking (>15 cig/day) in a women over 35. Relative contraindications include poorly controlled hypertension, migraine headaches with aura, and women on anticonvulsants. For women on anticonvulsants, consideration should be given to the possibility of decreased efficacy of either the OC or the anticonvulsant, as both are metabolized by the same P450 system liver microsomal enzymes.

PROGESTINS

Progestins are also effective for the treatment of endometriosis, likely due to suppression of the hypothalamic pituitary axis and estrogen levels, as well as by promoting decidualization and atrophy of endometrium. The uterine endometrium in women with endometriosis has somewhat reduced sensitivity to endogenous progesterone[129,159] resulting in a pro-inflammatory cascade and dysregulation or altered expression of matrix metaloproteinases (MMP). MMP are important for breaking down the extracellular matrix and to such cellular processes as angiogenesis, tissue repair, and metastasis. Dysregulation of these processes may foster abnormal endometrial cell growth or degradation of extracellular matrix, leading to invasion of the endometrial cells. However, progestins in high doses have anti-angiogenic, anti-inflammatory, and immunomodulatory effects on endometrium[127] such that both in situ and ectopic endometrium (implants) are fundamentally altered and become decidualized. These effects serve to inhibit implantation and growth of endometrium that reaches the peritoneal cavity via retrograde menstrual flow.[127]

Progestins alone have been shown to effectively treat endometriosis in clinical trials with over 80% obtaining partial or complete relief of pain.[151,160] This therapy has fewer risks than gonadoropin-releasing hormone (GnRH) agonists but has been shown to be equally effective in decreasing dysmenorrhea, dyspareunia, and pelvic pain at 12 month follow-up.[161] Additionally, there may be some decrease in the size of lesions on treatment.[162] Traditionally, progestin therapy was given for 6–12 months, but if the regimen is effective and well tolerated, it may be extended indefinitely. Side effects are common and include weight gain, irregular uterine bleeding, mood changes, nausea, breast tenderness, and depression. There is some concern for bone loss in patients with risk factors for osteoporosis when given high doses of medroxyprgesterone acetate; however, bone density improves when estrogen levels return to normal. Adverse effects on HDL and LDL are sometimes seen with long-term use of norethindrone acetate. Bone density and/or lipids should be monitored in patients on long-term progestin therapy. Neither bone loss nor lipid abnormalities have been observed with use of the levonorgestrel-releasing intrauterine device (IUD).[163]

The levonorgestrel-releasing IUD causes decidualization, glandular atrophy, increased apoptosis, and down-regulation of cell proliferation of the endometrium and has been shown in small studies to be effective in improving the pain symptoms of endometriosis.[164-168] To date, there is not sufficient evidence to recommend its use as a first-line therapy, but many providers use it as a second-line therapy or to prevent recurrence of symptoms after surgical destruction/excision of lesions.[169]

Due to the efficacy, safety, low cost, and tolerability of OCs and progestins, these are generally recommended as first-line therapies. When these agents are ineffective or not tolerated, second medical therapy with GnRH analogs, danazol, or high-dose progestins is often effective. However, these are more costly and have a broader, more severe side effect profile (Table 11.1).

GONADOTROPIN-RELEASING HORMONE AGONISTS

Trials of GnRH agonists have found effectiveness for treatment of pain in women with endometriosis that is at least as beneficial as other therapies in alleviating pain and decreasing the size of implants and is more effective for dysmenorrhea.[170] Initially GnRH agonists bind to receptors that stimulate the pituitary to produce luteinizing hormone (LH) and follicle-stimulating hormone (FSH); however, longer treatment leads to a down-regulation of receptors, pituitary desensitization, and a fall in LH and FSH levels. This results in suppression of ovarian function and simulates a menopausal state with very low levels of circulating estrogens and progesterone. Many clinicians will give a trial of GnRH agonists to patients prior to laparoscopic surgery and presume that if symptoms are relieved then the diagnosis of endometriosis is highly likely; however, if continued for a full 6-month course, GnRH agonists may obviate the need for surgery. Side effects of GnRH agonists are similar to menopause and include amenorrhea (some women will bleed heavily 2 weeks after treatment initiation before becoming amenorrheaic), hot flushes and night sweats, mood changes, headaches, insomnia, urogenital atrophy, and bone loss.[171] Due to these concerns, GnRH agonists are approved for a 6-month course but can be administered safely for 2 years when low-dose add-back estrogen and progestin or progestin-only therapy is administered for bone protection. Norethindrone acetate (5 mg) is recommended as first line for add-back therapy as it has been shown to preserve bone density levels while still providing effective relief from vasomotor side effects. Selective serotonin reuptake inhibitors (SSRIs) and serotonin norepinepherine reuptake inhibitors (SNRIs) are useful for mood and hot flashes. Safety of GnRH agonists has not been established for young women (under 25) who have not yet reached peak bone mineral density.[172–175] Symptoms resolve when treatment is finished and bone density improves when estrogen levels return to normal. It is interesting to note that many women with chronic pelvic pain who do not have endometriosis can also experience pain relief with GnRH agonists.[176,177]

DANAZOL

Danazol has been shown to be effective in treating the painful symptoms of endometriosis and in reducing the size of endometriotic implants.[152] Danazol has progestin-like effects and is a derivative of 19-nortestosterone. It inhibits pituitary gonadotropin release, inhibits endometriotic implant growth, and decreases ovarian estrogen production. Side effects can be severe and are dose dependent. They include weight gain, muscle cramps, decreased breast size, acne, hirsutism, oily skin, hot flashes, mood changes, depression, decreased HDL, and increased liver enzymes, which can be treated by lowering the dose. Unlike GnRH agonists, add-back therapy is not useful for minimizing side effects. Due to the high side effect profile, danazol use is not as popular as other treatment modalities. More recently, lower doses of danazol have been used intravaginally (100–200 mg per day) and have shown promise for treatment of deeply infiltrating endometriosis without the high side effect profile associated with oral use.[178,179]

AROMATASE INHIBITORS

In endometrial tissue (including implants) of women with endometriosis, prostaglandin E2 stimulates aromatase activity and overexpression, leading to the conversion of androgens to excess estrogens. This creates a positive feedback loop as estrogen further stimulates prostaglandin E2 production.[180] Aromatase inhibitors (AIs) regulate local formation of estrogen within endometriotic lesions by inhibiting the overstimulated aromatase enzyme as well as by decreasing estrogen production in the ovary, brain, and periphery. AIs have been shown to significantly decrease pelvic pain from endometriosis to reduce lesion size[181] and may also be effective in women with refractory endometriosis pain.[180,182] Because AIs stimulate FSH release, they can cause multifollicular cyst development; they require ovarian suppression by another hormonal agent such as an OC, progestin, or GnRH agonist.[181] They can also cause bone loss with prolonged use. Combining AI use with GnRH agonists results in significantly more pain reduction and improved patient outcomes compared with GnRH agonists alone.[183]

OTHER HORMONAL MODULATORS

Selective progesterone receptor modulators have been shown to diminish the pain of endometriosis, but they cannot be administered for longer than 3–4 months and there is concern for endometrial thickening and histological changes.[184,185] The selective estrogen receptor modulator (SERM), raloxifene, was shown to be ineffective for controlling endometriosis and unexpectedly shortened the time to return of pain symptoms after surgical excision of endometriosis.[186] Other SERMs and selective progesterone receptor modulators are under study and may prove useful in the future. Similarly, antiprogestins (such as mifepristone) have demonstrated promise as therapy for endometriosis, but use has not become widespread.[151,187]

NOVEL THERAPY

Novel therapies focus on immune modulation. Endometriosis is associated with increased numbers of peritoneal macrophages and local inflammation as discussed next.[31,145,188] Novel therapies target angiogenesis, TNF-α, and peroxisome proliferators-activated receptors gamma.[61,189–193] TNF-α has been studied in one clinical trial and found to be ineffective.[101,191] Chinese herbal therapy, such as Gui Zhi Fu Ling[194] (which is composed of five ingredients, including cinnamon twig, white peony root, and china root), has shown efficacy in some clinical trials[195] and appears to function by inhibiting immunological and inflammatory factors as suggested by vitro studies.[196,197]

SURGICAL THERAPY

Removal of all lesions to treat endometriosis-related CPP is based on oncologic principles. However, even with optimal surgical resection, pain recurrence and reoperation rates are high (50%–60% within 1 year).[37,198,199] In practice, the surgery is often merely a debulking procedure because all visible lesions are not completely removed due to depth, extent, or location on the ureter or bowel. In many patients, however, no endometriosis is found at the time of the second surgery, suggesting independent central neural or other mechanisms contributing to recurrence of the pain.[37] Reoperation rates have been found to be lower after hysterectomy than laparoscopy, indicating that removal of the uterus may contribute to the therapeutic effect of the surgery.[199,200] Removal of both ovaries and the uterus resulted in the lowest rate of reoperation at 7 years (8.3%) compared with hysterectomy alone (23%). However, interestingly, women between the ages of 30–39 did not appear to benefit from removal of the ovaries in terms of preventing further surgery.[199] In patients under 30 years of age, up to 70% undergo further surgery within 7 years, thereby leading one to question the utility of surgical intervention in this age group.[199] When the ovaries are preserved, it is important to prevent ovulation in order to decrease the incidence of pain recurrence, preserve fertility, and avoid reoperation; many advocate for the use of medical therapy after surgery.[201] When the ovaries are removed, low-dose hormone replacement therapy (HRT) may be given to prevent bone loss and vasomotor side effects. There is a low likelihood of symptom recurrence with HRT in women who had all endometriosis resected (3.5%).[202]

The only well-designed, randomized clinical trials of surgical intervention for endometriosis have been limited by brief follow-up, small numbers, and loss to follow-up, [59,203,204] although many observational and retrospective studies have demonstrated favorable results. Some studies report the earlier return of symptoms in patients with minimal or mild disease than those with moderate or severe lesions, while others state that disease stage is not correlated with time to pain recurrence.[60,205] The variability in lesion size, location, and appearance across studies and the lack of methods to document that all disease has been treated make the results difficult to interpret. Prospective, randomized controlled studies are clearly needed.

Studies demonstrate that up to 20% of patients do not have relief of pain with surgery and that this is more likely in those who are found to have minimal or mild disease, perhaps because the endometriosis is not the sole cause of the pain. "Endometriosis-related pain syndrome" has been coined as a term to reflect the situation in which the pain may not be directly due to endometriosis implants but may still be related to the complex CNS changes associated with the disease.[2,59,203,204,206] Other culprits include bladder pain syndrome/interstitial cystitis, irritable bowel syndrome, myofascial pain (abdominal wall, lower back, or pelvic floor), fibromyalgia, or neuropathy.

Another important unstudied area involves the surgical technique used to treat lesions, that is, ablation or excision. While technically easier, ablation may lead to formation of adhesions and result in scarring that is misinterpreted as endometriotic lesions at future surgeries and may not reach the full extent of DIE lesions. The timing of surgery with respect to the menstrual cycle may also be important as peritoneal healing requires 3–5 days and if retrograde menstruation occurs during the healing process, endometriosis and/or adhesion formation may be promoted.[207] This concept has been demonstrated with in vitro models.[208] Adhesion formation after surgery further complicates the clinical picture with respect to fertility outcome, as reformation after surgery and in the presence of endometriosis is common; however, the impact of adhesions on the return of pain symptoms is not known.[49] Other surgical strategies, including removal of all pelvic peritoneum to excise "microscopic" endometriosis,[209] uterine nerve ablation, presacral neurectomy,[14,210,211] and conscious pain mapping,[212,213] have demonstrated limited success. Larger, well-designed prospective clinical trials to further delineate the role of various surgical interventions to treat the pain associated with endometriosis are warranted.

At the current time, it is not possible to predict which patients will respond well to surgical therapy, hormonal therapy, or analgesic therapy, and regimens must be tried until a suitable treatment is found. A multidisciplinary approach, including a psychologist and a physical therapist, is often required. Red flags that suggest the need for a multidisciplinary team include severe unremitting acyclic pain; depression; anxiety; disability; history of physical, sexual, or emotional trauma; substance or ethanol abuse; multiple visceral and somatic pain symptoms; and failure of traditional medical or surgical therapy to improve the pain.

SUMMARY

Endometriosis is a complex chronic condition, affecting women throughout their reproductive years. Symptoms include severe dysmenorrhea, dyspareunia, dyschezia, irregular or heavy vaginal bleeding, and in a sizeable proportion of cases, constant, debilitating pelvic pain. Some women may be asymptomatic and first receive the diagnosis during an evaluation for infertility. Endometriosis is often associated with other chronic visceral and somatic pain conditions. The experience of pain in endometriosis is influenced by ovarian sex steroids and menstruation, the peritoneal environment, lesion characteristics, innervations, and CNS modulation. During the reproductive years, women with endometriosis will generally require various pharmacologic and surgical therapies. Pain management can be challenging and early inclusion of a multidisciplinary therapeutic approach is warranted.

The chronic pain that develops in patients with endometriosis results from a complex interplay of many different factors beginning with an initial endometriotic lesion that leads to peripheral sensitization of the sensory and sympathetic fibers, central sensitization, central modification, and/or creation of memory and resulting ultimately in chronic pain that may be completely independent of the initiating lesion. These effects can each be modulated by the presence of estradiol. CNS interconnectivity may allow for cross-talk between organs and lead to related pain syndromes such as painful bladder, irritable bowel syndrome, or other systemic syndromes such as fibromyalgia. Continued research of the role of the peripheral and central nervous system, and the neuroendocrine and immune systems may result in the identification of more effective prevention and treatment strategies targeting the chronic pelvic pain associated with endometriosis.

Given the current knowledge of endometriosis, the evidence-based approach for management of women with chronic pelvic pain from this disease may be guided by the following:

1. Endometriosis is often suspected clinically and should be initially treated without a definitive diagnosis. Definitive diagnosis of endometriosis requires histological confirmation of disease at the time of surgery.
2. The mainstay of therapy for endometriosis should be hormonal suppression of the ovulation, reducing or eliminating menstrual flow, and lowering of endogenous estrogen levels using hormonal contraceptives, continuous progestins, or GnRH agonists. This treatment modality has the greatest likelihood of providing pain relief and preventing disease progression.
3. When medical management is inadequate, surgical exploration is warranted. Excision of all visible disease is likely to result in the highest level of pain relief; however, the surgery should be considered as a "debulking" procedure and not a "cure" for this chronic disease. Repetitive surgeries are not indicated.
4. Removal of visible endometriosis and both ovaries and uterus constitutes the most successful surgical approach. However, relief of pain in a woman under 40 years of age must be balanced with her fertility desires and overall health, as hormone replacement therapy is often not tolerated, prescribed, or taken as directed.
5. Endometriosis is prevalent but often is not the cause of all or most of the patient's pelvic

pain. Thoroughly investigate other disorders that can contribute to the pelvic pain, such as nerve entrapment or up-regulation of neural processing, myofascial pain, bladder pain syndrome, irritable bowel syndrome, and/or psychosocial conditions.

6. A multidisciplinary therapeutic approach should be considered for all women with persistent, chronic pelvic pain. This may include cognitive-behavioral pain management, physical therapy, local anesthetic nerve blocks, and other complementary approache,s including meditation, yoga, or acupuncture. Data on most of these approaches are currently lacking.

REFERENCES

1. Mathias SD, Kuppermann M, Liberman RF, Lipschutz RC, Steege JF. Chronic pelvic pain: prevalence, health-related quality of life, and economic correlates. *Obstet Gynecol* 1996;87:321–7.
2. Stratton P, Berkley KJ. Chronic pelvic pain and endometriosis: translational evidence of the relationship and implications. *Hum Reprod Update* 2010;17:327–46.
3. Burnett MA, Antao V, Black A, et al. Prevalence of primary dysmenorrhea in Canada. *J Obstet Gynaecol Can* 2005;27:765–70.
4. Dawood MY. Dysmenorrhea. *Clin Obstet Gynecol* 1990;33:168–78.
5. Howard FM. Chronic pelvic pain. *Obstet Gynecol* 2003;101:594–611.
6. Jabbour HN, Sales KJ. Prostaglandin receptor signalling and function in human endometrial pathology. *Trends Endocrinol Metab* 2004;15:398–404.
7. Dawood MY. Primary dysmenorrhea: advances in pathogenesis and management. *Obstet Gynecol* 2006;108:428–41.
8. Marjoribanks J, Proctor ML, Farquhar C. Nonsteroidal anti-inflammatory drugs for primary dysmenorrhoea. *Cochrane Database Syst Rev* 2003;(4):CD001751.
9. Proctor ML, Roberts H, Farquhar CM. Combined oral contraceptive pill (OCP) as treatment for primary dysmenorrhoea. *Cochrane Database Syst Rev* 2001;(4):CD002120.
10. Edelman AB, Gallo MF, Jensen JT, Nichols MD, Schulz KF, Grimes DA. Continuous or extended cycle vs. cyclic use of combined oral contraceptives for contraception. *Cochrane Database Syst Rev* 2005;(3):CD004695.
11. White AR. A review of controlled trials of acupuncture for women's reproductive health care. *J Fam Plann Reprod Health Care* 2003;29:233–6.
12. Proctor ML, Smith CA, Farquhar CM, Stones RW. Transcutaneous electrical nerve stimulation and acupuncture for primary dysmenorrhoea. *Cochrane Database Syst Rev* 2002;(1):CD002123.
13. Akin MD, Weingand KW, Hengehold DA, Goodale MB, Hinkle RT, Smith RP. Continuous low-level topical heat in the treatment of dysmenorrhea. *Obstet Gynecol* 2001;97:343–9.
14. Proctor ML, Latthe PM, Farquhar CM, Khan KS, Johnson NP. Surgical interruption of pelvic nerve pathways for primary and secondary dysmenorrhoea. *Cochrane Database Syst Rev* 2005;(4):CD001896.
15. Vercellini P, Parazzini F, Oldani S, Panazza S, Bramante T, Crosignani PG. Adenomyosis at hysterectomy: a study on frequency distribution and patient characteristics. *Hum Reprod* 1995;10:1160–2.
16. Templeman C, Marshall SF, Ursin G, et al. Adenomyosis and endometriosis in the California Teachers Study. *Fertil Steril* 2008;90:415–24.
17. Lee NC, Dicker RC, Rubin GL, Ory HW. Confirmation of the preoperative diagnoses for hysterectomy. *Am J Obstet Gynecol* 1984;150:283–7.
18. Levgur M. Diagnosis of adenomyosis: a review. *J Reprod Med* 2007;52:177–93.
19. Kim MD, Kim S, Kim NK, et al.. Long-term results of uterine artery embolization for symptomatic adenomyosis. *Am J Roentgenol* 2007;188:176–81.
20. Takayama K, Zeitoun K, Gunby RT, Sasano H, Carr BR, Bulun SE. Treatment of severe postmenopausal endometriosis with an aromatase inhibitor. *Fertil Steril* 1998;69:709–13.
21. Goodman HM, Kredentser D, Deligdisch L. Postmenopausal endometriosis associated with hormone replacement therapy. A case report. *J Reprod Med* 1989;34:231–3.
22. Missmer SA, Hankinson SE, Spiegelman D, et al. Reproductive history and endometriosis among premenopausal women. *Obstet Gynecol* 2004;104:965–74.
23. Cumiskey J, Whyte P, Kelehan P, Gibbons D. A detailed morphologic and immunohistochemical comparison of pre- and postmenopausal endometriosis. *J Clin Pathol* 2008;61:455–9.
24. Gao X, Outley J, Botteman M, Spalding J, Simon JA, Pashos CL. Economic burden of endometriosis. *Fertil Steril* 2006;86:1561–72.
25. Simoens S, Hummelshoj L, D'Hooghe T. Endometriosis: cost estimates and methodological perspective. *Hum Reprod Update* 2007;13:395–404.

26. Howard FM. Endometriosis and mechanisms of pelvic pain. *J Minim Invasive Gynecol* 2009;16:540–50.

27. Missmer SA, Hankinson SE, Spiegelman D, Barbieri RL, Marshall LM, Hunter DJ. Incidence of laparoscopically confirmed endometriosis by demographic, anthropometric, and lifestyle factors. *Am J Epidemiol* 2004;160:784–96.

28. Chatman DL, Ward AB. Endometriosis in adolescents. *J Reprod Med* 1982;27:156–60.

29. Treloar SA, Bell TA, Nagle CM, Purdie DM, Green AC. Early menstrual characteristics associated with subsequent diagnosis of endometriosis. *Am J Obstet Gynecol* 202:534 e531–6.

30. Hediger ML, Hartnett HJ, Louis GM. Association of endometriosis with body size and figure. *Fertil Steril* 2005;84:1366–74.

31. Bulun SE. Endometriosis. *N Engl J Med* 2009;360: 268–79.

32. Olive DL, Henderson DY. Endometriosis and mullerian anomalies. *Obstet Gynecol* 1987;69:412–5.

33. Brosens I, Donnez J, Benagiano G. Improving the classification of endometriosis. *Hum Reprod* 1993;8:1792–5.

34. Koninckx PR, Oosterlynck D, D'Hooghe T, Meuleman C. Deeply infiltrating endometriosis is a disease whereas mild endometriosis could be considered a non-disease. *Ann NY Acad Sci* 1994;734:333–41.

35. Nisolle M, Donnez J. Peritoneal endometriosis, ovarian endometriosis, and adenomyotic nodules of the rectovaginal septum are three different entities. *Fertil Steril* 1997;68:585–96.

36. Kennedy S, Bergqvist A, Chapron C, et al. ESHRE guideline for the diagnosis and treatment of endometriosis. *Hum Reprod* 2005;20:2698–704.

37. Vercellini P, Crosignani PG, Abbiati A, Somigliana E, Vigano P, Fedele L. The effect of surgery for symptomatic endometriosis: the other side of the story. *Hum Reprod Update* 2009;15:177–88.

38. Marcoux S, Maheux R, Berube S. Laparoscopic surgery in infertile women with minimal or mild endometriosis. Canadian Collaborative Group on Endometriosis. *N Engl J Med* 1997;337:217–22.

39. Martin DC, Hubert GD, Vander Zwaag R, el-Zeky FA. Laparoscopic appearances of peritoneal endometriosis. *Fertil Steril* 1989;51:63–7.

40. Vercellini P, Trespidi L, De Giorgi O, Cortesi I, Parazzini F, Crosignani PG. Endometriosis and pelvic pain: relation to disease stage and localization. *Fertil Steril* 1996;65:299–304.

41. Vercellini P, Fedele L, Aimi G, Pietropaolo G, Consonni D, Crosignani PG. Association between endometriosis stage, lesion type, patient characteristics and severity of pelvic pain symptoms: a multivariate analysis of over 1000 patients. *Hum Reprod* 2007;22:266–71.

42. Chapron C, Fauconnier A, Dubuisson JB, Barakat H, Vieira M, Breart G. Deep infiltrating endometriosis: relation between severity of dysmenorrhoea and extent of disease. *Hum Reprod* 2003;18:760–6.

43. Fauconnier A, Chapron C. Endometriosis and pelvic pain: epidemiological evidence of the relationship and implications. *Hum Reprod Update* 2005;11:595–606.

44. Chopin N, Ballester M, Borghese B, et al. Relation between severity of dysmenorrhea and endometrioma. *Acta Obstet Gynecol Scand* 2006;85:1375–80.

45. Chapron C, Pietin-Vialle C, Borghese B, Davy C, Foulot H, Chopin N. Associated ovarian endometrioma is a marker for greater severity of deeply infiltrating endometriosis. *Fertil Steril* 2009;92:453–7.

46. Fauconnier A, Chapron C, Dubuisson JB, Vieira M, Dousset B, Breart G. Relation between pain symptoms and the anatomic location of deep infiltrating endometriosis. *Fertil Steril* 2002;78:719–26.

47. Parazzini F, Mais V, Cipriani S. Adhesions and pain in women with first diagnosis of endometriosis: results from a cross-sectional study. *J Minim Invasive Gynecol* 2006;13:49–54.

48. Parker JD, Sinaii N, Segars JH, Godoy H, Winkel C, Stratton P. Adhesion formation after laparoscopic excision of endometriosis and lysis of adhesions. *Fertil Steril* 2005;84:1457–61.

49. Rapkin AJ. Adhesions and pelvic pain: a retrospective study. *Obstet Gynecol* 1986;68:13–15.

50. Yeung PP, Jr., Shwayder J, Pasic RP. Laparoscopic management of endometriosis: comprehensive review of best evidence. *J Minim Invasive Gynecol* 2009;16:269–81.

51. Peters AA, Van den Tillaart SA. The difficult patient in gastroenterology: chronic pelvic pain, adhesions, and sub occlusive episodes. *Best Pract Res Clin Gastroenterol* 2007;21:445–63.

52. Berkley KJ, Rapkin AJ, Papka RE. The pains of endometriosis. *Science* 2005;308:1587–9.

53. Bedaiwy MA, Falcone T. Laboratory testing for endometriosis. *Clin Chim Acta* 2004;340:41–56.

54. Vercellini P, Fedele L, Aimi G, De Giorgi O, Consonni D, Crosignani PG. Reproductive performance, pain recurrence and disease relapse after conservative surgical treatment for endometriosis: the predictive value of the current classification system. *Hum Reprod* 2006;21:2679–85.

55. Dworkin RH, Turk DC, Farrar JT, et al. Core outcome measures for chronic pain clinical trials: IMMPACT recommendations. *Pain* 2005;113:9–19.

56. Vincent K, Kennedy S, Stratton P. Pain scoring in endometriosis: entry criteria and outcome measures for clinical trials. Report from the Art and Science of Endometriosis meeting. *Fertil Steril* 2008;93:62–7.

57. Vercellini P, Somigliana E, Vigano P, Abbiati A, Barbara G, Fedele L. Chronic pelvic pain in women: etiology, pathogenesis and diagnostic approach. *Gynecol Endocrinol* 2009;25:149–58.

58. Sinaii N, Cleary SD, Ballweg ML, Nieman LK, Stratton P. High rates of autoimmune and endocrine disorders, fibromyalgia, chronic fatigue syndrome and atopic diseases among women with endometriosis: a survey analysis. *Hum Reprod* 2002;17:2715–24.

59. Abbott J, Hawe J, Hunter D, Holmes M, Finn P, Garry R. Laparoscopic excision of endometriosis: a randomized, placebo-controlled trial. *Fertil Steril* 2004;82:878–84.

60. Sutton CJ, Ewen SP, Whitelaw N, Haines P. Prospective, randomized, double-blind, controlled trial of laser laparoscopy in the treatment of pelvic pain associated with minimal, mild, and moderate endometriosis. *Fertil Steril* 1994;62:696–700.

61. May K, Becker CM. Endometriosis and angiogenesis. *Minerva Ginecol* 2008;60:245–54.

62. Burnstock G. Autonomic neurotransmission: 60 years since sir Henry Dale. *Annu Rev Pharmacol Toxicol* 2009;49:1–30.

63. Raab S, Plate KH. Different networks, common growth factors: shared growth factors and receptors of the vascular and the nervous system. *Acta Neuropathol* 2007;113:607–26.

64. Carmeliet P, Tessier-Lavigne M. Common mechanisms of nerve and blood vessel wiring. *Nature* 2005;436:193–200.

65. Jones CA, Li DY. Common cues regulate neural and vascular patterning. *Curr Opin Genet Dev* 2007;17:332–6.

66. Berkley KJ, Dmitrieva N, Curtis KS, Papka RE. Innervation of ectopic endometrium in a rat model of endometriosis. *Proc Natl Acad Sci USA* 2004;101:11094–8.

67. Cason AM, Samuelsen CL, Berkley KJ. Estrous changes in vaginal nociception in a rat model of endometriosis. *Horm Behav* 2003;44:123–31.

68. Morrison TC, Dmitrieva N, Winnard KP, Berkley KJ. Opposing viscerovisceral effects of surgically induced endometriosis and a control abdominal surgery on the rat bladder. *Fertil Steril* 2006;86:1067–73.

69. Nagabukuro H, Berkley KJ. Influence of endometriosis on visceromotor and cardiovascular responses induced by vaginal distention in the rat. *Pain* 2007;132(Suppl 1):S96–103.

70. Mendell LM, Albers KM, Davis BM. Neurotrophins, nociceptors, and pain. *Microsc Res Tech* 1999;45:252–61.

71. Mechsner S, Kaiser A, Kopf A, Gericke C, Ebert A, Bartley J. A pilot study to evaluate the clinical relevance of endometriosis-associated nerve fibers in peritoneal endometriotic lesions. *Fertil Steril* 2009;92:1856–61.

72. Anaf V, Simon P, El Nakadi I, et al. Relationship between endometriotic foci and nerves in rectovaginal endometriotic nodules. *Hum Reprod* 2000;15:1744–50.

73. Wang G, Tokushige N, Markham R, Fraser IS. Rich innervation of deep infiltrating endometriosis. *Hum Reprod* 2009;24:827–34.

74. Fraser IS, Tokushige N, Markham R, Russell P. Sensory nerve endings and endometriotic implants. *Fertil Steril* 2008;89:1847.

75. Tokushige N, Markham R, Russell P, Fraser IS. Nerve fibres in peritoneal endometriosis. *Hum Reprod* 2006;21:3001–7.

76. Tokushige N, Russell P, Black K, et al. Nerve fibers in ovarian endometriomas. *Fertil Steril*94:1944–7.

77. Wang G, Tokushige N, Russell P, Dubinovsky S, Markham R, Fraser IS. Hyperinnervation in intestinal deep infiltrating endometriosis. *J Minim Invasive Gynecol* 2009;16:713–9.

78. Anaf V, El Nakadi I, De Moor V, Chapron C, Pistofidis G, Noel JC. Increased nerve density in deep infiltrating endometriotic nodules. *Gynecol Obstet Invest*71:112–7.

79. Anaf V, Chapron C, El Nakadi I, De Moor V, Simonart T, Noel JC. Pain, mast cells, and nerves in peritoneal, ovarian, and deep infiltrating endometriosis. *Fertil Steril* 2006;86:1336–43.

80. Tulandi T, Chen MF, Al-Took S, Watkin K. A study of nerve fibers and histopathology of postsurgical, postinfectious, and endometriosis-related adhesions. *Obstet Gynecol* 1998;92:766–8.

81. Tulandi T, Felemban A, Chen MF. Nerve fibers and histopathology of endometriosis-harboring peritoneum. *J Am Assoc Gynecol Laparosc* 2001;8:95–8.

82. Woolf CJ. Phenotypic modification of primary sensory neurons: the role of nerve growth factor in the production of persistent pain. *Philos Trans R Soc Lond B Biol Sci* 1996;351:441–8.

83. Ramer MS, Bisby MA. Adrenergic innervation of rat sensory ganglia following proximal or distal painful sciatic neuropathy: distinct mechanisms

revealed by anti-NGF treatment. *Eur J Neurosci* 1999;11:837–46.

84. Tokushige N, Markham R, Russell P, Fraser IS. Different types of small nerve fibers in eutopic endometrium and myometrium in women with endometriosis. *Fertil Steril* 2007;88:795–803.

85. Al-Jefout M, Andreadis N, Tokushige N, Markham R, Fraser I. A pilot study to evaluate the relative efficacy of endometrial biopsy and full curettage in making a diagnosis of endometriosis by the detection of endometrial nerve fibers. *Am J Obstet Gynecol* 2007;197:578 e571–4.

86. Al-Jefout M, Dezarnaulds G, Cooper M, et al. Diagnosis of endometriosis by detection of nerve fibres in an endometrial biopsy: a double blind study. *Hum Reprod* 2009;24:3019–24.

87. Woolf CJ. Evidence for a central component of post-injury pain hypersensitivity. *Nature* 1983;306:686–8.

88. Woolf CJ, Salter MW. Neuronal plasticity: increasing the gain in pain. *Science* 2000;288:1765–9.

89. Melzack R, Coderre TJ, Katz J, Vaccarino AL. Central neuroplasticity and pathological pain. *Ann NY Acad Sci* 2001;933:157–74.

90. McAllister SL, McGinty KA, Resuehr D, Berkley KJ. Endometriosis-induced vaginal hyperalgesia in the rat: role of the ectopic growths and their innervation. *Pain* 2009;147:255–64.

91. Bajaj P, Madsen H, Arendt-Nielsen L. Endometriosis is associated with central sensitization: a psychophysical controlled study. *J Pain* 2003;4:372–80.

92. Giamberardino MA, Berkley KJ, Affaitati G, et al. Influence of endometriosis on pain behaviors and muscle hyperalgesia induced by a ureteral calculosis in female rats. *Pain* 2002;95:247–57.

93. Li J, Micevych P, McDonald J, Rapkin A, Chaban V. Inflammation in the uterus induces phosphorylated extracellular signal-regulated kinase and substance P immunoreactivity in dorsal root ganglia neurons innervating both uterus and colon in rats. *J Neurosci Res* 2008;86:2746–52.

94. Ustinova EE, Fraser MO, Pezzone MA. Cross-talk and sensitization of bladder afferent nerves. *Neurourol Urodyn* 2010;29:77–81.

95. Asante A, Taylor RN. Endometriosis: the role of neuroangiogenesis. *Annu Rev Physiol* 2011;73: 163–82.

96. Machado D, Abrao M, Berardo P, Takiya C, Nasciutti L. Vascular density and distribution of vascular endothelial growth factor (VEGF) and its receptor VEGFR-2 (Flk-1) are significantly higher in patients with deeply infiltrating endometriosis affecting the rectum. *Fertil Steril* 2008;90:148–55.

97. Wieseler-Frank J, Maier SF, Watkins LR. Central proinflammatory cytokines and pain enhancement. *Neurosignals* 2005;14: 166–74.

98. Koninckx PR, Kennedy SH, Barlow DH. Endometriotic disease: the role of peritoneal fluid. *Hum Reprod Update* 1998;4:741–51.

99. Coelho A, Fioramonti J, Bueno L. Brain interleukin-1beta and tumor necrosis factor-alpha are involved in lipopolysaccharide-induced delayed rectal allodynia in awake rats. *Brain Res Bull* 2000;52:223–8.

100. Maier SF, Watkins LR. Immune-to-central nervous system communication and its role in modulating pain and cognition: implications for cancer and cancer treatment. *Brain Behav Immun* 2003;17(Suppl 1):S125–31.

101. Lv D, Song H, Shi G. Anti-TNF-alpha treatment for pelvic pain associated with endometriosis. *Cochrane Database Syst Rev* 2010;(3):CD008088.

102. Cheng JK, Ji RR. Intracellular signaling in primary sensory neurons and persistent pain. *Neurochem Res* 2008;33:1970–8.

103. Tamburro S, Canis M, Albuisson E, Dechelotte P, Darcha C, Mage G. Expression of transforming growth factor beta1 in nerve fibers is related to dysmenorrhea and laparoscopic appearance of endometriotic implants. *Fertil Steril* 2003;80:1131–6.

104. Zhang G, Dmitrieva N, Liu Y, McGinty KA, Berkley KJ. Endometriosis as a neurovascular condition: estrous variations in innervation, vascularization, and growth factor content of ectopic endometrial cysts in the rat. *Am J Physiol Regul Integr Comp Physiol* 2008;294:R162–71.

105. Sofroniew MV, Howe CL, Mobley WC. Nerve growth factor signaling, neuroprotection, and neural repair. *Annu Rev Neurosci* 2001;24:1217–81.

106. Possover M, Tersiev P, Angelov DN. Comparative study of the neuropeptide-Y sympathetic nerves in endometriotic involved and noninvolved sacrouterine ligaments in women with pelvic endometriosis. *J Minim Invasive Gynecol* 2009;16:340–3.

107. Zhang X, Yao H, Huang X, Lu B, Xu H, Zhou C. Nerve fibres in ovarian endometriotic lesions in women with ovarian endometriosis. *Hum Reprod* 2010;25:392–7.

108. Cervero F, Janig W. Visceral nociceptors: a new world order? *Trends Neurosci* 1992;15:374–8.

109. Michaelis M, Habler HJ, Jaenig W. Silent afferents: a separate class of primary afferents? *Clin Exp Pharmacol Physiol* 1996;23:99–105.

110. Holzer P. Neurogenic vasodilatation and plasma leakage in the skin. *Gen Pharmacol* 1998; 30:5–11.

111. Szolcsanyi J. Forty years in capsaicin research for sensory pharmacology and physiology. *Neuropeptides* 2004;38:377–84.

112. Gebhart GF. Peripheral contributions to visceral hyperalgesia. *Can J Gastroenterol* 1999;13(Suppl A):37A–41A.

113. Taylor BK, Akana SF, Peterson MA, Dallman MF, Basbaum AI. Pituitary-adrenocortical responses to persistent noxious stimuli in the awake rat: endogenous corticosterone does not reduce nociception in the formalin test. *Endocrinology* 1998;139:2407–13.

114. Blackburn-Munro G, Blackburn-Munro R. Pain in the brain: are hormones to blame? *Trends Endocrinol Metab* 2003;14:20–7.

115. Crofford LJ. The hypothalamic-pituitary-adrenal axis in the pathogenesis of rheumatic diseases. *Endocrinol Metab Clin North Am* 2002;31: 1–13.

116. Torpy DJ, Papanicolaou DA, Lotsikas AJ, Wilder RL, Chrousos GP, Pillemer SR. Responses of the sympathetic nervous system and the hypothalamic-pituitary-adrenal axis to interleukin-6: a pilot study in fibromyalgia. *Arthritis Rheum* 2000;43:872–80.

117. Huang HY. Medical treatment of endometriosis. *Chang Gung Med J* 2008;31:431–40.

118. Fedele L, Somigliana E, Frontino G, Benaglia L, Vigano P. New drugs in development for the treatment of endometriosis. *Expert Opin Investig Drugs* 2008;17:1187–202.

119. Kaur G, Janik J, Isaacson LG, Callahan P. Estrogen regulation of neurotrophin expression in sympathetic neurons and vascular targets. *Brain Res* 2007;1139:6–14.

120. Craft RM, Mogil JS, Aloisi AM. Sex differences in pain and analgesia: the role of gonadal hormones. *Eur J Pain* 2004;8:397–411.

121. Greenspan JD, Craft RM, LeResche L, et al. Studying sex and gender differences in pain and analgesia: a consensus report. *Pain* 2007;132(Suppl 1):S26–45.

122. Reed WR, Chadha HK, Hubscher CH. Effects of 17beta-estradiol on responses of viscerosomatic convergent thalamic neurons in the ovariectomized female rat. *J Neurophysiol* 2009;102:1062–74.

123. Berkley KJ, McAllister SL, Accius BE, Winnard KP. Endometriosis-induced vaginal hyperalgesia in the rat: effect of estropause, ovariectomy, and estradiol replacement. *Pain* 2007;132(Suppl 1):S150–9.

124. Salamonsen LA, Zhang J, Brasted M. Leukocyte networks and human endometrial remodelling. *J Reprod Immunol* 2002;57:95–108.

125. Jabbour HN, Kelly RW, Fraser HM, Critchley HO. Endocrine regulation of menstruation. *Endocr Rev* 2006;27:17–46.

126. Critchley HO, Kelly RW, Baird DT, Brenner RM. Regulation of human endometrial function: mechanisms relevant to uterine bleeding. *Reprod Biol Endocrinol* 2006;4(Suppl 1):S5.

127. Vercellini P, Fedele L, Pietropaolo G, Frontino G, Somigliana E, Crosignani PG. Progestogens for endometriosis: forward to the past. *Hum Reprod Update* 2003;9:387–96.

128. Giudice LC, Kao LC. Endometriosis. *Lancet* 2004;364:1789–99.

129. Osteen KG, Bruner-Tran KL, Eisenberg E. Reduced progesterone action during endometrial maturation: a potential risk factor for the development of endometriosis. *Fertil Steril* 2005;83:529–37.

130. Tokushige N, Markham R, Russell P, Fraser IS. High density of small nerve fibres in the functional layer of the endometrium in women with endometriosis. *Hum Reprod* 2006;21:782–7.

131. Tokushige N, Markham R, Russell P, Fraser IS. Effects of hormonal treatment on nerve fibers in endometrium and myometrium in women with endometriosis. *Fertil Steril* 2008;90:1589–98.

132. Baird DT, Cameron ST, Critchley HO, et al. Prostaglandins and menstruation. *Eur J Obstet Gynecol Reprod Biol* 1996;70:15–7.

133. Nawroth F, Rahimi G, Nawroth C, Foth D, Ludwig M, Schmidt T. Is there an association between septate uterus and endometriosis? *Hum Reprod* 2006;21:542–4.

134. Sanfilippo JS, Wakim NG, Schikler KN, Yussman MA. Endometriosis in association with uterine anomaly. *Am J Obstet Gynecol* 1986;154:39–43.

135. Bulletti C, D DEZ, Setti PL, Cicinelli E, Polli V, Flamigni C. The patterns of uterine contractility in normal menstruating women: from physiology to pathology. *Ann NY Acad Sci* 2004;1034:64–83.

136. Maslow KD, Lyons EA. Effect of prostaglandin and antiprostaglandin on midcycle myometrial contractions. *Fertil Steril* 2004;82:511–3.

137. Kido A, Togashi K, Kataoka M, et al. The effect of oral contraceptives on uterine contractility and menstrual pain: an assessment with cine MR imaging. *Hum Reprod* 2007;22:2066–71.

138. Salamanca A, Beltran E. Subendometrial contractility in menstrual phase visualized

by transvaginal sonography in patients with endometriosis. *Fertil Steril* 1995;64:193–5.

139. Bulletti C, Rossi S, Albonetti A, et al. Uterine contractility in patients with endometriosis. *J Am Assoc Gynecol Laparosc* 1996;3:S5.

140. Buscher U, Chen FC, Kentenich H, Schmiady H. Cytokines in the follicular fluid of stimulated and non-stimulated human ovaries; is ovulation a suppressed inflammatory reaction? *Hum Reprod* 1999;14:162–6.

141. Townson DH, Liptak AR. Chemokines in the corpus luteum: implications of leukocyte chemotaxis. *Reprod Biol Endocrinol* 2003;1:94.

142. Baird DT, Fraser IS. Blood production and ovarian secretion rates of estradiol-17 beta and estrone in women throughout the menstrual cycle. *J Clin Endocrinol Metab* 1974;38:1009–17.

143. Scheenjes E, te Velde ER, Kremer J. Inspection of the ovaries and steroids in serum and peritoneal fluid at various time intervals after ovulation in fertile women: implications for the luteinized unruptured follicle syndrome. *Fertil Steril* 1990;54:38–41.

144. Kim-Bjorklund T, Landgren BM, Hamberger L. Peritoneal fluid volume and levels of steroid hormones and gonadotrophins in peritoneal fluid of normal and norethisterone-treated women. *Hum Reprod* 1991;6:1233–7.

145. Weinberg JB, Haney AF, Xu FJ, Ramakrishnan S. Peritoneal fluid and plasma levels of human macrophage colony-stimulating factor in relation to peritoneal fluid macrophage content. *Blood* 1991;78:513–6.

146. Katsuki Y, Takano Y, Futamura Y, et al. Effects of dienogest, a synthetic steroid, on experimental endometriosis in rats. *Eur J Endocrinol* 1998;138:216–26.

147. Nakamura M, Katsuki Y, Shibutani Y, Oikawa T. Dienogest, a synthetic steroid, suppresses both embryonic and tumor-cell-induced angiogenesis. *Eur J Pharmacol* 1999;386:33–40.

148. Allen C, Hopewell S, Prentice A, Gregory D. Nonsteroidal anti-inflammatory drugs for pain in women with endometriosis. *Cochrane Database Syst Rev* 2009;(2):CD004753.

149. Rapkin AJ, Kames LD. The pain management approach to chronic pelvic pain. *J Reprod Med* 1987;32:323–7.

150. Rapkin A J, Hartshorn T G, P P. Pain management. *Clinical Updates Women's Health Care* 2011;10:1–158.

151. Prentice A, Deary AJ, Bland E. Progestagens and anti-progestagens for pain associated with endometriosis. *Cochrane Database Syst Rev* 2000;(2):CD002122.

152. Selak V, Farquhar C, Prentice A, Singla A. Danazol for pelvic pain associated with endometriosis. *Cochrane Database Syst Rev* 2007;(4):CD000068.

153. Davis L, Kennedy SS, Moore J, Prentice A. Modern combined oral contraceptives for pain associated with endometriosis. *Cochrane Database Syst Rev* 2007;(3):CD001019.

154. Nisolle-Pochet M, Casanas-Roux F, Donnez J. Histologic study of ovarian endometriosis after hormonal therapy. *Fertil Steril* 1988;49:423–6.

155. Grow DR, Iromloo K. Oral contraceptives maintain a very thin endometrium before operative hysteroscopy. *Fertil Steril* 2006;85:204–7.

156. Harada T, Momoeda M, Taketani Y, Hoshiai H, Terakawa N. Low-dose oral contraceptive pill for dysmenorrhea associated with endometriosis: a placebo-controlled, double-blind, randomized trial. *Fertil Steril* 2008;90:1583–8.

157. Hughes E, Brown J, Collins JJ, Farquhar C, Fedorkow DM, Vandekerckhove P: Ovulation suppression for endometriosis. *Cochrane Database Syst Rev* 2007;(3):CD000155.

158. Maguire K, Westhoff C. The state of hormonal contraception today: established and emerging noncontraceptive health benefits. *Am J Obstet Gynecol* 2011;205(4 Suppl):S4–8.

159. Igarashi TM, Bruner-Tran KL, Yeaman GR, et al. Reduced expression of progesterone receptor-B in the endometrium of women with endometriosis and in cocultures of endometrial cells exposed to 2,3,7,8-tetrachlorodibenzo-p-dioxin. *Fertil Steril* 2005;84:67–74.

160. Luciano AA, Turksoy RN, Carleo J. Evaluation of oral medroxyprogesterone acetate in the treatment of endometriosis. *Obstet Gynecol* 1988;72:323–7.

161. Crosignani PG, Luciano A, Ray A, Bergqvist A. Subcutaneous depot medroxyprogesterone acetate versus leuprolide acetate in the treatment of endometriosis-associated pain. *Hum Reprod* 2006;21:248–56.

162. Telimaa S, Ronnberg L, Kauppila A. Placebo-controlled comparison of danazol and high-dose medroxyprogesterone acetate in the treatment of endometriosis after conservative surgery. *Gynecol Endocrinol* 1987;1:363–71.

163. Mansour D. The benefits and risks of using a levonorgestrel-releasing intrauterine system for contraception. *Contraception* 2012;85(3):224–34.

164. Vercellini P, Vigano P, Somigliana E. The role of the levonorgestrel-releasing intrauterine device in the management of symptomatic endometriosis. *Curr Opin Obstet Gynecol* 2005;17:359–65.

165. Vercellini P, Aimi G, Panazza S, De Giorgi O, Pesole A, Crosignani PG. A levonorgestrel-releasing intrauterine system for the treatment of dysmenorrhea associated with endometriosis: a pilot study. *Fertil Steril* 1999;72:505–8.

166. Vercellini P, Frontino G, De Giorgi O, Aimi G, Zaina B, Crosignani PG. Comparison of a levonorgestrel-releasing intrauterine device versus expectant management after conservative surgery for symptomatic endometriosis: a pilot study. *Fertil Steril* 2003;80:305–9.

167. Lockhat FB, Emembolu JO, Konje JC. The evaluation of the effectiveness of an intrauterine-administered progestogen (levonorgestrel) in the symptomatic treatment of endometriosis and in the staging of the disease. *Hum Reprod* 2004;19:179–84.

168. Lockhat FB, Emembolu JO, Konje JC. The efficacy, side-effects and continuation rates in women with symptomatic endometriosis undergoing treatment with an intra-uterine administered progestogen (levonorgestrel): a 3 year follow-up. *Hum Reprod* 2005;20:789–93.

169. Abou-Setta AM, Al-Inany HG, Farquhar CM. Levonorgestrel-releasing intrauterine device (LNG-IUD) for symptomatic endometriosis following surgery. *Cochrane Database Syst Rev* 2006;(4):CD005072.

170. Brown J, Pan A, Hart RJ. Gonadotrophin-releasing hormone analogues for pain associated with endometriosis. *Cochrane Database Syst Rev* 2010;(3):CD008475.

171. Dlugi AM, Miller JD, Knittle J. Lupron depot (leuprolide acetate for depot suspension) in the treatment of endometriosis: a randomized, placebo-controlled, double-blind study. Lupron Study Group. *Fertil Steril* 1990;54:419–27.

172. Surrey ES. Add-back therapy and gonadotropin-releasing hormone agonists in the treatment of patients with endometriosis: can a consensus be reached? Add-Back Consensus Working Group. *Fertil Steril* 1999;71:420–4.

173. Surrey ES, Hornstein MD. Prolonged GnRH agonist and add-back therapy for symptomatic endometriosis: long-term follow-up. *Obstet Gynecol* 2002;99:709–19.

174. Divasta AD, Laufer MR, Gordon CM. Bone density in adolescents treated with a GnRH agonist and add-back therapy for endometriosis. *J Pediatr Adolesc Gynecol* 2007;20:293–7.

175. Laufer MR. Current approaches to optimizing the treatment of endometriosis in adolescents. *Gynecol Obstet Invest* 2008;66(Suppl 1):19–27.

176. Ling FW. Randomized controlled trial of depot leuprolide in patients with chronic pelvic pain and clinically suspected endometriosis. Pelvic Pain Study Group. *Obstet Gynecol* 1999;93:51–8.

177. Jenkins TR, Liu CY, White J. Does response to hormonal therapy predict presence or absence of endometriosis? *J Minim Invasive Gynecol* 2008;15:82–6.

178. Razzi S, Luisi S, Calonaci F, Altomare A, Bocchi C, Petraglia F. Efficacy of vaginal danazol treatment in women with recurrent deeply infiltrating endometriosis. *Fertil Steril* 2007;88:789–94.

179. Ferrero S, Tramalloni D, Venturini PL, Remorgida V. Vaginal danazol for women with rectovaginal endometriosis and pain symptoms persisting after insertion of a levonorgestrel-releasing intrauterine device. *Int J Gynaecol Obstet* 2011; 113:116–9.

180. Bulun SE, Zeitoun K, Takayama K, et al. Estrogen production in endometriosis and use of aromatase inhibitors to treat endometriosis. *Endocr Relat Cancer* 1999;6:293–301.

181. Attar E, Bulun SE. Aromatase inhibitors: the next generation of therapeutics for endometriosis? *Fertil Steril* 2006;85:1307–18.

182. Amsterdam LL, Gentry W, Jobanputra S, Wolf M, Rubin SD, Bulun SE. Anastrazole and oral contraceptives: a novel treatment for endometriosis. *Fertil Steril* 2005;84:300–4.

183. Nawathe A, Patwardhan S, Yates D, Harrison GR, Khan KS. Systematic review of the effects of aromatase inhibitors on pain associated with endometriosis. *BJOG* 2008;115:818–22.

184. Chwalisz K, Perez MC, Demanno D, Winkel C, Schubert G, Elger W. Selective progesterone receptor modulator development and use in the treatment of leiomyomata and endometriosis. *Endocr Rev* 2005;26:423–38.

185. Spitz IM. Clinical utility of progesterone receptor modulators and their effect on the endometrium. *Curr Opin Obstet Gynecol* 2009;21: 318–24.

186. Stratton P, Sinaii N, Segars J, et al. Return of chronic pelvic pain from endometriosis after raloxifene treatment: a randomized controlled trial. *Obstet Gynecol* 2008;111:88–96.

187. Kettel LM, Murphy AA, Morales AJ, Yen SS. Preliminary report on the treatment of endometriosis with low-dose mifepristone (RU 486). *Am J Obstet Gynecol* 1998;178: 1151–6.

188. Taylor RN, Ryan IP, Moore ES, Hornung D, Shifren JL, Tseng JF. Angiogenesis and macrophage activation in endometriosis. *Ann NY Acad Sci* 1997;828:194–207.

189. Becker CM, D'Amato RJ. Angiogenesis and antiangiogenic therapy in endometriosis. *Microvasc Res* 2007;74:121–30.

190. Barrier BF, Bates GW, Leland MM, Leach DA, Robinson RD, Propst AM. Efficacy of anti-tumor necrosis factor therapy in the treatment of spontaneous endometriosis in baboons. *Fertil Steril* 2004;81(Suppl 1):775–9.

191. Koninckx PR, Craessaerts M, Timmerman D, Cornillie F, Kennedy S. Anti-TNF-alpha treatment for deep endometriosis-associated pain: a randomized placebo-controlled trial. *Hum Reprod* 2008;23:2017–23.

192. Pritts EA, Zhao D, Ricke E, Waite L, Taylor RN. PPAR-gamma decreases endometrial stromal cell transcription and translation of RANTES in vitro. *J Clin Endocrinol Metab* 2002;87:1841–44.

193. Tee MK, Vigne JL, Taylor RN. All-trans retinoic acid inhibits vascular endothelial growth factor expression in a cell model of neutrophil activation. *Endocrinology* 2006;147:1264–70.

194. Ji X, Gao J, Cai X, et al. Immunological regulation of Chinese herb guizhi fuling capsule on rat endometriosis model. *J Ethnopharmacol* 2011;134:624–9.

195. Flower A, Liu JP, Chen S, Lewith G, Little P. Chinese herbal medicine for endometriosis. *Cochrane Database Syst Rev* 2009;(5):CD006568.

196. Wieser F, Yu J, Park J, et al. A botanical extract from channel flow inhibits cell proliferation, induces apoptosis, and suppresses CCL5 in human endometriotic stromal cells. *Biol Reprod* 2009;81:371–7.

197. Wieser F, Cohen M, Gaeddert A, et al. Evolution of medical treatment for endometriosis: back to the roots? *Hum Reprod Update* 2007;13:487–99.

198. Cheong Y, Tay P, Luk F, Gan HC, Li TC, Cooke I. Laparoscopic surgery for endometriosis: how often do we need to re-operate? *J Obstet Gynaecol* 2008;28:82–5.

199. Shakiba K, Bena JF, McGill KM, Minger J, Falcone T. Surgical treatment of endometriosis: a 7-year follow-up on the requirement for further surgery. *Obstet Gynecol* 2008;111:1285–92.

200. Sinaii N, Cleary SD, Younes N, Ballweg ML, Stratton P. Treatment utilization for endometriosis symptoms: a cross-sectional survey study of lifetime experience. *Fertil Steril* 2007;87:1277–86.

201. Vercellini P, Somigliana E, Vigano P, De Matteis S, Barbara G, Fedele L. Post-operative endometriosis recurrence: a plea for prevention based on pathogenetic, epidemiological and clinical evidence. *Reprod Biomed Online* 2010;21:259–65.

202. Matorras R, Elorriaga MA, Pijoan JI, Ramon O, Rodriguez-Escudero FJ. Recurrence of endometriosis in women with bilateral adnexectomy (with or without total hysterectomy) who received hormone replacement therapy. *Fertil Steril* 2002;77:303–8.

203. Sutton CJ, Pooley AS, Ewen SP, Haines P. Follow-up report on a randomized controlled trial of laser laparoscopy in the treatment of pelvic pain associated with minimal to moderate endometriosis. *Fertil Steril* 1997;68:1070–4.

204. Jones KD, Haines P, Sutton CJ. Long-term follow-up of a controlled trial of laser laparoscopy for pelvic pain. *JSLS* 2001;5:111–5.

205. Jarrell J, Brant R, Leung W, Taenzer P. Women's pain experience predicts future surgery for pain associated with endometriosis. *J Obstet Gynaecol Can* 2007;29:988–91.

206. Woolf CJ. Central sensitization: implications for the diagnosis and treatment of pain. *Pain Biennial Rev Suppl* 2011;152:S2–15.

207. Schweppe KW, Ring D. Peritoneal defects and the development of endometriosis in relation to the timing of endoscopic surgery during the menstrual cycle. *Fertil Steril* 2002;78:763–6.

208. Witz CA, Dechaud H, Montoya-Rodriguez IA, et al. An in vitro model to study the pathogenesis of the early endometriosis lesion. *Ann NY Acad Sci* 2002;955:296–307; discussion 340–292, 396–406.

209. Redwine DB. Aggressive laparoscopic excision of endometriosis of the cul-de-sac and uterosacral ligaments. *J Am Assoc Gynecol Laparosc* 1997;4:540–1.

210. Gambone JC, Mittman BS, Munro MG, Scialli AR, Winkel CA. Consensus statement for the management of chronic pelvic pain and endometriosis: proceedings of an expert-panel consensus process. *Fertil Steril* 2002;78:961–72.

211. Daniels J, Gray R, Hills RK, et al. Laparoscopic uterosacral nerve ablation for alleviating chronic pelvic pain: a randomized controlled trial. *JAMA* 2009;302:955–61.

212. Howard FM, El-Minawi AM, Sanchez RA. Conscious pain mapping by laparoscopy in women with chronic pelvic pain. *Obstet Gynecol* 2000;96:934–9.

213. Steege JF. Clinical utility of pelvic pain mapping. *J Am Assoc Gynecol Laparosc* 2001;8:263–6.

12

VULVODYNIA

Ursula Wesselmann and Peter Czakanski

INTRODUCTION

This chapter will discuss the neurobiology, etiology, clinical presentation, diagnosis, and clinical management of vulvodynia, a chronic vulvar pain syndrome. Chronic nonmalignant pain syndromes (longer than 6 months duration) of urogenital origin are well described but poorly understood focal pain syndromes.[1] In the female patient these pain syndromes include vulvar dysesthesia, clitoral pain, urethral syndrome, coccygodynia, and generalized perineal pain, and the "counterparts" in the male patient are orchialgia, prostatodynia, and chronic penile pain, as well as coccygodynia and generalized perineal pain. While the focus of the chapter is on vulvodynia, it is important to recognize that chronic vulvar pain is one of the clinical presentations of the chronic nonmalignant urogenital pain syndromes. This concept will guide the health care provider in making the diagnosis of a chronic pain syndrome and the researcher in understanding vulvodynia in the context of complex changes in pain modulation.

DEFINITIONS AND TAXONOMY

The term *vulvodynia* (Latin: vulva; Greek: -odynia, pain) is a modern word for an age-old pain condition. Historically, vulvar pain cannot be separated from the earlier description of painful intercourse: dyspareunia.[2] The first recorded reference to vulvar pain is embedded in the ancient Egyptian Ramesseum Papyrus over 2,000 years ago.[3] The phenomenon was not described in medical texts until the 19th century, where it was variably called vulvar hyperesthesia, vulvar "supersensitiveness," and heightened vulvar "sensitivity."[4]

Surprisingly, despite early detailed reports, chronic vulvar dysesthesia disappeared to a large extent from the medical literature until the mid 1970s. The first attempt to develop formal terminology for vulvar pain occurred in 1976, when the International Society for the Study of Vulvovaginal Disease (ISSVD) identified idiopathic vulvar pain as a unique entity and introduced the term "burning vulva syndrome," based on the observation that most women describe the pain as a hot, burning sensation. The ISSVD subsequently coined the term *vulvodynia* (defined as chronic vulvar discomfort, especially that characterized by the patient's complaint of burning, and sometimes stinging, irritation, or rawness) to describe this disorder.[5] The ISSVD stated that vulvodynia was a symptom rather than a diagnosis and that multiple etiologies might be possible. Subsequently two subsets of vulvodynia were identified. One subgroup of patients complained about entrance dyspareunia (pain with tampon insertion and pain at vaginal penetration during sexual intercourse), rather than diffuse vulvar pain. The term *vulvar vestibulitis* was introduced for this subset of vulvodynia and the following diagnostic criteria were established: (1) presence of severe pain on vestibular touch or attempted vaginal entry, (2) tenderness to pressure localized within the vulvar vestibule, and (3) physical findings confined to vestibular erythema of various degrees.[6] The other main subgroup of patients with vulvodynia presented with generalized, spontaneous vulvar pain occurring in the absence of physical findings. The term *dysesthetic (or essential) vulvodynia* was suggested for this symptom complex. Clinically two different groups of patients with vulvar vestibulitis have been described: *primary vulvar vestibulitis* is defined as dyspareunia from the first attempt of sexual intercourse, whereas in *secondary vulvar vestibulitis* the dyspareunia appears after a period of pain-free sexual intercourse. It has been suggested that these two subgroups differ in etiological, clinical, and genetic variables.[7-11] Based on the concern that the suffix "-itis" in vulvar vestibulitis incorrectly implies an inflammatory etiology, the term *vestibulodynia* has been suggested (see ref. 5 for review). The most recent revision of the ISSVD of the terminology of vulvodynia has been published in 2004.[5] This classification suggests categorizing a generalized and a localized (*vestibulodynia*, clitorodynia, hemivulvodynia, etc.) form of vulvodynia and to differentiate subgroups within those two categories based on the observation whether the vulvar pain is provoked, unprovoked, or mixed (provoked and unprovoked).

Similar to other chronic pain syndromes, vulvodynia has an impact on patient's psychological well-being and quality of life, but unlike many other pain syndromes, this pain condition has a significant impact on the patient's sexual functioning. Recommendations for the upcoming *Diagnosis and Statistical Manual of Mental Disorders-V* suggest a single diagnostic entity called genito-pelvic pain/penetration disorder, which includes vulvodynia in the context of the sexual pain disorders.[12] Similar to other areas in the health sciences, where multiple disciplines are involved, developing a uniform and comprehensive terminology that improves clinical communication and enhances research efforts into the etiology of the disease remains a challenge.

EPIDEMIOLOGY

Community studies suggest that vulvar pain is common, but the prevalence rates vary widely from 3% to 18%.[13-16] A survey of sexual dysfunction, analyzing data from the National Health and Social Life Survey, reported that 16% of women between the ages of 18 and 59 years living in households throughout the United States experience pain during sex.[17] Epidemiological studies have confirmed that localized provoked vulvodynia is the most common vulvodynia subtype in pre-menopausal women.[14,15] Goetsch[18] reported that 15% of all patients seen in her general gynecological private practice fulfilled the definition of localized provoked vulvodynia. Fifty percent of these patients had always experienced entry dyspareunia and pain with inserting tampons, most since their teenage years. They had often wondered whether they were unique or had a hidden emotional aversion to sex. Initial reports postulated that vulvodynia affects primarily women of Caucasian origin[12,18]; however, a survey in the United States of ethnically diverse women showed that Hispanic women were 80% more likely to experience chronic vulvar pain than were white and African American women.[15] A small study done in Ghana in 2005 revealed a prevalence rate of 20% in an all-black population.[19] Vulvodynia affects women of all age groups. The incidence of symptom onset is highest between ages 18 and 25, decreases through age 44, and then remains fairly constant.[15] Several widely divergent estimates have been postulated for the lifetime cumulative incidence of vulvar pain syndrome ranging between 200,000 and 14 million women in the United States.[15]

The frequency of vulvodynia is likely to be underestimated, because women are often reluctant to discuss their symptoms, since the area where they experience pain is considered taboo and they are afraid that the chronic pain will be dismissed as "being all in the head." In addition, health care providers, who are not familiar with the disease, sometimes dismiss the problem as being psychological and unimportant. As vulvodynia receives increased attention by both the medical profession and the media, more women are seeking care for their vulvar pain, and the increased frequency of vulvodynia is being realized.[20]

UROGENITAL NEUROBIOLOGY AND VULVAR PAIN—CLINICALLY RELEVANT DATA

Pain arising from within the pelvis and pelvic floor involve diverse neuronal mechanisms (Fig. 12.1), although there are some general characteristics. In general, sensations from the pelvic viscera are conveyed within the sacral afferent parasympathetic system, with a far lesser afferent supply from thoracolumbar sympathetic origin.[21] Receptive fields in the perineum are understood to be carried out primarily by sensory-motor discharges associated with pudendal nerve afferents.[21,22] Entrapment of the pudendal nerve has been considered as one of the causes of urogenital pain.[23] While the interactions of sensory afferents are quite complex, likely possibilities by which these pathways exert effects on autonomic efferent function include mediatory effects on spinal cord reflexes and modulatory effects on efferent release in peripheral autonomic ganglia and in peripheral organs.

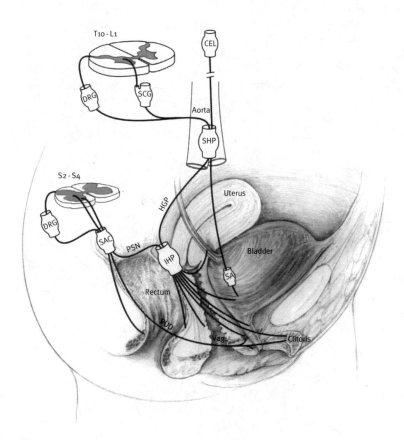

FIGURE 12.1   Innervation of the urogenital area in females. Although this diagram attempts to show the innervation in humans, much of the anatomic information is derived from animal data. CEL, celiac plexus; DRG, dorsal root ganglion; HGP, hypogastric plexus; IHP, inferior hypogastric plexus; PSN, pelvic splanchnic nerve; PUD, pudendal nerve; SA, short adrenergic projections; SAC, sacral plexus; SCG, sympathetic chain ganglion; SHP, superior hypogastric plexus; Vag, vagina. (Reproduced from Wesselmann U, Burnett AL, Heinberg LJ. The urogenital and rectal pain syndromes. *Pain* 1997;73[3]:269–94, with permission of the International Association for the Study of Pain).

Most studies on vulvar/vaginal innervation have been derived from animal studies.[1,24] Compared to other areas of neuroscience, little is known about the functional neural correlates that signal the wide range of sensations from the vulvar and vaginal area ranging from pleasure to pain. The vulva is densely innervated by branches of the pudendal nerves (somatic nerves), conveying information about gentle and intense mechanical stimulation to the sacral spinal cord (S2–S4). The vagina is innervated by the pelvic nerves (parasympathetic nerves). The cervix and adjacent fornix region of the vagina are innervated more densely than the rest of the vagina by the pelvic and hypogastric nerves. Information arriving from the vulva, vagina, and cervix is conveyed to widespread regions of the central nervous system, implying that stimulation of these regions can affect a wide range of physiological and perceptual functions.[25-28] Fibers innervating the vagina are activated by both gentle and intense mechanical stimulation, including noxious stimuli.[25,27] Mechanical probing (non-noxious stimuli) of the vagina and/or cervix has produced anti-nociceptive effects in rats and analgesia in women.[29,30] The urogenital sinus of the embryo differentiates into the adult urachus, bladder, urethra, and vestibule, which in the adult comprises a shallow funnel of endodermal origin, sandwiched in between the (ectodermally derived) vulva and vagina proper.[31-34] In no other anatomic region, in either gender, do epithelia derived from each of the trilaminar embryonic cell lines (ectoderm, endoderm, and mesoderm) juxtapose more closely than in the vulvovaginal region. The vulvar vestibule bears a closer resemblance to the lower urinary tract than to the external vulva or vagina.[35] In the clinical context, two urogenital pain syndromes are often observed together: interstitital cystitis and vulvodynia, which could in part be explained by the common embryological background.[36] The human vulvar vestibule contains free nerve endings but has no specialized nerve endings such as Meissner's or Pacinian corpuscles.[37] The first survey of the innervation pattern in the human vagina using a pan-axonal marker was published in 1995.[38] Free intraepithelial nerve endings were only detected in the introitus vaginae region. These very superficial free nerve endings are considered to be nociceptive or thermoceptive.[39] Studies in rats have demonstrated that the extent of the vaginal innervation varies as a function of the gonadal hormonal status.[40] This plasticity of the innervation is not restricted to the vagina, but it has been reported in other parts of the female reproductive tract as well: remodeling of the innervation has been described in the rodent and human uterus during the estrous cycle and during gestation. Estrogen seems to be a major factor, but not the only one, determining the level of innervation during the reproductive cycle.[41] Interestingly, four independent studies reported vestibular neural hyperplasia in women with vulvar vestibulitis, which might provide a morphological explanation for the vestibular hyperalgesia reported by these patients.[33,42-44]

Surprisingly, there had been little focus on neurotransmitters in the vulvo-vaginal area. In rabbits, hypothalamic neuropeptides have a contractile and relaxant effect on vaginal strips and arteries.[45] In female rats estradiol down-regulates estrogen-receptor alpha and up-regulates progesterone-receptor expression in the vagina.[46] Several studies have focused on steroid receptor expression in the vaginal epithelium and in the vulvar vestibular mucosa as a function of hormonal contraceptives and the menstrual cycle.[47,48] Estrogen-receptor beta was more abundant in the vulvar vestibular mucosa of women using combined oral contraceptives (COC) than in women without COC use. During the menstrual cycle, progesterone-receptor B was more abundant in the stromal tissue of the vulvar vestibular mucosa in the follicular phase than in the luteal phase in healthy women. In women with vulvodynia, there was a higher expression in estrogen-receptor alpha in the vulvar vestibular mucosa, but the epithelial morphology seemed unaffected.[49] CGRP, a neuropeptide known to exist in nociceptive afferent nerves, was the only neuropeptide detected in the superficial nerves of the vestibular epithelium in an earlier study by Bohm-Starke et al.[50] Studies using vestibular biopsy tissue from patients with localized provoked vulvodynia have demonstrated an increase in vanilloid receptor TRPV1 (a receptor expressed by nociceptors) innervation as compared to controls.[51]

Increased vulvar innervation could conceivably enhance transmission of painful sensation, particularly in the presence of local inflammation that can sensitize nerve endings, and contribute to peripheral sensitization of vulvar nociceptors.

PATHOPHYSIOLOGICAL MECHANISMS

The etiology of vulvodynia is considered multifactorial. Systemic factors that facilitate abnormal inflammatory processes have been hypothesized. In vitro and in vivo evidence of enhanced vulvar and systemic inflammatory responses to pathogens and allergens suggests that vulvar pain may be symptomatic of an abnormal inflammatory response. T-cell lymphocytes make up most of the inflammatory cells present in vulvar biopsies obtained from women with vulvodynia. Two studies on pro-inflammatory mediators have been published with conflicting results. Foster and Hasday found elevated tissue levels of interleukin I-ß (IL-1) and tumor necrosis factor alpha in vulvar tissue of patients with vulvodynia, but these pro-inflammatory mediators were actually at higher levels in the surrounding vulvar tissue than in the area of inflammation, confirming the clinical finding of a wider area of involvement beyond the area of erythema.[52] These results were not supported in a study by Eva et al., who found no difference in these mediators between patients and controls.[53]

There is increasing evidence of genetic polymorphisms that are found more often in women with localized provoked vulvodynia (including genes for mannose-binding lectin, cytokines, Interleukin-1 receptor antagonist, and Interleukin-1 beta), indicating that in some women, the over- or underexpression of certain pro-inflammatory cytokines could underlie abnormal physiological mechanisms driving vulvar pain.[54] In such cases, the magnitude or duration of the inflammatory response may be altered in response to otherwise innocuous levels of stimulation. However, equivocal findings of occasional redness and inflammatory infiltrate in vulvar biopsy tissue of women with provoked vulvar pain have called this inflammatory hypothesis into question.[55] It has been hypothesized that a subgroup of women experience vulvodynia of an inflammatory origin, yet the existence of such a subgroup has not been confirmed or rejected by clinical phenotyping efforts.

A possible etiological correlation between oral contraceptives (OCs) and provoked localized vulvodynia has been investigated in epidemiological studies. In a clinic-based study from 2002, the results showed a relative risk of vulvar vestibulitis of 6.6 (95% confidence interval, 2.5–17.4) for ever users compared to non-users. When OCs were used before age 16, the relative risk reached 9.3 and increased with duration of OC use up to 2–4 years. The relative risk was higher when the pill used was of high progestogenic, high androgenic, and low on estrogenic potency.[56] These findings were, however, not confirmed by a population-based case-control study from 2008.[57] The vestibular mucosa of healthy women on OCs undergoes changes compared to non-users.[48] The dermal papillae become shallower and sparser, which might result in a more fragile and sensitive mucosa.[58] Women without dyspareunia, using OCs, have lower vestibular pain thresholds to mechanical stimuli.[59] These findings are thought to be a gestagenic effect and support the data of an increased risk of developing vestibular pain using OCs with gestagenic potency. However, more data are needed and the current recommendation is to continue to prescribe the pill when it is needed, but both users and prescribers should be aware of side effects such as dryness, soreness, and pain.[58]

Vulvar allodynia and hyperalgesia can be assessed in the laboratory using quantitative sensory testing. Women with vulvodynia have reduced touch detection and mechanical pain thresholds in the genital area compared to age-matched controls,[60] as well as heightened pain sensitivity at nongenital body sites.[60-62] Thus, in some women, vulvar pain may not simply be a local sensory phenomenon, but central pain modulatory mechanisms might be involved. It is unclear whether heightened body sensitivity is a predisposing factor to vulvar pain, or whether it is the result. Notably, some evidence suggests symptomatic overlap between vulvodynia and systemic pain disorders like fibromyalgia.[63]

Evidence of central alterations in women with vulvodynia is mixed. Central abnormalities in pain processing were first suspected when women with provoked vulvar pain were found to have altered mechanical and thermal sensitivity in unaffected dermatomes.[55] A lack of an abnormal diffuse noxious inhibitory control response in women with vulvodynia indicates that such changes do not reflect descending control.[64] Magnetic resonance imaging studies of the brain indicated that women diagnosed with vulvodynia have significantly higher activation levels in the insular and frontal cortical regions than did control women during pressure applied to the posterior portion of the vulvar vestibule.[65] These results imply that women with vulvodynia exhibit an augmentation of genital sensory processing which is similar to that observed for a variety of syndromes causing hypersensitivity, including fibromyalgia, irritable bowel syndrome, and neuropathic pain. Increased regional gray matter volume in the parahippocampal gyrus/hippocampus and basal ganglia in the brains of women with vulvodynia suggests that the experience of vulvar pain may alter brain structure.[66] However, these brain regions participate in the processing of a broad range of cognitive and sensorimotor information that far surpasses the experience of vulvar pain.

Increased prevalence of comorbid psychopathology has been reported in women with vulvodynia. However, from an etiological standpoint it is not clear how this finding relates to vulvodynia, since this may be considered either a cause or a consequence for different women.[2] Higher rates of depression and anxiety disorders have been found in women with provoked vulvodynia, both using structured interviews and self-report instruments. Personality characteristics in women with provoked vulvodynia include higher levels of trait anxiety, shyness, hysterical personality, perfectionism, reward dependency, low self-esteem, fear of negative evaluation, and harm avoidance, as compared to healthy female controls. Higher pain ratings in women with vulvodynia were associated with lower marital adjustment and with higher levels of harm avoidance and reward dependence. Although women with vulvodynia, not surprisingly, report negative feelings about sexual contact with their partner, their relationship satisfaction regarding non-sexual aspects did not differ from controls.

CLINICAL PRESENTATIONS AND TREATMENT APPROACHES

Vulvodynia is a diagnosis of exclusion and established largely through history and clinical examination.[2,20] On physical examination patients with vulvodynia usually present with no visible abnormalities. Other causes of burning and irritation must be ruled out, including genital infections (candidiasis, human papillomavirus, herpes simplex virus, bacterial vaginosis), vulvar dermatoses, vulvar dysplasia, and urogenital atrophy. Local agents applied to the vulvar region can cause irritant reactions, which resolve after discontinuation of the irritant agent. Depending on the location of the pain, a diagnosis of generalized or localized vulvar dysesthesia is made. In patients with localized vulvar pain, it can easily be elicited or exacerbated by a simple "Q-tip test"; touching the dysesthetic area with a moist cotton swab results in sharp, burning pain.

Because the pathophysiological mechanisms of vulvodynia are not yet known, targeted therapy is not available at present. Treatment approaches are empirical only and target presumed etiologies. Multiple treatments have been used for vulvodynia,[67,68] including vulvar care measures: topical, oral, and injectable medications, which have been used for other chronic pain conditions; biofeedback; physical therapy; low oxalate diet and calcium citrate supplements; surgery (perineoplasty and pudendal nerve release); implantable nerve stimulation (Interstim); acupuncture; nitroglycerin; hypnotherapy; and botulinum toxin injections.

To identify women where entrapment of the pudendal nerve[23] or pudendal neuralgia,[69] a painful neuropathic condition, might be the cause of their vulvar pain, a pudendal nerve block has been suggested both as a diagnostic and therapeutic test.[23,70,71] Subsequent medical and surgical treatment has been advocated, with physical therapy as a key component to all aspects of the treatment.[23,69–71] While there is a subgroup of women with vulvar pain, who seem to experience pain relief with pudendal nerve blocks and surgical decompression of the pudendal nerve, identifying women who might benefit from this invasive approach remains difficult. Historically, the objective of these interventions was to block pain transmission from the site of origin to the brain. However, as concepts of neuropathic pain and central sensitization are becoming more clearly understood, we are beginning to appreciate the limitations of such a simplistic approach.[72,73]

Haefner et al.[68] reviewed the literature and provided guidelines based on expert opinion regarding the treatment of vulvodynia (Fig. 12.2). While no single treatment is successful for all women suffering from vulvodynia, the algorithm may be helpful to the patient and the health care provider in dealing with this condition. It is important for both the patient and the health care provider to acknowledge that sexual pain involves physical, psychological, and relationship aspects. A multidisciplinary

and multidimensional approach is advocated, including sexual counseling, psychological approaches, and couples counseling.[68]

Few studies have examined treatment approaches to vulvodynia in a randomized controlled trial. A recent trial assessing the efficacy of oral desipramine and topical lidocaine, as monotherapy or in combination, failed to reduce vulvodynia pain more than placebo.[74] A randomized comparison of vaginal biofeedback, group cognitive-behavioral therapy, and vestibulectomy found similar treatment outcomes for all modalities.[75]

THE FUTURE: CHALLENGES AND OPPORTUNITIES

Vulvodynia is a poorly defined and understudied chronic pain syndrome in women, and there is an urgent need to expand both basic science as well as clinic research in this field.[76] The long-term goal in treatment of lower genital tract pain

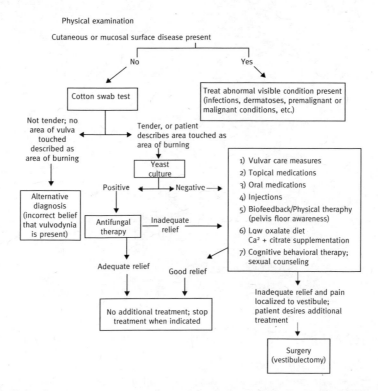

FIGURE 12.2 Vulvodynia assessment and treatment algorithm. (Reproduced from Haefner HK, Collins ME, Davis GD, et al. The vulvodynia guideline. *J Low Genit Tract Dis* 2005;9[1]:40–51, with permission of the American Society for Colposcopy and Cervical Pathology.)

will be the development of a mechanism-based classification of the disease and treatment based upon the most effective treatment against the identified mechanism. Further development of in vitro cell culture bioassays and/or animal models will be required to identify and target peripheral and central pathophysiological mechanisms. Recent studies on neurochemical substrates in the female urogenital area may provide a basis for future research on peripheral neurochemical mechanisms involved in the etiology of the sexual pain and sexual arousal disorders. There is already an impressive body of literature on visceral nociceptive processing and potential novel drugs,[77] and future studies could extend these findings to sexual pain disorders, which might lead to the identification of peripheral targets for treatment. The rapidly evolving field of vulvodynia research is increasingly focusing on multidisciplinary, concurrent assessment and treatment for vulvar pain, combining biomedical efforts with pelvic floor physical therapy and cognitive pain management approaches. There is a growing body of literature demonstrating that several chronic pain syndromes, including vulvodynia, often occur together in the same patient.[78] Efforts to understand the pathophysiology of chronic pain syndromes have shifted from an organ-based approach to a more global, systemic approach. Vulvar pain is increasingly studied in relation to (1) the surrounding structures (pelvic floor musculature, adjacent visceral organs), (2) the mind that must react and adapt to the repeated presence of pain, and (3) the intimate partners who are affected by the psychological and behavioral consequences of vulvar pain. Before industry-funded research is likely to proceed, researchers will need to clearly answer the questions of prevalence, proportions of phenotypically characterized subsets, and long-term morbidity of chronic vulvar pain.

ACKNOWLEDGEMENTS

Ursula Wesselmann's research program is supported by National Institutes of Health grants DK066641 (NIDDK) and HD39699 (NICHD, Office of Research for Women's Health).

RESOURCES FOR HEALTH CARE PROVIDERS, PATIENTS, AND RESEARCHERS

American College of Obstetricians and Gynecologists (ACOG)

Vulvodynia. Patient Education Pamphlet FAQ127, May 2011
http://www.acog.org/For_Patients

International Association for the Study of Pain (Iasp)

Global Year against Pain in Women (vulvodynia fact sheets)
111 Queen Anne Ave N. Suite 501
Seattle, WA 98105-4955
Tel: 206-238-0311
Website: http://www.iasp-pain.org

National Vulvodynia Association (NVA)

PO Box 4491
Silver Spring, MD 20914-4491
Tel: 301-299-0775
Website: http://www.nva.org

Office of Research on Women's Health (ORWH)

Vulvodynia
http://orwh.od.nih.gov/resources/health/research-andyourhealth/index.asp

REFERENCES

1. Wesselmann U, Burnett AL, Heinberg LJ. The urogenital and rectal pain syndromes. *Pain* 1997;73(3):269–94.
2. van Lankveld JJ, Granot M, Weijmar Schultz WC, et al. Women's sexual pain disorders. *J Sex Med* 2010;7(1 Pt 2):615–31.
3. Farmer MA, Kukkonen T, Binik YM. Female genital pain and its treatment. In: Rowland DL, Inrocci L, eds. *Handbook of Sexual and Identity Disorders*. Hoboken, NJ: John Wiley & Sons; 2008: 220–50.
4. Amalraj P, Kelly S, Bachmann GA. Historical perspective of vulvodynia. In: Goldstein AT, Pukall CF, Goldstein I, eds. *Female Sexual Pain*

Disorders: Evaluation and Management. New York: Wiley-Blackwell; 2008: 1–3.

5. Moyal-Barracco M, Lynch PJ. 2003 ISSVD terminology and classification of vulvodynia: a historical perspective. *J Reprod Med* 2004;49(10): 772–7.

6. Friedrich EG. Vulvar vestibulitis syndrome. *J Reprod Med* 1987;32(2):110–4.

7. Babula O, Linhares IM, Bongiovanni AM, Ledger WJ, Witkin SS. Association between primary vulvar vestibulitis syndrome, defective induction of tumor necrosis factor-alpha, and carriage of the mannose-binding lectin codon 54 gene polymorphism. *Am J Obstet Gynecol* 2008;198(1):101 e101–4.

8. Bornstein J, Maman M, Abramovici H. "Primary" versus "secondary" vulvar vestibulitis: one disease, two variants. *Am J Obstet Gynecol* 2001;184(2):28–31.

9. Granot M, Friedman M, Yarnitsky D, Tamir A, Zimmer EZ. Primary and secondary vulvar vestibulitis syndrome: systemic pain perception and psychophysical characteristics. *Am J Obstet Gynecol* 2004;191(1):138–42.

10. Witkin SS, Gerber S, Ledger WJ. Differential characterization of women with vulvar vestibulitis syndrome. *Am J Obstet Gynecol* 2002;187(3):589–94.

11. Zolnoun D, Park EM, Moore CG, Liebert CA, Tu FF, As-Sanie S. Somatization and psychological distress among women with vulvar vestibulitis syndrome. *Int J Gynaecol Obstet* 2008;103(1):38–43.

12. Bergeron S, Rosen NO, Morin M. Genital pain in women: beyond interference with intercourse. *Pain* 2011;152(6):1223–5.

13. Arnold LD, Bachmann GA, Rosen R, Rhoads GG. Assessment of vulvodynia symptoms in a sample of US women: a prevalence survey with a nested case control study. *Am J Obstet Gynecol* 2007;196(2):128 e121–6.

14. Harlow BL, Wise LA, Stewart EG. Prevalence and predictors of chronic lower genital tract discomfort. *Am J Obstet Gynecol* 2001;185(3):545–50.

15. Harlow BL, Stewart EG. A population-based assessment of chronic unexplained vulvar pain: have we underestimated the prevalence of vulvodynia? *J Am Med Womens Assoc* 2003;58(2):82–8.

16. Reed BD, Crawford S, Couper M, Cave C, Haefner HK. Pain at the vulvar vestibule: a web-based survey. *J Low Genit Tract Dis* 2004;8(1):48–57.

17. Laumann EO, Paik A, Rosen RC. Sexual dysfunction in the United States: prevalence and predictors. *JAMA* 1999;281(6):537–44.

18. Goetsch MF. Vulvar vestibulitis: prevalence and historic features in a general gynecologic practice population. *Am J Obstet Gynecol* 1991;164(6 Pt 1):1609–14; discussion 1614–16.

19. Adanu RM, Haefner HK, Reed BD. Vulvar pain in women attending a general medical clinic in Accra, Ghana. *J Reprod Med* 2005;50(2):130–4.

20. Edwards L. New concepts in vulvodynia. *Am J Obstet Gynecol* 2003;189(3 Suppl):S24–30.

21. Janig W, Koltzenberg M. Pain arising from the urogenital tract. In: Maggi CA, ed. *Nervous Control of the Urogenital System.* Chur, Switzerland: Harwood Academic Publishers; 1993: 525–78.

22. De Groat WC, Booth AM. Synaptic transmission in pelvic ganglia. In: Maggi CA, ed. *Nervous Control of the Urogenital System.* Chur, Switzerland: Harwood Academic Publishers; 1993: 91–347.

23. Labat JJ, Riant T, Robert R, Amarenco G, Lefaucheur JP, Rigaud J. Diagnostic criteria for pudendal neuralgia by pudendal nerve entrapment (Nantes criteria). *Neurourol Urodyn* 2008;27(4):306–10.

24. Burnett AL, Saito S, Maguire MP, Yamaguchi H, Chang TS, Hanley DF. Localization of nitric oxide synthase in spinal nuclei innervating pelvic ganglia. *J Urol* 1995;153(1):212–7.

25. Berkley KJ, Hubscher CH, Wall PD. Neuronal responses to stimulation of the cervix, uterus, colon, and skin in the rat spinal cord. *J Neurophysiol* 1993;69(2):545–56.

26. Berkley KJ, Benoist JM, Gautron M, Guilbaud G. Responses of neurons in the caudal intralaminar thalamic complex of the rat to stimulation of the uterus, vagina, cervix, colon and skin. *Brain Res* 1995;695(1):92–5.

27. Berkley KJ, Wood E, Scofield SL, Little M. Behavioral responses to uterine or vaginal distension in the rat. *Pain* 1995;61(1):121–31.

28. Bradshaw HB, Berkley KJ. Estrous changes in responses of rat gracile nucleus neurons to stimulation of skin and pelvic viscera. *J Neurosci* 2000;20(20):7722–7.

29. Komisaruk BR, Larsson K. Suppression of a spinal and a cranial nerve reflex by vaginal or rectal probing in rats. *Brain Res* 1971;35(1):231–5.

30. Komisaruk BR, Whipple B. The suppression of pain by genital stimulation in females. *Ann Rev Sex Res* 1995;6:151–86.

31. Friedrich EG, Jr. The vulvar vestibule. *J Reprod Med* 1983;28(11):773–7.

32. Marinoff SC, Turner ML. Vulvar vestibulitis syndrome. *Dermatol Clin* 1992;10(2):435–44.

33. Westrom LV, Willen R. Vestibular nerve fiber proliferation in vulvar vestibulitis syndrome. *Obstet Gynecol* 1998;91(4):572–6.

34. Woodruff JD, Friedrich EG, Jr. The vestibule. *Clin Obstet Gynecol* 1985;28(1):134–41.

35. Robboy SJ, Ross JS, Prat J, Keh PC, Welch WR. Urogenital sinus origin of mucinous and ciliated cysts of the vulva. *Obstet Gynecol* 1978;51(3):347–51.

36. McCormack WM. Two urogenital sinus syndromes. Interstitial cystitis and focal vulvitis. *J Reprod Med* 1990;35(9):873–6.

37. Krantz KE. Innervation of the human vulva and vagina; a microscopic study. *Obstet Gynecol* 1958;12(4):382–96.

38. Hilliges M, Falconer C, Ekman-Ordeberg G, Johansson O. Innervation of the human vaginal mucosa as revealed by PGP 9.5 immunohistochemistry. *Acta Anat (Basel)* 1995;153(2):119–26.

39. Iggo A, Andres KH. Morphology of cutaneous receptors. *Annu Rev Neurosci* 1982; 5:1–31.

40. Ting AY, Blacklock AD, Smith PG. Estrogen regulates vaginal sensory and autonomic nerve density in the rat. *Biol Reprod* 2004;71(4):1397–404.

41. Latini C, Frontini A, Morroni M, Marzioni D, Castellucci M, Smith PG. Remodeling of uterine innervation. *Cell Tissue Res* 2008;334(1):1–6.

42. Bohm-Starke N, Hilliges M, Falconer C, Rylander E. Increased intraepithelial innervation in women with vulvar vestibulitis syndrome. *Gynecol Obstet Invest* 1998;46(4):256–60.

43. Halperin R, Zehavi S, Vaknin Z, Ben-Ami I, Pansky M, Schneider D. The major histopathologic characteristics in the vulvar vestibulitis syndrome. *Gynecol Obstet Invest* 2005;59(2):75–9.

44. Tympanidis P, Terenghi G, Dowd P. Increased innervation of the vulval vestibule in patients with vulvodynia. *Br J Dermatol* 2003;148(5):1021–7.

45. Aughton KL, Hamilton-Smith K, Gupta J, Morton JS, Wayman CP, Jackson VM. Pharmacological profiling of neuropeptides on rabbit vaginal wall and vaginal artery smooth muscle in vitro. *Br J Pharmacol* 2008;155(2):236–43.

46. Pessina MA, Hoyt RF, Jr., Goldstein I, Traish AM. Differential regulation of the expression of estrogen, progesterone, and androgen receptors by sex steroid hormones in the vagina: immunohistochemical studies. *J Sex Med* 2006;3(5):804–14.

47. Ildgruben A, Sjoberg I, Hammarstrom ML, Backstrom T. Steroid receptor expression in vaginal epithelium of healthy fertile women and influences of hormonal contraceptive usage. *Contraception* 2005;72(5):383–92.

48. Johannesson U, Sahlin L, Masironi B, Rylander E, Bohm-Starke N. Steroid receptor expression in the vulvar vestibular mucosa—effects of oral contraceptives and menstrual cycle. *Contraception* 2007;76(4):319–25.

49. Johannesson U, Sahlin L, Masironi B, et al. Steroid receptor expression and morphology in provoked vestibulodynia. *Am J Obstet Gynecol* 2008;198(3):e311–6.

50. Bohm-Starke N, Hilliges M, Falconer C, Rylander E. Neurochemical characterization of the vestibular nerves in women with vulvar vestibulitis syndrome. *Gynecol Obstet Invest* 1999;48(4):270–5.

51. Tympanidis P, Casula MA, Yiangou Y, Terenghi G, Dowd P, Anand P. Increased vanilloid receptor VR1 innervation in vulvodynia. *Eur J Pain* 2004;8(2):129–33.

52. Foster DC, Hasday JD. Elevated tissue levels of interleukin-1 beta and tumor necrosis factor-alpha in vulvar vestibulitis. *Obstet Gynecol* 1997;89(2):291–6.

53. Eva LJ, Rolfe KJ, MacLean AB, et al. Is localized, provoked vulvodynia an inflammatory condition? *J Reprod Med* 2007; 52(5):379–84.

54. Gerber S, Witkin SS, Stucki D. Immunological and genetic characterization of women with vulvodynia. *J Med Life* 2008;1(4):432–8.

55. Bohm-Starke N. Medical and physical predictors of localized provoked vulvodynia. *Acta Obstet Gynecol Scand* 2010;89(12):1504–10.

56. Bouchard C, Brisson J, Fortier M, Morin C, Blanchette C. Use of oral contraceptive pills and vulvar vestibulitis: a case-control study. *Am J Epidemiol* 2002;156(3):254–61.

57. Harlow BL, Vitonis AF, Stewart EG. Influence of oral contraceptive use on the risk of adult-onset vulvodynia. *J Reprod Med* 2008;53(2):102–10.

58. Johannesson U, Blomgren B, Hilliges M, Rylander E, Bohm-Starke N. The vulval vestibular mucosa-morphological effects of oral contraceptives and menstrual cycle. *Br J Dermatol* 2007;157(3):487–93.

59. Bohm-Starke N, Johannesson U, Hilliges M, Rylander E, Torebjork E. Decreased mechanical pain threshold in the vestibular mucosa of women using oral contraceptives: a contributing factor in vulvar vestibulitis? *J Reprod Med* 2004;49(11):888–92.

60. Pukall CF, Binik YM, Khalife S, Amsel R, Abbott FV. Vestibular tactile and pain thresholds in women with vulvar vestibulitis syndrome. *Pain* 2002;96(1–2):163–75.

61. Giesecke J, Reed BD, Haefner HK, Giesecke T, Clauw DJ, Gracely RH. Quantitative sensory testing in vulvodynia patients and increased peripheral pressure pain sensitivity. *Obstet Gynecol* 2004;104(1):126–33.

62. Granot M, Friedman M, Yarnitsky D, Zimmer EZ. Enhancement of the perception of systemic pain in women with vulvar vestibulitis. *BJOG* 2002;109(8):863–6.

63. Pukall CF, Baron M, Amsel R, Khalife S, Binik YM. Tender point examination in women with vulvar vestibulitis syndrome. *Clin J Pain* 2006;22(7):601–9.

64. Johannesson U, de Boussard CN, Brodda Jansen G, Bohm-Starke N. Evidence of diffuse noxious inhibitory controls (DNIC) elicited by cold noxious stimulation in patients with provoked vestibulodynia. *Pain* 2007;130(1–2):31–9.

65. Pukall CF, Strigo IA, Binik YM, Amsel R, Khalife S, Bushnell MC. Neural correlates of painful genital touch in women with vulvar vestibulitis syndrome. *Pain* 2005;115(1–2):118–27.

66. Schweinhardt P, Kuchinad A, Pukall CF, Bushnell MC. Increased gray matter density in young women with chronic vulvar pain. *Pain* 2008;140(3):411–9.

67. Goldstein AT, Burrows L. Vulvodynia. *J Sex Med* 2008;5(1):5–14.

68. Haefner HK, Collins ME, Davis GD, et al. The vulvodynia guideline. *J Low Genit Tract Dis* 2005;9(1):40–51.

69. Hibner M, Desai N, Robertson LJ, Nour M. Pudendal neuralgia. *J Minim Invasive Gynecol* 2010;17(2):148–53.

70. Rigaud J, Delavierre D, Sibert L, Labat JJ. [Treatment algorithms for the management of chronic pelvic and perineal pain: from syndrome to treatment]. *Prog Urol* 2010;20(12):1132–8.

71. Shafik A. Pudendal canal syndrome as a cause of vulvodynia and its treatment by pudendal nerve decompression. *Eur J Obstet Gynecol Reprod Biol* 1998;80(2):215–20.

72. Dickson DE, Humphrey VR. Nerve Blocks in Urogenital Pain. In: Baranowski AP, Abrams P, Fall M, eds. *Urogenital Pain in Clinical Practice*. New York: Informa Healthcare USA; 2008: 451–69.

73. Woolf CJ. Central sensitization: implications for the diagnosis and treatment of pain. *Pain* 2011;152(3 Suppl):S2–15.

74. Foster DC, Kotok MB, Huang LS, et al. Oral desipramine and topical lidocaine for vulvodynia: a randomized controlled trial. *Obstet Gynecol* 2010;116(3):583–93.

75. Bergeron S, Binik YM, Khalife S, et al. A randomized comparison of group cognitive—behavioral therapy, surface electromyographic biofeedback, and vestibulectomy in the treatment of dyspareunia resulting from vulvar vestibulitis. *Pain* 2001;91(3):297–306.

76. Bachmann GA, Rosen R, Pinn VW, et al. Vulvodynia: a state-of-the-art consensus on definitions, diagnosis and management. *J Reprod Med* 2006;51(6):447–56.

77. Wesselmann U, Baranowski AP, Borjesson M, et al. Emerging therapies and novel approaches to visceral pain. *Drug Discov Today Ther Strateg* 2009;6(3):89–95.

78. Rodriguez MA, Afari N, Buchwald DS. Evidence for overlap between urological and nonurological unexplained clinical conditions. *J Urol* 2009;182(5):2123–31.

13

PERSISTENT PAIN AFTER BREAST CANCER TREATMENT

Kenneth Geving Andersen and Henrik Kehlet

INTRODUCTION

The incidence of breast cancer is about 1.4 million new cases annually, it accounts for 460,000 deaths per year worldwide, and it is the most frequent malignant disease among women.[1] Improvements in oncologic treatment have increased survival, and in the Nordic countries and the United States the 5-year survival is now 79%–90%,[2,3] emphasizing the need for more attention on the late sequelae of the treatment. Persistent pain following surgery has been established as a significant problem in several surgical procedures,[4–6] including breast cancer treatment.[7] Risk factors that may contribute to the development of persistent pain are as follows: age, preoperative pain, nerve injury, acute postoperative pain, psychosocial factors, type of surgery, adjuvant treatment, sex, type of analgesia, and genetics, and they are often divided into pre-, intra-, and postoperative risk factors.[4] Many of these risk factors are common across different surgical procedures, whereas others may only apply for patients treated for breast cancer. A review of persistent pain following breast cancer treatment (PPBCT) has recently been published.[7] This chapter is an updated overview of the pre-, intra-, and postoperative risk factors for the development of PPBCT as well as the areas that need more research.

DEVELOPMENTS IN BREAST CANCER TREATMENT

Until the 1970s, breast cancer treatment was based on the Halstedian concept of aggressive local surgical treatment,[8] with extensive removal of breast, lymph nodes, muscles, and ribs. Development of radiation therapy, and especially chemotherapeutic drugs and endocrine therapy, has changed the understanding of breast cancer as a more systemic disease.[9] This has led to less invasive surgery, and modern breast cancer surgery consists today of two different surgical procedures in the breast area (mastectomy and breast conservative surgery [BCS]) and two procedures for the axilla (sentinel lymph node biopsy [SLNB] and axillary lymph node dissection [ALND]). Adjuvant treatment is indicated for most patients, and it consists of radiation therapy, chemotherapy, and endocrine therapy (see Table 13.1). All treatment modalities may modify the risk of developing persistent pain and should thus be taken into consideration when treating patients or planning a study on PPBCT.

DEFINITIONS

The condition of pain following breast cancer treatment has formerly been termed postmastectomy pain syndrome (PMPS).[7] This was defined

Table 13.1   Overview of Breast Cancer Treatment Modalities

TREATMENT MODALITY	PROCEDURE	SUBGROUPS	DESCRIPTION
Surgery, breast	Mastectomy	Radical mastectomy	Removal of skin, breast pectoral muscles, and rib
		Modified radical mastectomy	Removal of breast
	Breast conserving surgery		Excision of tumor
Surgery, axilla			
	SLNB		Removal of average 1–4 lymph nodes
	ALND	Level 1	Removal of lymph nodes lateral to the minor pectoral muscle
		Level 1–2	Removal of lymph nodes in level 1 and behind the minor pectoral muscle
		Level 1–3	Complete removal of all lymph nodes
		Delayed ALND	SLNB followed by ALND in a separate procedure
Radiation therapy	BRT		Radiation field over residual breast tissue or anterior thoracic wall
	ATRT		Radiation field over anterior thoracic wall
	LRRT		Radiation field over periclavicular, axillary level 3 nodes. For right-side cancers may also include the internal mammary nodes
Chemotherapy	CMF	+/– Trasuztumab	Cyclophosphamide Methotrexate Fluoruracil
	FAC	+/– Trasuztumab	Cyclophosphamide Anthracycline Fluoruracil
	TAC	+/– Trasuztumab	Cyclophosphamide Anthracycline Taxanes
Endocrine therapy	TAM		Tamoxifen
	AI		Aromatase inhibitor

ALND, axillary lymph node dissection; ATRT, anterior thoracic radiation therapy; BCS, breast-conserving surgery; BRT, breast radiation therapy (residual breast tissue); LRRT, locoregional radiation therapy; SNLB, sentinel lymph node biopsy.

as a typical neuropathic pain condition with unpleasant sensations described as numbness, pins and needles, burning, or stabbing. The pain is located in the axilla, arm, shoulder, or chest wall on the side of surgery, and it may last more than 3 months after surgery.[10] This definition was criticized by Jung et al., who proposed four distinct neuropathic pain syndromes.[11] Although neuropathic pain may account for a large part of PPBCT, clear evidence for the pathogenic mechanisms is still missing in the literature.[7] This, taken together with the recent discussions on the definition of neuropathic pain,[12] argues for a more pragmatic definition of PPBCT. Radiation and chemotherapy are treatments that induce several side effects, such as chemotherapy-induced neuropathy.[13] Thus, a static point of time of 3 months after surgery may be artificial, as pain in this period may be one of the accepted side effects from adjuvant therapy. Therefore, a more realistic definition would be to take this into account and define PPBCT as pain 3 months after therapy has ended. Since this was not taken into consideration in any study, PPBCT in this chapter refers to patients with persistent pain 3 months after surgery.

EPIDEMIOLOGY

Surgical and adjuvant treatment, as well as definition, measurement method, and anatomical localization, have influence on the prevalence of PPBCT. Studies using the PMPS definition report the prevalence to be around 25%, and studies using the IASP definition report prevalence around 50% across all treatments.[7] A large nationwide study, where patients were divided into 12 well-defined treatment groups, found the prevalence vary from 25% in the lower end (patients treated with mastectomy, sentinel lymph node biopsy without chemo or radiation therapy) to 60% in the upper end (patients treated with BCS, axillary lymph node dissection, and a radiation field extending to the periclavicular lymph nodes).[14]

PREOPERATIVE RISK FACTORS

Preoperative risk factors are patient-related factors that upon identification may be used in preventive measures.

Age

Across several surgical procedures age is a consistent risk factor for the development of persistent pain after surgery,[4] including breast cancer treatment,[7] and younger patients are at a higher risk of developing PPBCT. In a large nationwide study, patients treated with BCS aged 18–39 years have an odds ratio of 3.62 of developing PPBCT compared with patients aged 60–69 years.[14] It is not clear whether this is due to an age-dependent pathophysiologic reduction in pain perception, a change in the subjective pain acceptance and expression, or whether it is due to a general decrease in mobility. There are indications of a relationship between age and psychosocial factors; that is, younger patients also report more psychological distress after the treatment.[15–17] The association between age and PPBCT could also be of interest in therapeutic trials, that is, trying more aggressive analgesic regimens as well as a closer psychological support in patients of younger age.

Psychosocial Factors

Psychological morbidity such as anxiety,[18] depression,[19] fear of pain, and catastrophizing[20] are known to influence pain perception. Several studies have examined this in breast cancer patients, who show an association of PPBCT and psychological morbidity.[7] However, the causality relationship between psychosocial factors and PPBCT remains unclear due to a lack of sufficiently designed prospective studies taking all risk factors into consideration.

Preoperative Pain in the Breast

Preoperative pain in the area of surgery is a known risk factor for persistent pain after other surgical procedures.[4,5,18] This potential risk factor is not well examined in breast cancer patients, due to the lack of prospective studies.[7] Preoperative pain could be an indication of a higher nociceptive response, which in experimental studies has been shown to be a risk factor for acute and persistent postsurgical pain.[5,21] This could prove a useful tool to predict PPBCT, and it should be included in future studies.

Pain in Other Locations in the Body

Pain located outside the area of surgery, shoulder, side of chest, and arm on the side of surgery are common in the breast cancer population. In a Danish nationwide study 40% of the patients reported unspecific pain complaints in the joints and muscles, such as headache, neck-shoulder pain, and low-back pain. This was found to be associated with an increased risk of reporting PPBCT,[14] which is consistent with studies made in other surgical procedures.[22–24] In the general population these complaints in the same age group are around 20%.[25] Furthermore, joint and muscle pain are a known side effect of the endocrine treatment, especially for the recently introduced aromatase inhibitors.[26] It is unclear whether the pathophysiological mechanisms for the relationship between PPBCT and pain in other locations are due to higher pain sensitivity or a higher pain reporting in patients experiencing these pains.

Other Potential Preoperative Risk Factors

Obesity may constitute a risk factor because of two mechanisms. Obese patients have a higher risk of developing lymphedema,[27] which also contributes to PPBCT. Furthermore, axillary surgery may be more challenging in obese patients, possibly leading to a higher incidence of nerve damage and therefore a higher risk of PPBCT. The considerable interindividual difference of pain perception may be related to specific genotypes,[28] and several genes have been proposed as candidates. So far only one gene, *CACNG2*, has been assessed in the breast cancer population,[29] but not all the risk factors had been taken into consideration. Despite intensive research in this area, progress in genetic research in pain pathophysiology has been hindered by problems in the methodology and availability of large well-defined phenotype groups.[7,30]

INTRAOPERATIVE RISK FACTORS

Surgery

Nerve injury is considered an important contributing factor in breast cancer surgery in the development of persistent postoperative pain.[4] During axillary dissection the intercostobrachial nerve (ICBN) may be injured. The ICBN is a sensory nerve that innervates the axilla, medial upper arm, and lateral chest. Unfortunately, the studies on preservation of this nerve are poor and inconclusive.[7] However, comparisons between axillary lymph node dissection (ALND) and sentinel lymph node biopsy (SLNB) show a consistently higher prevalence of pain and pain intensity among patients operated with ALND,[7] which suggests that ICBN injury may play an important role in persistent pain in these patients.

The extent of breast surgery per se may potentially influence the prevalence of PPBCT. For instance, in a large nationwide study, more patients who underwent mastectomy experienced severe PPBCT than patients treated with BCS.[14] However, patients who undergo BCS also receive radiation therapy, which may in turn contribute to persistent pain, thereby confounding the interpretation of PPBCT in these patients.

Preventive Analgesia

Preventive analgesia is an interesting hypothesis, where administration of analgesics is commenced before and throughout the period of time during which nociceptive input may lead to central neuroplastic changes.[31] This hypothesis was tested in the breast cancer population, but with small and heterogeneous study samples, as well as a limited treatment time, no conclusions can be drawn.[7] In a recent trial where patients were randomized to gabapentin 300 mg/d, venlafaxine 37.5 mg/d, or placebo, the group treated with venlafaxine had a lower prevalence of PPBCT, pain intensity, and need for analgesics than the other two groups.[32] Preventive analgesia is an interesting concept that may yield a new strategy to prevent PPBCT. However, this study lacks details of enrollment of patients and breast cancer treatment, and it should therefore be interpreted with caution. Future studies in PPBCT should include risk factors when interpreting their findings.

POSTOPERATIVE RISK FACTORS

Adjuvant Therapy

Patients treated with BCS also undergo *radiation therapy* on residual breast tissue. Mastectomy patients receive radiation on the anterior thoracic wall if there is invasive growth in the muscle. The radiation field may be more extensive if the nodes are positive and are not all removed or if the tumor is large. Potential side effects of radiation therapy include cardiotoxicity, lung fibrosis, lymphedema, reduced shoulder mobility, and neurotoxicity.[33,34] Several studies have found radiation therapy to be a risk factor for developing PPBCT.[7] Radiation therapy may cause demyelination and thereby neuropathic pain.[34] Furthermore, radiation therapy is associated with an increased risk of lymphedema and fibrosis in the axilla, both of which may also cause pain. A recent study comparing intraoperative radiation therapy (which targets and limits the radiation to the area where the tumour was excised) to conventional radiation therapy suggests equivalent results.[35] Our own results from a study comparing intraoperative radiation therapy and conventional radiation therapy suggest a potential favourable effect of intraoperative radiation therapy on PPBCT[36]; however, studies looking at a larger number of patients are needed.

Chemotherapy may also be a risk factor for developing PPBCT, depending on the regimen used. Treatment with cyclophosfamide, epirubicine and fluoruracil may not be associated with a risk of PPBCT.[14] Taxanes, platinum agents, and vinca alkaloids are known to be neurotoxic and may induce chemotherapy-induced peripheral neuropathy (CIPN),[37] which is identified as a risk factor for neuropathic pain.[38] Taxanes improve survival in breast cancer,[39,40] and currently paclitaxel and docetaxel are used in breast cancer treatment. Hershman et al. evaluated patients treated with paclitaxel using questionnaires and quantitative sensory testing.[41] Numbness and discomfort in the hands were common for up to 2 years after treatment and were associated to increased thresholds for vibration. Six months after treatment 25% of the patients rated numbness and discomfort as severe.[41] Neurotoxicity associated with taxanes is dose dependent and differs between paclitaxel and docetaxel. The second-generation taxane docetacel is associated with a lower incidence of CIPN, and sensory symptoms are milder.[37] However, it is not known how taxanes influence development of PPBCT.

Endocrine treatment with *tamoxifen* or *aromatase inhibitors* is notable for causing musculoskeletal pain.[26] Large randomized studies that have evaluated musculoskeletal as a safety issue have insufficient methodology to allow an analysis in relation to PPBCT.[26] In summary, adjuvant systemic treatment may constitute an important factor in the pathophysiologic mechanisms in PPBCT.

Early Postoperative Pain

Some of the studies on PPBCT indicate that early postoperative pain increases the risk of PPBCT[7]; however, most studies examined this issue retrospectively and are thus susceptible to recall bias. A recent prospective study found that patients that developed PPBCT reported higher pain ratings before discharge.[42] The correlation of acute postoperative pain and PPBCT is interesting in light of studies showing a predictive value of preoperative nociceptive stimuli on acute and persistent postoperative pain.[18,21] Further prospective studies are needed to further define whether acute postoperative pain poses an increased risk for PPBCT.

Lymphedema

Lymphedema is a significant problem in the breast cancer population and has a negative impact on the quality of life.[43] Prevalences are reported to be between 4% and 49%, depending on means of measurement and breast cancer treatment modalities.[44] Unlike other arm symptoms, such as arm functioning and arm pain, the prevalence of lymphedema is reported to increase over time.[45] In a large review Tsai et al. found that mastectomy, the extent of axillary dissection, use of radiation therapy, and the presence of positive nodes all pose as risk factors for developing lymphedema.[44] In a large nationwide questionnaire study, a young age, ALND, and radiotherapy were found to be risk factors.[46] Cross-sectional questionnaire studies indicate that PPBCT and lymphedema may share similar risk factors.[46] Self-reported lymphedema varies between 13% and 65%, depending on breast cancer treatment,[46] whereas studies objectively assessing lymphedema reports a prevalence of around 13%.[27,45]

Those patients who do not present with lymphedema clinically but report the discomfort and a sensation of heaviness associated with lymphedema may be reporting discomfort caused by PPBCT and nerve damage. A large prospective study is needed to establish the relationship between PPBCT and lymphedema.

TIME COURSE

Pain is dynamic in its nature and the evidence on temporal development or resolution of PPBCT is inconclusive. Most studies are retrospective with no well-defined time period for follow-up.[7] On the other hand, two studies with a follow-up time of greater than 5 years showed a decrease in PPBCT prevalence.[47,48] More information on the course of PPBCT over time in well-defined cohorts is needed to further understand the pathophysiological mechanisms and should be studied in a large prospective trials.

THE PATHOPHYSIOLOGY OF PERSISTENT PAIN FOLLOWING BREAST CANCER TREATMENT

Since there are many different risk factors associated with PPBCT, the pathophysiology is likely complex and inconclusive. Three mechanisms stand out as most probable and they may interact synergistically: neuropathic pain, central sensitization, and lymphedema.

Neuropathic pain is supported by evidence that sensory disturbances are a prominent feature in PPBCT.[11,14] The prevalence for sensory disturbances may range from 31% to 85% depending on the treatment,[14] with patients treated with BCS, SLNB, and radiation therapy on residual breast at the lower end, and patients treated with BCS, ALND, and radiation therapy toward the axilla at the higher end. This pattern is consistent with pain measurements and supports the type of surgery and radiation therapy as possible pathogenic mechanisms. However, the same pattern follows lymphedema, and it may affect reporting of pain and sensory disturbances. Quantitative sensory testing (QST)[49,50] has been performed to a limited degree in the breast cancer population.[51,52] Two studies have examined the surgical area with QST. Gottrup et al. performed QST on 15 pain patients and

11 pain-free controls and found lower pressure pain thresholds and higher evoked pain to repetitive stimuli.[51] Vilholm et al. examined 55 patients with pain and 27 patients without pain, and they found higher thermal thresholds in both groups but with a larger difference in the pain group, as well as higher evoked pain to repetitive stimuli.[52] Methodological issues due to inclusion of relatively few patients and with different treatment modalities preclude a conclusion but argue for neuropathic features in PPBCT.

Central sensitization is a prominent feature of chronic pain states, in which peripheral input modulates pain processing centrally.[53] Recent studies report that myofascial pain syndrome is a prominent part of PPBCT, and widespread tender points may serve as an indication of peripheral and central sensitization.[54-56] These studies are of small size, and specific points on the treatment modalites are not reported. However, since the endocrine treatment may induce musculoskeletal pain,[26] this may also contribute to central sensitization.

TREATMENT

There are few studies on pain treatment of PPBCT, most of which are small and on heterogeneous populations.[7] Unfortunately, there is no evidence to recommend specific treatments for PPBCT. In view of the large number of patients affected by this problem, PPBCT should be a major area of focus for future research. Treatment may be based on the proposed mechanisms involved in PPBCT. The treatment of neuropathic pain in and of itself is challenging, and there is a general lack of evidence in the area of postsurgical neuropathic pain.[57] Patients suffering from PPBCT may prove a reasonable model to study the effect of neuropathic pain medications, if information on the other possible risk factors are taken in consideration, and the population is carefully limited to the patients most likely suffering from neuropathic pain. Until such research results are available, we suggest using the best evidence-based treatment principles for neuropathic pain[57] as listed in Table 13.2. Lymphedema may be treated with various forms of conservative therapy, including compression, exercise, massage, and

Table 13.2 Published Randomized Placebo-Controlled Trials in Neuropathic Pain after Peripheral Nerve Injury

	POSITIVE TRIALS	NEGATIVE TRIALS	NNT	95% CI
TCA	1	1		
SNRI		1		
Gabapentin	1	2		
Pregabalin	1		NS	
Levetiracetam		1		
Opioids	2		5.1	(2.7–36)
Tramadol	1		NA	
Cannabinoids	1		NS	
Topical lidocaine	1	1		
NMDA antagonists		2		
Mexiletine		2		
Topical capsaicin	1	1		

Note: The table indicates positive and negative trials and numbers needed to treat (NNT) to obtain one patient with more than 50% pain relief. Derived from Finnerup et al.[57]

NA, data not available; NS, absolute risk difference not significant; SNRI, serotonin noradrenaline reuptake inhibitor; TCA, tricyclic antidepressants.

skin hygiene.[58] Surgery to re-establish lymph circulation has been tried, but the results are inconclusive.[58] Lymphedema treatment has not changed much the past years, but promising results in preclinical models, such as inducing growth of new lymph capillaries,[59] may give us new therapies in the future. Preventive analgesia may have a role in preventing PPBCT, but careful consideration of study design is of outmost importance to prove any role for this in preventing PPBCT.[31] Finally, reducing psychological distress may also be helpful to those patients who are emotionally vulnerable.[60]

DIRECTIONS FOR FUTURE RESEARCH

The relative role of the different pathogenic mechanisms of PPBCT is not completely understood,[7] which makes research in this field challenging Important factors to be considered in prospective studies are outlined in Table 13.3. Future studies should focus on acquiring more precise epidemiological information, including the time course of PPBCT, improvement in the surgical handling of the ICBN, the role of

preventive analgesia in reducing PPBCT, and the role of chemotherapy and radiation therapy in the development of PPBCT. Furthermore, sensory disturbances should be assessed by methods such as QST and skin biopsies,[61] to evaluate the neuropathic component in PPBCT. Lymphedema should be assessed separately and preferably with interventions to alleviate lymphedema to help understand the relationship of lymphedema and PPBCT. Pain measurements should be done according to the recommendation by the Initative in Methods, Measurement, and Pain Assessment in Clinical Trials (IMMPACT)[62] with emphasis on pain in movement as well as the consequences of pain on physical function.[63] Questionnaires should be procedure specific to the breast cancer population to improve comparability within the population and to define the specific functional and psychosocial consequences of PPBCT. Finally, blood samples should be taken and stored for genetic studies.

SUMMARY

Persistent pain after breast cancer treatment is a significant clinical problem, and it affects

Table 13.3 Proposed Factors and Confounders to Be Included in Future Studies of Persistent Pain Following Breast Cancer Treatment

	ITEM	DESCRIPTION
Design	Method	Prospective/retrospective/RCT
	Questionnaire	Procedure-specific questionnaire
	Clinical examination	Protocol for questions and examinations
	Follow-up	>3 months, details on time
	Pain evaluation:	• NRS/VRS
		• Pain characteristics
		• Anatomical localization
		• Pain in rest
		• Pain in movement
		• Pain-related functional impairment
Exclusion criteria	Recurrent cancer	Systematic examination
	Metastasis	Systematic examination
	Previous surgery in area	Medical records, clinical examination
	Breast reconstruction	
Preoperative	Demographics:	Included in analysis
	• Age	TNM, receptor status
	• BMI	Analgesics, psychotherapeutic agents
	• Socioeconomic	
	• Ethnicity	Neuropathy, cardiac disease
	Disease status	NRS
	Preoperative medication	Muscle and joint pain, location and intensity
	Comorbidity	
	Nociceptive function	Validated instrument (e.g., HADS)
	Pain in breast area	
	Pain other locations	
	Psychological assessment	
	Blood sample for genetic analysis	
Intraoperative	Surgical procedure on breast	Description of procedure
	Surgical procedure on axilla	Description of procedure, concomitant with or separate from breast procedure
	Handling of nerves	
	Analgesics	Preservation of ICBN
		Preemptive analgesia

(continued)

Table 13.3 *(Continued)*

	ITEM	DESCRIPTION
Postoperative	Early postoperative pain	NRS
	Analgesics	Postsurgical pain regimen
	Adjuvant therapy:	• Radiotherapy
	Lymphedema	- Radiation field
	Complications	- Radiation dose
	Sensory disturbances	- Timing
	Social/physical consequences	• Chemotherapy
		- Regime
		- Cumulative dose
		- Timing
		• Endocrine therapy
		- Regime
		- Dose
		- Timing
		Subjective/clinical examination
		Seroma, hematoma, infection
		Subjective/clinical examination/ QST
		Validated instrument

BMI, body mass index; ICBN, intercostobrachial nerve; NRS, numberical rating scale; QST, quantitative sensory testing; RCT, randomized controlled trial; VRS, verbal rating scale.

between 25% and 60% of the patients, depending of treatment. The pathophysiology is complex and consists of several pre-, intra-, and postoperative risk factors. To date, we have identified young age, extensive surgery in the axilla, radiation therapy, lymphedema, and pain located elsewhere in the body as risk factors. Well-designed prospective studies that include potential risk factors are required to help develop preventive strategies as well as treatment for PPBCT.

ACKNOWLEDGMENTS

This study was funded by a grant from the Danish Cancer Society, and the research leading to this work is part of the Europain Collaboration, which has received support from the Innovative Medicines Initiative Joint Undertaking, under grant agreement no 115007, resources of which are composed of financial contribution from the European Union's Seventh Framework Programme (FP7/2007–2013) and EFPIA companies' in kind contribution.

REFERENCES

1. Internation al agency for research on cancer, Globocan 2008. Available at: http://www.globo-can.iarc.fr. [accessed on December 5, 2011].
2. National Cancer Institute. Surveillance epidemiology and end results. Cancer statistics. Available at: http://www.seer.cancer.gov/statistics. [accessed on December 5, 2011].
3. Tryggvadottir L, Gislum M, Bray F, et al. Trends in the survival of patients diagnosed with breast cancer in the Nordic countries 1964–2003 followed up to the end of 2006. *Acta Oncol* 2010;49(5):624–31.
4. Kehlet H, Jensen TS, Woolf CJ. Persistent postsurgical pain: risk factors and prevention. *Lancet* 2006;367(9522):1618–25.

5. Aasvang EK, Gmaehle E, Hansen JB, et al. Predictive risk factors for persistent postherniotomy pain. *Anesthesiology* 2010;112(4):957–69.

6. Wildgaard K, Ravn J, Kehlet H. Chronic post-thoracotomy pain: a critical review of pathogenic mechanisms and strategies for prevention. *Eur J Cardiothorac Surg* 2009;36(1):170–80.

7. Andersen KG, Kehlet H. Persistent pain after breast cancer treatment: a critical review of risk factors and strategies for prevention. *J Pain* 2011;12(7):725–46.

8. Sakorafas GH, Safioleas M. Breast cancer surgery: an historical narrative. Part II. 18th and 19th centuries. *Eur J Cancer Care (Engl)* 2010;19(1):6–29.

9. Sakorafas GH, Safioleas M. Breast cancer surgery: an historical narrative. Part III. From the sunset of the 19th to the dawn of the 21st century. *Eur J Cancer Care (Engl)* 2010;19(2):145–66.

10. Smith WC, Bourne D, Squair J, Phillips DO, Chambers WA. A retrospective cohort study of post mastectomy pain syndrome. *Pain* 1999;83(1):91–5.

11. Jung BF, Ahrendt GM, Oaklander AL, Dworkin RH. Neuropathic pain following breast cancer surgery: proposed classification and research update. *Pain* 2003;104(1–2):1–13.

12. Haanpaa M, Attal N, Backonja M, et al. NeuPSIG guidelines on neuropathic pain assessment. *Pain* 2011;152(1):14–27.

13. Jung BF, Herrmann D, Griggs J, Oaklander AL, Dworkin RH. Neuropathic pain associated with non-surgical treatment of breast cancer. *Pain* 2005;118(1–2):10–14.

14. Gartner R, Jensen MB, Nielsen J, Ewertz M, Kroman N, Kehlet H. Prevalence of and factors associated with persistent pain following breast cancer surgery. *JAMA* 2009;302(18):1985–92.

15. Tasmuth T, von SK, Kalso E. Pain and other symptoms during the first year after radical and conservative surgery for breast cancer. *Br J Cancer* 1996;74(12):2024–31.

16. Kudel I, Edwards RR, Kozachik S, et al. Predictors and consequences of multiple persistent postmastectomy pains. *J Pain Symptom Manage* 2007;34(6):619–27.

17. Hack TF, Cohen L, Katz J, Robson LS, Goss P. Physical and psychological morbidity after axillary lymph node dissection for breast cancer. *J Clin Oncol* 1999;17(1):143–9.

18. Ip HY, Abrishami A, Peng PW, Wong J, Chung F. Predictors of postoperative pain and analgesic consumption: a qualitative systematic review. *Anesthesiology* 2009;111(3):657–77.

19. Bair MJ, Robinson RL, Katon W, Kroenke K. Depression and pain comorbidity: a literature review. *Arch Intern Med* 2003;163(20):2433–45.

20. Hirsh AT, George SZ, Bialosky JE, Robinson ME. Fear of pain, pain catastrophizing, and acute pain perception: relative prediction and timing of assessment. *J Pain* 2008;9(9):806–12.

21. Werner MU, Mjobo HN, Nielsen PR, Rudin A. Prediction of postoperative pain: a systematic review of predictive experimental pain studies. *Anesthesiology* 2010;112(6):1494–1502.

22. Wildgaard K, Ravn J, Nikolajsen L, Jakobsen E, Jensen TS, Kehlet H. Consequences of persistent pain after lung cancer surgery: a nationwide questionnaire study. *Acta Anaesthesiol Scand* 2011;55(1):60–8.

23. Brandsborg B, Nikolajsen L, Hansen CT, Kehlet H, Jensen TS. Risk factors for chronic pain after hysterectomy: a nationwide questionnaire and database study. *Anesthesiology* 2007;106(5):1003–12.

24. Aasvang E, Kehlet H. Chronic postoperative pain: the case of inguinal herniorrhaphy. *Br J Anaesth* 2005;95(1):69–76.

25. Eriksen J, Jensen MK, Sjogren P, Ekholm O, Rasmussen NK. Epidemiology of chronic non-malignant pain in Denmark. *Pain* 2003;106(3):221–8.

26. Din OS, Dodwell D, Wakefield RJ, Coleman RE. Aromatase inhibitor-induced arthralgia in early breast cancer: what do we know and how can we find out more? *Breast Cancer Res Treat* 2010;120(3):525–38.

27. Kwan ML, Darbinian J, Schmitz KH, et al. Risk factors for lymphedema in a prospective breast cancer survivorship study: the Pathways Study. *Arch Surg* 2010;145(11):1055–63.

28. Lacroix-Fralish ML, Mogil JS. Progress in genetic studies of pain and analgesia. *Annu Rev Pharmacol Toxicol* 2009;49:97–121.

29. Nissenbaum J, Devor M, Seltzer Z, et al. Susceptibility to chronic pain following nerve injury is genetically affected by CACNG2. *Genome Res* 2010;20(9):1180–90.

30. Belfer I, Dai F. Phenotyping and genotyping neuropathic pain. *Curr Pain Headache Rep* 2010;14(3):203–12.

31. Dahl JB, Kehlet H. Preventive analgesia. *Curr Opin Anaesthesiol* 2011;24(3):331–8.

32. Amr YM, Yousef AA. Evaluation of efficacy of the perioperative administration of venlafaxine or gabapentin on acute and chronic postmastectomy pain. *Clin J Pain* 2010;26(5):381–5.

33. Rutqvist LE, Rose C, Cavallin-Stahl E. A systematic overview of radiation therapy effects in breast cancer. *Acta Oncol* 2003;42(5–6):532–45.

34. Cross NE, Glantz MJ. Neurologic complications of radiation therapy. *Neurol Clin* 2003;21(1):249–77.

35. Vaidya JS, Joseph DJ, Tobias JS, et al. Targeted intraoperative radiotherapy versus whole breast radiotherapy for breast cancer (TARGIT-A trial): an international, prospective, randomised, non-inferiority phase 3 trial. *Lancet* 2010;376(9735):91–102.

36. Andersen KG, Gartner R, Kroman N, Flyger H, Kehlet H. Persistent pain after targeted intraoperative radiotherapy (TARGIT) or external breast radiotherapy for breast cancer: a randomized trial. *Breast* 2012;21(1):46–9.

37. Balayssac D, Ferrier J, Descoeur J, et al. Chemotherapy-induced peripheral neuropathies: from clinical relevance to preclinical evidence. *Expert Opin Drug Saf* 2011;10(3):407–17.

38. Reyes-Gibby CC, Morrow PK, Buzdar A, Shete S. Chemotherapy-induced peripheral neuropathy as a predictor of neuropathic pain in breast cancer patients previously treated with paclitaxel. *J Pain* 2009;10(11):1146–50.

39. Martin M, Pienkowski T, Mackey J, et al. Adjuvant docetaxel for node-positive breast cancer. *N Engl J Med* 2005;352(22):2302–13.

40. Martin M, Segui MA, Anton A, et al. Adjuvant docetaxel for high-risk, node-negative breast cancer. *N Engl J Med* 2010;363(23):2200–10.

41. Hershman DL, Weimer LH, Wang A, et al. Association between patient reported outcomes and quantitative sensory tests for measuring long-term neurotoxicity in breast cancer survivors treated with adjuvant paclitaxel chemotherapy. *Breast Cancer Res Treat* 2011;125(3):767–74.

42. Hickey OT, Burke SM, Hafeez P, Mudrakouski AL, Hayes ID, Shorten GD. Severity of acute pain after breast surgery is associated with the likelihood of subsequently developing persistent pain. *Clin J Pain* 2010;26(7):556–60.

43. Ahmed RL, Prizment A, Lazovich D, Schmitz KH, Folsom AR. Lymphedema and quality of life in breast cancer survivors: the Iowa Women's Health Study. *J Clin Oncol* 2008;26(35):5689–96.

44. Tsai RJ, Dennis LK, Lynch CF, Snetselaar LG, Zamba GK, Scott-Conner C. The risk of developing arm lymphedema among breast cancer survivors: a meta-analysis of treatment factors. *Ann Surg Oncol* 2009;16(7):1959–72.

45. Sagen A, Karesen R, Sandvik L, Risberg MA. Changes in arm morbidities and health-related quality of life after breast cancer surgery—a five-year follow-up study. *Acta Oncol* 2009;48(8):1111–8.

46. Gartner R, Jensen MB, Kronborg L, Ewertz M, Kehlet H, Kroman N. Self-reported arm-lymphedema and functional impairment after breast cancer treatment—a nationwide study of prevalence and associated factors. *Breast* 2010;19(6):506–15.

47. Macdonald L, Bruce J, Scott NW, Smith WC, Chambers WA. Long-term follow-up of breast cancer survivors with post-mastectomy pain syndrome. *Br J Cancer* 2005;92(2):225–30.

48. Peuckmann V, Ekholm O, Rasmussen NK, et al. Chronic pain and other sequelae in long-term breast cancer survivors: nationwide survey in Denmark. *Eur J Pain* 2009;13(5):478–85.

49. Walk D, Sehgal N, Moeller-Bertram T, et al. Quantitative sensory testing and mapping: a review of nonautomated quantitative methods for examination of the patient with neuropathic pain. *Clin J Pain* 2009;25(7):632–40.

50. Backonja MM, Walk D, Edwards RR, et al. Quantitative sensory testing in measurement of neuropathic pain phenomena and other sensory abnormalities. *Clin J Pain* 2009;25(7):641–7.

51. Gottrup H, Andersen J, rendt-Nielsen L, Jensen TS. Psychophysical examination in patients with post-mastectomy pain. *Pain* 2000;87(3):275–84.

52. Vilholm OJ, Cold S, Rasmussen L, Sindrup SH. Sensory function and pain in a population of patients treated for breast cancer. *Acta Anaesthesiol Scand* 2009;53(6):800–6.

53. Woolf CJ. Central sensitization: implications for the diagnosis and treatment of pain. *Pain* 2011;152(3 Suppl):S2–15.

54. Fernandez-Lao C, Cantarero-Villanueva I, Fernandez-DE-Las-Penas C, Del-Moral-Avila R, rendt-Nielsen L, Arroyo-Morales M. Myofascial trigger points in neck and shoulder muscles and widespread pressure pain hypersensitivtiy in patients with postmastectomy pain: evidence of peripheral and central sensitization. *Clin J Pain* 2010;26(9):798–806.

55. Fernandez-Lao C, Cantarero-Villanueva I, Fernandez-DE-Las-Penas C, Del-Moral-Avila R, Menjon-Beltran S, Arroyo-Morales M. Widespread mechanical pain hypersensitivity as a sign of central sensitization after breast cancer surgery: comparison between mastectomy and lumpectomy. *Pain Med* 2011;12(1):72–8.

56. Torres LM, Mayoral del MO, Coperias Zazo JL, Gerwin RD, Goni AZ. Incidence of myofascial pain syndrome in breast cancer surgery: a prospective study. *Clin J Pain* 2010;26(4):320–5.

57. Finnerup NB, Sindrup SH, Jensen TS. The evidence for pharmacological treatment of neuropathic pain. *Pain* 2010;150(3):573–81.

58. Warren AG, Brorson H, Borud LJ, Slavin SA. Lymphedema: a comprehensive review. *Ann Plast Surg* 2007;59(4):464–72.

59. Tammela T, Alitalo K. Lymphangiogenesis: molecular mechanisms and future promise. *Cell* 2010;140(4):460–76.
60. Bidstrup PE, Mertz BG, Dalton SO, et al. Accuracy of the Danish version of the "distress thermometer." *Psychooncology* 2011;21(4):436–43.
61. Walk D. Role of skin biopsy in the diagnosis of peripheral neuropathic pain. *Curr Pain Headache Rep* 2009;13(3):191–6.
62. Dworkin RH, Turk DC, Farrar JT, et al. Core outcome measures for chronic pain clinical trials: IMMPACT recommendations. *Pain* 2005; 113(1–2):9–19.
63. Srikandarajah S, Gilron I. Systematic review of movement-evoked pain versus pain at rest in postsurgical clinical trials and meta-analyses: A fundamental distinction requiring standardized measurement. *Pain* 2011;152(8):1734–9.

14

INTERVENTIONAL TECHNIQUES FOR PELVIC CANCER PAIN

Kari Kopko Bancroft and Oscar A. de Leon-Casasola

INTRODUCTION

Visceral, somatic, and neuropathic pain pathways are involved in the transmission of pain arising from the bladder, uterus, rectum, vagina, and prostate. Although visceral pain is typically present in the early stages of disease, invasion of adjacent structures by tumor growth will result in somatic and/or neuropathic pain. Likewise, invasion of lymph nodes, or tumor metastasis to the paravertebral areas, may result in nerve root involvement by tumor with the generation of neuropathic pain. Moreover, patients undergoing pelvic radiation may develop postradiation cystitis and/or enteritis or proctitis. Even though the initial pain is visceral in origin, chronic untreated visceral pain may lead to central hyperalgesia (secondary hyperalgesia), and these patients may present with characteristics of neuropathic pain. Careful assessment of the pain presentation and a mechanistic analysis are important when diagnosing and treating these patients in order to determine the best way to treat their pain.

It is noteworthy that pelvic pain associated with cancer will respond to comprehensive pharmacological therapy in 90%–95% of the cases. Consequently, 5%–10% of these patients will require more aggressive and invasive techniques to treat their pain. Neurolytic blocks of the sympathetic axis, such as superior hypogastric plexus block and ganglion impar neurolysis, are effective in treating visceral pain. When there is a somatic or neuropathic component present, intrathecal therapy with an opioid, clonidine, and bupivacaine at low doses may be more effective. This chapter will address the use of these interventional techniques in optimizing the management of pelvic pain in cancer patients.

TREATING VISCERAL PAIN

Invasive tumors can stretch, compress, and distend visceral structures, resulting in poorly localized visceral pain, which is often described as vague, deep, squeezing, crampy, or colicky. Other signs and symptoms may include referred pain, for instance, pain in the medial aspect of the thigh. Neurolytic blocks of the superior hypogastric plexus are effective in controlling pelvic visceral pain due to cancer and should be considered as important adjuncts to pharmacologic therapy for the relief of severe visceral pain experienced by cancer patients. These blocks do not eliminate the cancer pain entirely because patients frequently experience coexisting somatic and neuropathic pain. Therefore, oral pharmacologic therapy must be continued in the majority of the cases, albeit at lower doses, or intrathecal analgesic techniques may be needed. The goal of performing a neurolytic block is to maximize the analgesic effects of opioid or nonopioid analgesics, preferably at lower daily doses of these agents, to reduce the incidence and the severity of side effects.

SUPERIOR HYPOGASTRIC PLEXUS BLOCK

Cancer patients with tumors circumscribed within the capsule of the organs of the pelvis, with no evidence of metastases, may experience severe pain that is unresponsive to oral or parenteral opioids. Moreover, excessive sedation or other side effects may limit the acceptability and usefulness of oral opioid therapy and/or adjuvants. Therefore, an invasive approach is needed to control pain and improve the quality of life of these patients.

Clinical Uses

Visceral pelvic pain associated with cancer and chronic nonmalignant conditions may be alleviated by blocking the superior hypogastric plexus.[1,2] The afferent fibers innervating the organs in the pelvis travel with the sympathetic nerves, trunks, ganglia, and rami. Thus, a sympathectomy for visceral pain is akin to a peripheral neurectomy or dorsal rhizotomy for somatic pain. A recent study[2] suggests that visceral pain is an important component of the cancer pain syndrome experienced by patients with cancer of the pelvis, even in advanced stages. Thus, percutaneous neurolytic blocks of the superior hypogastric plexus should be considered when treating patients with advanced stages of pelvic cancer.

Anatomy

The superior hypogastric plexus is situated in the retroperitoneum and extends bilaterally from the lower third of the fifth lumbar vertebral body to the upper third of the first sacral vertebral body. This plexus receives fibers from the inferior hypogastric plexus, which in turn receives all the afferent fibers from the pelvic organs. The inferior hypogastric plexus is not a well-defined structure, which can be easily targeted and blocked. Conversely, the superior hypogastric plexus has two well-defined ganglia, making it more feasible to block.

Technique

Patients are placed in the prone position with a pillow under the pelvis to flatten the lumbar lordosis. Two Chiba needles (15 cm, 22 gauge) are inserted with the bevel directed medially, 45 degrees and 30 degrees caudad so that the tips lay anterolateral to the L5-S1 intervertebral disc space. Aspiration is important to avoid injection into the iliac vessels. If blood is aspirated, a transvascular approach can be used (with potential complications). The accurate placement of needle is verified via biplanar fluoroscopy. Anterior-posterior (AP) views should reveal the tip of the needle at the level of the junction of the L5 and S1 vertebral bodies. Lateral views will confirm placement of the needle's tip just beyond the vertebral body's anterolateral margin. The injection of 3–5 mL of water-soluble contrast medium is used to verify accurate needle placement and to rule out intravascular injection. In the AP view, the spread of contrast should be confined to the midline region. In the lateral view, a smooth posterior contour corresponding to the anterior psoas fascia indicates that the needle is at the appropriate depth.

Alternatively, a transdiscal approach at the L5-S1 level could be used. Under these circumstances a 25-gauge needle is inserted into the disc under fluoroscopy seen here in an oblique view of the lumbosacral spine (Fig. 14.1). The needle is then advanced under fluoroscopy guidance in the lateral view until it exits the anterior border of the disc. Three to five milliliters of water-soluble contrast medium is injected at this point and fluoroscopic corroboration of the agent's spread is done in the lateral and AP views (Figs. 14.2 and 14.3).

For a prognostic hypogastric plexus blockade, local anesthetic alone is used (bupivacaine 0.25%). For therapeutic purposes in patients with cancer-related pain, 4–6 mL of 6%–10% phenol is typically used as the neurolytic solution.

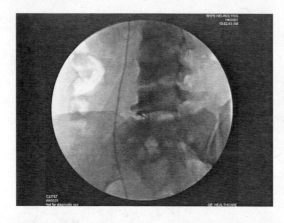

FIGURE 14.1 Oblique view of lumbar spine with a 25-gauge needle inserted lateral to the superior articular process of S1 prior to advancing it into the intervertebral disc.

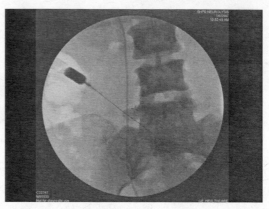

FIGURE 14.3 Anteroposterior view of the lumbosacral area with adequate contrast medium spread.

Efficacy

The effectiveness of the block was originally demonstrated by documenting a significant decrease in pain via visual analog pain scores (VAPS). In this study, Plancarte et al.[1] showed that this block was effective in reducing VAPS scores in 70% of the patients with pelvic pain associated with cancer. The majority of the enrolled patients had cervical cancer. In a subsequent study, 69% of the patients experienced a decrease in VAPS scores. Moreover, a mean

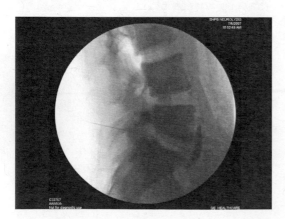

FIGURE 14.2 Lateral view of the lumbosacral spine with the tip of the needle adequately placed, just anterior to the intervertebral disc. Contrast medium is seen spreading anterior to the spine between L5 and S1.

daily opioid morphine reduction of 67% was seen in the success group (736 ± 633 reduced to 251 ± 191 mg/day), and 45% in the failure group (1,443 ± 703 reduced to 800 ± 345 mg/day).[2] In a multicenter study, 159 patients with pelvic pain associated with cancer were evaluated. Overall, 115 patients (72%) had satisfactory pain relief after one or two neurolytic procedures. Mean opioid use decreased by 40% from 58 ± 43 to 35 ± 18 equianalgesic mg/day of morphine 3 weeks after treatment in all the studied patients. This decrease in opioid consumption was significant for both the success group (56 ± 32 reduced to 32 ± 16 mg/day) and the failure group (65 ± 28 reduced to 48 ± 21 mg/day).[3] In these two studies, success was defined as a reduction in opioid consumption by at least 50% in the 3 weeks following the block and a decrease in the pain scores below 4/10 in the VAPS scores.[2,3]

In a recent case report, Rosenberg and colleagues[4] reported on the efficacy of this block in a patient with severe chronic nonmalignant penile pain after transurethral resection of the prostate. Although the patient did not receive a neurolytic agent, a diagnostic block performed with 0.25% bupivacaine and 20 mg of methylprednisolone acetate was effective in relieving the pain for more than 6 months. The usefulness of this block in chronic benign pain conditions has not been adequately documented in a large cohort of patients

Complications

The combined experience of more than 200 cases from the Mexican Institute of Cancer, Roswell Park Cancer Institute, and M.D. Anderson Cancer Center did not report any neurologic complications from this block.[3] However, imprecise needle placement may lead to catastrophic consequences. Thus, fluoroscopy with contrast medium is essential in order to demonstrate accurate needle placement *and* appropriate contrast medium spread.

There are only a limited number of reports detailing use of superior hypogastric plexus block and none have reported complications with this procedure. Due to the close proximity of the iliac vessels, intravascular injection may easily occur. In patients with evidence of atherosclerotic disease, there is risk of dislodging a plaque and producing a distal embolism.

GANGLION IMPAR BLOCK

The ganglion impar is a solitary retroperitoneal structure anterior to the sacro-coccygeal junction. Visceral pain in the perineal area associated with malignancies may be effectively treated with neurolysis of the ganglion impar (Walther's).[5] It has been argued that patients who will benefit from this block frequently present with a vague, poorly localized pain that is frequently accompanied by sensations of burning and urgency in the perineal region. However, the clinical value of this block is not clear as the published experience is limited. Moreover, in my personal experience the results of this block have been discouraging.

Anatomy

The ganglion impar marks the termination of the two sympathetic chains and is the only unpaired autonomic ganglion in the body. This ganglion has gray nerve-fiber communication from the ganglion to the spinal nerve, but it appears to lack white nerve fiber communication from the spinal nerves to the ganglia in the thoracic and upper lumbar regions.[6] Visceral afferents innervating the perineum, distal rectum, anus, distal urethra, vulva, and distal third of vagina converge at the ganglion impar.

The original technique for ganglion impar block was described by Plancarte and collaborators.[7] This technique calls for the patient to be positioned in the lateral decubitus position with the hips fully flexed. A standard 22-gauge, 3.5-inch spinal needle is bent 1 inch from its hub to form a 30-degree angle. The needle is then introduced under local anesthesia through the anococcygeal ligament with its concavity oriented posteriorly. Under fluoroscopic guidance, the needle is directed along the midline at or near the sacrococcygeal junction with a finger in the rectum to prevent puncturing this structure. Retroperitoneal location is verified by observation of the spread of 2 mL of water-soluble contrast medium. As an alternative the needle may be bent in the shape of an arc, as proposed by Nebab.[8]

Two alternative approaches for this block have been described. The first alternative is to place the patient in the lithotomy position.[9] This position straightens the path from the anococcygogeal ligament to the ganglion impar and eliminates the need to bend the needle. In the other approach, the trans-sacrococcygeal approach, the tip of the needle is directly placed in the retroperitoneal space by inserting a 20-gauge, 1.5-inch needle through the sacro-coccygeal ligament under fluoroscopy so that the tip of the needle is just anterior to the bone.[10] This technique avoids the invasion of more caudal structures with the needle and the need to insert a finger in the rectal lumen.

For diagnostic blocks, local anesthetic alone is used (bupivacaine 0.25%). For neurolytic blocks, 2–3 mL of 6% phenol is used. Cryoablation of the ganglion impar has been also described for repeated procedures via a trans-sacrococcygeal approach in a patient with chronic benign pain post abdomino-perineal resection.[11]

Efficacy

Three prospective, nonrandomized, noncontrolled studies evaluated the efficacy of the ganglion impar block. Plancarte and colleagues[7] evaluated 16 patients, 13 women and 3 men, ranging in age from 24 to 87, with advanced cancer (cervix, 9; colon, 2; bladder, 2; rectum, 1; endometrium 2) and persistent pain despite treatment (pharmacologic management resulted in a 30% global reduction in pain). Localized perineal pain was present in all cases and was characterized as burning in 8 patients and of mixed character in 8 patients. Pain was referred to the rectum (7 patients), perineum (6 patients), or vagina (3 patients). After a neurolytic block with a transanococcygeal approach, 8 patients reported complete pain relief, with the remainder experiencing significant pain reduction (60% to 90%). Blocks were repeated in 2 patients. Follow-up was carried out for 14–120 days depending on patient survival.

Swofford and Ratzman[12] reported on the efficacy of the transsacrococcygeal approach. Twenty patients, age ranging from 35 to 70, with perineal pain unresponsive to previous intervention were studied, 18 with a bupivacaine/steroid block and 2 with a neurolytic block. In the bupivacaine/steroid group, 5 patients reported complete (100%) pain relief, 10 patients reported >75% pain reduction, and 3 patients reported >50% pain reduction. Both neurolytic blocks resulted in complete pain relief. Duration of the pain relief was 4 weeks or greater.

Vranken and colleagues[13] studied the effect of the ganglion impar block in chronic, treatment-resistant coccygodynia. Twenty patients, 17 women and 3 men, with diagnosis of coccygodynia (spontaneous, 7; fracture, 3; injury, 10) received a 5 mL injection of 0.25% bupivacaine. There was no pain reduction or improvement of quality of life associated with the procedure. Thus, based on this study, it would appear that this block is not effective for the treatment of coccygodynia.

Complications

Although there is always the risk of injury to adjacent structures, there have been no complications reported from the ganglion impar block. Plancarte[14] has reported one case in which epidural spread of contrast within the caudal canal was observed. In this case, repositioning the needle resolved the problem. Although published experience is limited and criteria to predict success or failure is not available, patients with perineal pain, which may be poorly localized and burning in character, are considered candidates for this block. The procedure appears safe, and no complications have been reported.

INTRATHECAL ANALGESIA

Neuraxial analgesia is achieved by the epidural or intrathecal administration of an opioid alone (very rarely) or in combination with other agents such as bupivacaine and clonidine. With the use of neuraxial analgesia, pain relief is generally attained without motor or sympathetic blockade, which makes this analgesic modality highly adaptable to the home care environment. The mechanism of analgesia in neuraxial opioid therapy is due to the administration of small quantities of opioids in close proximity to their receptors in the substantia gelatinosa of the spinal cord to achieve high concentrations at these sites.[15,16] Thus, analgesia is superior to that achieved when opioids are administered by other routes, and since the total amount of drug administered is reduced, the side effects are minimized. Currently, the biggest advantage is the ability to use multiple agents to target multiple receptors resulting in better neuropathic, somatic, and visceral pain control while minimizing side effects.

In general, patients with survival expectancy greater than 3 months are candidates for intrathecal therapy with a permanent intraspinal catheter and an implanted subcutaneous pump. Conversely, those patients with survival expectancy less than 3 months are candidates for epidural therapy with an implanted system (such as the Sims® epidural port-a-cath), which will be connected to an external pump with PCA capabilities.[17]

Epidural Trial

When considering a patient for intrathecal therapy with a permanent intrathecal catheter and a subcutaneous pump, a trial with an epidural catheter will be necessary to (1) assess the need for intrathecal multimodal therapy, (2) estimate the doses of the opioid to be used, and (3) confirm the best site for catheter tip positioning. The tip of the epidural catheter is best placed at the site where nociception is being processed within the spinal cord.

We conduct this trial on an outpatient basis, and the goal is to achieve at least an 80% decrease in pain. If the trial is successful, we will proceed to implant the permanent device. For this purpose, we use the following protocol[18]:

- Epidural Catheter position: dermatomal specific for the area of nociception under fluoroscopy guidance (Fig. 14.4).
  1. Opioids:
     Morphine: 0.1 (60 mg)–0.2 (120 mg) mg/mL
     Hydromorphone: 0.03 (20 mg)–0.12 (80 mg) mg/mL
  2. Bupivacaine: 1–2 mg/mL (0.1–0.2%)
  3. Total volume: 600 mL
  4. If the patient's source of nociception is in the lower lumbar or sacral areas, thus precluding the use of high concentrations of bupivacaine, then we use a more diluted solution of bupivacaine (0.05%) to minimize the possibility of motor block and we compensate by adding clonidine: 3–5 mcg/mL
- Determining epidural opioid doses:
  1. If the patient is receiving > 300 mcg/h of Fentanyl or 1,200 mg/day of MS or 600 mg/day of oxycodone or 160 mg/day of methadone, or >300 mg/day of oxymorphone: Hydromorphone: 0.12 mg/mL
  2. If the patient is receiving between 100 and 300 mcg/h of fentanyl or an equivalent opioid dose:
     Hydromorphone: 0.06 mg/mL
  3. If the patient is receiving less than 100 mcg/h of fentanyl or equivalent dose: Hydromorphone: 0.03 mg/mL
- Basal infusion: 2 mL/h
- No bolus during the first 72 hours, then 2 mL q 10 min
- Trial for 7–14 days as an outpatient

If the patient had a successful trial, as defined earlier, we proceed to implant an intrathecal system. We suggest the following protocol to achieve more than 80% pain relief.

- Conditions for success:
  Place the tip of the intrathecal catheter in the dermatome corresponding to the area of nociception under fluoroscopy guidance. In patients with pelvic pain a retrograde approach will be needed (Fig. 14.5).
  For severe somatic pain, combinations of local anesthetics (at a low dose to avoid lower extremity weakness) and an opioid will be needed.
  For neuropathic pain: Since the tip of the catheter will be in the lumbosacral region, initial therapy with opioid + clonidine is used. If there is no adequate pain control despite clonidine dose titration, then bupivacaine is added at a dose no greater than 12 mg/day to avoid motor weakness of the lower extremities.

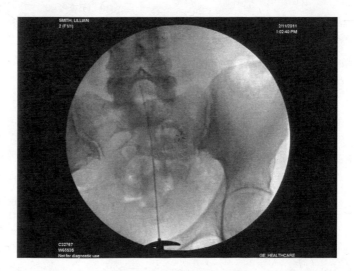

FIGURE 14.4   Epidural catheter placed via a caudal approach in the spinal area where nociception is being processed. Note the epidurogram showing adequate spread after 3 mL of Iohexol.

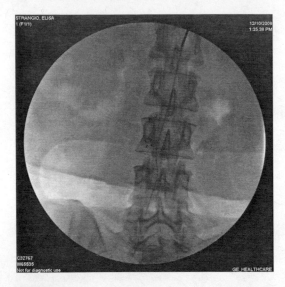

FIGURE 14.5 Intrathecal catheter placed via a retrograde approach for a patient with pelvic pain.

The doses and drugs that we use in our practice specifically for pelvic pain can be found in Table 14.1.

The steps that we use to implement the therapy are as follows:

• Step 1:
  Opioid + clonidine:
  • Clonidine: 250–2,000 µg/day
  Opioid + bupivacaine:
  • MS 3–25 mg/day or hydromorphone 0.5–15 mg/day

Table 14.1 Pharmacologic Management of Pelvic Pain

DRUG	RANGE OF DOSES
Morphine	1.0–20 mg/day
Hydromorphone	0.5–25 mg/day
Sufentanil	10–100 ug/day
Bupivacaine	6–12 mg/day
Clonidine	250–2,000 ug/day

Note: Compounding by a trained pharmacist will be needed. The goal is to concentrate these drugs to twice the daily dose, so that the 20 mL programmable pumps may be programmed to deliver 0.5 mL/h. In this way, patients may be able to minimize visits for pump refills to monthly or even longer periods.

**6 mg of MS/day = 1 mg of hydromorphone/day
  • Bupivacaine: 6–12 mg/day
• Step 2: Opioid + bupivacaine + clonidine

PUMP AND CATHETER MALFUNCTION

If triple therapy with an opioid, bupivacaine, and clonidine at optimal doses is not working, then evaluation for catheter obstruction, disconnection, catheter migration, or pump malfunction is a must. In doing so, consider the following possibilities.

Pump

Computer program analysis for volume and the volume present within the pump needs to be within 10% of each other; otherwise pump failure is suspected due to the following:

• Magnetic resonance imaging(MRI) effects (Medtronic Medical Device Correction, August 2008). There is a potential for a delay in the return of proper drug infusion after a MRI affecting *all* SyncroMed pumps. Moreover, with SynchroMed II pumps, there is the potential for a delay in the logging of motor stall events after MRI. Although the reported incidence of these phenomena is very low (0.014% and 0.11%, respectively), it is important to interrogate all pumps after the MRI, to spare patients from not receiving medication. This is particularly important for SynchroMed pumps, as a "Pump Memory Error" may be generated and the pump will *not* restart infusing unless it is reprogrammed. In contrast, the SynchroMed II may continue infusing even though the interrogation may show a stall state. In either case, the pump will alarm in the face of a stall phenomenon.
• Missing propellant within the pump: Synchromed® II Missing Propellant. Models affected: 8637–20, 8637–40 (Medtronic Medical Device Recall—May 2008)
• Synchromed® EL Pump Motor Stall Due to Gear Shaft Wear (Patient Management Information; Medtronic, August 2007)

Catheter

A myelogram performed through the diagnostic port of the pump will be needed to determine whether there is obstruction or disconnection (Medical Device Safety Alert—June 2008: Proper Connection of Sutureless Connector Intrathecal Catheters Models Affected: 8709SC, 8731SC, 8596SC, 8578), and the position of the tip of the catheter. When performing a myelogram through the diagnostic port of the pump, remember that this only accommodates a 25-gauge Huber needle. Moreover, consider the following:

A. The dead space of the catheter when injecting the contrast medium: 0.196 mL (89 cm total catheter length [81.4 cm for the spinal segment + 7.6 of the catheter interface with the sutureless connector] × 0.0022 mL/cm catheter volume for the model 8709 SC)
B. The need for a bolus dose after the study is completed, as the catheter will be filled with contrast medium. Consequently, at a programmed rate of 0.5 mL/hr, it will take 9.4 hours for the pump to clear all this volume, resulting in inadequate pain control and possibly opioid withdrawal symptoms.

When performing the pump's diagnostic port injections, one needs the following:

A. To withdraw enough amount of cerebrospinal fluid/therapeutic solution prior to injecting contrast medium to remove all the volume of the drug within the catheter and avoid giving the patient a bolus of the medications in use. If this was not performed, up to 0.196 mL of solution could be pushed alone with the contrast medium. Likewise, we suggest that one should aspirate the fluid with a 3 mL syringe at a very low negative pressure to avoid turbulent flow and the risk of leaving medication within the catheter (cavitations phenomenon). We usually aspirate a total of 3 mL of fluid, as this should contain all the medication left in the catheter's dead space and some cerebrospinal fluid.

B. A bolus dose should be programmed after the myelogram to clear the catheter's dead space containing contrast medium at this point. By doing so, one avoids leaving the patient without intrathecal treatment for periods of 16–20 hours depending on how much catheter was implanted.

SUMMARY

Neurolysis of the superior hypogastric plexus block and the ganglion impar may be used in patients with visceral pain of the pelvis and the perineal region, respectively. The incidence of complications reported in the literature is very low. However, they may occur. Thus, strict adherence to the technique is important to prevent potential problems. Moreover, the use of this technique for patients who do not have a significant visceral pain component is not warranted. Intrathecal therapy is indicated when somatic or neuropathic pain is present. With intrathecal analgesia, the steps toward successful therapy include (1) the use of an opioid in combination with bupivacaine and/or clonidine, (2) the positioning of the tip of the catheter in the area of nociception, and (3) an epidural trial.

REFERENCES

1. Plancarte R, Amescua C, Patt RB, et al. Superior hypogastric plexus block for pelvic cancer pain. *Anesthesiology* 1990;73:236–9.
2. de Leon-Casasola OA, Kent E, Lema MJ. Neurolytic superior hypogastric plexus block for chronic pelvic pain associated with cancer. *Pain* 1993;54:145–51.
3. Plancarte R, de Leon-Casasola OA, El-Helaly M, et al. Neurolytic superior hypogastric plexus block for chronic pelvic pain associated with cancer. *Regional Anesthesia* 1997;22:562–8.
4. Rosenberg SK, Tewari R, Boswell MV, et al. Superior hypogastric plexus block successfully treats severe penile pain after transurethral resection of the prostate. *Reg Anesthes Pain Med* 1998;23:618–20.
5. de Leon-Casasola OA. Superior hypogastric plexus block and ganglion impar neurolysis for pain associated with cancer. *Tech Reg Anesthes Pain Manage* 1997;1:31.
6. Gray H. *Gray's Anatomy*. Philadelphia Running Press 1974.

7. Plancarte R, Amescua C, Patt RB. Presacral blockade of the ganglion impar (ganglion of Walther). *Anesthesiology* 1990;73:A751.

8. Nebab EG, Florence IM. An alternative needle geometry for interruption of the ganglion impar. *Anesthesiology* 1997;86:1213–4.

9. Xue B, Lema MJ, de Leon-Casasola OA. Ganglion impar block. In: Benzon H, Srinivasa NR, Fishman SM, et al., eds. *Essentials of Pain Medicine and Regional Anesthesia*. Philadelphia, PA: Churchill Livingstone; 1999: 329–31.

10. Wemm KJ, Sabersky L. Modified approach to block the ganglion impar (ganglion of Walther). *Reg Anesthes* 1995;20:544–5.

11. Loev MA, Varklet VL, Wilsey BL. Cryoablation: a novel approach to neurolysis of the ganglion impar. *Anesthesiology* 1998;88:1391–3.

12. Swofford JB, Ratzman DM. A transarticular approach to blockade of the ganglion impar (ganglion of walther). *Reg Anesthes Pain Med* 1998;23(3 Suppl):103.

13. Vranken JH, Bannink IMJ, Zuurmond WWA. Invasive procedures in patients with coccygodynia: caudal epidural infiltration, pudendal nerve block and blockade of the ganglion impar. *Reg Anesthes Pain Med* 2000;25(2 Suppl):25.

14. Plancarte R, Velazquez R, Patt RB. Neurolytic blocks of the sympathetic axis. In: Patt RB, ed. *Cancer Pain*. Philadelphia, PA: Lippincott-Raven; 1993: 419.

15. Cousins MJ, Mather LE. Intrathecal and epidural administration of opioids. *Anesthesiology* 1984;61:276–310.

16. Yaksh TL. Spinal opiates: a review of their effect on spinal function with an emphasis on pain processing. *Acta Anaesthes Scand* 1987;31(Suppl 85):25.

17. Du Pen S, Kharasch ED, Williams A, et al. Chronic epidural bupivacaine-opioid infusion in intractable cancer pain. *Pain* 1992;49:293–300.

18. de Leon-Casasola OA, Yarussi A. Cancer pain management. In: Benzon H, Rathmell JP, Wu CL, Turk DC, Argoff CE, eds. *Raj's Practical Management of Pain*. 4th ed. Philadelphia, PA: Mosby/Elsevier; 2008: 413–26.

SECTION FOUR

PAINFUL CONDITIONS WITH FEMALE PREVALENCE

15

FIBROMYALGIA AND CHRONIC FATIGUE SYNDROME

Alethia Baldwin Sellers and Daniel Clauw

INTRODUCTION

This chapter provides an overview of some important aspects of fibromyalgia (FM) and chronic fatigue syndrome (CFS). These conditions are known to be closely associated with each other, as at least half of the individuals that meet diagnostic criteria for one of these conditions will also have met criteria for the other, and both entities are similarly related to conditions such as irritable bowel syndrome, interstitial cystitis, temporomandibular disorder, and headache.[1] These conditions have a strong familial and genetic predisposition.[2] They occur more commonly in females than males, but in the case of FM this is largely an artifact of the original case definition for FM that required a certain degree of tenderness. Our understanding of the underlying pathophysiology and current treatment options for these patients have been improved by research focusing on genetics, psychophysiology, brain imaging, and drug trials. Like other chronic pain conditions, it is probable that different mechanisms contribute differently to the clinical picture (in individual patients). Similarly, the effect of any single drug examined in isolation (i.e., 50% improvement in pain in 30%–40% of patients treated) is modest, at least in groups of individuals. This is no different than other analgesics in other chronic pain states— nonsteroidal anti-inflammatory drugs (NSAIDs) and opioids have comparable modest efficacy in conditions

such as osteoarthritis or chronic low back pain.[3] This stresses the need for combined pharmacotherapies and incorporation of pharmacotherapy into a broader program of education (and other nonpharmacologic therapies). It needs to be acknowledged that the majority of CFS and FM patients have unmet needs other than widespread pain, including mood disorders, dyscognitive symptoms, sexual dysfunction, and a lack of sociomedical acceptance—aspects that have a deep impact on quality of life and that need to be addressed by future research. As such, CFS and FM remain a scientific and clinical challenge.

DEFINITION AND EPIDEMIOLOGY OF CHRONIC FATIGUE SYNDROME

Diagnostic criteria established by the Centers for Disease Control and Prevention (CDC) have helped classify CFS as an overlap of fatigue with behavioral and biological components.[4] The criteria require the presence of fatigue for more than 6 months associated with a diminution of functional activity and somatic symptoms and pain not attributable to a specific diagnosis or disease. In addition, four of the following criteria need to be present: sore throat, impaired memory or cognition, unrefreshing sleep, postexertional fatigue, tender glands, aching stiff muscles, joint pain, and headaches. Five of these "minor" criteria are pain in diffuse widespread body areas, which partly accounts significant overlap with FM. Medical conditions that may explain the prolonged fatigue (e.g., congestive heart failure, hypothyroidism) as well as a number of psychiatric diagnoses (e.g., eating disorders, psychotic disorders, bipolar disorder, melancholic depression, and substance abuse within 2 years of the onset of fatigue) exclude a patient from the diagnosis of CFS. A notable feature of the CDC case definition is that many nonpsychotic disorders are not exclusionary for the diagnosis of CFS. Those who do not meet the fatigue severity or symptom criteria can be given a diagnosis of idiopathic chronic fatigue (ICF). Both the prevalence rates of CFS at 0.5% to 3% and ICF at 5% to 10% are remarkably consistent in urban and rural settings and in different cultures and countries.[5-9] Community surveys have found that whites have a lower risk of CFS compared with Latino, African American, and Native American subjects. This suggests that the increased prevalence of CFS among white subjects found in clinic populations is most likely the result of a disparity attributable to health care access and use.

DEFINITION AND EPIDEMIOLOGY OF FIBROMYALGIA

The previous American College of Rheumatology (ACR) criteria for FM, put forth in 1990, required that an individual has both a history of chronic widespread pain (CWP), pain above and below the waist involving the left and right sides of the body and the axial skeleton, and the finding of 11 (or greater) of 18 possible tender points on examination.[10] Tender points are located in nine paired predefined regions of the body, often over musculotendinous insertions. If an individual reports pain when a region is palpated with 4 kilograms of pressure, this is considered a positive tender point (see Fig. 15.1). Between 25% and 50% of individuals who have CWP (primarily women—since they are generally more tender) will also have 11 or greater tender points, and thus meet criteria for FM. Using these diagnostic criteria, the prevalence of FM is currently estimated to be 2%–5%, and like CFS this rate is remarkably consistent and just as high in rural or nonindustrialized societies as it is in countries such as the United States. The new ACR diagnostic criteria for FM, put forth in 2010, allow the diagnosis of FM without performing a tender point examination, since they focus on identifying the core symptoms of FM, including not only pain but also fatigue, unrefreshed sleep, and/or cognitive symptoms.[11] These symptom-based or screening diagnostic criteria for FM are expected to define far more males as FM patients than the older criteria because of eliminating the requirement of 11 tender points (in population-based studies women are 10 times more likely than men to have 11 tender points[12]) and thus the prevalence will likely be correspondingly higher.

UNIQUE CHARACTERISTICS OF THE FATIGUE ASSOCIATED WITH CHRONIC FATIGUE SYNDROME

There is nothing unique about the fatigue associated with CFS, except that it is chronic and severe enough to be functionally disabling. The best indicator of whether fatigue is associated with CFS rather than another condition is literally "the company it keeps." In the overwhelming majority of patients with CFS, the fatigue is accompanied by multifocal pain, sleep disturbances, and/or cognitive difficulties, also a hallmark of FM as well as the other "allied" conditions such as irritable bowel syndrome, temporomandibular disorder, and interstitial cystitis. These symptoms are encompassed within the eight "minor" criteria for the CFS diagnosis. Many patients with CFS also experience anorexia, nausea, night sweats, a subjective sense of fevers, frequent dizziness, and intolerance to alcohol and medications.

From this point forward, the chapter will be discussing mainly topics related to FM because there is more information available. However, at the end there will be further reference to CFS.

TENDER POINTS IN FIBROMYALGIA

At the time the ACR criteria were published, it was thought that there may be some unique significance to the locations of tender points. In fact, a term "control points" was coined to describe areas of the body that should not

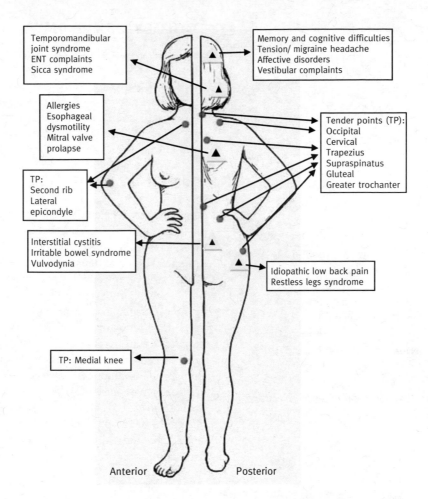

Temporomandibular
joint syndrome
ENT complaints
Sicca syndrome

Memory and cognitive difficulties
Tension/ migraine headache
Affective disorders
Vestibular complaints

Allergies
Esophageal
dysmotility
Mitral valve
prolapse

Tender points (TP):
Occipital
Cervical
Trapezius
Supraspinatus
Gluteal
Greater trochanter

TP:
Second rib
Lateral
epicondyle

Interstitial cystitis
Irritable bowel syndrome
Vulvodynia

Idiopathic low back pain
Restless legs syndrome

TP: Medial knee

Anterior   Posterior

FIGURE 15.1   Circles represent tender points in fibromyalgia. Triangles represents regional or localized syndromes that overlap with fibromyalgia in prevalence, mechanisms, and treatment. (Adapted from Clauw, DJ, *Etiology of Fibromyalgia*, edited by McCarberg and Clauw. Fibromyalgia, p. 5. 2009, Informa Healthcare USA, Inc.)

be tender in fibromyalgia. Individuals were assumed to have a psychological cause for their pain if they were tender in these regions. Since then, we have learned that the tenderness in fibromyalgia extends throughout the entire body. Relative to the pain threshold that a normal non-fibromyalgia patient would experience at the same points, "control" regions of the body such as the thumbnail and forehead are just as tender as in fibromyalgia tender points.[13] To assess tenderness in clinical practice, the practitioner can apply pressure anywhere, and as long as he or she performs this exam with the same pressure in a series of patients, the practitioner can get a good sense of the overall pain threshold of any individual patient. Even

in chronic pain patients who do not have FM or CFS, finding diffuse hyperalgesia on exam, as well as a history of pain in multiple body regions, fatigue, and sleep disturbances, can be an important clue that the individual's pain has "centralized," and that he or she is more likely to respond to centrally rather than peripherally mediated therapies.

THE PROBLEM WITH TENDER POINTS

The tender point requirement in the ACR criteria not only misrepresents the nature of the tenderness in this condition (i.e., local rather than widespread) but also strongly influenced the demographic and psychological characteristics of FM. Requiring a certain number of tender points turned FM into an almost exclusively female disease. Another unintended consequence of requiring both CWP and at least 11 tender points to be diagnosed with FM is that many individuals with fibromyalgia will have high levels of distress. Wolfe has described tender points as a "sedimentation rate for distress" because of population-based studies showing that tender points are more common in distressed individuals. Distress is usually considered as a combination of somatic symptoms and symptoms of anxiety and/or depression.[14] Until recently, many assumed that because *tender points* were associated with distress, that *tenderness* (an individual's sensitivity to mechanical pressure) was associated with distress. However, recent evidence suggests that this latter association is probably due to the standard tender point technique, which consists of applying steadily increasing pressure until reaching 4 kg.

In this situation, individuals who are anxious or "expectant" have a tendency to "bail out" and report tenderness. Recently, more sophisticated measures of tenderness have been developed that give stimuli in a random, unpredictable fashion, and the results of these tests are independent of psychological status.[15] Thus, since tender points are associated with high levels of distress, requiring 11 or greater tender points in order to diagnose someone with CWP with FM dramatically increases the likelihood that these individuals will be female and/or distressed, compared to individuals with CWP and fewer than 11 tender points. Although many clinicians uniquely associate fibromyalgia with women who display high levels of distress, much of this is an artifact of (1) the ACR criteria that require 11 tender points, and (2) the fact that most studies of FM have originated from clinical samples from tertiary care centers, where health care–seeking behaviors lead to the fact that psychological and psychiatric comorbidities are much higher.[16] When all these biases are eliminated by examining CWP in population-based studies, a clearer picture of fibromyalgia can be seen, and chronic widespread pain becomes much like chronic musculoskeletal pain in any other region of the body.

ETIOLOGY OF FIBROMYALGIA

Research has indicated a strong familial component to the development of fibromyalgia. First-degree relatives of individuals with fibromyalgia display an eight-fold greater risk of developing fibromyalgia than those in the general population.[2] Approximately half of the risk of developing FM and related conditions appears to be due to genetic factors, and the other half of the risk is due to environmental factors.[17] Environmental "stressors" temporally associated with the development of either fibromyalgia or chronic fatigue syndrome include physical trauma (especially involving the trunk), certain infections (such as hepatitis C and Epstein Barr virus), and emotional stress (Fig. 15.2). Of note, each of these stressors only leads to CWP or fibromyalgia in approximately 5%–10% of individuals who are exposed; the overwhelming majority of individuals who experience these same infections or other stressful events regain their baseline state of health. War may be an environment where individuals are simultaneously exposed to a multitude of stressors, triggering the development of this type of illness in susceptible individuals.[18,19] The disorder is also associated with other regional pain conditions or autoimmune disorders (Fig. 15.1). As many as 25% of patients correctly diagnosed with generalized inflammatory disorders such as systemic lupus erythematosus (SLE) and rheumatoid arthritis (RA) will also fulfill criteria for FM.[20] In this setting when comorbid FM goes unrecognized, patients are often unnecessarily treated more aggressively with toxic immunosuppressive drugs.

ROLE OF STRESS AND STRESSORS

Is being "stressed" a risk factor for FM? It appears to depend in part on the type of stress and context, and even then, only weakly so. Population-based studies show that individuals with high levels of distress, but without pain, are approximately 2–2.5 times as likely to develop CWP within the next year as those in the population without stress.[21] Having stressful events occur early in life, such as the death of a mother, prolonged hospitalization, or being involved in a

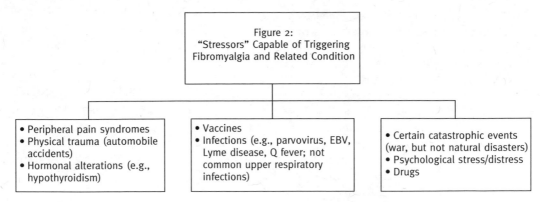

FIGURE 15.2   "Stressors" capable of triggering fibromyalgia and related condition. EBV, Epstein-Barr virus.

motor traffic accident, increase the risk of developing CWP by 50%–100% later in life.[22]

Because of this link between exposure to "stressors" and the subsequent development of fibromyalgia, the human stress systems have been extensively studied in this condition. These studies have generally shown alterations of the hypothalamic pituitary adrenal axis (HPA) and the sympathetic nervous system in fibromyalgia and related conditions.[19] Although these studies often note either hypo- or hyperactivity of both the HPA axis and sympathetic nervous system in individuals with fibromyalgia and related conditions, the precise abnormality varies from study to study. These studies only find "abnormal" HPA or autonomic function in a very small percentage of patients, and there is tremendous overlap between patients and controls in these studies. A recent meta-analysis suggests that individuals with CFS or FM with more prominent fatigue may be most likely to display HPA hypoactivity. But it is clear that early life trauma and an individual's pain level markedly affect these measures.[23–25] With respect to the autonomic nervous system, the most consistent findings are an attenuated response to stressors, with low parasympathetic tone (which may be partly due to deconditioning) and high sympathetic tone, especially at night.[26,27]

AUGMENTED PAIN AND SENSORY PROCESSING IN FIBROMYALGIA

The underlying mechanism that has the most support in FM as well as a number of other chronic pain states is that there is centrally mediated pain and sensory augmentation that can be noted even in the absence of psychological factors. Because tender points are a measure of pressure pain threshold, this is the measure of tenderness that has been most often assessed in FM. A variety of studies have shown that individuals with FM are diffusely tender in all bodily regions (tender points are merely regions where everyone is more tender), even when experimental pain testing paradigms are used that minimize or eliminate the potential role of psychological factors (e.g., hypervigilance, expectancy).[13,28,29] FM patients are more responsive to nearly any other type of stimuli as well, including decreased pain thresholds to heat, cold, and electrical stimuli, as well as increased sensitivity to hypertonic saline infusion. Interestingly other studies have shown that FM patients display sensitivity to a number of other sensory modalities, such as the brightness of light or loudness of auditory tones. This suggests that in many individuals this may be a more global problem with sensory processing rather than specific abnormality in pain processing.[30,31]

Experimental pain testing has also identified at least one potential reason for the widespread pain sensitivity (i.e., diffuse hyperalgesia) in individuals with FM: attenuated descending inhibitory or antinociceptive activity. In healthy humans the application of an intense painful stimulus produces an increase in pain thresholds (in body regions remote from the initial site of nociceptive stimulation). This analgesic effect, termed diffuse noxious inhibitory control

(DNIC), has been consistently observed to be attenuated in groups of FM patients, as compared to healthy controls. It has also been frequently noted to be abnormal in other chronic pain states.[32-34] A decrease in DNIC is seen in many other chronic pain conditions, but not in patients with major depressive disorder.[35] The DNIC response in humans relies on (probably several different) descending antinociceptive systems (opioidergic and noradrenergic/serotonergic), projecting from the brainstem (periaqueductal gray, rostroventromedial medulla, nucleus cuneiformis) to the spine and controlling or down-regulating peripheral/nociceptive input to the dorsal horn. These systems are in turn under the influence of various forebrain structures such as the anterior cingulate cortex (ACC, pre- and subgenual part), amygdala, and frontopolar cortex. It is thought that a certain amount of nociceptive signaling (via C and Aδ fibers), possibly present even physiologically, is suppressed on the spinal level in healthy humans but gains access to the brain in FM patients due to impaired inhibitory control.

Evidence from functional magnetic resonance imaging (fMRI) supports these findings by showing individuals with FM having increased neuronal activation in pain processing regions of the brain when otherwise innocuous stimuli are applied.[36-38] Just as with experimental pain testing studies, these studies have shown that this augmented pain processing in sensory processing regions of the brain is largely independent of the presence of psychiatric factors such as depression.[37]

Other brain imaging studies investigating FM patients have reported a hypoperfusion of the striatum and thalamus at rest, as well as changes in the size of brain structure in the cingulate cortex, insular cortex, striatum, and thalamus.[39-41] Although some of these changes may be due to comorbid depression and other psychiatric comorbidities,[42] these findings suggest functional and morphological changes in the forebrain, especially in structures known to be part of the human pain system. However, it is yet to be determined whether these changes follow an increased nociceptive input (possibly promoting the process of pain chronification), or whether they actually constitute the primary pathophysiology.

POSSIBLE REASONS FOR AUGMENTED PAIN AND SENSORY PROCESSING

Current evidence suggests that genetic factors are at least 50% responsible for overall sensitivity to experimental pain. There are at least four sets of genes that change an individual's pain sensitivity and increase one's likelihood of developing one or more chronic pain states: COMT, a number of sodium channel mutations, GTP cyclohydroxylase, and a potassium channel gene (KCNS).[43-46] Family members of FM patients have a much higher risk of any type of chronic pain, and they are also more tender than the family members of controls.[2] They also have higher rates of psychiatric comorbidity, but this overall risk is approximately two times that of controls whereas the excess rate of pain disorders is much higher. A number of genetics studies, especially twin studies, nicely demonstrate that there are two somewhat independent but overlapping sets of traits: one that is related to pain and sensory sensitivity and the other related to psychiatric comorbidity.[17,47,48] Furthermore, different groups have described specific genetic polymorphisms associated with an increased risk of developing FM, the most important of which pertain to the serotonin and catecholamine metabolism, which also confer an increased risk of a developing a mood disorder. An example is the serotonin 2a receptor gene, which meta-analyses suggest is different in FM patients and healthy controls.[49,50] Of note, a number of serotonergic genes have also been found to occur more frequently in patients with depressive disorders, suggesting one reason why there may be higher rates of mood disorders in FM patients and their family members. Similarly, many studies have implicated the catecholamine-O-methyl-transferase (COMT) polymorphisms or haplotype in FM and other pain states, and this same gene has been associated with features of several mood disorders, especially the sex differences in expression of these disorders.[51-54] Several recent studies have also implicated beta-2 adrenergic receptor abnormalities in FM.[55,56]

Low levels (or low activity) of neurotransmitters such as serotonin, norepinephrine, and dopamine may play a role in FM. This assertion

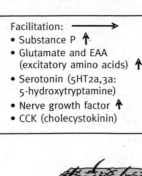
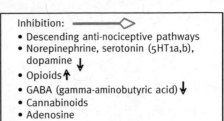

Facilitation: ⟶
- Substance P ↑
- Glutamate and EAA (excitatory amino acids) ↑
- Serotonin (5HT2a,3a: 5-hydroxytryptamine)
- Nerve growth factor ↑
- CCK (cholecystokinin)

Inhibition: ⟶◇
- Descending anti-nociceptive pathways
- Norepinephrine, serotonin (5HT1a,b), dopamine ↓
- Opioids ↑
- GABA (gamma-aminobutyric acid) ↓
- Cannabinoids
- Adenosine

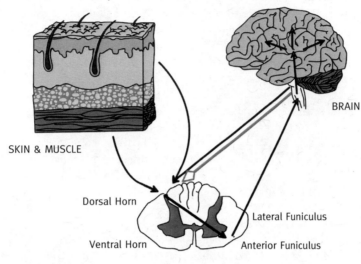

SKIN & MUSCLE

BRAIN

Dorsal Horn

Lateral Funiculus

Ventral Horn

Anterior Funiculus

SPINAL CORD

FIGURE 15.3 Neurotransmitters that are known to play either faciliatory (generally increase pain transmission in the spinal cord) or inhibitory (decreasing pain transmission) roles in the central nervous system. The arrows indicate the direction of the abnormality that has been identified in fibromyalgia, showing that the only neurotransmitter system that has been studied in fibromyalgia that has not been found to be abnormal in a direction that would cause hyperalgesia/allodynia is the opioidergic system, which may explain why this class of drugs is not very efficacious in fibromyalgia. (Adapted from Clauw, D.J., *Etiology of Fibromyalgia*, edited by McCarberg and Clauw. Fibromyalgia, p. 12. 2009, Informa Healthcare USA, Inc.)

is supported and extended by finding changes of these and other neurotransmitter concentrations capable of altering sensory processing, either in the cerebrospinal fluid (CSF) or brain, which are depicted in Figure 15.3. Many of the neurotransmitters known to facilitate central nervous system (CNS) transmission of pain, such as substance P, glutamate, and nerve growth factor, have been shown to be increased in the CSF of individuals with FM. However, levels of metabolites of neurotransmitters that typically inhibit pain transmission, such as serotonin, norepinepinephrine, and dopamine, are reduced.[57–63] The only paradoxical direction for the abnormality of a neurotransmitter that

modulates pain occurs in the endogenous opioid system, where CSF levels of enkephalins have been shown to be elevated in FM patients.[64] This finding is in line with a positron emission tomography (PET) study showing decreased mu-opioid receptor availability in the nucleus accumbens and cingulate gyrus in FM patients demonstrating an increased baseline occupancy of opioid receptors.[65] It has been hypothesized that elevated enkephalin levels might result from an ongoing attempt to control nociception in FM patients, and thus this might explain the anecdotal experience that giving exogenous opioids (i.e., opiate analgesics) to individuals with FM is (at least anecdotally) often of no benefit.

The idea that the diffuse hyperalgesia, sleep abnormalities, memory problems, and mood disturbances seen in individuals with FM and CFS may have common neurotransmitter underpinnings is currently the most acceptable theory for the pathogenesis of these conditions.[66] All of the neurotransmitter systems that have been shown to be abnormal in FM control more than simply pain and sensory processing. They have broad effects in controlling alertness, sleep, memory, and mood. Moreover, as is discussed later, all of the currently FDA-approved treatments for FM, as well as other nonapproved classes such as tricyclic drugs and sodium oxybate, lead to simultaneous improvement in more than one symptom domain.

PERIPHERAL ABNORMALITIES IN FIBROMYALGIA

Although a few studies have found mild abnormalities in the skeletal muscles of FM patients, these findings have been inconsistent and may be due to deconditioning rather than the illness itself.[67] However, there are a few studies that suggest there may be subsets of FM patients with damage to small nerve fibers in the skin, as has been seen with other chronic pain states.[68] Although FM, irritable bowel syndrome, and other central pain states were originally felt to be autoimmune or inflammatory diseases and then later felt not to be, recent findings are leading to a reconsideration of whether subtle inflammatory changes may be responsible for some of the symptoms seen.[69] Immunological cascades have a role in the maintenance of central sensitivity and chronic pain, which is enhanced through the release of pro-inflammatory cytokines by CNS glial cells; thus, the traditional paradigm regarding inflammatory versus noninflammatory pain may gradually become less of a dichotomy. A delicate apparatus of checks and balances is at work in the spinal transmission of pain as may be expected in any complex biological system. Multiple inhibitory transmitters act at the spinal level to reduce the "volume" of pain transmission. Serotonin, norepinephrine, enkephalins, dopamine, and gamma-amino-butyric acid (GABA) are among the better known players in this balance.

Furthermore, studies suggest that maintenance of central augmentation requires persistent noxious peripheral input, even in syndromes such as irritable bowel sydrome and FM, which are characterized by the absence of well-defined, localized, pain-causing lesions.[70] In fact, a recent study of 68 fibromyalgia patients with myofascial pain syndromes and 56 fibromyalgia patients with regional joint pain showed that peripheral trigger point injections and hydroelectrophoresis ameliorate fibromyalgia pain and increase pain thresholds at sites distant from the therapeutic interventions, providing further evidence that painful peripheral stimuli contribute to the perpetuation of central augmentation interventions.[71] In summary, these data suggest that FM is a "mixed pain state" like almost all other chronic pain states, with some contribution of peripheral factors in some individuals.

SLEEP AND ACTIVITY IN FIBROMYALGIA

In addition to pain, other symptoms very commonly seen in FM include disturbed sleep and poor physical function. One of the first biological findings in FM was that selective sleep deprivation led to symptoms of FM in healthy individuals, and these findings have subsequently been replicated by several groups.[72] However, the electroencephalogram abnormalities that were noted in this first study and initially thought to be a marker for FM, so-called alpha intrusions, have subsequently been found to be present in normals and in individuals with other conditions. More recent findings on polysomnography that occur more commonly in FM include demonstration of fewer sleep spindles, an increase in cyclic alternating pattern rate, upper airway resistance syndrome, and/or poor sleep efficiency.[73] There is no evidence that individuals should be screened for these disorders unless they have symptoms or risk factors suggesting a sleep disorder.

PSYCHIATRIC AND PSYCHOLOGICAL COMORBIDITIES

Psychological and behavioral factors also play a role in symptom expression in many FM patients. The rate of current psychiatric comorbidity in patients with FM may be as high as 30% to 60% in tertiary care settings, and the rate of lifetime psychiatric disorders even higher.[74] Depression and anxiety disorders are the most commonly seen. However, these rates may be artifactually elevated by virtue of the fact that most of these studies have been performed in tertiary care centers. Individuals who meet ACR criteria for FM who are identified in the general population do not generally have nearly quite this high a rate of identifiable psychiatric conditions.

As already noted, population-based studies have demonstrated that the relationship between pain and distress is complex and that distress is both a cause and consequence of pain. In this latter instance, a typical pattern is that as a result of pain and other symptoms of FM, individuals begin to function less well in their various roles. They may have difficulties with spouses and/or children, and work inside or outside the home, which can exacerbate symptoms and lead to maladaptive illness behaviors. These include isolation, cessation of pleasurable activities, reductions in activity and exercise, and so on. In the worst cases, patients become involved with disability and compensation systems that almost ensure that they will not improve.

The complex interaction of biological, psychological, and behavioral mechanisms is not, however, unique to FM. Nonbiological factors play a prominent role in symptom expression in all chronic pain states. In fact, in conditions such as rheumatoid arthritis and osteoarthritis, nonbiological factors such as level of formal education, coping strategies, and socioeconomic variables account for more of the variance in pain report and disability than biologic factors, such as the joint space width or sedimentation rate.[75] There are also clearly subgroups of patients that can be identified with differential psychological factors playing a role in their symptom expression, including patients in whom it appears as though they are psychologically "resilient" and who may be "buffering" the functional impact of their symptoms.[76,77]

fMRI studies have also investigated how comorbid mood disorders or an individual's thoughts about his or her pain may be influencing pain processing in FM. One fMRI study found that the level of depressive symptomatology did not influence the degree of neuronal activation in brain regions responsible for coding for the sensory intensity of pain, the primary and secondary somatosensory cortices. But it did affect neuronal activation in the affective pain processing regions of the brain, such as the amygdala and anterior insula.[78] Another study with similar methodology examined how the presence or absence of catastrophizing might influence pain report in FM.[79] In contrast to the results noted earlier, the presence of catastrophizing was associated with increased neuronal activations in the sensory coding regions. These studies thus provide empirical evidence for the value of treatments such as cognitive-behavioral therapy. This is especially the case if individuals exhibit cognitions such as catastrophizing, which, independent of other factors, may be capable of increasing pain intensity.

THE EVALUATION OF INDIVIDUALS WITH CHRONIC WIDESPREAD PAIN

The evaluation of an individual with chronic pain is a complex process. Unlike most other medical problems, simply arriving at a "diagnosis" is typically insufficient to guide treatment. This is because within any given pain diagnosis, there is tremendous heterogeneity with respect to the underlying causes and contributors to symptoms, and the most effective treatments. In particular, individuals with chronic pain can have greater or lesser peripheral nociceptive (i.e., tissue damage, inflammation) and central nonnociceptive (i.e., pain amplification, psychological factors) contributions to their pain. Therefore, the differential diagnosis of chronic pain involves identifying which of these factors are present in which individuals, so that the appropriate pharmacologic, procedural, and psychological therapies can be administered.

A careful musculoskeletal history and examination remains the most important diagnostic test for musculoskeletal pain. In other fields of medicine, advances in diagnostic testing have largely rendered a physical examination obsolete. However, in musculoskeletal medicine, technology confuses as much as it helps.

Therefore, the musculoskeletal history and examination must allow the clinician to arrive at the diagnosis (or at worst a very narrow differential diagnosis), and then if necessary, further diagnostic testing should be used to confirm these findings.

DIAGNOSTIC CRITERIA OF FIBROMYALGIA

The ACR criteria for fibromyalgia were never intended to be used as strict diagnostic criteria for use in clinical practice. Many individuals who clearly have fibromyalgia will not have pain throughout their entire body or not have 11 tender points. Moreover, pain and tenderness occur across a continuum in the population. It is impossible to know where to draw the line between an individual with symptoms and someone with an illness.

PAIN-RELATED SYMPTOMS

In clinical practice, one should suspect fibromyalgia in individuals with multifocal pain that cannot be fully explained on the basis of damage or inflammation in those regions of the body. In most cases, musculoskeletal pain is the most prominent feature, but because pain pathways throughout the body are amplified, pain can be perceived more generally. Thus, chronic headaches, sore throats, chest pain, abdominal pain, and pelvic pain are very common in individuals with fibromyalgia, and patients with chronic regional pain in any of these locations are more likely to have fibromyalgia.

Because pain is a defining feature of fibromyalgia, it is helpful to focus on the features of the pain that can help distinguish it from other disorders. The pain of fibromyalgia is typically diffuse or multifocal, often waxes and wanes, and is frequently migratory in nature. Patients may complain of discomfort when they are touched or when wearing tight clothing, and they may experience dysesthesias or paresthesias that accompany the pain.

NON-PAIN SYMPTOMS

Aside from the pain, a number of seemingly nonrelated symptoms may develop and persist. These include fatigue (and thus the significant overlap between FM and CFS), sleep difficulties, weakness, problems with attention or memory, unexplainable weight fluctuations, and heat and cold intolerance. "Allergies" are reported much more commonly in fibromyalgia patients, although these excess symptoms are better considered hypersensitivities rather than true IgE-mediated immunological reactions. These patients are also more prone to nonallergic rhinitis, sinus and nasal congestion, and lower respiratory symptoms, all of which again may primarily be attributable to neural mechanisms. Distortions in hearing, vision, and vestibular symptoms are often reported, as are sicca symptoms (sometimes so prominent that these individuals will overlap with those with Sjogren's syndrome).

"Functional disorders" involving visceral organs have long been noted to be more common in fibromyalgia. These include noncardiac chest pain, heartburn and palpitations, and the frequent comorbidity of irritable bowel syndrome. Thus, there are reports of increased echocardiographic evidence of mitral valve prolapse and esophageal dysmotility, and reduced static inspiratory and expiratory pressure on pulmonary function tests. The latter might be explained by pain in respiratory muscles. Syncope and hypotension are symptoms that may occur in FM, and in some cases will be accompanied by neurally mediated hypotension or postural orthostatic tachycardia. Pelvic complaints are common, including not only pain but also urinary frequency and urgency. In females the frequent comorbid diagnoses are dysmenorrhea, interstitial cystitis, endometriosis, and sensitivity disorders like vulvar vestibulitis and vulvodynia. In males, these same symptoms are sometimes diagnosed as chronic or nonbacterial prostatitis (see Fig. 15.1).

PHYSICAL EXAMINATION AND LABORATORY INVESTIGATIONS

Physical examination is often unremarkable, except for the presence of tenderness. As previously discussed, tenderness may be generalized and thus present anywhere in the body. Laboratory testing is generally not useful, except for the purpose of differential diagnosis. The length of time the patient has had symptoms is one factor that can help guide the intensity of the diagnostic workup. If the patient's symptoms have persisted for several years, minimal testing is required, whereas a more aggressive strategy should be employed for acute or subacute onset of symptoms. If the patient's symptoms correlate with the use of statin therapy, myalgias may result as a side effect. The statin should be discontinued before diagnosing a patient with FM. Simple testing should be limited to complete blood count and routine serum chemistries, along with TSH and erythrocyte sedimentation rate and/or C-reactive protein. Serologic studies such as antinuclear antibody and rheumatoid factor assays should generally be avoided unless there are historical features not seen in FM or abnormalities on physical examination. This represents a problem in clinical practice, because several autoimmune disorders share overlapping symptomatology with FM. These include not only fatigue, arthralgias, and myalgias but also such symptoms as morning stiffness and subjective swelling of the hands and feet. Certain dermatologic features commonly seen in FM, including malar flushing, livedo reticularis, and Raynaud's-like reddening of the hands, also mimic symptoms of autoimmune disorders. This sometimes results in patients with FM being misdiagnosed as having an autoimmune disorder such as systemic lupus erythematosus.

TREATMENT OF FIBROMYALGIA

Once a physician rules out other potential disorders, an important and at times controversial step in the management of FM is asserting the diagnosis. Despite some assumptions that being "labeled" with FM may adversely affect patients, several studies have shown that labeling an individual with FM actually increases health satisfaction and reduces overall medical costs (primarily by reducing subspecialty referral and diagnostic testing).[80,81] However, in certain select individuals, that is, adolescents or young adults, or overtly anxious persons, the preferred route may still be not to label. Regardless, diagnosis confirmation should be ideally coupled to patient education, an inter-vention shown to be effective in randomized controlled trials.

Pharmacologic Therapy

It is important to use symptom-based pharmacologic therapy together with nonpharmacologic therapies because medications typically target symptoms, whereas nonpharmacologic therapies target dysfunction/functional decline (see Table 15.1).[82]

TRICYCLIC ANTIDEPRESSANTS

The most frequently studied pharmacologic therapy for FM is low doses of tricyclic compounds. Most TCAs increase the concentrations of serotonin and/or norepinephrine (noradrenaline) by directly blocking their respective reuptake. The effectiveness of TCAs, particularly amitriptyline and cyclobenzaprine, in treating the symptoms of pain, poor sleep, and fatigue associated with fibromyalgia is supported by several randomized, controlled trials.[83,84] Tolerability is a problem but can be improved by beginning at very low doses (e.g., 10 mg of amitriptyline or 5 mg of cyclobenzaprine), giving the dose a few hours before bedtime, and very slowly escalating the dose.

SELECTIVE SEROTONIN REUPTAKE INHIBITORS

Because of a better side effect profile, newer antidepressants (i.e., selective serotonin reuptake inhibitors; SSRIs) are frequently used in fibromyalgia. The SSRIs fluoxetine, citalopram, and paroxetine have each been evaluated in randomized, placebo-controlled trials. The newer "highly selective" serotonin reuptake inhibitors, for example, citalopram, seem to be less efficacious than the older SSRIs, which have some noradrenergic activity at higher doses.[85] For example, although several studies have examined the efficacy of fluoxetine in FM, the one that used the highest doses (an average of 45 mg/day) showed the greatest efficacy, perhaps because at this dose the drug has significant noradrenergic as well as serotonergic effects.[86]

Table 15.1   Pharmacologic Therapies

STRONG EVIDENCE	MODEST EVIDENCE	WEAK EVIDENCE	NOT SHOWN EFFECTIVE
Tricyclics (amitriptyline, cyclobenzaprine)	Tramadol	Growth hormone	Opioids, NSAIDs, corticosteroids
Dual-reuptake inhibitors (SNRI/NSRI—duloxetine, milnacipran)	Selective serotonin reuptake inhibitors (SSRIs)	5-hydroxytryptamine	Benzodiazepine and nonbenzodiazepine hypnotics, melatonin
Alpha-2-delta ligands (pregabalin, gabapentin)	Dopamine agonists	Tropisetron	Melatonin, guanifenesin
	Gamma hydroxybutyrate (GHB)	S-adenosyl-L-methionine (SAMe)	Dehydroepiandrosterone

NSAIDs, nonsteroidal anti-inflammatory drugs; SNRI/NSRI, serotonin-NE and NE-serotonin reuptake inhibitors.

DUAL REUPTAKE INHIBITORS

Because of the salutary effects of TCAs and high doses of certain "SSRIs," it was logical to conclude that the dual receptor inhibitors such as serotonin-NE and NE-serotonin reuptake inhibitors (SNRIs and NSRIs) may be of more benefit than pure serotonergic drugs. These drugs are pharmacologically similar to some TCAs in their ability to inhibit the reuptake of both serotonin and NE, but they differ from TCAs in being generally devoid of significant activity at other receptor systems. This selectivity results in diminished side effects and enhanced tolerability. The first available SNRI, venlafaxine, has some data to support its use in conditions such as fibromyalgia, again especially at higher doses.[87] Desvenlafaxine is the major metabolite of venlafaxine with similar activity. With the reduced risk for pharmacokinetic drug interactions, it may have a potential advantage over its parent compound.[88] There are considerably better data to support the use of duloxetine and milnacipran, both of which are approved by the FDA for use in FM.[89–92] In the studies evaluating milnacipran, statistically significant differences were noted in overall improvement, physical functioning, level of fatigue, and degree of reported physical impairment. In the trials of duloxetine, compared to placebo participants treated with duloxetine had decreased self-reported pain and stiffness, and a reduced number of tender points. In both studies, benefits were shown to be independent of the drug effect on mood. This suggests that the analgesic and other positive effects of this class of drugs in fibromyalgia are not simply due to their antidepressant effects. Both of these drugs are better tolerated if taken with food. Patients should be told about likely initial nausea and counseled that this typically resolves in a week or so; if not, then they should discontinue the drug. The maximum approved dose of duloxetine is 60 mg per day, but it was studied in trials at doses up to 120 mg and shown to be safe, and similarly the initial dose of milnacipran is 100 mg but some patients will benefit from increasing the dose as high as 200 mg.

OTHER CENTRAL NERVOUS SYSTEM ACTING DRUGS

Antiepileptic drugs are widely used in the treatment of various chronic pain conditions, including postherpetic neuralgia and painful diabetic neuropathy. Pregabalin and gabapentin have the same mechanism of action and bind to the alpha-2-delta subunit of calcium channels. Both are approved for the treatment of neuropathic pain as well as several other indications. Several studies have shown the efficacy of pregabalin against pain, sleep disturbances, and fatigue as compared to placebo in fibromyalgia, leading to approval of this drug in the United States for use in this condition.[90,93] Gabapentin has been shown to have very similar efficacy and side effect profile in FM, and it has been approved for a number of other chronic pain states as well.[94,95] The tolerability of these drugs can be dramatically enhanced by beginning at a low dose, and giving either two-thirds of the dose, or the entire dose, at bedtime. The maximally approved dose of pregabalin is 450 mg, but in trials it was studied at doses as high as 600 mg and shown to be safe and efficacious. Another antiepileptic compound, clonazepam, has demonstrated efficacy in treating temporal mandibular disorder and associated jaw pain and is useful in the treatment of restless leg syndrome and may be of value in FM.[96]

Sedative-hypnotic compounds are widely used by FM patients. A handful of studies have been published on the use of certain nonbenzodiazepine hypnotics in FM, such as zopiclone and zolpidem. These reports have suggested that these agents can improve the sleep and, perhaps, fatigue of FM patients, though they had no significant effects upon pain. On the other hand, gamma-hydroxybutyrate (also known as sodium oxabate), a precursor of GABA with powerful sedative properties, was recently shown to be very useful in simultaneously improving fatigue, pain, and sleep architecture in patients with FM.[97] This strongly suggests that GABA deficiency may be playing a role in FM. Note, however, that this agent is a scheduled substance due to its abuse potential.

Pramipexole is a dopamine agonist indicated for Parkinson's disease that has shown also shown utility in the treatment of periodic leg movement disorder. Although some studies have suggested that this class of drug can have utility in FM, subsequent studies have yielded conflicting results, and many practitioners reserve this agent for individuals with FM or CFS who have comorbid periodic leg movement disorder.[98]

Tizanidine is a centrally acting alpha-2 adrenergic agonist approved by the FDA for the treatment of muscle spasticity associated with multiple sclerosis and stroke. Literature suggests that this agent is a useful adjunct in treating several chronic pain conditions, including chronic daily headaches and low back pain. A recent trial reported significant improvements in several parameters in FM, including sleep, pain, and measures of quality of life.[99] Of particular interest was the demonstration that treatment with tizanidine resulted in a reduction in substance P levels within the CSF of patients with FM.

There have been no adequate, randomized controlled clinical trials of opiates in FM. Many in the field (including the authors) have not found this class of compounds to be effective in anecdotal experience. Tramadol is a compound that has some opioid activity (weak mu agonist activity) combined with serotonin/NE reuptake inhibition. This compound does appear to be somewhat efficacious in the management of FM, as both an isolated compound and as fixed-dose combination with acetaminophen.[100]

A large number of FM patients use NSAIDs and acetaminophen. Although numerous studies have failed to confirm their effectiveness as analgesics in FM, there is limited evidence that patients may experience enhanced analgesia when treated with combinations of NSAIDs and other agents. This phenomenon may be a result of concurrent "peripheral" pain (i.e., due to damage or inflammation of tissues, e.g., osteoarthritis, rheumatoid arthritis) conditions that may be present, and/or that these comorbid peripheral pain generators might lead to worsening of "central" pain.

NONPHARMACOLOGIC THERAPY

The two best-studied nonpharmacologic therapies are cognitive-behavioral therapy (CBT) and exercise (Table 15.2). Both of these therapies have been shown to be efficacious in the treatment of fibromyalgia, as well as a plethora of other medical conditions.[101-104] Both of these treatments can lead to sustained (e.g., greater than 1 year) improvements and are

Table 15.2 Nonpharmacologic Therapies

STRONG EVIDENCE	MODEST EVIDENCE	WEAK EVIDENCE	NO EVIDENCE
Cardiovascular exercise	Strength training	Acupuncture	Tender (trigger) point injections
Cognitive-behavioral therapy	Acupuncture	Manual and massage therapy	Flexibility exercise
Patient education	Hypnotherapy	Chiropractic	
Multidisciplinary therapy	Biofeedback, balneotherapy	Electrotherapy, ultrasound	

very effective when an individual complies with therapy. These therapies are particularly attractive because they are likely working better on domains that are not as well treated with drugs in FM and CFS. For example, exercise appears to be a better treatment for fatigue and functional status than most drugs that are in routine use. Recent studies have shown that even increasing an individual's activity (without getting to "exercise) can have a beneficial effect. This is particularly helpful as a first step for individuals with chronic pain or fatigue than for individuals who have become very sedentary and deconditioned.[105,106] Other studies have taken alternative approaches to classic CBT that have been shown to be successful, including incorporating motivational interviewing, addressing early life trauma via emotional awareness, and delivering these interventions via the Internet.[107–109]

Alternative therapies have been explored by patients managing their own illness, as well as health care providers. As with other diseases, there are few controlled trials to advocate their general use. Trigger-point injections, chiropractic manipulation, acupuncture, and myofascial release therapy are among the more commonly used modalities, which achieve varying levels of success. Trials of acupuncture have yielded inconsistent results when compared to sham acupuncture, but this may be because PET studies have indicated that although both active and sham acupuncture are associated with similar clinical improvements in pain, the effects of these two treatments on CNS mu-opioid activity are quite different, with the effects of sham appearing similar to previous studies

of the placebo effect.[110,111] Tai chi and yoga have been shown to be efficacious in some studies.[112] There is some evidence that in addition to direct benefits, the use of alternative therapies gives patients a greater sense of control over their illness. Even when efficacy of a complementary or alternative therapy is not proven, in instances where these therapies are safe and this sense of control is accompanied by an improved clinical state, the decision to use these therapies is between physicians and patients themselves.

TREATMENT OF CHRONIC FATIGUE SYNDROME

There is much overlap in the pathophysiology of CFS with FM, as mentioned earlier. Some hallmarks of CFS may be correlations between inflammation and infection, augmented sensory processing, abnormalities of neurotransmitters, nerve growth factors, low levels of serotonin and norepinephrine, abnormalities of homeostasis of the stress system, and autonomic dysfunction. The relative contributions of each of these abnormalities to the profound fatigue associated with CFS need to be explored further to better evaluate and treat the syndrome. There is much less known overall about the etiology of CFS. Many factors play a role: stress, augmented nociceptive and sensory processing, genetic factors, neurotransmitter levels, peripheral abnormalities, psychiatric comorbidities, and sleep and activity. More common to CFS include a possible clear relation of infection to trigger the illness. Although there is overwhelming support for the notion that CFS (or FM) can be "triggered" by an infectious illness, a much more controversial area remains whether there is a subset of CFS patients whose symptoms are *caused* by an ongoing active infectious illness.[18,113,114] The history of the condition now known as CFS is littered with infectious agents that were originally thought to cause the illness, which were later refuted. The latest appears to be the retrovirus XMRV.[115] Initial studies showing this virus in a high proportion of individuals with CFS were generally not replicated by other groups, and the most recent studies show that this was highly likely to be due to a contaminant.[116]

Although in general there has been far more high-quality research in FM, there are many areas where CFS has been better studied than FM. For example, cognitive dysfunction (common in FM and sometimes referred to by patients as fibrofog) has been well studied in CFS, with studies showing decreased speeds of motor and information processing, working memory, and attentional tasks are common complaints in CFS.[117-119]

Exercise and activity level are important. Couch potatoes rarely develop CFS. Having high premorbid levels of activity and/or a lower body mass in young adulthood were the strongest predictors of CFS later in life in a recent study.[120,121] Female patients were much more likely to have somatic symptoms when deprived of either sleep and/or exercise. Studies have not found personality to be abnormal in people with CFS, dispelling the misconception that these are type A individuals. But a recent study did show that some traits of neuroticism were associated with more severe symptoms in those with CFS.[122,123] Treatment in CFS is very similar to that of FM. Refer to the details of the treatment mentioned earlier and in Tables 15.1 and 15.2.

CONCLUSION

FM and CFS are similar entities but still different. FM is thought of as the prototypical "central" pain syndrome that occurs mainly because of spinal and supraspinal mechanisms involved in pain transmission, rather than due to peripheral inflammation. The same mechanisms thought to lead to centrally mediated pain also lead to other somatic symptoms such as fatigue in CFS. FM and CFS may likely be on a continuum of the same type of disease. At this time the current state-of-the-art treatment for both is the same. Thus, further research is needed to individualize pathophysiology and treatment.

REFERENCES

1. Aaron LA, Burke MM, Buchwald D. Overlapping conditions among patients with chronic fatigue syndrome, fibromyalgia, and temporomandibular disorder. *Arch Int Med* 2000; 160(2):221–7.
2. Arnold LM, Hudson JI, Hess EV, et al. Family study of fibromyalgia. *Arthritis Rheum* 2004;50(3): 944–52.
3. Clauw DJ. Pain management: Fibromyalgia drugs are "as good as it gets" in chronic pain. *Nat Rev Rheumatol* 2010;6(8): 439–40.
4. Fukuda K, Straus SE, Hickie I, Sharpe MC, Dobbins JG, Komaroff A. The chronic fatigue syndrome: a comprehensive approach to its definition and study. International Chronic Fatigue Syndrome Study Group. *Ann Int Med* 1994;121(12): 953–9.
5. van't Leven M, Zielhuis GA, van der Meer JW, Verbeek AL, Bleijenberg G. Fatigue and chronicfatigue syndrome-like complaints in the generalpopulation. *Eur J Public Health* 2010;20(3):251–7.
6. Reeves WC, Jones JF, Maloney E, et al. Prevalence of chronic fatigue syndrome in metropolitan, urban, and rural Georgia. *Popul Health Metr* 2007;5: 5.
7. Njoku MG, Jason LA, Torres-Harding SR. The prevalence of chronic fatigue syndrome in Nigeria. *J Health Psychol* 2007;12(3): 461–74.
8. Jason LA, Taylor RR, Kennedy CL, Song S, Johnson D, Torres S. Chronic fatigue syndrome: occupation, medical utilization, and subtypes in a community-based sample. *J Nervous Mental Dis* 2000;188(9): 568–76.
9. Jason LA, Taylor RR, Carrico AW. A community-based study of chronic fatigue syndrome. *Arch Int Med* 1999;159(18): 2129–37.
10. Wolfe F, Smythe HA, Yunus MB, et al. The American College of Rheumatology 1990 criteria for the classification of fibromyalgia. Report of the Multicenter Criteria Committee. *Arthritis Rheum* 1990;33(2):160–72.
11. Wolfe F, Clauw DJ, Fitzcharles MA, et al. The American College of Rheumatology preliminary diagnostic criteria for fibromyalgia and measurement of symptom severity. *Arthritis Care Res (Hoboken)* 2010;62(5): 600–10.

12. Wolfe F, Ross K, Anderson J, Russell IJ, Hebert L. The prevalence and characteristics of fibromyalgia in the general population. *Arthritis Rheum* 1995;38(1):19–28.

13. Granges G, Littlejohn G. Pressure pain threshold in pain-free subjects, in patients with chronic regional pain syndromes, and in patients with fibromyalgia syndrome. *Arthritis Rheum* 1993;36(5):642–6.

14. Wolfe F. The relation between tender points and fibromyalgia symptom variables: evidence that fibromyalgia is not a discrete disorder in the clinic. *Ann Rheumatic Dis*, 1997;56(4):268–71.

15. Petzke F, Gracely RH, Park KM, Ambrose K, Clauw DJ. What do tender points measure? Influence of distress on 4 measures of tenderness. *J Rheumatol* 2003;30(3):567–74.

16. Aaron LA, Bradley LA, Alarcon GS, et al, Psychiatric diagnoses in patients with fibromyalgia are related to health care-seeking behavior rather than to illness. *Arthritis Rheum* 1996;39(3):436–45.

17. Kato K, Sullivan PF, Evengård B, Pedersen NL. A population-based twin study of functional somatic syndromes. *Psychol Med* 2009; 39(3):497–505.

18. Ablin K, Clauw DJ. From fibrositis to functional somatic syndromes to a bell-shaped curve of pain and sensory sensitivity: evolution of a clinical construct. *Rheum Dis Clin North Am* 2009;35(2):233–51.

19. Hassett AL, Clauw DJ. The role of stress in rheumatic diseases. *Arthritis Res Ther* 2010. 12(3):123.

20. Clauw DJ, Katz P. The overlap between fibromyalgia and inflammatory rheumatic disease: when and why does it occur? *J Clin Rheumatol* 1995;1(6):335–42.

21. McBeth J, Macfarlane GJ, Hunt IM, Silman AJ. Risk factors for persistent chronic widespread pain: a community-based study. *Rheumatology (Oxford)* 2001;40(1):95–101.

22. Jones GT, Power C, Macfarlane GJ. Adverse events in childhood and chronic widespread pain in adult life: results from the 1958 British Birth Cohort Study. *Pain* 2009;143(1–2):92–6.

23. Tak LM, Cleare AJ, Ormel J, et al. Meta-analysis and meta-regression of hypothalamic-pituitary-adrenal axis activity in functional somatic disorders. *Biol Psychol* 2011;87(2): 183–94

24. McLean SA, Williams DA, Stein PK, et al. Cerebrospinal fluid corticotropin-releasing factor concentration is associated with pain but not fatigue symptoms in patients with fibromyalgia. *Neuropsychopharmacology* 2006; 31(12):2776–82.

25. McLean SA,Williams DA, Harris RE, et al. Momentary relationship between cortisol secretion and symptoms in patients with fibromyalgia. *Arthritis Rheum* 2005;52(11):3660–9.

26. Clauw DJ, Chrousos GP. Chronic pain and fatigue syndromes: overlapping clinical and neuroendocrine features and potential pathogenic mechanisms. *Neuroimmunomodulation* 1997;4(3):134–53.

27. Martinez-Lavin M, Hermosillo AG, Rosas M, Soto ME. Circadian studies of autonomic nervous balance in patients with fibromyalgia: a heart rate variability analysis. *Arthritis Rheum* 1998;41(11):1966–71.

28. Gibson SJ, et al. Increased thermal pain sensitivity in patients with fibromyalgia syndrome. In: Bromm B, Desmedt JE, eds. *Pain and the Brain.* New York: Raven Press; 1995: 401–11.

29. Petzke F, Clauw DJ, Ambrose K, Khine A, Gracely RH. Increased pain sensitivity in fibromyalgia: effects of stimulus type and mode of presentation. *Pain* 2003;105(3):403–13.

30. Geisser ME, Glass JM, Rajcevska LD, et al. A psychophysical study of auditory and pressure sensitivity in patients with fibromyalgia and healthy controls. *J Pain* 2008;9(5):417–22.

31. Geisser ME, Strader Donnell C, Petzke F, Gracely RH, Clauw DJ, Williams DA. Comorbid somatic symptoms and functional status in patients with fibromyalgia and chronic fatigue syndrome: sensory amplification as a common mechanism. *Psychosomatics* 2008;49(3):235–42.

32. Kosek E, Hansson P. Modulatory influence on somatosensory perception from vibration and heterotopic noxious conditioning stimulation (HNCS) in fibromyalgia patients and healthy subjects. *Pain* 1997;70(1):41–51.

33. Lautenbacher S, Rollman GB. Possible deficiencies of pain modulation in fibromyalgia. *Clin J Pain* 1997;13(3):189–96.

34. Julien N, Goffaux P, Arsenault P, Marchand S. Widespread pain in fibromyalgia is related to a deficit of endogenous pain inhibition. *Pain* 2005;114(1–2):295–302.

35. Normand E, Potvin S, Gaumond I, Cloutier G, Corbin JF, Marchand S. Pain inhibition is deficient in chronic widespread pain but normal in major depressive disorder. *J Clin Psychiatry* 2011;72(2):219–24.

36. Gracely RH, Petzke F, Wolf JM, Clauw DJ. Functional magnetic resonance imaging evidence of augmented pain processing in fibromyalgia. *Arthritis Rheum* 2002;46(5):1333–43.

37. Giesecke T, Gracely RH, Williams DA, Geisser ME, Petzke FW, Clauw DJ. The relationship between depression, clinical pain, and experimental pain in a chronic pain cohort. *Arthritis Rheum* 2005;52(5):1577–84.

38. Cook DB, Lange G, Ciccone DS, Liu WC, Steffener J, Natelson BH. Functional imaging of pain in patients with primary fibromyalgia. *J Rheumatol* 2004;31(2):364–78.

39. Mountz JM, Bradley LA, Modell JG, et al. Fibromyalgia in women. Abnormalities of regional cerebral blood flow in the thalamus and the caudate nucleus are associated with low pain threshold levels. *Arthritis Rheum* 1995;38(7):926–38.

40. Schmidt-Wilcke T, Luerding R, Weigand T, et al. Striatal grey matter increase in patients suffering from fibromyalgia—a voxel-based morphometry study. *Pain* 2007;132(Suppl 1):S109–16.

41. Kuchinad A, Schweinhardt P, Seminowicz DA, Wood PB, Chizh BA, Bushnell MC. Accelerated brain gray matter loss in fibromyalgia patients: premature aging of the brain? *J Neurosci* 2007;27(15):4004–7.

42. Hsu MC, Harris RE, Sundgren PC, et al. No consistent difference in gray matter volume between individuals with fibromyalgia and age-matched healthy subjects when controlling for affective disorder. *Pain* 2009;143(3):262–7.

43. Costigan M, Belfer I, Griffin RS, et al. Multiple chronic pain states are associated with a common amino acid-changing allele in KCNS1. *Brain* 2010;133(9):2519–27.

44. Tegeder I, Adolph J, Schmidt H, Woolf CJ, Geisslinger G, Lötsch J. Reduced hyperalgesia in homozygous carriers of a GTP cyclohydrolase 1 haplotype. *Eur J Pain* 2008;12(8):1069–77.

45. Diatchenko L, Nackley AG, Slade GD, et al. Catechol-O-methyltransferase gene polymorphisms are associated with multiple pain-evoking stimuli. *Pain* 2006;125(3):216–24.

46. Zubieta JK, Heitzeg MM, Smith YR, et al. COMT val158met genotype affects mu-opioid neurotransmitter responses to a pain stressor. *Science* 2003;299(5610):1240–3.

47. Kato K, Sullivan PF, Evengård B, Pedersen NL. A population-based twin study of functional somatic syndromes. *Psychol Med* 2009;39(3):497–505.

48. Diatchenko L, Nackley AG, Tchivileva IE, Shabalina SA, Maixner W. Genetic architecture of human pain perception. *Trends Genet* 2007;23(12):605–13.

49. Cohen H, Buskila D, Neumann L, Ebstein RP. Confirmation of an association between fibromyalgia and serotonin transporter promoter region (5- HTTLPR) polymorphism, and relationship to anxiety-related personality traits. *Arthritis Rheum* 2002;46(3):845–7.

50. Lee YH, Choi SJ, Ji JD, Song GG. Candidate gene studies of fibromyalgia: a systematic review and meta-analysis. *Rheumatol Int* 2010;32(2):417–26.

51. Nackley AG, Diatchenko L. Assessing potential functionality of catechol-O-methyltransferase (COMT) polymorphisms associated with pain sensitivity and temporomandibular joint disorders. *Methods Mol Biol* 2010;617:375–93.

52. McLean SA, Diatchenko L, Lee YM, et al. Catechol O-methyltransferase haplotype predicts immediate musculoskeletal neck pain and psychological symptoms after motor vehicle collision. *J Pain* 2011;12(1):101–7.

53. Matsuda JB, Barbosa FR, Morel LJ, et al. Serotonin receptor (5-HT 2A) and catechol-O-methyltransferase (COMT) gene polymorphisms: triggers of fibromyalgia? *Rev Bras Reumatol* 2010;50(2):141–9.

54. Harrison PJ, Tunbridge EM. Catechol-O-Methyltransferase (COMT): a gene contributing to sex differences in brain function, and to sexual dimorphism in the predisposition to psychiatric disorders. *Neuropsychopharmacology* 2008;33(13):3037–45.

55. Xiao Y, He W, Russell IJ, Genetic polymorphisms of the {beta}2-adrenergic receptor relate to guanosine protein-coupled stimulator receptor dysfunction in fibromyalgia syndrome. *J Rheumatol* 2011;38(6):1095–103.

56. Light AR, Bateman L, Jo D, et al., Gene expression alterations at baseline and following moderate exercise in patients with chronic fatigue syndrome and fibromyalgia syndrome. *J Int Med* 2012;271(1):64–81.

57. Giovengo SL, Russell IJ, Larson AA. Increased concentrations of nerve growth factor in cerebrospinal fluid of patients with fibromyalgia. *J Rheumatol* 1999;26(7):1564–9.

58. Russell IJ, Vaeroy H, Javors M, Nyberg F. Cerebrospinal fluid biogenic amine metabolites in fibromyalgia/fibrositis syndrome and rheumatoid arthritis. *Arthritis Rheum* 1992;35(5):550–6.

59. Russell IJ, et al. Characteristics of spinal fluid (CSF) substance p (SP) and calcitonin gene related peptide (CGRP) in fibromyalgia syndrome (FMS). *Arthritis Rheum* 1996;39(9 Suppl):S275.

60. Sarchielli P, Di Filippo M, Nardi K, Calabresi P. Sensitization, glutamate, and the link between

migraine and fibromyalgia. *Curr Pain Headache Rep* 2007;11(5):343–51.

61. Wood PB, Patterson JC, II, Sunderland JJ, Tainter KH, Glabus MF, Lilien DL. Reduced presynaptic dopamine activity in fibromyalgia syndrome demonstrated with positron emission tomography: a pilot study. *J Pain* 2007;8(1):51–8.

62. Harris RE, Sundgren PC, Craig AD, et al. Elevated insular glutamate in fibromyalgia is associated with experimental pain. *Arthritis Rheum* 2009;60(10):3146–52.

63. Harris RE, Sundgren PC, Pang Y, et al. Dynamic levels of glutamate within the insula are associated with improvements in multiple pain domains in fibromyalgia. *Arthritis Rheum* 2008;58(3):903–7.

64. Baraniuk JN, Whalen G, Cunningham J, Clauw DJ. Cerebrospinal fluid levels of opioid peptides in fibromyalgia and chronic low back pain. *BMC Musculoskelet Disord* 2004;5:48.

65. Harris RE, Clauw DJ, Scott DJ, McLean SA, Gracely RH, Zubieta JK. Decreased central mu-opioid receptor availability in fibromyalgia. *J Neurosci* 2007;27(37):10000–6.

66. Schmidt-Wilcke T, Clauw DJ. Pharmacotherapy in fibromyalgia (FM)—Implications for the underlying pathophysiology. *Pharmacol Ther* 2010;127(3):283–94.

67. Simms RW. Fibromyalgia is not a muscle disorder. *Am J Med Sci* 1998;315(6):346–50.

68. Kim SH, Kim DH, Oh DH, Clauw DJ. Characteristic electron microscopic findings in the skin of patients with fibromyalgia—preliminary study. *Clin Rheumatol* 2008;27(3):407–11.

69. Wallace DJ, Linker-Israeli M, Hallegua D, Silverman S, Silver D, Weisman MH. et al. Cytokines play an aetiopathogenic role in fibromyalgia: a hypothesis and pilot study. Rheumatology (Oxford) 2001; 40(7): 743–749

70. Staud R. Is it all central sensitization? Role of peripheral tissue nociception in chronic musculoskeletal pain. *Curr Rheumatol Rep* 2010;12(6):448–54.

71. Affaitati G, Costantini R, Fabrizio A, Lapenna D, Tafuri E, Giamberardino MA. Effects of treatment of peripheral pain generators in fibromyalgia patients. *Eur J Pain* 2011;15(1):61–9.

72. Moldofsky H. The significance of dysfunctions of the sleeping/waking brain to the pathogenesis and treatment of fibromyalgia syndrome. *Rheum Dis Clin North Am* 2009;35(2):275–83.

73. Spitzer AR, Broadman M. A retrospective review of the sleep characteristics in patients with chronic fatigue syndrome and fibromyalgia. *Pain Pract* 2010;10(4):294–300.

74. Epstein SA, Kay G, Clauw D, et al. Psychiatric disorders in patients with fibromyalgia. A multicenter investigation. *Psychosomatics* 1999;40(1):57–63.

75. Wolfe F, Rasker JJ. The Symptom Intensity Scale, fibromyalgia, and the meaning of fibromyalgia-like symptoms. *J Rheumatol* 2006;33(11):2291–9.

76. Turk DC. The potential of treatment matching for subgroups of patients with chronic pain: lumping versus splitting. *Clin J Pain* 2005;21(1):44–55.

77. Giesecke T, Williams DA, Harris RE, et al. Subgrouping of fibromyalgia patients on the basis of pressure-pain thresholds and psychological factors. *Arthritis Rheum* 2003;48(10):2916–22.

78. Giesecke T, Gracely RH, Williams DA, Geisser ME, Petzke FW, Clauw DJ. The relationship between depression, clinical pain, and experimental pain in a chronic pain cohort. *Arthritis Rheum* 2005;52:1577–84.

79. Gracely RH, Geisser ME, Giesecke T, et al. Pain catastrophizing and neural responses to pain among persons with fibromyalgia. *Brain* 2004;127(Pt 4):835–43.

80. White KP, Nielson WR, Harth M, Ostbye T, Speechley M. Does the label "fibromyalgia" alter health status, function, and health service utilization? A prospective, within-group comparison in a community cohort of adults with chronic widespread pain. *Arthritis Rheum* 2002;47(3):260–5.

81. Annemans L, Wessely S, Spaepen E, et al. Health economic consequences related to the diagnosis of fibromyalgia syndrome. *Arthritis Rheum* 2008;58(3):895–902.

82. Goldenberg DL, Burckhardt C, Crofford L. Management of fibromyalgia syndrome. *JAMA* 2004;292:2388–95

83. Carette S, Bell MJ, Reynolds WJ, et al. Comparison of amitriptyline, cyclobenzaprine, and placebo in the treatment of fibromyalgia. A randomized, double-blind clinical trial. *Arthritis Rheum* 1994;37(1):32–40.

84. Häuser W, Bernardy K, Uçeyler N, Sommer C. Treatment of fibromyalgia syndrome with antidepressants: a meta-analysis. *JAMA* 2009;301(2):198–209.

85. Fishbain DA, Cutler R, Rosomoff HL, et al. Evidence-based data from animal and human experimental studies on pain relief with antidepressants: a structured review. *Pain Med* 2000;1:310–6.

86. Arnold LM, Hess EV, Hudson JI, Welge JA, Berno SE, Keck PE, Jr. A randomized, placebo-controlled,

double-blind, flexible-dose study of fluoxetine in the treatment of women with fibromyalgia. *Am J Med* 2002. 112(3):191–7.

87. Dharmshaktu P, Tayal V, Kalra BS. Efficacy of antidepressants as analgesics: a review. *J Clin Pharmacol* 2012;52(1):6–17.

88. Sproule BA, Hazra M, Pollock BG. Desvenlafaxine succinate for major depressive disorder. *Drugs Today (Barc)* 2008;44(7):475–87.

89. Häuser W, Petzke F, Üçeyler N, Sommer C. Comparative efficacy and acceptability of amitriptyline, duloxetine and milnacipran in fibromyalgia syndrome: a systematic review with meta-analysis. *Rheumatology (Oxford)* 2011;50(3):532–43.

90. Hauser W, Petzke F, Sommer C. Comparative efficacy and harms of duloxetine, milnacipran, and pregabalin in fibromyalgia syndrome. *J Pain* 2010;11(6):505–21.

91. Arnold LM, Lu Y, Crofford LJ, et al. *A double-blind, multicenter trial comparing duloxetine with placebo in the treatment of fibromyalgia patients with or without major depressive disorder. Arthritis Rheum* 2004;50(9):2974–84.

92. Gendreau RM, Thorn MD, Gendreau JF, et al. Efficacy of milnacipran in patients with fibromyalgia. *J Rheumatol* 2005;32(10):1975–85.

93. Crofford LJ, Rowbotham MC, Mease PJ, et al. Pregabalin for the treatment of fibromyalgia syndrome: results of a randomized, double-blind, placebo-controlled trial. *Arthritis Rheum* 2005;52(4):1264–73.

94. Moore RA, Wiffen PJ, Derry S, McQuay HJ. Gabapentin for chronic neuropathic pain and fibromyalgia in adults. *Cochrane Database Syst Rev* 2011;3:CD007938.

95. Arnold LM, Goldenberg DL, Stanford SB, et al. Gabapentin in the treatment of fibromyalgia: a randomized, double-blind, placebo-controlled, multicenter trial. *Arthritis Rheum* 2007;56(4):1336–44.

96. Wiffen P, Collins S, McQuay H, Carroll D, Jadad A, Moore A. Anticonvulsant drugs for acute and chronic pain. *Cochrane Database Syst Rev* 2000;(3):CD001133.

97. Russell IJ, Perkins AT, Michalek JE. Sodium oxybate relieves pain and improves function in fibromyalgia syndrome: a randomized, double-blind, placebo-controlled, multicenter clinical trial. *Arthritis Rheum* 2009;60(1):299–309.

98. Holman AJ, Myers RR. A randomized, double-blind, placebo-controlled trial of pramipexole, a dopamine agonist, in patients with fibromyalgia receiving concomitant medications. *Arthritis Rheum* 2005;52(8):2495–505.

99. Russell IJ,, Michaelek JE, Ziao Y, Haynes W, Vertiz R, Lawrence RA et al. Therapy with a central alpha 2-adrenergic agonist (tizanidine) decreases cerebrospinal fluid substance P, and may reduce serum hyaluronic acid as it improves the clinical symptoms of the fibromyalgia syndrome. *Arthritis Rheum* 2002; 46(9):S614.

100. Russell IJ, Kamin M, Bennett RM, Schnitzer TJ, Green JA, Katz WA. Efficacy of tramadol in treatment of pain in fibromyalgia. *J Clin Rheumatol* 2000;6:250–7.

101. Bernardy K, Füber N, Köllner V, Häuser W. Efficacy of cognitive-behavioral therapies in fibromyalgia syndrome—a systematic review and metaanalysis of randomized controlled trials. *J Rheumatol* 2010;37(10):1991–2005.

102. van Koulil S, van Lankveld W, Kraaimaat FW, et al. Tailored cognitive-behavioral therapy and exercise training for high-risk patients with fibromyalgia. *Arthritis Care Res (Hoboken)* 2010;62(10):1377–85.

103. Sañudo B, Galiano D, Carrasco L, de Hoyo M, McVeigh JG. Effects of a prolonged exercise program on key health outcomes in women with fibromyalgia: A randomized controlled trial. *J Rehabil Med* 2011;43(6):521–6.

104. Cazzola M, Atzeni F, Salaffi F, Stisi S, Cassisi G, Sarzi-Puttini P. Which kind of exercise is best in fibromyalgia therapeutic programmes? A practical review. *Clin Exp Rheumatol* 2010; 28(6 Suppl 63):S117–24.

105. Fontaine KR, Conn L, Clauw DJ. Effects of lifestyle physical activity in adults with fibromyalgia: results at follow-up. *J Clin Rheumatol* 2011;17(2):64–8.

106. Fontaine KR, Conn L, Clauw DJ. Effects of lifestyle physical activity on perceived symptoms and physical function in adults with fibromyalgia: results of a randomized trial. *Arthritis Res Ther* 2010;12(2):R55.

107. Williams DA, Kuper D, Segar M, Mohan N, Sheth M, Clauw DJ. Internet-enhanced management of fibromyalgia: a randomized controlled trial. *Pain* 2010;151(3):694–702.

108. Hsu MC, Schubiner H, Lumley MA, Stracks JS, Clauw DJ, Williams DA. Sustained pain reduction through affective self-awareness in fibromyalgia: a randomized controlled trial. *J Gen Intern Med* 2010;25(10):1064–70.

109. Ang DC, Kaleth AS, Bigatti S, et al. Research to Encourage Exercise for Fibromyalgia (REEF): use of motivational interviewing design and method. *Contemp Clin Trials* 2011;32(1):59–68.

110. Cao H, Liu J, Lewith GT. Traditional Chinese medicine for treatment of fibromyalgia: a systematic review of randomized controlled trials. *J Altern Complement Med* 2010;16(4):397–409.

111. Harris RE, Zubieta JK, Scott DJ, Napadow V, Gracely RH, Clauw DJ. Traditional Chinese acupuncture and placebo (sham) acupuncture are differentiated by their effects on mu-opioid receptors (MORs). *Neuroimage* 2009;47(3):1077–85.

112. Wang C, Schmid CH, Rones R, et al. A randomized trial of tai chi for fibromyalgia. *N Engl J Med* 2010;363(8):743–54.

113. Hickie I, Davenport T, Wakefield D, et al. Post-infective and chronic fatigue syndromes precipitated by viral and non-viral pathogens: prospective cohort study. *BMJ* 2006; 333(7568):575.

114. Buchwald D, Freedman AS, Ablashi DV, et al. A chronic "postinfectious" fatigue syndrome associated with benign lymphoproliferation, B-cell proliferation, and active replication of human herpesvirus-6. *J Clin Immunol* 1990;10(6):335–44.

115. Lombardi VC, Ruscetti FW, Gupta JD, et al. Detection of an infectious retrovirus, XMRV, in blood cells of patients with chronic fatigue syndrome. *Science* 2009;326(5952):585–9.

116. Knox K, Carrigan D, Simmons G, et al. No evidence of murine-like gamma retroviruses in CFS patients previously identified as XMRV-infected. *Science* 2011;333:94–7

117. Haig-Ferguson A, Tucker P, Eaton N, Hunt L, Crawley E. Memory and attention problems in children with chronic fatigue syndrome or myalgic encephalopathy. *Arch Dis Child* 2009;94(10):757–62.

118. Majer M, Welberg LA, Capuron L, Miller AH, Pagnoni G, Reeves WC. Neuropsychological performance in persons with chronic fatigue syndrome: results from a population-based study. *Psychosom Med* 2008;70(7):829–36.

119. DeLuca J, Johnson SK, Ellis SP, Natelson BH. Cognitive functioning is impaired in patients with chronic fatigue syndrome devoid of psychiatric disease. *J Neurol Neurosurg Psychiatry* 1997;62(2):151–5.

120. Riley MS, O'Brien CJ, McCluskey DR, et al. Aerobic work capacity in patients with chronic fatigue syndrome. *BMJ* 1990;301:953–6.

121. Harvey SB, Wadsworth M, Wessely S, et al. Etiology of chronic fatigue syndrome: testing popular hypotheses using a national birth cohort study. *Psychosom Med* 2008;70:488–95.

122. Harvey SB, Wadsworth M, Wessely S, et al. The relationship between prior psychiatric disorder and chronic fatigue: evidence from a national birth cohort study. *Psychol Med* 2008;38:933–40.

123. Fukuda S, Kuratsune H, Tajima S, et al. Premorbid personality in chronic fatigue syndrome as determined by the Temperament and Character Inventory. *Compr Psychiatry* 2010;51:78–85.

16

COMPLEX REGIONAL PAIN SYNDROME

Marissa de Mos and Frank J. P. M. Huygen

INTRODUCTION

The complex regional pain syndrome (CRPS) has long been marked with controversy and mystery. It was first described in 1634 by Ambroise Paré, who reported that King Charles IX suffered from persistent pain and contractures following a bloodletting procedure.[1] The next descriptions stem from the American Civil War, where the military physician Silas Weir Mitchell writes, "Long after every other trace of the effects of a wound has gone, these neuralgic symptoms are apt to linger, and too many carry with them throughout long years this final reminder of the battlefield."[2] Its various forms of disease presentation, the absence of one obvious pathophysiological substrate, and the sometimes impressive serious disease course have led to wide speculations about its etiology. This is reflected by the many different names that have been used in the past to address this disorder; the Anglo-Saxon literature alone reveals more than 70 different names, for example, Sudeck's dystrophy (after the German surgeon Paul Sudeck who issued the first scientific publication about the disorder), posttraumatic dystrophy, or sympathetic reflex dystrophy. In 1992 the International Association for the Study of Pain (IASP) decided to end the taxonomic diversity by introducing a new name that was based on description rather than on speculated etiology: complex regional pain syndrome.

CLINICAL FEATURES

CRPS is a painful condition that affects one or more body extremities and that has a wide variety of symptoms, including sensory, vasomotor, sudomotor, motortrophic, and neurologic disturbances (see Table 16.1).[3,4] It has a wide differential diagnosis (see Table 16.2). Some distinguish CRPS type 1 (without evidence of nerve injury) from CRPS type 2 (with evidence of nerve injury), but this is clinically not relevant. Primarily warm and primarily cold CRPS are also distinguished, which refers to whether the affected extremity feels either warm or cold compared to the contralateral side at the onset of the disease. Overall, the clinical presentation of CRPS is very heterogeneous and complaints may vary depending on the time of the day. Likely there are more subtypes to be distinguished, but they remain to be classified.

The onset of CRPS is usually preceded by a physical injury of the extremity that becomes affected later. In most cases this is a fracture or a surgery, but nearly all types of injury have been reported. The upper extremity is more frequently affected than the lower. The typical precipitating injury is a wrist fracture, with a reported occurrence of CRPS of 1%–37%. The initial injury may be very mild, such as a minor sprain or cut. CRPS may even occur spontaneously without identifiable initiating injury, although this is considered rare and in these cases the validity of the CRPS diagnosis is

Table 16.1 Regional Characteristics of Complex Regional Pain Syndrome

SENSORY	VASOMOTOR	SUDOMOTOR	MOTORTROPHIC	OTHER
Spontaneous pain	Warmth	Swelling/edema	Limited range of motion	Disturbed coordination
Hyperesthesia	Coldness	Increased transpiration	Paresis	Tremor
Hyperalgesia	Discoloration	Dryness	Dystonia	Involuntary movements
Allodynia			Altered hair growth	Paralysis
Hyperpathy			Altered nail growth	Muscle atrophy
Paresthesias			Skin atrophy	
Hypoesthesia				

Table 16.2 Differential Diagnosis for Complex Regional Pain Syndrome

Neuropathic pain syndromes

Peripheral neuropathy, nerve entrapment, radiculopathy, post herpetic neuralgia, post CVA deafferentation pain

Myofascial pain syndromes

Strain, repetitive strain injury, disuse, fibromyalgia, myofascial pain not otherwise specified

Degenerative disorders

(Pseudo)arthrosis, tendinosis, malposition or disunion after fracture

Inflammation

Epicondylitis, bursitis, tendinitis, erysipelas, seronegative arthritis, rheumatoid arthritis

Vascular diseases

Thrombosis, artherosclerosis, acrocyanosis, Reynaud's phenomenon, erythromelalgia, Charcot's disease

Psychogenic disorders

Somatoform disorders, Munchuasen's syndrome

subject to debate (see diagnostic criteria). The same accounts for reported cases of CRPS after central body events, such as myocardial infarction or stroke.

Usually, complaints are localized to the distal parts of an affected extremity and follow a sock or glove type pattern. Although the name of the disorder suggests that the complaints are regionally restricted, some suggest that CRPS is also associated with generalized complaints, such as extreme fatigue, headaches, and visceral and bowel disturbances. Moreover, the regional disturbances in CRPS may spread from one extremity to another (9%–32%).[5]

Spread to the contralateral limb (hand-hand or foot-foot) is most common, followed by ipsilateral spread (hand-foot on same side). Diagonal spread is rare and is usually precipitated by a new injury.[6]

The diagnosis of CRPS is based on the evaluation of specific symptoms (subjective or anamnestic) and signs (objective or by physical examination). New diagnostic criteria were introduced by the IASP in 1995,[7] based on expert consensus, and addressed as the "IASP diagnostic criteria for CRPS" (see Table 16.3). Another set of diagnostic criteria was developed by Bruehl and Harden, based on factor

Table 16.3 Two Diagnostic Criteria Sets for Complex Regional Pain Syndrome

IASP criteria

1. Develops after an initiating noxious event (type I) or after a nerve injury (type II)
2. Spontaneous pain or allodynia/hyperalgesia that is not limited to the territory of a single peripheral nerve and is disproportional to the inciting event
3. There is or has been evidence of edema, skin blood flow abnormality, or abnormal sudomotor activity in the region of the pain since the inciting event
4. This diagnosis is excluded by the existence of conditions that would otherwise account for the degree of pain and dysfunction

Budapest criteria

1. Continuing pain that is disproportionate to any event
2. Must report at least one symptom in *three of the four* following categories:

   Sensory: reports of hyperesthesia and/or allodynia

   Vasomotor: reports of temperature asymmetry and/or skin color changes and/or skin color asymmetry

   Sudomotor/edema: reports of edema and/or sweating changes and or sweating asymmetry

   Motor/trophic: reports of decreased range of motion and or motor dysfunction (weakness, tremor, dystonia) and/or trophic changes
3. Must display at least one sign **at time of evaluation** in *two or more* of the following categories:

   Sensory: evidence of hyperalgesia (to pinprick) and/or allodynia (to light touch and/or temperature sensation and/or deep somatic pressure and/or joint movement)

   Vasomotor: reports of temperature asymmetry (>1°C) and/or skin color changes and/or skin color asymmetry

   Sudomotor/edema: reports of edema and/or sweating changes and or sweating asymmetry

   Motor/trophic: reports of decreased range of motion and or motor dysfunction (weakness, tremor, dystonia) and/or trophic changes
4. There is no other diagnosis that better explains the signs and symptoms

For research purposes, diagnostic decision rule should be at least one symptom in all four symptom categories and at least one sign (observed at evaluation) in two or more sign categories

---

analyses of the symptoms and signs in a cohort of 123 CRPS patients. These criteria were modified during a consensus meeting held in Budapest in 2003[8] and have been subsequently referred to as the "Budapest criteria for CRPS" (see Table 16.3). Recent evaluation of both criteria sets[9] in 113 CRPS patients and 47 non-CRPS neuropathic pain patients showed that the IASP criteria lack specificity in comparison to the Budapest criteria. The Budapest criteria are further divided into *clinical* criteria, characterized by high sensitivity (0.99) and less specificity (0.68), and *research* criteria, characterized by less sensitivity (0.78) and higher specificity (0.79). An important difference between the IASP criteria and the Budapest criteria is that the former set does not discriminate between symptoms (subjective) and signs (objective). Remarkable is also that both criteria sets leave discussions about exceptional cases unsolved. Strictly applied, the IASP criteria deny the existence of spontaneous CRPS, since they require an initiating noxious event to confirm the diagnoses. The Budapest criteria rule out another presentation of debate, namely presumed CRPS with all the characteristics of CRPS except spontaneous pain. Although X-radiography, videothermography, nerve conduction tests, and skin biopsies all have demonstrated abnormal findings in CRPS patients, none of them have been sensitive or specific enough to be applied as diagnostic markers. However, they may be indicated in the diagnostic workup to rule out alternative diagnoses that can account for the patient's persistent complaints.

EPIDEMIOLOGY

Two population-based studies have investigated the incidence rate of CRPS, one North American[10] and one European.[11] The first study, in which both case identification and evaluation were performed using an electronic medical file system, yielded an incidence rate of 5.5 per 100,000 person years. The second study, which used an electronic general practitioners' database for case finding, then relied on medical specialist letters and patient visits for diagnostic evaluation and yielded a much higher incidence rate of 20–26 per 100,000 person years. The four- to five-fold difference between these studies may be a result of difference in population characteristics (rural versus urban), ethnicity, or differences in health care insurance systems. However, it is also the result of a difference in diagnosis evaluation strategy, which reflects the problems that arise when a diagnosis is fully based on clinical criteria. Considering the results of the second (European) study, CRPS is not a rare disorder: it has an incidence rate that is higher than, for example, multiple sclerosis and systemic lupus erythematosus. Both studies show a strong female predominance for CRPS: women are three to four times more often affected than men. Although CRPS can occur at any age, even in childhood, the peak incidence rate occurs between the fifth and seventh decade of life, suggesting an increasing risk after menopause. Sexual hormones, especially estrogens, have been suggested to be of importance in the pathophysiology of CRPS; this has been suggested for several autoimmune and chronic inflammatory disorders that show the same female predominance (for example, rheumatoid arthritis and multiple sclerosis). However, similar to these disorders, it seems difficult to unravel the actual relation between CRPS and sex hormones because the available research is scarce. The only study that investigated the association between CRPS and measures of cumulative and actual exposure to both endogenous and exogenous estrogens showed negative results, but it was much limited by its small size.[12] It is remarkable that CRPS patients often have a history of menstrual cycle–related complaints (metro/menorrhagia, dysmenorhea) and also of osteoporosis and migraine, disorders that are recognized to be sex hormone related.[13]

The major risk factor for CRPS is a physical injury to an extremity. By many this is considered a sine qua non for establishing the diagnosis. Severity of the initial injury is not related to the risk of CRPS; neither is the number of fracture repositions or treatment with external fixation. During cast immobilization, increased pressure and early complaints of tightness are predictive factors. A Dutch case-control study on the medical history of CRPS patients revealed that they suffer more frequently from asthma, migraine, osteoporosis, menstrual cycle–related disorders, and neuropathies than controls.[13] Associations with any specific psychiatric or psychogenic disorder were not observed in this study or in many others, although in the past CRPS has often been ascribed to depression, anxiety, and somatization.[14] Case reports describe the co-occurrence of CRPS with chronic inflammatory disorders,[15-21] amyotrophic lateral sclerosis,[22] and Ehlers Danlos syndrome.[23] Moreover, antecedent viral and bacterial infection have been identified as risk factors, including Parvo B19,[24,25] Herpes simplex,[26] Campylobacter jejuni,[27] Borelia burgdorferi,[28,29] and spirochetes,[30] as well as Hepatitis[31] and Rubella[32] vaccination. However, these associations were derived from case reports or very small-sized studies and need further investigation. Finally, there is wide interest for a potential genetic predisposition for CRPS. Associations with several HLA polymorphisms have been found in highly powered studies, although mainly performed in subgroups of CRPS patients with dystonia as a predominant feature.[33] There are families with multiple affected members, but most CRPS cases are sporadic. Siblings of CRPS patients are not at increased risk, unless they are below 50 years of age.[34] There are indications that familial CRPS patients have a younger age at onset, have a longer disease duration, more often show spread to other extremities, and are more often spontaneously affected.[5] This suggests that genetic predisposition for CRPS exists, although it is probably not relevant in the majority of cases.

PATHOPHYSIOLOGY

The disease mechanisms underlying CRPS have been a matter of debate since its first description by Sudeck, who called it an inflammatory disease, and the discussion is still ongoing. The main controversies relate to the inflammatory versus neuropathic nature of the disease and the central versus peripheral primary site of pathology. In the past, CRPS has often been considered an entirely pseudoneurological disease or as a somatoform disorder, but nowadays this narrow view is disregarded by most. Basically, there are five main theoretical disease mechanisms involved in CRPS, including (1) autonomic (sympathetic) nervous system dysfunction; (2) somatic nervous system dysfunction; (3) inflammation; (4) local hypoxia; and (5) psychological factors.[35] In the following paragraphs each mechanism will be addressed separately and then their interactions will be discussed.

Autonomic Nervous System

One of the former names of CRPS was reflex sympathetic dystrophy (RSD), referring to the signs of sympathetic dysregulation. A phenomenon called sympathetically maintained pain (SMP) was considered to cover almost the entire clinical presentation of CRPS. SMP is the description of pain that increases with increased sympathetic outflow, for example, with stress, coldness, or exercise. Nowadays, SMP is no longer regarded as synonymous to CRPS, although it can be one of the features. Not all CRPS patients show SMP, but some do. SMP can be treated by chemically blocking the sympathetic nerve plexus proximal to the affected area, thereby diminishing the sympathetic outflow.[36] After sympathetic suppression, the affected limb will become warm due to vasodilatation and in some cases the pain is successfully relieved. In experimental settings, injections of noradrenaline[37] or

phenylephrine,[38] both direct α-adrenergic receptor agonists, have been shown to increase the hyperalgesia in CRPS patients, even when there is no clear vasoconstriction. The mechanism underlying SMP is postulated to be some kind of coupling between the sympathetic and sensory system, whereby α-adrenergic receptors are expressed on primary afferent nerve endings or on their surrounding support cells.[39] In the presence of this coupling, SMP may result from increased sympathetic outflow itself or from increased local sensitivity to catecholamines, or from a combination of both. The sympathetic hyperactivity in its turn may be caused by inherent hyperactivity or by the loss of spinal inhibitory mechanisms. The hypersensitivity for cathecholamines may be the result of upregulation of α-adrenergic receptors or of receptor alterations that increase their sensitivity. The involvement of such mechanisms in CRPS is supported by the observation of a large density of α-adrenergic receptors in biopsies of the hyperalgesic skin of CRPS patients.[40] Moreover, systemic catecholamine levels in CRPS patients have been measured to be low,[41] which might indicate a local hypersensitivity.

Although there are indications that, in some CRPS patients, sympathetic-afferent coupling is responsible for the pain, it is unclear what initiates this process. There are speculations that small nerve injury can lead to α-adrenergic receptor up-regulation together with increased regional sympathetic nerve sprouting.[39] This may be the response to a temporary depletion of local catecholamines or may be caused by an inflammatory cascade when immune cells invade the injured site. It is clear that much research remains to be done to further elucidate this topic.

Somatic Nervous System

An intriguing feature of CRPS has always been that it shows many characteristics of a neuropathic pain syndrome, while in most patients there is no history of nerve injury or nerve injury demonstrable using neuronal conduction tests. Only a minority of patients (approximately 3%) display CRPS type 2, the subtype that develops after a typical nerve injury.

However, histopathological studies in skin biopsies of CRPS type 1 affected limbs do show neuronal derangements, such as a substantial loss of the normal C and Aδ fibers along with the presence of aberrantly branched fiber endings.[40] In one study the axonal density was reduced by 29% compared to healthy controls, although this varied widely per CRPS patient.[41] Therefore, although major nerve lesions may be absent in CRPS type 1, there are indications that small fiber damage may be of relevance.[42] Small fibers include small-diameter unmyelinated and thinly myelinated axons, and their pathology usually leads to pain and sensory disturbances that are restricted to the area of a single peripheral nerve, but it can also cause microvascular dysregulation, which may be apparent in the vasomotor symptoms and signs of CRPS. Some argue that the injuries that typically precede CRPS, such as bony fractures and soft tissue injury, are just the types of injuries that cause small fiber axon damage because bone and periosteum are densely innervated by such fibers. This is opposite to the clear nerve injuries that specifically affect one large fiber bundle and cause pain that typically follows the innervation area of the damaged nerve.

As with other neuropathic pains, the sensory disturbances in CRPS are not only related to pathology at the affected site itself but also relate to disturbances at the spinal and supraspinal levels of the somatic nervous system. Spinal sensitization comprises a state of hyperexcitability and disinhibition leading to a decreased stimulation threshold, whereby a normally nonpainful stimulus becomes painful. This sensitization is the result of neuronal neuroplasticity,[43] which is the ability of neurons to adapt their phenotype and function in response to altered stimulation patterns, for example, as a consequence of altered afferent input by damaged peripheral nerves. The mechanisms are complicated and not well studied for CRPS in particular, but they likely include the action of neurotransmitters on postsynaptic receptors, such as NMDA, AMPA, and Neurokinin-1 receptors. Finally, the ongoing cortical stimulation can lead to cortical reorganization with altered thalamic blood flow,[44,45] brain activation patterns,[46,47] and sensory mapping,[48,49] objectified in brain imaging and

functional magnetic resonance imaging studies performed in CRPS patients. This leads to perception disturbances, such as impaired tactile discrimination,[52] referred sensations[53,54] and body perception disturbances.[55,57]

Although pain and sensory disturbances are usually considered the major features of CRPS, the motor systems are also affected. Decreased range of motion is common and often not explained by pain alone. In some cases the motor signs are even predominant, such as in patients who develop severe dystonia.[58,59] In study settings, CRPS patients show impaired postsynaptic motor reflex inhibition,[60] hyperexcitability of the motor cortex,[61,62] and cortical reorganization of motor units that correlates with the extent of motor dysfunction.[63,64]

Neurogenic Inflammation

Many features of CRPS are similar to those observed during inflammation, such as pain, redness, warmth, and swelling. In his initial description of CRPS, Sudeck suggested that CRPS might be some kind of acute inflammation of the bone. However, this inflammation theory became abandoned because CRPS patients never displayed systemic signs of inflammation, such as a fever, increased sedimentation rate, C-reactive protein, or leucocytosis. However, treatment with corticosteroids, strong nonspecific inhibitors of inflammation, has been reported effective.[65] Moreover, it was found recently that specific inflammatory mediators are involved in CRPS. There is a proinflammatory cytokine expression profile in fluid derived from artificially produced blistered on CRPS affected limbs compared to the contralateral side, including overexpression of tryptase (a mast cell product), interleukin 6 (IL6), and tumor necrosis factor α (TNFα).[66–68] Similar observations were found in cerebrospinal fluid,[69,70] wherein levels of IL1β and TNFα were elevated compared to controls, and later also in blood,[71,72] wherein the mRNA for IL2 and TNFα was increased together with a decrease in levels of the anti-inflammatory cytokines IL4 and IL6. Furthermore, in plasma there have been found altered expressions of arginine (endothelium related amino acid) and glutamate (NMDA receptor–related amino acid), as well as increased taurine and serotonin levels.[73,74] The levels of at least some inflammatory mediators seem to decrease with long disease duration; however, this was not related to the severity of clinical signs.[75]

The inflammatory response that is likely to occur in CRPS is often referred to as neurogenic inflammation. Neurogenic inflammation is initiated by so-called neuropeptides, which can be excreted by peripheral nociceptive C fibers in response to various triggers, for example, mechanical injury. Such excretory C fibers are mainly located in the distal parts of extremities, the typical location for CRPS. These neuropeptides possess vasoactive and proinflammatory properties and are involved in central and peripheral sensitization. Neuropeptides that have been found elevated in CRPS patients are calcitonin gene-related protein (CGRP) and substance P (SP), as well as bradykinin.[76-78] Many of the inflammatory signs of CRPS could be explained as neuropeptide effects, including vasodilatation (warmth), long-lasting erythema, and plasma protein extravasation (swelling). Even some noninflammatory signs of CRPS could be attributed to neurotransmitters; for example, CGRP promotes hair growth and increased sweating.

CRPS patients show the tendency to develop neuroinflammatory responses more easily than normal. For example, microdialysis with a solution that contains SP evokes a stronger local response (plasma protein extravasation) in CRPS patients than in controls, in the affected as well as the unaffected limbs of CRPS patients.[79,80] The question this observation raises is whether this is an innate characteristic that predisposes someone to develop CRPS, or whether it is a systemic alteration that is caused by the CRPS itself. Compared to the general population, CRPS patients more often have a history of asthma and migraine, both disorders in which neuropeptide effects are involved.[13] Additionally, the use of angiotensin converting enzyme (ACE) inhibitors has been associated with an increased risk of CRPS.[81] ACE metabolizes neuropeptides by degradation, and the lack of its activity can result in neuropeptide accumulation. Such findings argue in favor of the idea that either an increased production and/or a decreased degradation of neuropeptides may predispose a person to develop CRPS after an injury.

Hypoxia

Studies using an animal model for CRPS, the so-called chronic postischemia pain (CPIP) model, suggest that local ischemia and reperfusion (I-R) injury may play a role in the pathogenesis of CRPS.[82,83] In this model, rats develop pain and hyperalgesia but also swelling and discoloration of their hind paw after 3 hours of tourniquet binding. Electron microscopic analysis showed that there was no major nerve injury in these rats; however, similar to human CRPS patients, there was a reduced density of small sensory fibers. Additionally, there were microvascular changes consistent with capillary slow flow/no reflow, resulting in local hypoperfusion and hypoxia, confirmed by increased tissue lactate levels and signs of free oxygen radical accumulation.

I-R injury is a phenomenon mostly described in heart muscle after coronary infarction. It may induce an inflammatory response, arteriolar vasospasms due to imbalanced nitric oxide (NO) and endothelin-1 (ET-1) release, capillary occlusions due to free radical damage to endothelial cells, and small nerve fiber injury due to endoneuronal vessel damage. This whole cascade is enhanced by interactions and positive feedback loops augmenting the inflammation and local ischemia. The developers of the CPIP model state that I-R injury may be relevant in CRPS, at least in some cases. Deep tissue injury can induce edema, causing a local compartment syndrome with tissue perfusion impairments leading to ischemia and reperfusion and its consequences.

Signs of oxidative stress in local tissues have been found in human CRPS patients, such as increased lactate levels,[84] muscle acidosis,[85] and histopathological characteristics that are consistent with hypoxia.[86] Moreover, decreased capillary oxygenation in skin is observed using micro-lightguide spectroscopy[87] and an altered NO/ET-1 balance compared to the unaffected side.[88] Hypoxia and the following acidosis and free radical formation are potent nociceptive triggers, as are inflammatory chemokines. Eventually, this chronic nociceptive stimulation may give rise to sensitization and lead to pain and sensory disturbances.

Psychological Factors

The role of psychological factors is often emphasized for chronic pains in general and for CRPS in particular. Some have suggested the existence of a "CRPS personality," implying that CRPS patients are typically women who show somatizing behavior and may have a secondary gain by their chronic impairments. However, all methodologically well-performed studies have found no clear association between CRPS onset and psychiatric or psychological disturbances[13,89–92] and so the current opinion is that CRPS is not a mainly psychogenic disorder. However, there are two possible explanations for this formerly long-lasting belief. First, before the official diagnostic criteria were published by the IASP, CRPS was diagnosed by the judgment of the treating physician. Often CRPS was used as final explanation for the patient's complaints when all other possible diagnoses were excluded. Likely, the CRPS diagnosis has frequently been given wrongly to patients with atypical limb pains that should have been assigned to a somatoform disorder. Thus, the population of CRPS patients became mixed up with somatoform disorder patients, who display typical somatizing behaviors. A second explanation might be that, similar to other chronic diseases, chronic CRPS patients may develop depression, anxiety, and other psychological complaints. This explanation may be relevant for CRPS patients in particular, since these patients had to cope with the frustrating burden of having severe chronic pains and impairments, for which there was no clear explanation or identifiable somatic substrate.

Although psychological factors do not seem to influence the onset of CRPS, there are indications that specific behaviors may influence the course of the disease, once it has started. Extreme fear of the pain caused by CRPS can lead to kinesiophobia and disuse, which prolong immobilization of the affected extremity, thereby negatively affecting nutritive blood flow and resulting in rigidity and muscle atrophy.[93] Additionally, emotional distress increases the release of catecholamines that cause vasoconstriction and enhance sympathetically maintained pain.[94]

The Complete Picture of Complex Regional Pain Syndrome: Interactions between the Separate Disease Mechanisms

For all the aforementioned mechanisms there is evidence for their involvement in CRPS. Moreover, many mediators involved in one mechanism are known to interact with mediators that are involved in one or more of the other mechanisms (see Fig. 16.1). Likely, CRPS results from a complex cascade of events. The exact starting point is unclear. Since a peripheral injury is usually the trigger, it can be assumed that local damage, via mechanisms as hypoxia and neurogenic inflammation, leads to spinal and supraspinal alterations in sensory and motor processing, resulting in pain and functional impairments. In early CRPS the inflammatory signs are often predominant, while later on they often, but not always, diminish and the neuropathic pain becomes more prominent. However, this does not account for all cases. For example, in some patients the affected extremity is cold instead of warm (inflammatory) from the beginning and signs of sympathetic dysregulation are the predominant features. The clinical picture can differ so broadly between patients that it would be reasonable to classify them into subtypes, according to their main clinical features and associated mechanisms. However, this appears difficult, since there is much overlap in clinical features and there are no routine clinical tests to indicate the underlying processes easily, such as neurogenic inflammation, sensitization, or sympathetic dysregulation. The clinical relevance of subtype classification would be that it could lead to mechanism-based treatment, tailored to the specific disease characteristics of one patient, instead of generalized treatment that may not fully cover the predominant mechanisms.

An important question remains why some persons develop CRPS after an injury, while most persons do not. Even more remarkable is that one person can experience major injury without developing CRPS but does

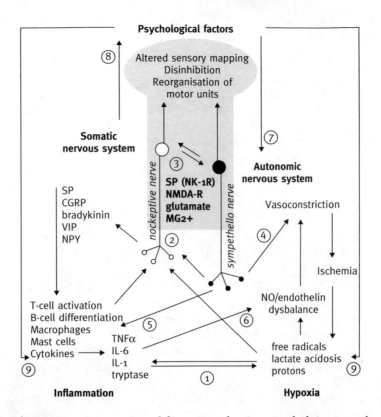

FIGURE 16.1 Schematic representation of disease mechanisms underlying complex regional pain syndrome and how they interact with each other through their mediators. *1*: Hypoxia may trigger inflammatory responses *(hypoxia ↔ inflammation)*; *2*: Continuous nociceptive input by hypoxia, inflammation, or sympathic stimulation may lead to sensitization and alterations in cortical organization of sensory and motor units *(hypoxia, inflammation, and autonomic dysfunction ↔ somatic neuronal dysfunction [sensitization and cortical reorganization])*; *3*: Neuropeptides (SP) released in the dorsal horn may facilitate sensitization trough interaction with NK-1 and NMDA receptors *(inflammation ↔ somatic neuronal dysfunction [sensitization])*; *4*: Sympathic dysfunction (either central sympathic hyperactivity or increased peripheral adrenergic receptor hypersensitivity) may cause hypoxia due to impaired nutritive blood flow *(autonomic dysfunction ↔ hypoxia)*; *5*: Adrenergic receptors can be expressed on immune cells and catecholamines can modulate cellular immunity, while it also has been speculated that inflammation may change sensitivity or expression of α-adrenergic receptors on nociceptive fibers *(autonomic dysfunction ↔ inflammation)*; *6*: Cytokines influence the NO/endothelin balance *(inflammation ↔ hypoxia)*; *7*: Psychological distress may influence sympathetic outflow and levels of catecholamines *(psychopathology ↔ autonomic dysfunction)*; *8*: Severe chronic pain and disability may cause psychological distress *(somatic neuronal dysfunction [sensitization] ↔ psychopathology)*; *9*: Fear of movement may result in the accumulation of inflammatory mediators and free radicals, and prevent desensitization *(psychopathology ↔ inflammation and hypoxia and somatic neuronal dysfunction)*. (Figure extracted with permission from de Mos M, Sturkenboom MC, Huygen FJ. Current understandings on complex regional pain syndrome. *Pain Pract* Mar-Apr 2009;9[2]:86–99.)

develop CRPS after a minor injury at another point in time. Many factors have been studied for their association with CRPS. Presumably intrinsic, extrinsic, and environmental factors all together contribute to a condition wherein a (minor) injury can be the trigger to start the cascade of events. However, at present there is no model or score available that can predict the odds for an injured person to develop CRPS.

TREATMENT

Many different treatments for CRPS are currently applied, often with limited evidence for their effectiveness. This is because clinical trials concerning CRPS are often hampered by the small sizes of their study populations and diagnostic difficulties in patient selection. In daily clinical practice CRPS patients often receive limited benefits to treatments that were successful in trials. An explanation for this may be that the positive results in such trials are attributable to only a specific subset of CRPS patients. Since CRPS is a disease with a very complex etiology that may vary between patients, one generalized standard treatment will be successful in only a subgroup of the patients. Better results may be achieved when patients are classified into subgroups and therefore would receive more tailored treatment. The aim for the future therefore is to classify patients by their predominant underlying disease mechanism and treat them accordingly. At present, the only available source of information for this classification is the clinical features of the patients, such as signs of inflammation, impaired blood flow, neuropathic pain, or motor disturbances. The clinical signs that are most predominant in a particular patient should therefore determine the choice of therapy. The general assumption is that the earlier the therapy is started, the better is the result. Although it has never been demonstrated in a study, this seems reasonable, since early attenuation of inflammatory and hypoxic injury to the nerve will prevent later nerve damage and sensitization.

The use of nonspecific inflammatory inhibitors has yielded limited success in the treatment of CRPS. Corticosteroids have been effective in a few small-sized studies,[65,95] but their use is not common practice in CRPS, probably due to their wide range of adverse effects. Nonsteroidal anti-inflammatory drugs (NSAIDs) have never been proven effective but are prescribed broadly to CRPS patients as analgesics.[96] The effect of specific inflammatory inhibitors, such as anti-TNFα, is under study.[97] Capsaicin, a red pepper substrate, depletes neurons of substance P and is described effective for CRPS in case reports.[98] Free radical scavengers have also been demonstrated effective in both treatment and prevention of CRPS in one French and two Dutch studies.[99-101] Currently, free radical scavengers, including vitamin C, N-acetylcysteine, and dimethylsulfoxide, are the standard treatment for CRPS in the Netherlands, although elsewhere their use is less common. Bisphosphonates also have anti-inflammatory and free radical scavenging properties and have been applied with beneficial effects.[102,103] Mannitol drips have also frequently been administered to CRPS patients, but nowadays they are considered useless and potentially harmful.[104]

All CRPS patients, but especially the ones with motor disturbances, should receive physiotherapy.[53,105] The purpose of this treatment is to improve blood flow, to prevent muscle athrophy, contractures, and kinesiophobia, and to restore function. It is not uncommon that pain and other complaints of CRPS worsen during or within the first hours after a therapy session. It should be explained to the patient that this is unpleasant, but not harmful. Only when the increase in complaints is persistent until the next day should the therapy be resumed at a level of lower intensity.

To improve blood flow, vasodilating drugs can be applied systemically, such as verapamil, ketanserin,[106] or topically as in a cream containing nitric oxide.[107] This is done frequently based on clinical rationale, although there exist no randomized controlled trials to support this treatment with evidence. When strong vasoconstriction is prominent, together with sympathetically maintained pain, a sympathetic block can be applied.[36] Usually, the effect of a test block is evaluated before a permanent block is given.

The neuropathic pains are treated with conventional analgesics and with "coanalgesics," including anti-epileptic and anti-depressant drugs, similar to the treatment of neuropathic pains with other origins. Esketamine is an NMDA receptor antagonist that may prevent or even undo central sensitization and has been administered to CRPS patients both systemically in different infusion regimes and locally by cream or iontophoresis.[108,109] Transcutaneous electrical neurostimulation is a noninvasive and often effective treatment, whereby the electric stimuli overrule the painful sensations. It can be applied for all sorts of (neuropathic) pains and may be effective as an analgesic in some CRPS patients. In extreme therapy-resistant cases with severe disabling pain, insertion of an epidural spinal electronic stimulator device can be considered.[110] This is a highly specialized treatment that is usually performed only in pain clinics and requires lifestyle adjustments and full cooperation of the patient. In cases of dystonia, spasmolytics can be prescribed. Intrathecal baclofen administration has been successful in CRPS patients with otherwise therapy-resistant dystonia, but it carries the risk of complications.[111]

The general opinion is that CRPS patients, especially those with severe and long-lasting disease, gain most benefit by treatment in a multidisciplinary setting, wherein pharmacotherapy, invasive treatment, physiotherapy, ergotherapy, and psychotherapy all together are combined to achieve maximal functional recovery. Currently, there is no standardized, evidence-based treatment protocol available, although local protocols exist. A treatment strategy as provided in Table 16.4 is used in the Pain Treatment Center of Erasmus University Medical Center in the Netherlands. Not all treatment steps are evidence-based due to a lack of double-blinded randomized controlled trials. However, it is meant to provide a practical guideline until more evidence is available. The choice of therapy is based on clinical characteristics of the patient. All patients receive the same basic treatment, namely a free radical scavenger in the form of vitamin C, the only drug that in the Netherlands is considered effective with a high level of evidence, combined with physiotherapy. Further treatment is based on specific clinical features, such as warmth, coldness, dystonia, or severe neuropathic pain.

When a person with a history of CRPS experiences a new physical injury or has to undergo limb surgery, prophylactic treatment should be considered. In the Erasmus Medical Center this is provided by the prescription of vitamin C, once daily 1,000 mg, at the moment of injury or starting 2 days before the scheduled surgery, continuing for at least 5 days after the injury/surgery. Moreover, with limb surgery it is advised to perform regional blocks (for example, a brachial plexus or femoral block) in order to attenuate painful stimuli as much as possible, preventing central sensitization.

PROGNOSIS

Similar to many other aspects of CRPS, the prognosis of the disease is a subject of controversy. It has been stated by some that the majority of patients recover completely within 1 year, even without therapy. However, this opinion is in contrast with other studies that have followed CRPS patients for 1 year or more and report severe remaining complaints, despite intensive therapy. In a Dutch study 102 CRPS patients were visited at, on average, 5.8 years after their CRPS onset and inquired about their ongoing complaints and impairments.[3] A striking observation was that three-quarters of the study population still reported sensory and motortrophic disturbances, while vasomotor and sudomotor disturbances were also prevalent.

Clustering on the remaining symptoms and signs revealed three outcome groups: best (62%), moderate (25%), and poor (13%). In the best outcome group most patients considered themselves recovered or at lease stabilized in their complaints. In the poor outcome group most patients reported to suffer from progressive disease and none of them was able to resume former working activities. The study was too small to identify strong risk factors for poor outcome, although it seemed that poor outcome was associated with CRPS in the upper extremity, cold CRPS, and CRPS that was developed after an "untypical event" (not a fracture).

CRPS patients in the Netherlands consulted, on average, 2.4 different medical specialties, among whom most often consisted of the general practitioner, an anesthesiologist, and a rehabilitation physician.[96] Almost all patients received treatment with oral or topical medication and physiotherapy. Half of the patients additionally received intravenous drug treatment or sympathetic blocks, treatments that require hospital admittance. Twenty-seven percent of the patients were still receiving treatment at the time of study (6 years after disease onset). A third of all patients had completely abandoned their job because of the

Table 16.4 Treatment Strategy for Complex Regional Pain Syndrome as Used in the Erasmus Medical Center, the Netherlands, Based on Clinical Presentation

	WARMTH	COLDNESS	NEUROPATHIC PAIN	DYSTONIA
Step 1	**Vitamin C** once daily 1,000 mg orally **Physiotherapy** twice weekly: activation/ mobilization **DMSO cream** four daily 50% in vaseline/ cetomacrogel	**Vitamin C** once daily 1,000 mg orally **Physiotherapy** twice weekly: activation/mobilization **N-Acetylcysteine** thrice daily 600 mg orally **Verapamil SR** once daily 240 mg **Or** **Ketanserin** Start twice daily 20 mg, increase to 40 mg	**Vitamin C** once daily 1,000 mg orally **Physiotherapy** twice weekly: activation/mobilization **Pregabalin** start once daily 75 mg, increase per 4 days with 75 mg until a maximum dose of twice daily 300 mg	**Vitamin C** once daily 1,000 mg orally **Physiotherapy** twice weekly: activation/ mobilization **Magnesium sulphate** Thrice daily 200 mg orally
Step 2	**Capsaïcin creme** instead of DMSO, four daily 0.075% in vaseline/ cetomacrogel, maximum duration of use 2 weeks, combine with EMLA cream 30 minutes in advance	**add Isosorbidedinitrate cream** 1%, local application four times daily	**add Amitriptyline** Start once daily 25 mg, increase until a maximum dose of thrice daily 25 mg **Or** **add Duloxetine** Start once daily 30 mg, increase until a maximum dose of twice daily 30 mg	**add Clonazepam** Start once daily 2 mg, increase until a maximum dose of twice daily 4 mg
Step 3	**Bisphophonates** Pandromic acid once monthly 60 mg intravenously for 3 months	**add a sympathic block** first a test block; if effective, then a permanent block	**transcutaneous electric neuronal stimulation (TENS)**	**add Baclofen** Start thrice daily 5 mg, increase every 3 days with thrice 5 mg until a maximum dose of thrice daily 25 mg
Step 4	**Infliximab** 1–3 times within 1 month 3–5 mg/kg intravenously		**Opioids**	**add Tizanidine** Start thrice daily 2 mg, increase until a maximum dose of thrice daily 8 mg
Step 5			**epidural spinal electric stimulation**	**intrathecal Baclofen**

impairments produced by CRPS and another 28% had changed their working activities or hours.

CONCLUDING REMARKS

CRPS has long been regarded as a rare disease with a high psychological component that is self-limiting within a not too long period of time. After all the research that has been performed, especially over the past two decades, the opposite seems real: the etiology of CRPS involves a very complex interaction between inflammation, hypoxia, and neuronal damage. Unraveling of the entire pathogenesis has just been started, and much work remains concerning the identification of subtypes with specific underlying pathology. The socioeconomic burden of CRPS is underlined by the relative high incidence and the high prevalence of remaining impairments and work leave, despite intensive and expensive treatment. This justifies further intensive research in the field of CRPS and the search for new mechanism-based treatments.

REFERENCES

1. Dommerholt J. Complex regional pain syndrome-1: history, diagnostic criteria and etiology. *Journal of Bodywork and Movement Therapies* 2004;8:167–77.
2. Mitchell S. Gunshot Wounds and Other Injuries of Nerves. Lippincott, Philadelphia, 1984.
3. de Mos M, Huygen FJ, van der Hoeven-Borgman M, Dieleman JP, Ch Stricker BH, Sturkenboom MC. Outcome of the complex regional pain syndrome. *Clin J Pain* 2009;25(7):590–597.
4. Veldman PH, Reynen HM, Arntz IE, Goris RJ. Signs and symptoms of reflex sympathetic dystrophy: prospective study of 829 patients. *Lancet* 1993;342(8878):1012–6.
5. de Rooij AM, de Mos M, Sturkenboom MC, Marinus J, van den Maagdenberg AM, van Hilten JJ. Familial occurrence of complex regional pain syndrome. *Eur J Pain* 2009;13(2):171–7.
6. van Rijn MA, Marinus J, Putter H, Bosselaar SR, Moseley GL, van Hilten JJ. Spreading of complex regional pain syndrome: not a random process. *J Neural Transm* 2011;118(9):1301–9.
7. Stanton-Hicks M, Janig W, Hassenbusch S, Haddox JD, Boas R, Wilson P. Reflex sympathetic dystrophy: changing concepts and taxonomy. *Pain* 1995;63(1):127–33.
8. Harden RN, Bruehl S, Stanton-Hicks M, Wilson PR. Proposed new diagnostic criteria for complex regional pain syndrome. *Pain Med* 2007; 8(4):326–31.
9. Harden RN, Bruehl S, Perez RS, et al. Validation of proposed diagnostic criteria (the "Budapest Criteria") for complex regional pain syndrome. *Pain* 2010;150(2):268–74.
10. Sandroni P, Benrud-Larson LM, McClelland RL, Low PA. Complex regional pain syndrome type I: incidence and prevalence in Olmsted county, a population-based study. *Pain* 2003; 103(1–2):199–207.
11. de Mos M, de Bruijn AG, Huygen FJ, Dieleman JP, Stricker BH, Sturkenboom MC. The incidence of complex regional pain syndrome: a population-based study. *Pain* 2007;129(1–2): 12–20.
12. de Mos M, Huygen FJ, Stricker BH, Dieleman JP, Sturkenboom MC. Estrogens and the risk of complex regional pain syndrome (CRPS). *Pharmacoepidemiol Drug Saf* 2009;18(1):44–52.
13. de Mos M, Huygen FJ, Dieleman JP, Koopman JS, Stricker BH, Sturkenboom MC. Medical history and the onset of complex regional pain syndrome (CRPS). *Pain* 2008;139(2):458–66.
14. Beerthuizen A, van 't Spijker A, Huygen FJ, Klein J, de Wit R. Is there an association between psychological factors and the complex regional pain syndrome type 1 (CRPS1) in adults? A systematic review. *Pain* 2009;145(1–2):52–9.
15. Bordin G, Atzeni F, Bettazzi L, Beyene NB, Carrabba M, Sarzi-Puttini P. Unilateral polymyalgia rheumatica with controlateral sympathetic dystrophy syndrome. A case of asymmetrical involvement due to pre-existing peripheral palsy. *Rheumatology (Oxford)* 2006;45(12):1578–80.
16. Das A, Puvanendran K. Syringomyelia and complex regional pain syndrome as complications of multiple sclerosis. *Arch Neurol* 1999; 56(8):1021–4.
17. Moroz A, Lee MH, Clark J. Reflex sympathetic dystrophy with hidradenitis suppurativa exacerbation: a case report. *Arch Phys Med Rehabil* 2001;82(3):412–4.
18. Bodur H, Gunduz OH, Yucel M. Reflex sympathetic dystrophy arising in a patient with familial Mediterranean fever. *Rheumatol Int* 1999; 19(1–2):69–70.
19. Wysenbeek AJ, Calabrese LH, Scherbel AL. Reflex sympathetic dystrophy syndrome complicating polymyalgia rheumatica. *Arthritis Rheum* 1981;24(6):863–4.
20. Tsutsumi A, Horita T, Ohmuro J, et al. Reflex sympathetic dystrophy in a patient

with the antiphospholipid syndrome. *Lupus* 1999;8(6):471–3.

21. Ostrov BE, Eichenfield AH, Goldsmith DP, Schumacher HR. Recurrent reflex sympathetic dystrophy as a manifestation of systemic lupus erythematosus. *J Rheumatol* 1993; 20(10):1774–6.

22. de Carvalho M, Nogueira A, Pinto A, Miguens J, Sales Luis ML. Reflex sympathetic dystrophy associated with amyotrophic lateral sclerosis. *J Neurol Sci* 1999;169(1–2):80–3.

23. Stoler JM, Oaklander AL. Patients with Ehlers Danlos syndrome and CRPS: a possible association? *Pain* 2006;123(1–2):204–9.

24. Gross O, Tschernatsch M, Brau ME, et al. Increased seroprevalence of parvovirus B 19 IgG in complex regional pain syndrome is not associated with antiendothelial autoimmunity. *Eur J Pain* 2007;11(2):237–40.

25. van de Vusse AC, Goossens VJ, Kemler MA, Weber WE. Screening of patients with complex regional pain syndrome for antecedent infections. *Clin J Pain* 2001;17(2):110–4.

26. Muneshige H, Toda K, Kimura H, Asou T. Does a viral infection cause complex regional pain syndrome? *Acupunct Electrother Res* 2003; 28(3–4):183–92.

27. Goebel A, Vogel H, Caneris O, et al. Immune responses to Campylobacter and serum autoantibodies in patients with complex regional pain syndrome. *J Neuroimmunol* 2005;162(1–2): 184–9.

28. Bruckbauer HR, Preac Mursic V, Herzer P, Hofmann H. Sudeck's atrophy in Lyme borreliosis. *Infection* 1997;25(6):372–6.

29. Sibanc B, Lesnicar G. Complex regional pain syndrome and lyme borreliosis: two different diseases? *Infection* 2002;30(6):396–9.

30. Neumann RA, Aberer E, Stanek G. Evidence for spirochetal origin of Sudeck's atrophy (algodystrophy, reflex sympathetic dystrophy). *Arch Orthop Trauma Surg* 1989;108(5):314–6.

31. Jastaniah WA, Dobson S, Lugsdin JG, Petty RE. Complex regional pain syndrome after hepatitis B vaccine. *J Pediatr* 2003;143(6):802–4.

32. Genc H, Karagoz A, Saracoglu M, Sert E, Erdem HR. Complex regional pain syndrome type-I after rubella vaccine. *Eur J Pain* 2005;9(5):517–20.

33. de Rooij AM, Florencia Gosso M, Haasnoot GW, et al. HLA-B62 and HLA-DQ8 are associated with complex regional pain syndrome with fixed dystonia. *Pain* 2009;145(1–2):82–5.

34. de Rooij AM, de Mos M, van Hilten JJ, et al. Increased risk of complex regional pain syndrome in siblings of patients? *J Pain* 2009; 10(12):1250–5.

35. de Mos M, Sturkenboom MC, Huygen FJ. Current understandings on complex regional pain syndrome. *Pain Pract* 2009;9(2):86–99.

36. Cepeda MS, Lau J, Carr DB. Defining the therapeutic role of local anesthetic sympathetic blockade in complex regional pain syndrome: a narrative and systematic review. *Clin J Pain* 2002;18(4):216–33.

37. Ali Z, Raja SN, Wesselmann U, Fuchs PN, Meyer RA, Campbell JN. Intradermal injection of norepinephrine evokes pain in patients with sympathetically maintained pain. *Pain* 2000; 88(2):161–8.

38. Mailis-Gagnon A, Bennett GJ. Abnormal contralateral pain responses from an intradermal injection of phenylephrine in a subset of patients with complex regional pain syndrome (CRPS). *Pain* 2004;111(3):378–84.

39. Gibbs GF, Drummond PD, Finch PM, Phillips JK. Unravelling the Pathophysiology of complex regional pain syndrome: focus on sympathetically maintained pain. *Clin Exp Pharmacol Physiol* 2008;35(7):717–24.

40. Drummond PD. Involvement of the sympathetic nervous system in complex regional pain syndrome. *Int J Low Extrem Wounds* 2004; 3(1):35–42.

41. Wasner G, Heckmann K, Maier C, Baron R. Vascular abnormalities in acute reflex sympathetic dystrophy (CRPS I): complete inhibition of sympathetic nerve activity with recovery. *Arch Neurol* 1999;56(5):613–20.

42. Albrecht PJ, Hines S, Eisenberg E, et al. Pathologic alterations of cutaneous innervation and vasculature in affected limbs from patients with complex regional pain syndrome. *Pain* 2006;120(3):244–66.

43. Oaklander AL, Rissmiller JG, Gelman LB, Zheng L, Chang Y, Gott R. Evidence of focal small-fiber axonal degeneration in complex regional pain syndrome-I (reflex sympathetic dystrophy). *Pain* 2006;120(3):235–43.

44. Oaklander AL. Role of minimal distal nerve injury in complex regional pain syndrome-I. *Pain Med* 2010;11(8):1251–6.

45. Woolf CJ. Central sensitization: uncovering the relation between pain and plasticity. *Anesthesiology* 2007;106(4):864–7.

46. Fukumoto M, Ushida T, Zinchuk VS, Yamamoto H, Yoshida S. Contralateral thalamic perfusion in patients with reflex sympathetic dystrophy syndrome. *Lancet* 1999;354(9192):1790–1.

47. Wu CT, Fan YM, Sun CM, et al. Correlation between changes in regional cerebral blood flow and pain relief in complex regional pain syndrome type 1. *Clin Nucl Med* 2006;31(6):317–20.

48. Maihofner C, Forster C, Birklein F, Neundorfer B, Handwerker HO. Brain processing during mechanical hyperalgesia in complex regional pain syndrome: a functional MRI study. *Pain* 2005;114(1–2):93–103.

49. Krause P, Foerderreuther S, Straube A. Effects of conditioning peripheral repetitive magnetic stimulation in patients with complex regional pain syndrome. *Neurol Res* 2005;27(4): 412–7.

50. Maihofner C, Handwerker HO, Neundorfer B, Birklein F. Patterns of cortical reorganization in complex regional pain syndrome. *Neurology* 2003;61(12):1707–15.

51. Pleger B, Ragert P, Schwenkreis P, et al. Patterns of cortical reorganization parallel impaired tactile discrimination and pain intensity in complex regional pain syndrome. *Neuroimage* 2006;32(2):503–10.

52. Pleger B, Tegenthoff M, Ragert P, et al. Sensorimotor retuning [corrected] in complex regional pain syndrome parallels pain reduction. *Ann Neurol* 2005;57(3):425–9.

53. McCabe CS, Haigh RC, Halligan PW, Blake DR. Referred sensations in patients with complex regional pain syndrome type 1. *Rheumatology (Oxford)* 2003;42(9):1067–73.

54. Maihofner C, Neundorfer B, Birklein F, Handwerker HO. Mislocalization of tactile stimulation in patients with complex regional pain syndrome. *J Neurol* 2006;253(6):772–9.

55. Lewis JS, Kersten P, McCabe CS, McPherson KM, Blake DR. Body perception disturbance: a contribution to pain in complex regional pain syndrome (CRPS). *Pain* 15 2007;133(1–3):111–9.

56. Moseley GL. Distorted body image in complex regional pain syndrome. *Neurology* 13 2005; 65(5):773.

57. Forderreuther S, Sailer U, Straube A. Impaired self-perception of the hand in complex regional pain syndrome (CRPS). *Pain* 2004; 110(3):756–61.

58. Morelet A, Gagneux-Lemoussu L, Brochot P, et al. Tonic dystonia: an uncommon complication of reflex sympathetic dystrophy syndrome. A review of five cases. *Joint Bone Spine* 2005;72(3):260–2.

59. van Rijn MA, Marinus J, Putter H, van Hilten JJ. Onset and progression of dystonia in complex regional pain syndrome. *Pain* 2007;130(3):287–93.

60. Schouten AC, Van de Beek WJ, Van Hilten JJ, Van der Helm FC. Proprioceptive reflexes in patients with reflex sympathetic dystrophy. *Exp Brain Res* 2003;151(1):1–8.

61. Schwenkreis P, Janssen F, Rommel O, et al. Bilateral motor cortex disinhibition in complex regional pain syndrome (CRPS) type I of the hand. *Neurology* 2003;61(4):515–9.

62. Eisenberg E, Chistyakov AV, Yudashkin M, Kaplan B, Hafner H, Feinsod M. Evidence for cortical hyperexcitability of the affected limb representation area in CRPS: a psychophysical and transcranial magnetic stimulation study. *Pain* 2005;113(1–2):99–105.

63. Maihofner C, Baron R, DeCol R, et al. The motor system shows adaptive changes in complex regional pain syndrome. *Brain* 2007;130 (Pt 10):2671–87.

64. Krause P, Forderreuther S, Straube A. TMS motor cortical brain mapping in patients with complex regional pain syndrome type I. *Clin Neurophysiol* 2006;117(1):169–76.

65. Kalita J, Vajpayee A, Misra UK. Comparison of prednisolone with piroxicam in complex regional pain syndrome following stroke: a randomized controlled trial. *QJM* 2006;99(2):89–95.

66. Huygen FJ, De Bruijn AG, De Bruin MT, Groeneweg JG, Klein J, Zijlstra FJ. Evidence for local inflammation in complex regional pain syndrome type 1. *Mediators Inflamm* 2002; 11(1):47–51.

57. Munnikes RJ, Muis C, Boersma M, Heijmans-Antonissen C, Zijlstra FJ, Huygen FJ. Intermediate stage complex regional pain syndrome type 1 is unrelated to proinflammatory cytokines. *Mediators Inflamm* 2005;2005(6): 366–72.

68. Heijmans-Antonissen C, Wesseldijk F, Munnikes RJ, et al. Multiplex bead array assay for detection of 25 soluble cytokines in blister fluid of patients with complex regional pain syndrome type 1. *Mediators Inflamm* 2006;2006(1):28398.

69. Alexander GM, van Rijn MA, van Hilten JJ, Perreault MJ, Schwartzman RJ. Changes in cerebrospinal fluid levels of pro-inflammatory cytokines in CRPS. *Pain* 2005;116(3):213–9.

70. Alexander GM, Perreault MJ, Reichenberger ER, Schwartzman RJ. Changes in immune and glial markers in the CSF of patients with complex regional pain syndrome. *Brain Behav Immun* 2007;21(5):668–76.

71. Uceyler N, Eberle T, Rolke R, Birklein F, Sommer C. Differential expression patterns of cytokines in complex regional pain syndrome. *Pain* 2007;132(1–2):195–205.

72. Maihofner C, Handwerker HO, Neundorfer B, Birklein F. Mechanical hyperalgesia in complex regional pain syndrome: a role for TNF-alpha? *Neurology* 2005;65(2):311–3.

73. Wesseldijk F, Fekkes D, Huygen FJ, Bogaerts-Taal E, Zijlstra FJ. Increased plasma serotonin in complex regional pain syndrome type 1. *Anesth Analg* 2008;106(6):1862–7.

74. Wesseldijk F, Fekkes D, Huygen FJ, van de Heide-Mulder M, Zijlstra FJ. Increased plasma glutamate, glycine, and arginine levels in complex regional pain syndrome type 1. *Acta Anaesthesiol Scand* 2008;52(5):688–94.

75. Wesseldijk F, Huygen FJ, Heijmans-Antonissen C, Niehof SP, Zijlstra FJ. Six years follow-up of the levels of TNF-alpha and IL-6 in patients with complex regional pain syndrome type 1. *Mediators Inflamm* 2008;2008:469439.

76. Schinkel C, Gaertner A, Zaspel J, Zedler S, Faist E, Schuermann M. Inflammatory mediators are altered in the acute phase of post-traumatic complex regional pain syndrome. *Clin J Pain* 2006;22(3):235–9.

77. Birklein F, Schmelz M, Schifter S, Weber M. The important role of neuropeptides in complex regional pain syndrome. *Neurology* 2001;57(12):2179–84.

78. Blair SJ, Chinthagada M, Hoppenstehdt D, Kijowski R, Fareed J. Role of neuropeptides in pathogenesis of reflex sympathetic dystrophy. *Acta Orthop Belg* 1998;64(4):448–51.

79. Leis S, Weber M, Schmelz M, Birklein F. Facilitated neurogenic inflammation in unaffected limbs of patients with complex regional pain syndrome. *Neurosci Lett* 2004;359(3):163–6.

80. Weber M, Birklein F, Neundorfer B, Schmelz M. Facilitated neurogenic inflammation in complex regional pain syndrome. *Pain* 2001;91(3):251–7.

81. de Mos M, Huygen FJ, Stricker BH, Dieleman JP, Sturkenboom MC. The association between ACE inhibitors and the complex regional pain syndrome: suggestions for a neuro-inflammatory pathogenesis of CRPS. *Pain* 2009;142(3):218–24.

82. Coderre TJ, Bennett GJ. A hypothesis for the cause of complex regional pain syndrome-type I (reflex sympathetic dystrophy): pain due to deep-tissue microvascular pathology. *Pain Med* 2010;11(8):1224–38.

83. Millecamps M, Coderre TJ. Rats with chronic post-ischemia pain exhibit an analgesic sensitivity profile similar to human patients with complex regional pain syndrome—type I. *Eur J Pharmacol* 2008;583(1):97–102.

84. Birklein F, Weber M, Neundorfer B. Increased skin lactate in complex regional pain syndrome: evidence for tissue hypoxia? *Neurology* 2000;55(8):1213–5.

85. Heerschap A, den Hollander JA, Reynen H, Goris RJ. Metabolic changes in reflex sympathetic dystrophy: a 31P NMR spectroscopy study. *Muscle Nerve* 1993;16(4):367–73.

86. van der Laan L, ter Laak HJ, Gabreels-Festen A, Gabreels F, Goris RJ. Complex regional pain syndrome type I (RSD): pathology of skeletal muscle and peripheral nerve. *Neurology* 1998;51(1):20–5.

87. Koban M, Leis S, Schultze-Mosgau S, Birklein F. Tissue hypoxia in complex regional pain syndrome. *Pain* 2003;104(1–2):149–57.

88. Groeneweg JG, Huygen FJ, Heijmans-Antonissen C, Niehof S, Zijlstra FJ. Increased endothelin-1 and diminished nitric oxide levels in blister fluids of patients with intermediate cold type complex regional pain syndrome type 1. *BMC Musculoskelet Disord* 2006;7:91.

89. Geertzen JH, de Bruijn H, de Bruijn-Kofman AT, Arendzen JH. Reflex sympathetic dystrophy: early treatment and psychological aspects. *Arch Phys Med Rehabil* 1994;75(4):442–6.

90. Geertzen JH, Dijkstra PU, Groothoff JW, ten Duis HJ, Eisma WH. Reflex sympathetic dystrophy of the upper extremity—a 5.5-year follow-up. Part II. Social life events, general health and changes in occupation. *Acta Orthop Scand Suppl* 1998;279:19–23.

91. Nelson DV, Novy DM. Psychological characteristics of reflex sympathetic dystrophy versus myofascial pain syndromes. *Reg Anesth* 1996;21(3):202–8.

92. Reedijk WJ, van Rijn MA, Roelofs K, Tuijl JP, Marinus J, van Hilten JJ. Psychological features of patients with complex regional pain syndrome type I related dystonia. *Mov Disorders* 2008;23(11):1551–9.

93. Singh HP, Davis TR. The effect of short-term dependency and immobility on skin temperature and colour in the hand. *J Hand Surg [Br]* 2006;31(6):611–5.

94. Harden RN, Rudin NJ, Bruehl S, et al. Increased systemic catecholamines in complex regional pain syndrome and relationship to psychological factors: a pilot study. *Anesth Analg* 2004;99(5):1478–85; table of contents.

95. Christensen K, Jensen EM, Noer I. The reflex dystrophy syndrome response to treatment with systemic corticosteroids. *Acta Chir Scand* 1982;148(8):653–5.

96. de Mos M, Huygen FJ, M VDH-B, Dieleman JP, Stricker BH, Sturkenboom MC. Referral and treatment patterns for complex regional pain syndrome in the Netherlands. *Acta Anaesthesiol Scand* 2009;53(6):816–25.

97. Huygen FJ, Niehof S, Zijlstra FJ, van Hagen PM, van Daele PL. Successful treatment of CRPS 1 with anti-TNF. *J Pain Symptom Manage* 2004;27(2):101–3.

98. Ribbers GM, Stam HJ. Complex regional pain syndrome type I treated with topical capsaicin: a case report. *Arch Phys Med Rehabil* 2001;82(6):851–2.

99. Zollinger PE, Tuinebreijer WE, Kreis RW, Breederveld RS. Effect of vitamin C on frequency of reflex sympathetic dystrophy in wrist fractures: a randomised trial. *Lancet* 1999; 354(9195):2025–8.

100. Perez RS, Zuurmond WW, Bezemer PD, et al. The treatment of complex regional pain syndrome type I with free radical scavengers: a randomized controlled study. *Pain* 2003; 102(3):297–307.

101. Cazeneuve JF, Leborgne JM, Kermad K, Hassan Y. [Vitamin C and prevention of reflex sympathetic dystrophy following surgical management of distal radius fractures]. *Acta Orthop Belg* 2002;68(5):481–4.

102. Forouzanfar T, Koke AJ, van Kleef M, Weber WE. Treatment of complex regional pain syndrome type I. *Eur J Pain* 2002;6(2):105–22.

103. Manicourt DH, Brasseur JP, Boutsen Y, Depreseux G, Devogelaer JP. Role of alendronate in therapy for posttraumatic complex regional pain syndrome type I of the lower extremity. *Arthritis Rheum* 2004;50(11):3690–7.

104. Perez RS, Pragt E, Geurts J, Zuurmond WW, Patijn J, van Kleef M. Treatment of patients with complex regional pain syndrome type I with Mannitol: a prospective, randomized, placebo-controlled, double-blinded study. *J Pain* 2008;9(8):678–86.

105. Oerlemans HM, Oostendorp RA, de Boo T, Goris RJ. Pain and reduced mobility in complex regional pain syndrome I: outcome of a prospective randomised controlled clinical trial of adjuvant physical therapy versus occupational therapy. *Pain* 1999;83(1):77–83.

106. Kingery WS. A critical review of controlled clinical trials for peripheral neuropathic pain and complex regional pain syndromes. *Pain* 1997;73(2):123–39.

107. Groeneweg G, Niehof S, Wesseldijk F, Huygen FJ, Zijlstra FJ. Vasodilative effect of isosorbide dinitrate ointment in complex regional pain syndrome type 1. *Clin J Pain* 2008;24(1):89–92.

108. Finch PM, Knudsen L, Drummond PD. Reduction of allodynia in patients with complex regional pain syndrome: a double-blind placebo-controlled trial of topical ketamine. *Pain* 2009;146(1–2):18–25.

109. Sigtermans MJ, van Hilten JJ, Bauer MC, et al. Ketamine produces effective and long-term pain relief in patients with complex regional pain syndrome type 1. *Pain* 2009;145(3): 304–11.

110. Kemler MA, Raphael JH, Bentley A, Taylor RS. The cost-effectiveness of spinal cord stimulation for complex regional pain syndrome. *Value Health* 2010;13(6):735–42.

111. van Rijn MA, Munts AG, Marinus J, et al. Intrathecal baclofen for dystonia of complex regional pain syndrome. *Pain* 2009;143(1–2): 41–7.

17

IRRITABLE BOWEL SYNDROME

Margaret D. Eugenio, Monica E. Jarrett, and Margaret M. Heitkemper

INTRODUCTION

Irritable bowel syndrome (IBS) is a chronic functional gastrointestinal (GI) disorder that disproportionately affects women as compared to men.[1] Currently, no known noninvasive biomarker is predictive or diagnostic for IBS. However, lack of a noninvasive biomarker contributes to the number of diagnostic procedures performed and the clinical burden of this common condition. Functional GI disorders, including IBS, are among the most common and costly health care problems in the United States as well as Europe and Asia.[2–8] Estimates of the prevalence range from 8% to 15%. A recent US survey notes that there is a growing number of reported functional GI disorders, including, IBS in both active duty and returning veterans.[7] The impact of IBS has been quantified by the significant amount of health care resources used (e.g., 8–10 doctor visits; 5 million prescriptions per year).[6,8,9] Costs associated with IBS are affected by disease severity, recent exacerbation of bowel symptoms, and number of health care visits. In several studies, excess surgeries were among the health care events associated with an IBS diagnosis.[10–13] In a survey of over 4,000 IBS patients within a US health maintenance organization, 33% of women with IBS had a history of hysterectomy as compared to 17% in the matched non-IBS group.[12] Also, more hysterectomies were reported in women with IBS in the United Kingdom.[13] However, another US study of African Americans and Caucasians failed to find an increase in abdominal and pelvic surgery in patients with IBS.[14] There are numerous published reports about the negative impact of IBS on quality of life as well as work and school performance.[15,16] A survey in the general population in Sweden reported that GI symptoms, including abdominal pain, affect daily work life of both men and women with IBS.[12] Of the over 3 million people identified in the US National Health Interview Survey as having IBS, 34% rated their health as fair to poor, had an average of 30 sick days a year, and over 20% reported limitations in their activity.[17]

A HETEROGENOUS CONDITION

A constellation of GI symptoms, referred to as the Rome III criteria, is used as the diagnostic criteria for IBS. Specifically, the IBS diagnostic criteria include abdominal pain or discomfort with two of three of the following at least 3 days per month: relief of pain by a bowel movement or pain associated with changes in stool form or frequency. For research, the criteria is pain/discomfort frequency of at least 2 days a week during screening evaluation.[1] As reflected by these criteria, IBS is a heterogeneous condition as evidenced by differences in bowel predominant symptoms (e.g., constipation, diarrhea, alternating stool pattern), symptom frequency (e.g., daily versus weekly), and symptom severity (mild to very severe). To understand the complexity of pain in a heterogeneous condition such as IBS, IBS needs to be viewed within a biopsychosocial framework that considers gender and sex, sociocultural factors, genetics, diet, early childhood adverse events, infection/inflammation, motility, and daily and lifetime psychological distress. This model for IBS originally proposed by Drossman in the 1980s recognizes the contributions of these person and environment factors to patient outcomes, including symptom relief.[18] IBS is likely a multi-component disorder characterized by dysfunctions in GI motor activity, visceral sensation, increased inflammation and intestinal permeability, imbalanced autonomic nervous system, and/or altered processing of internal and external information by the central nervous system. As a functional pain condition, IBS has been linked to other pain-related conditions such as fibromyalgia, migraine headache, and chronic vulvar pain, which have unknown etiology. It may be that for some patients, IBS is part of a chronic widespread pain disorder possibly linked to stress.[19]

GENDER AND IRRITABLE BOWEL SYNDROME

In the United States and other Western and Eastern industrial countries, more women than men seek health care services for IBS.[2,5,20–24] Studies from Asian countries provide equivocal evidence for a gender difference in IBS; that is, some demonstrate a female predominance while others do not.[25–31] The reasons for the gender difference in IBS in the United States remains poorly understood. Gender differences exist in types of GI symptoms (e.g., women report greater problems with constipation while men more frequently report diarrhea) as well as other extraintestinal symptoms.[31] A prospective study of adults with IBS (diagnosed using Rome I criteria) noted that the female to male ratio for IBS could be accounted for by the severity of constipation reported by women.[32]

In a meta-analysis of 22 studies (Fig. 17.1) in which gender differences were examined, Adeyemo and colleagues [33] concluded that gender differences in IBS symptoms exist but that these differences were modest. In the majority of studies reviewed, women were significantly more likely than men to report individual IBS symptoms, including abdominal discomfort. There is some evidence to suggest that gender

differences in symptoms are most pronounced during the peak reproductive years. Thus, it is logical to suspect that reproductive status, in particular ovarian hormones, influence pain/discomfort reporting in at least a subset of women with IBS. Sex differences in opioid, dopaminergic, and serotonergic pain-related systems may contribute to gender differences in symptoms. However, to determine the effect of reproductive status (e.g., menstrual cycle phase, perimenopause transition, postmenopause), it is necessary that, in addition to age, to carefully establish where the women are during their reproductive cycle at time of testing and whether hormone therapies are used. It is interesting to note that one study from Korea[34] found reductions in male hormones, such as testosterone, in men with IBS, suggesting that male hormones may "protect" against IBS. Associations between low testosterone levels and IBS symptoms have also been described.[35]

With regard to menstruating women, there is evidence of menstrual cycle influences on symptom reports with an amplification of bloating, abdominal pain, and looser stools near or at menses.[36–40] The link between menstrual cycle and abdominal discomfort/pain is not limited to IBS. A study of women with gastroparesis also found a rise in symptoms of increased satiety and nausea but no differences in abdominal pain during the luteal phase as compared to the follicular phase.[41] The specific component of the ovarian hormone fluctuations, that is, absolute levels or slope of hormone changes that are linked to menstrual cycle–linked variations in symptoms remains elusive. Receptors for both estrogen and progesterone are found on smooth muscle as well as sensory afferent fibers.[42,43]

Estrogen and progesterone may also influence gut motility, secretion, and pain perception via peripheral release of serotonin.[44] Approximately 95% of the body's serotonin (5-HT) comes from the GI tract, in particular the enterochromaffin cells. Limited data suggest there may be drug therapies directed at stimulating or antagonizing serotonergic receptors in the bowel influence motility and sensitivity. Early studies with alosetron, a 5-HT$_3$ receptor antagonist, revealed that women showed greater therapeutic response when compared

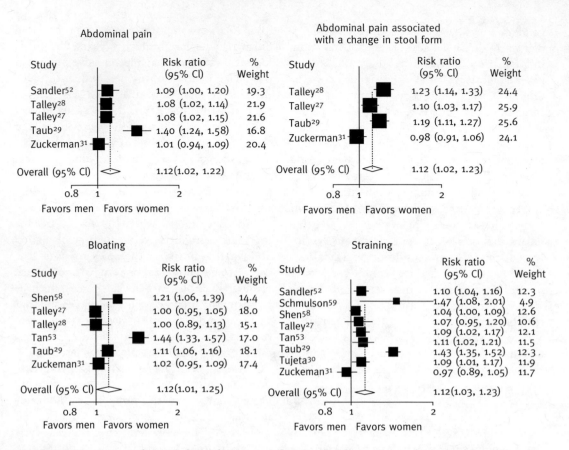

FIGURE 17.1   Forest plots of the risk ratios and 95% confidence intervals for gender differences in general population studies evaluating abdominal pain, bloating, and straining are shown. (From Adeyemo MA, Spiegel BMR, Chang L. Meta analysis: do irritable bowel syndrome symptoms vary between men and women? *Aliment Pharmacol Ther* 2010;32:738–55.)

to men. However, due to the low number of men enrolled in the clinical trials this was not statistically significant.[45] Gender differences in indicators of serotonin uptake into platelets have been reported.[46] Recently Houghton and colleagues demonstrated that patients with IBS diarrhea have higher platelet-depleted plasma (PDP) 5-HT concentrations than healthy controls under fasting and fed conditions.[47] This finding was more pronounced in men with IBS diarrhea as compared to women. Interestingly, in women with IBS the PDP 5-HT levels were higher when the ratio of progesterone to estrogen was elevated. When levels of progesterone and estrogen (menses) were low, the PDP levels were similar to healthy controls. Similar to IBS-D women with high progesterone/estrogen levels, IBS-D men also

have raised PDP 5-HT concentrations. It may be that fluctuations in serotonin concentration in concert with estrogen and progesterone levels across the menstrual cycle contribute to either enhanced intestinal transit or increased secretion in patients with IBS-D. Such findings linking ovarian hormone status with neurochemicals associated with both bowel function and pain sensitivity may be important for drug development as well as treatment protocols focused on women.[48,49]

IRRITABLE BOWEL SYNDROME CATEGORIES

Patients with IBS differ by predominant stool type, severity, and frequency of pain/discomfort; comorbidities, including psychological distress; and somatic complaints, as well as urogynecologic symptoms in women. The use of categories based on predominant bowel pattern (constipation-predominant, diarrhea-predominant, alternating or mixed; IBS-D, IBS-C, IBS-M, respectively; Rome III criteria) has received acceptance by most clinical investigators.[1] Indeed, this categorization commonly dictates drug testing and management. Despite the higher prevalence of IBS in women, a limited number of studies have examined bowel function (motility, transit) in concert with visceral pain perception across reproductive stages. Recent reviews reflect the importance of examining gender during drug development as well as mechanistic studies.[48,49]

In addition to bowel pattern symptoms, investigators have looked at abdominal pain/discomfort to also differentiate the response of patients to treatments. There is evidence that pain and discomfort are relevant to subtyping IBS as well as understanding mechanisms responsible for symptom reports. Women with medically diagnosed IBS report greater daily abdominal pain/discomfort, bloating, and intestinal gas than bowel pattern symptoms of constipation and diarrhea. In women with IBS abdominal pain/discomfort, symptoms correlate more strongly with reductions in quality of life and interference with work and school than bowel pattern (constipation, diarrhea) symptoms. Others have suggested that subgroups of patients with functional GI disorders based on bowel patterns alone may not sufficiently identify clinically distinct entities.[50,51] The severity of bowel and abdominal pain/discomfort symptoms range from mild to severe and disabling. The importance of symptom severity to the disease burden of IBS was recently addressed by Bond and Spiegel.[50,51]

In studies of IBS patient groups, symptom severity often distinguishes those who seek health care services, those at risk for psychiatric morbidity, and those who may need pharmacologic interventions.[51-54] In a Spanish study of 66 health care consulters, 70 nonconsulters, and 117 controls, Rey[15] found that while quality of life was reduced in all subgroups of patients with IBS the degree of impairment was dependent on symptom severity as well as psychological factors, for example, anxiety. Drossman[53] in a study of women with moderate-severe functional bowel disorders noted that women with severe symptoms had higher depression and psychological distress scores, poorer physical functioning and quality of life, poorer coping strategies, and greater health care utilization when compared to those with milder symptoms. In a large cohort study of IBS patients recruited at a university-based center, subjects were asked to complete a bowel symptom questionnaire, which asked "overall severity of GI symptoms," as measured on a 0–20 scale (20 = most severe). Six factors predicted severity, including abdominal pain rating; belief that "something serious is wrong with body"; straining with defecation; myalgias; urgency with defecation; and bloating.[50] Bond[51] using a 4-week diary, found that pain/discomfort, abdominal uneasiness, flatulence/distension, and incomplete evacuation correlated more highly with IBS symptom intensity and that these symptoms contributed the largest component as compared to diarrhea and constipation to the symptom burden in IBS patients. It is evident that within the population with IBS there is a range of symptom distress and that IBS symptom severity as opposed to simply the report of the symptom may be the important outcome variable.

Although there is a lack of clarity as to whether IBS symptom severity represents a distinct physiologic subgrouping in IBS, this possibility was suggested by Kanazawa.[55] Using the barostat, they found that in 44 IBS-diarrhea, 29 IBS-constipation, and 45 IBS-mixed patients, symptom severity was correlated with the pain thresholds. In addition, they noted that IBS-diarrhea and IBS-constipation patients' motility index and barostat baseline muscle tone differed, suggesting that combining severity with bowel type may provide more precision in looking for IBS mechanisms. Drossman[56] utilizing functional magnetic resonance imaging. noted marked differences in an IBS patient over a 16-year period. During severe illness, the patient had a low visceral pain threshold and activation of the midcingulate cortex, prefrontal area, and somatosensory cortex with rectal distention. When the patient improved clinically, there was no longer activation of these three brain areas along with increased tolerance of rectal distention. In healthy male volunteers Coen and colleagues[57] used brain imaging techniques and found that negative emotions induced by emotionally valent music affected the anterior cingulated gyrus and insula, areas involved in processing of painful visceral stimuli. Prior work has also demonstrated that symptom severity in combination with bowel symptom subgrouping is associated with an autonomic nervous system balance index (i.e., heart rate variability) in subgroups of women (age 18–46) with IBS.[58]

The report of abdominal pain/discomfort is a fundamental symptom in the diagnosis of IBS using the current Rome III criteria.[1] One study utilizing a 1-month daily diary found that premenopausal women with IBS (based on Rome II criteria) reported moderate to severe abdominal pain on 37% of days.[59] Although women in all three bowel pattern IBS subgroups (IBS-constipation, IBS-diarrhea, IBS-mixed constipation and diarrhea) reported abdominal pain/discomfort, the severity of abdominal pain/discomfort was not similar across bowel pattern subgroups. For example, the impact on IBS on quality of life was greater in the IBS-diarrhea group, who reported severe abdominal pain severity, while the quality of life impact in the IBS-constipation group occurred regardless of pain severity (Fig. 17.2). Those patients who report more frequent or severe abdominal pain/discomfort also report greater psychological distress, more negative cognitions about IBS, and more interruptions in daily activities. The study of abdominal pain/discomfort within distinct bowel pattern subgroups is challenged by the various methodological approaches that can be taken. Often in clinical practice or research protocols, retrospective questionnaires completed by patients or physician ratings are used. But this information may not capture the typical bowel pattern or pain reports. Digesu,[60] utilizing respondents from urogynecology, gynecology, and colorectal clinics, found that women had difficulty recalling bowel symptoms that had occurred even within a 6-month period. With retrospective measures there is the potential for recall bias to influence responses to bowel questionnaires.

PSYCHOLOGICAL DISTRESS AND IRRITABLE BOWEL SYNDROME

IBS patients are more likely to report psychological distress such as anxiety and depression and more bodily preoccupation relative to healthy individuals as well as patients with organic disease.[61-66] Comorbid psychological disorders are present in approximately 42%–61% of patients with IBS. The importance of psychological factors, for example, depression and anxiety in IBS patients, has been well established.[63-65] IBS patients with higher anxiety and depression scores also report greater impact of IBS symptoms on quality of life and more dysfunctional cognitions about their symptoms. In a recent Swedish study of a total of 268 patients with IBS, 24% of men and 32% of women met the criteria for a possible anxiety disorder using the Hospital Anxiety and Depression Scale (HADS). In this study a significant gender difference (men > women) was found in the depression scale.[69]

Psychological factors, including depression, generalized anxiety, and phobic disorders, influence not only the report of GI symptoms but also other symptoms (fatigue, muscle pain, temporomandiular pain) and may reflect a common theme with other pain-related conditions. Given the range of bowel pattern characteristics and pain/discomfort severity as well as other symptoms, it is not surprising that different etiologies may produce a variety of GI and extraintestinal symptom reports. For a significant number of patients the abdominal pain begins in childhood.[67] Recent attention has focused on the role of early childhood adverse experiences in addition to childhood trauma, for example, physical and sexual abuse, in IBS. Videlock and colleagues found that IBS patients with a history of adverse childhood events exhibited higher cortisol levels after a visceral stressor (sigmoidoscopy) compared to those without this history.[68] In a recent review of animal literature related to maternal separation, O'Mahony proposed that this represents an appropriate model for examination of the links among the microbiome, immune function, and hypothalamic-pituitary-adrenal axis.[69] Stress (both physical and psychological) is identified as eliciting acute and/or chronic

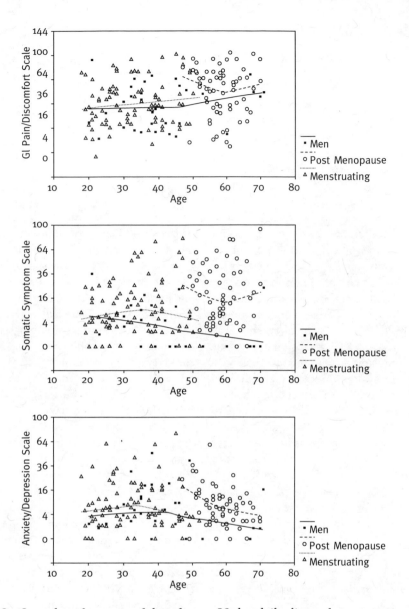

FIGURE 17.2 Scattplot of percent of days from a 28-day daily diary when symptom scales were rated as moderate to severe in men and women with irritable bowel syndrome. (*a*) Gastrointestinal (GI) pain/discomfort (abdominal pain, abdominal distension, bloating, intestinal gas) scale. (*b*) Somatic symptom (backache, headache, joint pain, muscle pain) scale. (*c*) Anxiety/depression (anger, anxiety, panic feelings, decreased desire to talk/move, depressed or blue, fatigue/tiredness, hard to concentrate, sleepiness during day, stressed) scale. (From Cain KC, Jarrett ME, Burr RL, et l. Gender differences in gastrointestinal, psychological, and somatic symptoms in irritable bowel syndrome. *Dig Dis Sci.* 2009;54:1542–49.)

alterations in GI function (e.g., increased intestinal permeability, heightened visceral sensitivity, accelerated intestinal transit). In a study of perceived social support with predominantly female sample (85%), Lackner and colleagues found that lack of social support was associated with pain.[70] The implications are that beyond the physiology of sex differences, the social environment influences symptom distress in patients with IBS.

VISCERAL SENSITIVITY

Enhanced visceral perception is linked to IBS in approximately 50%–80% of patients. Clinically the stimulation of GI visceral afferents via rectal balloon distention results in differential responses in IBS versus non-IBS individuals.[71-77] There are gender differences in visceral sensitivity measures; women exhibit decreased discomfort and lower pain thresholds.[76] Several descriptive, comparative studies assessed sex differences in lower GI perception in IBS patients, although menstrual cycle phase and hormonal therapy were not measured. Ragnarsson[78] in a study of 39 adult women and 13 men with a median age of 40 years reported that women had a more pronounced decrease in maximal tolerable rectal distention than men. Chang[77] compared 58 IBS (34 men, 24 women) and 26 controls (9 men, 17 women) with a mean age of 42 on perception of rectosigmoid stimuli. They found that women with IBS had the lowest discomfort thresholds for rectal stimuli compared with their men counterparts and healthy control women. In addition, they reported that although healthy women had reduced baseline perceptual responses (decreased sensitivity), women as a group, regardless of IBS diagnoses, when compared to men had evidence of sensitization after repeated noxious sigmoid stimulation. A study performed in Korea failed to find differences among IBS and controls or among men and women.[79] However, this study has been criticized for its use of a slow ramp distension paradigm, which has not been found to elicit differences in visceral perception between IBS and controls.

The work of Houghton and colleagues has provided insights into the potential contribution of menstrual cycle phase on visceral sensitivity. In a study of women with IBS, rectal sensitivity (induced by a rectal balloon controlled by a barostat) was increased at menses compared to other cycle phases.[80] Sex-based differences are also found in animal models.[78,79,81] Colorectal distention (CRD) stimulation has been utilized to evoke acute visceral pain as evidenced by avoidance behavior and pseudo-affective reflexes in awake rats.[80,82-84] The CRD behavioral response in animal models can be altered by electrical stimulation of the locus coeruleus/subcoeruleus, major sites of autonomic nervous system regulation.[85]

Visceral hypersensitivity may also explain the role of specific dietary substances in IBS symptoms. Sorbitol, fructose, and lactose intolerance are associated with increased gas production and may subsequently trigger abdominal discomfort secondary to bowel lumen distention.

CENTRAL NERVOUS SYSTEM AND IRRITABLE BOWEL SYNDROME

At the level of the central nervous system, gender differences in brain activation subsequent to visceral stimulation have been found. Female IBS patients show greater activation of limbic and paralimbic regions, including the amygdala and anterior cingulate cortex, whereas male IBS patients demonstrate greater activation of the insula.[85,86] Labus and colleagues[87] monitored startle eye blink reactivity and positrion emission tomography brain imaging and noted that most of the sex-related differences were found in the effective connectivity of the emotional–arousal network. There were fewer gender differences in the cortical-modulatory and homeostatic-afferent network. The investigators concluded that IBS patients with increased trait and state anxiety may allocate increased attention to gut-related symptoms in the absence of any noxious visceral stimuli. For example, women showed consistently stronger connectivity between the pons and the locus coeruleus complex and the medial orbital frontal cortex during all conditions, whereas males consistently showed much weaker engagement of this circuit.[88]

White and gray matter density differences between IBS and healthy controls have been reported. Blankstein described increased density of the hypothalamus in 15 female IBS patients relative to healthy controls.[89] This matches other literature related to alterations of the hypothalamic-pituitary adrenal axis in patients with IBS. Whether this is ultimately linked to increased pain sensitivity or chronic pain experiences of patients remains to be determined. Seminowicz,[90] who used magnetic resonance imaging–based techniques to compare gray matter density in IBS patients

$(n = 55)$ and healthy controls $(n = 48)$, found gender differences in specific brain regions (i.e., medial prefrontal and ventrolateral prefrontal cortex, posterior parietal cortex, ventral striatum, and thalamus) in the IBS patients. However, when anxiety and depression were controlled for, there were no significant gender differences in gray matter density in areas involved in affective processing.

A growing number of studies are focusing on central circuits as well as descending inhibitory influences on visceral pain/discomfort perception in patients with IBS. Using a measure of central processing of noxious stimuli, Heyman and colleagues noted that the female IBS patients exhibited a deficient diffuse noxious inhibitory control relative to controls.[91] This remained statistically significant with psychological state.

AUTONOMIC NERVOUS SYSTEM AND IRRITABLE BOWEL SYNDROME

Farmer and Aziz[92,93] recently highlighted the inconsistencies in the literature surrounding autonomic dysfunction in chronic pain conditions, including IBS, chronic fatigue, and fibromyalgia. Explanations for lack of consistency include the heterogeneity of the conditions (e.g., IBS-constipation, IBS-diarrhea), psychological factors, and different methodologies employed. Gender and age also contribute to innate differences in autonomic nervous system measures. History of abuse and current psychological distress may influence indices of autonomic nervous system function (i.e., reduce vagal tone measures) in women with IBS.[94]

POSTINFECTIOUS IRRITABLE BOWEL SYNDROME AND IMMUNE SYSTEM DYSREGULATION

At one time IBS was considered primarily a brain-gut motility disturbance. However, there is increasing evidence that immune system dysregulation may contribute to the pathophysiology of IBS in at least a subset of patients.[95–98] Examining colonic tissue biopsies, Cremon and colleagues found approximately 50% of the samples had evidence of increased infiltration of T cells and that these observations were gender specific.[95] Men demonstrated higher levels of CD3+ and CD8+ T cells and women greater mast cell infiltration. These histological findings were correlated with self-report of bloating and dyspepsia. Altered inflammatory markers such as the balance of IL-10 and higher levels of pro-inflammatory cytokines such as TNF-α, IL-1β, IL-5, IL-6, and IL-13, have been reported.[99] Other findings suggestive of an inflammatory component include the observation that in approximately 10% of patients, IBS develops following an episode of viral or bacterial gastroenteritis.[97] Visceral hypersensitivity has also been linked to infectious conditions creating the entity "postinfectious" IBS.[97] Gender may also influence the development of IBS following infectious gastroenteritis. In a follow-up study of individuals in the Walkerton Health Study who experienced an acute gastroenteritis due to municipal water contamination, it was found that being female was a risk for later development and persistence of IBS.[100]

SUMMARY

IBS is a common health care problem. Its etiology and pathophysiology are heterogeneous, which makes effective treatment challenging. There are subtle differences in specific GI symptoms as well extraintestinal symptoms. Women seek health care services more often than men, which may be explained by factors other than symptom severity. Gender-related differences in pain perception and processing, inflammatory responses, and autonomic nervous system reactivity may all contribute to the clinical presentation of IBS. In addition, gender role may contribute to overall symptom distress and health care–seeking behavior.[77] Additional research is needed to clarify the mechanisms for sex differences in pain and to develop new treatment modalities that improve pain management for both men and women.

REFERENCES

1. Drossman DA, Corazziari E, Delvaux M, et al. *Rome III the Functional Gastrointestinal Disorders.* McLean, VA: Degnon Associates; 2006.

2. Hillila MT, Farkkila NJ, Farkkila MA. Societal costs for irritable bowel syndrome—a population based study. *Scand J Gastroenterol* 2010;45:582–91.

3. Sandler RS. Epidemiology of irritable bowel syndrome in the United States. *Gastroenterology* 1990;99:409–15.

4. Agarwal N, Spiegel BM. The effect of irritable bowel syndrome on health-related quality of life and health care expenditures. *Gastroenterol Clin North Am* 2011;40:11–9.

5. Cremonini F, Talley NJ. Irritable bowel syndrome: epidemiology, natural history, health care seeking and emerging risk factors. *Gastroenterol Clin North Am* 2005;34:189–204.

6. Brun-Strang C, Dapoigny M, Lafuma A, et al. Irritable bowel syndrome in France: quality of life, medical management, and costs: the Encoli study. *Eur J Gastroenterol Hepatol* 2007;19:1097–103.

7. White DL, Savas LS, Daci K, et al. Trauma history and risk of the irritable bowel syndrome in women veterans. *Aliment Pharmacol Ther* 2010;32:551–61.

8. National Insitutes of Health. US Department of Health and Human Services. *Opportunities and Challenges in Digestive Diseases Research: Recommendations of the National Commission on Digestive Diseases*. Bethesda, MD: National Institue of Health; 2009.

9. Pare P, Gray J, Lam S, et al. Health-related quality of life, work productivity, and health care resource utilization of subjects with irritable bowel syndrome: baseline results from LOGIC (Longitudinal Outcomes Study of Gastrointestinal Symptoms in Canada), a naturalistic study. *Clin Ther* 2006;28:1726–35; discussion 10–11.

10. Cole JA, Yeaw JM, Cutone JA, et al. The incidence of abdominal and pelvic surgery among patients with irritable bowel syndrome. *Dig Dis Sci* 2005;50:2268–75.

11. Lu CL, Liu CC, Fuh JL, et al. Irritable bowel syndrome and negative appendectomy: a prospective multivariable investigation. *Gut* 2007;56:655–60.

12. Longstreth GF, Yao JF. Irritable bowel syndrome and surgery: a multivariable analysis. *Gastroenterology* 2004;126:1665–73.

13. Kennedy TM, Jones RH. The epidemiology of hysterectomy and irritable bowel syndrome in a UK population. *Int J Clin Pract* 2000;54:647–50.

14. Minocha A, Johnson WD, Wigington WC. Prevalence of abdominal and pelvic surgeries in patients with irritable bowel syndrome: comparison between Caucasian and African Americans. *Am J Med Sci* 2008;335:82–8.

15. Rey E, Garcia-Alonso MO, Moreno-Ortega M, et al. Determinants of quality of life in irritable bowel syndrome. *J Clin Gastroenterol* 2008;42:1003–9.

16. Dean BB, Aguilar D, Barghout V, et al. Impairment in work productivity and health-related quality of life in patients with IBS. *Am J Manag Care* 2005;11:S17–26.

17. Hahn BA, Saunders WB, Maier WC. Differences between individuals with self-reported irritable bowel syndrome (IBS) and IBS-like symptoms. *Dig Dis Sci* 1997;42:2585–90.

18. Tanaka Y, Kanazawa M, Fukudo S, et al. Biopsychosocial model of irritable bowel syndrome. *J Neurogastroenterol Motil* 2011;17:131–9.

19. Chen X, Green PG, Levine JD. Stress enhances muscle nociceptor activity in the rat. *Neuroscience* 2011;185:166–73.

20. Faresjo A, Grodzinsky E, Johansson S, et al. A population-based case-control study of work and psychosocial problems in patients with irritable bowel syndrome—women are more seriously affected than men. *Am J Gastroenterol* 2007;102:371–9.

21. Lee V, Guthrie E, Robinson A, et al. Functional bowel disorders in primary care: factors associated with health-related quality of life and doctor consultation. *J Psychosom Res* 2008;64:129–38.

22. Chang L, Toner BB, Fukudo S, et al. Gender, age, society, culture, and the patient's perspective in the functional gastrointestinal disorders. *Gastroenterology* 2006;130:1435–46.

23. Chang L, Heitkemper MM. Gender differences in irritable bowel syndrome. *Gastroenterology* 2002;123:1686–01.

24. Schmulson M, Adeyemo M, Gutierrez-Reyes G, et al. Differences in gastrointestinal symptoms according to gender in Rome II positive IBS and dyspepsia in a Latin American population. *Am J Gastroenterol* 2010;105:925–32.

25. Kubo M, Fujiwara Y, Shiba M, et al. Differences between risk factors among irritable bowel syndrome subtypes in Japanese adults. *Neurogastroenterol Motil* 2011;23:249–54.

26. Kim YJ, Ban DJ. Prevalence of irritable bowel syndrome, influence of lifestyle factors and bowel habits in Korean college students. *Int J Nurs Stud* 2005;42:247–54.

27. Lu CL, Chang FY, Chen CY, et al. Significance of Rome II-defined functional constipation in Taiwan and comparison with constipation-predominant

irritable bowel syndrome. *Aliment Pharmacol Ther* 2006;24:429–38.

28. Tan YM, Goh KL, Muhidayah R, et al. Prevalence of irritable bowel syndrome in young adult Malaysians: a survey among medical students. *J Gastroenterol Hepatol* 2003;18:1412–6.

29. Han SH, Lee OY, Bae SC, et al. Prevalence of irritable bowel syndrome in Korea: population-based survey using the Rome II criteria. *J Gastroenterol Hepatol* 2006;21:1687–92.

30. Gwee KA, Wee S, Wong ML, et al. The prevalence, symptom characteristics, and impact of irritable bowel syndrome in an asian urban community. *Am J Gastroenterol* 2004;99:924–31.

31. Lee OY, Mayer EA, Schmulson M, et al. Gender-related differences in IBS symptoms. *Am J Gastroenterol* 2001;96:2184–93.

32. Herman J, Pokkunuri V, Braham L, et al. Gender distribution in irritable bowel syndrome is proportional to the severity of constipation relative to diarrhea. *Gend Med* 2010;7:240–6.

33. Adeyemo MA, Spiegel BM, Chang L. Meta-analysis: do irritable bowel syndrome symptoms vary between men and women? *Aliment Pharmacol Ther* 2010;32:738–55.

34. Kim BJ, Rhee PL, Park JH, et al. Male sex hormones may influence the symptoms of irritable bowel syndrome in young men. *Digestion* 2008;78:88–92.

35. Houghton LA, Jackson NA, Whorwell PJ, et al. Do male sex hormones protect from irritable bowel syndrome? *Am J Gastroenterol* 2000;95:2296–300.

36. Heitkemper MM, Cain KC, Jarrett ME, et al. Symptoms across the menstrual cycle in women with irritable bowel syndrome. *Am J Gastroenterol* 2003;98:420–30.

37. Heitkemper MM, Jarrett M. Pattern of gastrointestinal and somatic symptoms across the menstrual cycle. *Gastroenterology* 1992;102:505–13.

38. Altman G, Cain KC, Motzer S, et al. Increased symptoms in female IBS patients with dysmenorrhea and PMS. *Gastroenterol Nurs* 2006;29:4–11.

39. Heitkemper MM, Cain KC, Jarrett ME, et al. Relationship of bloating to other GI and menstrual symptoms in women with irritable bowel syndrome. *Dig Dis Sci* 2004;49:88–95.

40. Crowell MD, Dubin NH, Robinson JC, et al. Functional bowel disorders in women with dysmenorrhea. *Am J Gastroenterol* 1994;89:1973–77.

41. Verrengia M, Sachdeva P, Gaughan J, et al. Variation of symptoms during the menstrual cycle in female patients with gastroparesis. *Neurogastroenterol Motil* 2011;23(7):625–e254.

42. Younes M, Honma N. Estrogen receptor beta. *Arch Pathol Lab Med* 2011;135:63–6.

43. Xiao ZL, Biancani P, Behar J. Effects of progesterone on motility and prostaglandin levels in the distal guinea pig colon. *Am J Physiol Gastrointest Liver Physiol* 2009;297:G886–93.

44. Martin VT. Ovarian hormones and pain response: a review of clinical and basic science studies. *Gend Med* 2009;6(Suppl 2):168–92.

45. Ford AC, Marwaha A, Lim A, et al. Systematic review and meta-analysis of the prevalence of irritable bowel syndrome in individuals with dyspepsia. *Clin Gastroenterol Hepatol* 2010; 8(5):401–9.

46. Franke L, Schmidtmann M, Riedl A, et al. Serotonin transporter activity and serotonin concentration in platelets of patients with irritable bowel syndrome: effect of gender. *J Gastroenterol* 2010;45:389–398.

47. Houghton LA, Brown H, Atkinson W, et al. 5-hydroxytryptamine signalling in irritable bowel syndrome with diarrhoea: effects of gender and menstrual status. *Aliment Pharmacol Ther* 2009;30:919–29.

48. Tsynman DN, Thor S, Kroser JA. Treatment of irritable bowel syndrome in women. *Gastroenterol Clin North Am* 2011;40:265–90.

49. Fisher JA, Ronald LM. Sex, gender, and pharmaceutical politics: from drug development to marketing. *Gend Med* 2010;7:357–70.

50. Spiegel B, Strickland A, Naliboff BD, et al. Predictors of patient-assessed illness severity in irritable bowel syndrome. *Am J Gastroenterol* 2008;103:2536–43.

51. Bond B, Quinlan J, Dukes GE, et al. Irritable bowel syndrome: more than abdominal pain and bowel habit abnormalities. *Clin Gastroenterol Hepatol* 2009;7:73–9.

52. Ringstrom G, Abrahamsson H, Strid H, et al. Why do subjects with irritable bowel syndrome seek health care for their symptoms? *Scand J Gastroenterol* 2007;42:1194–203.

53. Drossman DA, Whitehead WE, Toner BB, et al. What determines severity among patients with painful functional bowel disorders? *Am J Gastroenterol* 2000;95:974–80.

54. Creed F, Tomenson B, Guthrie E, et al. The relationship between somatisation and outcome in patients with severe irritable bowel syndrome. *J Psychosom Res* 2008;64:613–20.

55. Kanazawa M, Palsson OS, Thiwan SI, et al. Contributions of pain sensitivity and colonic motility to IBS symptom severity and

predominant bowel habits. *Am J Gastroenterol* 2008;103:2550–61.

56. Drossman DA, Ringel Y, Vogt BA, et al. Alterations of brain activity associated with resolution of emotional distress and pain in a case of severe irritable bowel syndrome. *Gastroenterology* 2003;124:754–61.

57. Coen SJ, Yaguez L, Aziz Q, et al. Negative mood affects brain processing of visceral sensation. *Gastroenterology* 2009;137:253–261, 61 e1–e2.

58. Cain KC, Jarrett ME, Burr RL, et al. Heart rate variability is related to pain severity and predominant bowel pattern in women with irritable bowel syndrome. *Neurogastroenterol Motil* 2007;19:110–18.

59. Cain KC, Jarrett ME, Burr RL, et al. Gender differences in gastrointestinal, psychological, and somatic symptoms in irritable bowel syndrome. *Dig Dis Sci* 2009;54:1542–9.

60. Digesu GA, Panayi D, Kundi N, et al. Validity of the Rome III Criteria in assessing constipation in women. *Int Urogynecol J Pelvic Floor Dysfunct* 2010;21:1185–93.

61. Jerndal P, Ringstrom G, Agerforz P, et al. Gastrointestinal-specific anxiety: an important factor for severity of GI symptoms and quality of life in IBS. *Neurogastroenterol Motil* 2010;22:646–e179.

62. Spiegel BM, Kanwal F, Naliboff B, et al. The impact of somatization on the use of gastrointestinal health-care resources in patients with irritable bowel syndrome. *Am J Gastroenterol* 2005;100:2262–73.

63. de Medeiros MT, Carvalho AF, de Oliveira Lima JW, et al. Impact of depressive symptoms on visceral sensitivity among patients with different subtypes of irritable bowel syndrome. *J Nerv Ment Dis* 2008;196:711–4.

64. Thijssen AY, Jonkers DM, Leue C, et al. Dysfunctional cognitions, anxiety and depression in irritable bowel syndrome. *J Clin Gastroenterol* 2010;44:e236–41.

65. Mykletun A, Jacka F, Williams L, et al. Prevalence of mood and anxiety disorder in self reported irritable bowel syndrome (IBS). An epidemiological population based study of women. *BMC Gastroenterol* 2010;10:88.

66. Choung RS, Locke GR, 3rd, Zinsmeister AR, et al. Psychosocial distress and somatic symptoms in community subjects with irritable bowel syndrome: a psychological component is the rule. *Am J Gastroenterol* 2009;104:1772–9.

67. Chitkara DK, Talley NJ, Schleck C, et al. Recollection of childhood abdominal pain in adults with functional gastrointestinal disorders. *Scand J Gastroenterol* 2009;44:301–7.

68. Videlock EJ, Adeyemo M, Licudine A, et al. Childhood trauma is associated with hypothalamic-pituitary-adrenal axis responsiveness in irritable bowel syndrome. *Gastroenterology* 2009;137:1954–62.

69. O'Mahony S, Chua AS, Quigley EM, et al. Evidence of an enhanced central 5HT response in irritable bowel syndrome and in the rat maternal separation model. *Neurogastroenterol Motil* 2008;20:680–8.

70. Lackner JM, Brasel AM, Quigley BM, et al. The ties that bind: perceived social support, stress, and IBS in severely affected patients. *Neurogastroenterol Motil* 2010;22:893–900.

71. Accarino AM, Azpiroz F, Malagelada JR. Attention and distraction: effects on gut perception. *Gastroenterology* 1997;113:415–22.

72. McKee DP, Quigley EMM. Intestinal motility in irritable bowel syndrome: is IBS a motility disorder? Part 2. Motility of the small bowel, esophagus, stomach, and gall-bladder. *Dig Dis Sci* 1993;38:1773–82.

73. Accarino AM, Azpiroz F, Malagelada JR. Selective dysfunction of mechanosensitive intestinal afferents in irritable bowel syndrome. *Gastroenterology* 1995;108:636–43.

74. Hu WH, Talley NJ. Visceral perception in functional gastro-intestinal disorders: disease marker or epiphenomenon? *Dig Dis* 1996;14:276–88.

75. Berman SM, Naliboff BD, Chang L, et al. Enhanced preattentive central nervous system reactivity in irritable bowel syndrome. *Am J Gastroenterol* 2002;97:2791–7.

76. Houghton LA, Calvert EL, Jackson NA, et al. Visceral sensation and emotion: a study using hypnosis. *Gut* 2002;51:701–4.

77. Lee OY, Mayer EA, Schmulson M, Chang L, Naliboff V. *Am J Gastroenterolog* 2001;96:2184–93.

78. Ragnarsson G HO, Bodemar G. Abdominal symptoms are not related to anorectal function in the irritable bowel syndrome. *Scand J Gastroenterol* 1999;34:250–8.

79. Kim HS, Rhee PL, Park J, et al. Gender-related differences in visceral perception in health and irritable bowel syndrome. *J Gastroenterol Hepatol* 2006;21:468–73.

80. Sanoja R, Cervero F. Estrogen-dependent changes in visceral afferent sensitivity. *Auton Neurosci* 2010;153:84–9.

81. Jackson N, Houghton L, Whorwel P. The menstrual cycle affects rectal sensitivity in patients with irritable bowel syndrome (IBS) but not healthy volunteers. *Gastroenterology* 1997;112:A1132.

82. Wang Z, Guo Y, Bradesi S, et al. Sex differences in functional brain activation during noxious visceral stimulation in rats. *Pain* 2009;145:120–8.

83. Murphy AZ, Suckow SK, Johns M, et al. Sex differences in the activation of the spinoparabrachial circuit by visceral pain. *Physiol Behav* 2009;97:205–12.

84. Liu L, Tsuruoka M, Maeda M, et al. Descending modulation of visceral nociceptive transmission from the locus coeruleus/subcoeruleus in the rat. *Brain Res Bull* 2008;76:616–25.

85. Myers B, Schulkin J, Greenwood-Van Meerveld B. Sex steroids localized to the amygdala increase pain responses to visceral stimulation in rats. *J Pain* 2011;12:486–94.

86. Kilpatrick LA, Ornitz E, Ibrahimovic H, et al. Sex-related differences in prepulse inhibition of startle in irritable bowel syndrome (IBS). *Biol Psychol* 2010;84:272–8.

87. Labus JS, Naliboff BN, Fallon J, et al. Sex differences in brain activity during aversive visceral stimulation and its expectation in patients with chronic abdominal pain: a network analysis. *Neuroimage* 2008;41:1032–43.

88. Tomasi D, Volkow ND. Gender differences in brain functional connectivity density. *Hum Brain Mapp* 2012;33(4):849–60.

89. Blankstein U, Chen J, Diamant NE, et al. Altered brain structure in irritable bowel syndrome: potential contributions of pre-existing and disease-driven factors. *Gastroenterology* 2010;138:1783–9.

90. Seminowicz DA, Labus JS, Bueller JA, et al. Regional gray matter density changes in brains of patients with irritable bowel syndrome. *Gastroenterology* 2011;139:48–57 e2.

91. Heymen S, Maixner W, Whitehead WE, et al. Central processing of noxious somatic stimuli in patients with irritable bowel syndrome compared with healthy controls. *Clin J Pain* 2010;26:104–9.

92. Farmer AD, Aziz Q. Visceral pain hypersensitivity in functional gastrointestinal disorders. *Br Med Bull* 2009;91:123–36.

93. Farmer AD, Aziz Q, Tack J, et al. The future of neuroscientific research in functional gastrointestinal disorders: integration towards multidimensional (visceral) pain endophenotypes? *J Psychosom Res* 2010;68:475–81.

94. Heitkemper MM, Cain KC, Burr RL, et al. Is childhood abuse or neglect associated with symptom reports and physiological measures in women with irritable bowel syndrome? *Biol Res Nurs* 2011;13(4):399–408.

95. Ghoshal UC, Kumar S, Mehrotra M, et al. Frequency of small intestinal bacterial overgrowth in patients with irritable bowel syndrome and chronic non-specific diarrhea. *J Neurogastroenterol Motil* 2010;16:40–6.

96. Cremon C, Gargano L, Morselli-Labate AM, et al. Mucosal immune activation in irritable bowel syndrome: gender-dependence and association with digestive symptoms. *Am J Gastroenterol* 2009;104:392–400.

97. Gwee KA, Leong YL, Graham C, et al. The role of psychological and biological factors in postinfective gut dysfunction. *Gut* 1999;44: 400–6.

98. Alonso C, Santos J. A closer look at mucosal inflammation in irritable bowel syndrome: sex- and gender-related disparities—quantity, quality, or both? *Am J Gastroenterol* 2009;104: 401–3.

99. O'Malley D, Quigley EM, Dinan TG, et al. Do interactions between stress and immune responses lead to symptom exacerbations in irritable bowel syndrome? *Brain Behav Immun* 2011;25(7):1333–41.

100. Marshall JK, Thabane M, Garg AX, et al. Eight year prognosis of postinfectious irritable bowel syndrome following waterborne bacterial dysentery. *Gut* 2010;59:605–11.

18

INTERSTITIAL CYSTITIS/BLADDER
PAIN SYNDROME

Meredith T. Robbins and Timothy J. Ness

INTRODUCTION

As defined by the International Association for the Study of Pain, pain is more than just a sensation but also a response to a sensation. A unique aspect of pain is that it can be modified by psychological factors such as stress and anxiety. When pain arises from particularly private sites or those associated with basic bodily functions, psychological factors become extremely important because they serve both as components of responses and as potential exacerbators of sensation. This is most certainly the case when pains arise in women from structures involved in the processes of reproduction and urination. There is increasing evidence that psychological factors also modify physiological responses to deep tissue stimuli, and this in turn makes the job of a diagnostic clinician challenging. Multiple pelvic structures have innervation that converges within the central nervous system, making symptoms alone inadequate as diagnostic tools. Even a precise history and meticulous physical examination may result in diagnostic ambiguity. Patients may contribute further to the ambiguity by omitting observations they find to be too embarrassing to describe or discuss.

The primary focus of this chapter will be a specific pelvic pain disorder, interstitial cystitis/bladder pain syndrome (IC/BPS), a chronic, debilitating visceral pain syndrome that is characterized by lower abdominal, pelvic and/

or vulvar pain, urinary urgency and frequency, and nocturia. The lack of a validated IC/BPS-specific marker and questions regarding etiology and pathophysiology have not only made the diagnosis and optimal management of IC/BPS particularly challenging but also made its prevalence difficult to determine. Some have put forward the concept of excluding "confusable diagnoses" as a necessary step to the assignment of the diagnosis of IC/BPS, but others have accepted that what is called IC/BPS is a symptomatic descriptive diagnosis that may have multiple etiologies.

FEMALE PREVALENCE

IC/BPS is more common in women than men and was first described in 1915 by Hunner,[1] who described female patients presenting with fibrotic, contracted bladders and distinct ulcers of the bladder epithelium. At that time, it was thought to be an extremely rare condition, but recent epidemiological studies coupled with changing clinical definitions result in quite a different picture. Several different methods of population-based prevalence studies have been utilized to determine the prevalence of IC/BPS. Two self-report studies performed in the 1980s/1990s, using the more stringent criteria of the time, asked participants whether they have ever been diagnosed with the condition; and they reported virtually identical prevalence estimates of approximately 83,000 men and

1,200,000 women across the United States. When symptom assessments are utilized to identify the presence of symptoms suggestive of IC/BPS such as in the 2004 version of the Nurses' Health Study of women ages 58 to 83 years, then the prevalence of IC/BPS appears to be 2.3% of the female population.[2] In that study, prevalence increased from 1.7% in women younger than 65 years to 4.0% in women 80 and older. Data from the Boston Area Community Health study identified that approximately 1% of males and 2% of females surveyed reported symptoms consistent with IC/BPS.[3] Surveying individuals who have been diagnosed with IC/BPS by a clinician is yet another way to estimate prevalence. Using this method, a review of the Nurses' Health Study indicated that the prevalence of IC/BPS was 52–67/100,000.[4] Administrative billing data of patients from the Kaiser Permanente Northwest managed care population suggest a prevalence of IC/BPS of 197/100,000 women and 41/100,000 men.[5] Despite the fact that using different methods results in varied prevalence estimates, it is clear from all of these reports that IC/BPS occurs much more often in women than in men.

CONFUSABLE DIAGNOSES

Pain localized to the lower abdomen, pelvic region, groin, and/or vulva of women falls within the practice of virtually every medical specialty but in particular the specialties of gynecology, urology, and gastroenterology. This kind of pain has multiple etiologies, numerous common comorbidities,[6,7] and the various painful disorders have profound similarities in presentation and examination findings.[8,9] Vulvar, groin, pelvic, and lower abdominal symptomatology constitute some of the most common presenting symptoms for the primary care physician as over 50% of females experience urinary symptoms in their lives and 15%–20% have recurrent vulvar pain (childbirth excluded) at some point in their lives. These pains may originate in the viscera but can also arise from pathology of the nervous system innervating those structures, vascular structures feeding those structures, or musculoskeletal-articular structures. Table 18.1 contains a list of "confusable diagnoses" put forward by the European

Society for the Study of Interstitial Cystitis (ESSIC). Unlike pains arising from the surface of the body, which are well localized and evoke localized motor responses, pains arising from deep structures tend to have relatively poor localization, leading to ambiguity related to the origin of the pain. These pains also tend to produce strong emotional responses, produce immobility coupled with tonic or "spastic" increases in muscle tone and evoke vigorous, nonspecific, autonomic responses such as heart rate changes, sweating, and abnormal bowel or bladder control. Stimuli that predict real or potential tissue damage (e.g., cutting, burning, pinching) always produce reports of pain when applied to the skin but unreliably evoke reports of pain when applied to pelvic organs. However, women use tissue damage-related descriptors (e.g., stabbing) when describing their deep pains, as a *perception* of tissue damage is present even if there is no objective evidence that tissue damage is occurring.

SENSORY PATHWAYS

In women, the peripheral nervous system pathways related to the lower urinary tract are complex, and this is no surprise when one examines the complex embryological development of this region of the body with modifications of structure leading to the formation of the organs utilized for urine formation, storage, and elimination.[10–12] The urinary bladder arises from structures that traversed the developing umbilicus and is still connected to that site by the residual urachus. Because of this, the bladder has an innervation that includes sensory inputs that extend up to the T10 level. Like all structures that physically open their orifices to sacral dermatomes like the bladder does with the urethra, dual spinal innervations exist with both local sacral inputs (pelvic and pudendal nerves; S2–4) and thoracolumbar inputs that "reach down" from those dorsal root ganglia (T10-L2) to travel with the efferent nerve fibers of the sympathetic nervous system through paravertebral ganglia (sympathetic chain). An apparent "gap" in the innervation of lower urinary tract structures is simply the absence of those nerves associated with somites that selectively grew to be the hindlimb

Table 18.1   Relevant Confusable Diseases for Interstitial Cystitis/Bladder Pain Syndrome and How They Can Be Excluded or Diagnosed

CONFUSABLE DISEASE	EXCLUDED OR DIAGNOSED BY
Malignancies	
Carcinoma	Cystoscopy and biopsy
Carcinoma in situ	Cystoscopy and biopsy
Cervical, uterine, ovarian cancer	Physical examination
Prostate cancer	Physical examination and prostate-specific antigen
Urinary tract infections	
Intestinal bacteria	Routine bacterial culture
Mycobacterium tuberculosis	Dipstick; if "sterile" pyuria culture for *M. tuberculosis*
Chlamydia trachomatis	Special culture
Ureaplasma urealyticum	Special culture
Mycoplasma hominis	Special culture
Mycoplasma genitalium	Special culture
Corynebacterium urealyticum	Special culture
Candida species	Special culture
Herpes simplex	Physical examination
Human papilloma virus	Physical examination
Other bladder conditions	
Overactive bladder	Medical history and urodynamics
Bladder neck obstruction	Flowmetry and ultrasound
Neurogenic outlet obstruction	Medical history, flowmetry, and ultrasound
Bladder stone	Imaging or cytoscopy
Lower ureteric stone	Medical history, haematuria, imaging
Bladder retention	Postvoid residual volume measurement
Gynecological conditions	
Endometriosis	Medical history and physical examination
Vaginal candidiasis	Medical history and physical examination
Cervical, uterine, ovarian cancer	Medical history and physical examination
Male diseases	
Prostate cancer	Physical examination and prostate-specific antigen
Benign prostate obstruction	Flowmetry and pressure-flow studies
Chronic nonbacterial prostatitis	Medical history, physical examination, culture
Chronic bacterial prostatitis	Medical history, physical examination, culture
Cystitis: other causes	
Drug-induced cystitis	Medical history
Radiation-induced cystitis	Medical history
Eosinophilic cystitis	
Various	
Pudendal nerve entrapment	Medical history, physical examination, nerve block
Pelvic floor muscle related pain	Medical history and physical examination
Urogenital prolapsed	Medical history and physical examination

Source: Adapted from Van de Merwe JP, Nordling J, Bouchelouche P, et al. Diagnositic criteria, classification and nomenclature for painful bladder syndrome/interstitial cystitis: an ESSIC proposal. *Eur Urol* 2008;53:60–7.

bud (L3-S1). Mixed with spinal innervations are the wandering inputs and outputs of the vagus nerve and an elaborate local ganglionic circuitry. Conglomerations of ganglionic material have been lumped together by anatomists and named the pelvic (inferior hypogastric) and superior hypogastric ganglia or plexuses. Numerous additional names have been utilized and pathways that traverse the celiac and superior mesenteric plexuses to high thoracic levels have been found extensively in other species. Furthermore, thoracolumbar afferents have been demonstrated to travel with sacral afferents via "contamination" of the pelvic nerve by inputs traversing the sympathetic chain. Simply put, the peripheral sensory innervation of urogenital structures is a weblike conglomerate of afferent nerves that travels by numerous paths through nerve plexuses in the pelvis and retroperitoneum to have its heaviest afferent input to the spinal cord at the T10-L2 and S2–4 spinal levels. Figure 18.1 is a schematic description of the innervation of the lower urinary tract. Because the bladder has a plethora of pathways, an attempt to ablate *all* afferent input from it by localized injections or radiofrequency treatments in the pelvis or retroperitoneal spaces is not a realistic goal, although a significant reduction in inputs from a specific structure can occur. Notably, most afferents to the spinal cord have cell bodies located in the dorsal root ganglia. Hence, peripheral ablations affect only axonal extensions of these neurons and spare cell bodies, which have a potential for regeneration, making attempts at permanent denervation difficult if not futile.

Central nervous system pathways related to lower urinary tract sensation have been roughly defined and include nontraditional pain pathways such as the dorsal columns of the spinal cord but also have components that follow the more traditional pathways of the anterolateral white matter (i.e., spinothalamic tract) of the spinal cord.[13,14] Clinical series have demonstrated effective treatment of pelvic organ cancers with dorsal midline ablations in humans,[15] but with only a few exceptions,[16,17] the effect of such lesions on chronic benign pains is yet to be demonstrated and so identical pathways cannot be absolutely inferred. Known sites of tertiary-level supraspinal processing include the thalamus, hypothalamus, mesencephalon, pons, and medulla,[18] and cortical sites of sensory processing related to the bladder, inferred from positron emission tomography and functional magnetic resonance imaging,[19] occur within the midcingulate cortex, bilaterally in the frontal and parietal regions and in the cerebellum. Basic science studies of sensory processing in nonhumans have demonstrated a profound overlap of the sites and substrates of central nervous system processing for multiple urogenital structures (viscero-visceral convergence) and nearby somatic structures (viscerosomatic convergence).

ETIOLOGY AND PATHOPHYSIOLOGY

At present, there is no universally accepted etiology or pathophysiology for IC/BPS. Theories related to its development have centered on various hypotheses that are not mutually exclusive, and a variety of etiologies have been proposed, including disruption of urinary bladder structure,[20] abnormal neuronal function,[21] mast cell activation,[22] presence of antiproliferative substances,[23] and occurrence of developmental insults.[24,25] Any one of these proposed etiologies may be the origin of IC/BPS for a particular patient.

There is good evidence that there is a disruption of the normal urothelial barrier in most if not all of IC/BPS patients as evidenced by the use of the potassium sensitivity test. In this test 40 ml of a potassium chloride solution (40 mEq in 100 ml water) is administered into the bladder by a catheter and responses are observed 3–5 minutes later. A positive test is pain/urgency evoked by the potassium solution, but minimal if any symptoms from water instilled into their bladder.[26] As a provocative diagnostic test for IC/BPS, the potassium test has good sensitivity (70%–90%), but it may lack specificity and so, at present, this test serves to demonstrate increased urothelial permeability that may accompany many painful conditions. Mukerji et al.[27] have proposed greater specificity with the use of ice water to evoke reports of pain from subjects with IC/BPS, but use of that test has not been extensive.

The etiology of the breakdown in the urothelial barrier in IC/BPS and the consequences of

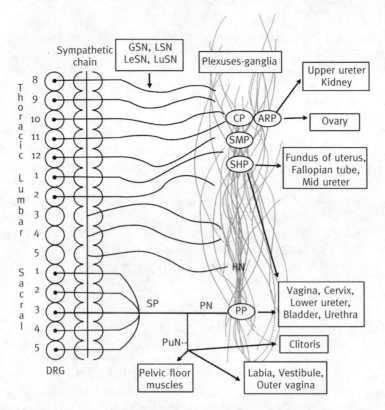

FIGURE 18.1   Schematic diagram of the innervation of urogenital structures in human females. At left, spinal segments of primary afferent entry. Dorsal root ganglia (DRG) with afferent cell bodies are located at thoracolumbar and sacral levels. Primary afferent axons extend through the sympathetic chain and sacral plexus (SP) to join the weblike plexuses of the abdomen via multiple connections, including the greater (GSN), lesser (LSN), least (LeSN), and lumbar (LuSN) splanchnic nerves. Within the abdominal plexus are multiple cellular and nerve fiber gatherings forming plexus-ganglia, including the celiac (CP), aortico-renal (ARP), superior mesenteric (SMP), superior hypogastric (SHP), and pelvic (PP) plexuses. The PP is also known as the inferior hypogastric plexus and is connected with the SHP by the hypogastric nerve (HN). The sacral plexus has multiple branches, including the pelvic nerve (PN), pudendal nerve (PuN) with branches to pelvic floor musculature. Not pictured, the vagus nerve also provides inputs into the abdominal plexus, and the genitofemoral nerve (from L1-L2) provides sensory input to the labia majora (female). Illustration by Emily Ness.

this breakdown are still an issue for debate. One theory proposes that the breakdown of the urothelial barrier is a failure to maintain adequate glycosaminoglycans that provide a protective coating to the urothelium. Other theories propose that IC/BPS is a systemic autoimmune disease presenting as a local manifestation or that abnormal mast cell activity exists within the bladder, which leads to local tissue and neurological effects.[28] Mast cells are present in mucosal, submucosal, and muscular tissues throughout the gastrointestinal system and urinary bladder.[29] Histological and

morphological studies have demonstrated the presence of mast cells in close proximity to sensory neurons, and it is understood that mast cells and nerves fibers engage in crosstalk.[30] Once activated, mast cells release various chemical mediators (degranulation), including vasoactive and pro-inflammatory substances, such as histamine, that can affect neuronal signaling and vascular permeability.[31] Increased mast cell degranulation and increased total numbers of mast cells have been observed in the mucosa of urinary bladder tissues of patients with IC/BPS.[32] Stimulators of mast cell activation/proliferation have been reported to be increased in damaged urothelial cells, as well as in IC/BPS patients, and a number of animal models of cystitis provide support for a role of mast cells in this painful cystitis.[33-35]

Increased levels of nerve growth factor have been noted to be present in the urine of subjects with the diagnosis of IC/BPS, suggesting a potential for neuropathological changes.[36] MicroRNAs have been proposed as epigenetic modifiers of bladder and neuronal tissues.[37] A mechanistic theory relates to the presence of a specific peptide present within the urine of IC/BPS patients that impairs urothelial regrowth.[38] Named APF, this low molecular weight peptide is present in bladder urine, but not renal pelvis urine of IC/BPS patients,[39] is present in over 90% of clinically diagnosed IC/BPS patients from different countries/cultures,[40] and is not present in other disorders. Whether this APF is due to rheumatological, immunological, infectious, genetic, or neurological causes has not been determined, but it has been demonstrated to produce a down-regulation of genes that stimulate epithelial proliferation and up-regulation of genes that inhibit cell growth.[23]

Independent of the specific reason for urothelial disruption, the simplest explanation of the consequences of this breakdown is that it allows an exposure of urinary constituents, bacterial products, and cell death products to bladder sensory nerves that normally are protected by an intact barrier. In addition, the same processes could alter the primary sensitivity of these same nerves. Some alteration of peripheral and/or central nervous system structures occurs in patients with IC/BPS since these subjects are hypersensitive to distending stimuli during cystometric testing,[41] prompting some to propose that IC/BPS also constitutes a type of neuropathic pain.

EFFECT OF PSYCHOLOGICAL FACTORS

It is has been observed that anxiety and stress may also initiate and worsen urinary symptoms in IC/BPS.[42,43] Stress-related mechanisms are associated with inflammatory processes within the bladder that sometimes accompany IC/BPS.[44] The majority of IC/BPS patients

self-report symptom exacerbation by stress.[45] A clinical study examining this relationship using a daily symptom diary demonstrated that IC/BPS patients report greater mean daily stress, as well as greater bladder pain, urgency, and nocturnal frequency, than healthy individuals.[46] The relationship between stress and symptom manifestation in this study became even more evident as severity of the disease increased. Exacerbation of IC/BPS symptoms by stress has also been demonstrated in laboratory studies in which acute mental stress increased urgency and pain.[47] The severe pain accompanying IC/BPS and worry over not having access to a toilet when needed may cause patients to become socially isolated. The fact that symptoms can be aggravated by sexual intercourse can also negatively affect patients' interpersonal relationships. The resulting decreases in social functioning can worsen anxiety and depression, creating a viscous cycle whereby stress and pain are perpetuated.

Stress-induced bladder hypersensitivity has also been demonstrated using animal models of acute and chronic stress. Chronic exposure to footshock and water avoidance stressors enhances abdominal contractions to a urinary bladder distension stimulus, indicating bladder hypersensitivity.[48,49] Acute restraint stress, in which animals are either wrapped with a soft wire mesh and adhesive tape or are placed in a plastic tube similar to the size of the animal for a period of time, activates bladder mast cells and produces morphological changes in the bladder that correlate with histopathological findings in bladder biopsies obtained from IC/BPS patients.[46,50] One particular stressor, neonatal maternal deprivation, has been used extensively as an animal model believed relevant to clinical disease. The neonatal period is often referred to as a stress hyporesponsive period characterized by diminished adrenocorticotropin and corticosterone responses to most stressors. However, this diminished response can be overcome by a severe stressor, such as prolonged maternal deprivation, resulting in permanent alterations in the hypothalamic-pituitary-adrenocortical (HPA) axis. Specifically, major stresses occurring in early childhood cause the HPA feedback loop to become stronger and stronger with each new stressful experience, producing an adult with an extremely sensitive stress circuit. The quality of early life environment helps shape an organism's response to psychological stressors and may increase the risk of maladaptive responses to stressors throughout life. These animal models of stress are being utilized to elucidate the mechanisms underlying stress-induced bladder pain and to gain a better understanding of the relationship between stress and IC/BPS symptom exacerbation.

Epidemiological studies in humans have reported a correlation between medical visits during infancy, particularly those associated with painful events, and associated chronic pains in adulthood.[51-53] Furthermore, adults who repeatedly endured painful procedures as infants have altered pain sensitivity when tested later in life.[54-56] Bladder infections are common during infancy, particularly in the female population, and epidemiologic studies have reported that a subset of adult women diagnosed with IC/BPS recall experiencing early-in-life bladder symptoms.[57]

A series of animals studies has demonstrated that that early-in-life exposure to bladder inflammation can lead to a hypersensitive bladder in adulthood[58,59] that is accompanied by functional changes in the urologic system (increased micturition frequency, reduced micturition volume thresholds) and increased neuropeptide content and neurogenic plasma extravasation in adult bladders, but without altering the structure of the bladder. The early neonatal period is a time of significant developmental plasticity; thus, exposure to painful stimuli or stress during this critical period can alter both somatic and visceral nociceptive pathways, predisposing an individual to various pathologies in adulthood. The adult bladder hypersensitivity induced by neonatal bladder inflammation may be a consequence of direct changes in the nervous system and/or a "priming" of either peripheral or central substrates, which causes the system to overrespond to otherwise benign stimuli later in life.

COMORBIDITIES

IC/BPS is frequently associated with other chronic diseases and pain syndromes such as inflammatory bowel disease, systemic lupus erythematosus, irritable bowel syndrome, "sensitive" skin, fibromyalgia, chronic fatigue syndrome, migraine, and allergies.[6,7] Many of these disorders are characterized as "unexplained nonurological conditions" due to a lack of clear physical or biological etiology or inconsistent demonstration of laboratory abnormalities.[60] Although the reason that IC/BPS often coexists with some of these other chronic conditions remains elusive, Rodriguez et al.[7] proposed a multidimensional model to help explain the overlap of some of these conditions. There are genetic and common environmental factors that predispose individuals to developing chronic syndromes. Initial inciting events (e.g., infection, trauma, and toxins) could lead to the development of one condition, such as IC/BPS, which can then, over time, alter central and autonomic nervous systems and HPA axis responsiveness. Consequently, this patient may develop IBS or other chronic pelvic pains due to enhancement in central nervous system processing of visceral nociceptive information and cross-organ sensitization.

That a majority of these chronic conditions primarily affect women, and clinical pain, such as that associated with IC/BPS, varies as a function of the menstrual cycle suggests obvious potential for the involvement of cyclical ovarian hormones such as estrogen.[61] Gender differences in human pain perception are well documented, and estrogen was postulated as the source of some of these differences.[62-65] To complement these findings in humans, numerous laboratory studies in animals clearly indicate a role for estrogen in nociceptive processing.[66-68] As discussed previously, stress exacerbates symptoms in various chronic conditions. Thus, prolonged stress in an individual with chronic fatigue syndrome, for example, may induce pathophysiological changes (e.g., inflammation, neuroendocrine abnormalities) that could potentially lead to the development of IC/BPS. Diagnosis and treatment of these comorbid conditions is a significant challenge for physicians, but investigations into the mechanisms that may predispose, precipitate, perpetuate, and predict these diseases and disorders will lead to a better understanding of the factors that contribute to IC/BPS.

DIAGNOSTIC WORKUP

As noted before, the diagnosis of IC/BPS is often complicated by the fact that patients frequently have a constellation of symptoms related to other pelvic organs. It is necessary to first rule out other diseases with a similar symptom profile as that of IC/BPS. These include urinary and genital tract infections, tumors of the urogenital and gastrointestinal tract, gynecological tumors, cancer, previous exposure to radiation and chemotherapeutic agents, and endometriosis. Thus, IC/BPS is often a diagnosis of exclusion.

The formal diagnostic criteria for IC/BPS have changed over time from somewhat restrictive to a broader diagnosis as depicted in Table 18.2. Initially, the only inclusion criterion apart from the presenting symptoms was cystoscopic evidence of a bladder mucosal ulceration (a Hunner's patch) or of submucosal petechial hemorrhages following hydrodistension (glomerulations). All other diagnostic criteria were exclusionary and generally done prior to or as part of cystoscopic examination. Using the 1990 NIDDK criteria,[69] Pontari et al.[70] proposed an approach for the evaluation and treatment of IC/BPS that includes urine cultures, pelvic and rectal examinations, cystometry, and cystoscopy prior to assignment of a diagnosis. In 2009 Nickel et al.[71] put forward the UPOINT phenotyping system to direct patients into specific paths for care that might be directed at psychological, infectious, neurological, or musculoskeletal components of the pain without requiring an exhaustive workup process. A broader diagnosis of IC/BPS advocated by the American Urological Association (AUA) in the United States in 2011 built on the guidelines proposed by the ESSIC. Using the more recent definitions, all that is required for the diagnosis of IC/BPS is a 6-week (AUA) or 6-month (ESSIC) or greater history of pain, pressure, or discomfort perceived to be related to the bladder and associated with lower urinary tract symptoms (e.g., urgency, frequency), which cannot be attributed to other causes such as infection, tumor, or structural abnormality. The AUA has put forth guidelines[72] for evaluation that progress from the minimally invasive to more invasive as dictated by responses to therapies that start conservatively and become more complex if there is a lack of response to treatment.

The use of intravesical potassium solutions as a provocative diagnostic test for IC/BPS has been advocated with a sensitivity of 75%. This test is rarely (≤4%) positive in control subjects who are devoid of other symptomatology, but it is positive in the presence of other forms of cystitis (infectious, postradiation), urethral syndrome,[73] and in gynecological patients who also carry the diagnoses of endometriosis, vulvodynia, and unspecified pelvic pain.[73,74] There is a high correlation of positive potassium tests with abnormal urodynamic studies suggestive of a hyperactive bladder.[75] The best evidence for a laboratory test for IC/BPS indicates that urinary levels of antiproliferative factor (APF) are the most sensitive and selective measures developed to date,[76] although this measure is still predominantly a research tool. APF, which inhibits the development of epithelial cells, was first isolated in the urine of a number of IC/BPS patients by Keay et al.[39]

The presence of a Hunner's patch separates IC/BPS patients into those with ulcerative versus nonulcerative types. Glomerulations are not unique to IC/BPS, but they occur in other forms of cystitis (e.g., radiation cystitis) and may be a normal variant since one study found that they were common in asymptomatic female subjects undergoing tubal ligation surgery.[77] The change in definition has and will lead to some confusion related to epidemiology of the disorders and responses to therapy, and there will likely be additional evolution of nomenclature.

TREATMENT

An algorithm of treatments for IC/BPS is given in Figure 18.2 and is an adaptation of the recommendations of the AUA.[72] First-line treatments include education, behavioral therapies (e.g., stress management), and self-care strategies such as timed voiding. Dietary modification to avoid foods that exacerbate symptoms (e.g., acidic foods such as cranberry juice) has much anecdotal support.[78] The working assumption of dietary restriction is that certain foods are excreted into urine, making it more "toxic" and therefore eliciting pain. Alkalinization of the urine has been utilized as an early therapeutic.

Table 18.2   Interstitial Cystitis/Bladder Pain Syndrome Diagnostic Criteria

CRITERIA	NIDDK WORKSHOP ON INTERSTITIAL CYSTITIS (WEIN ET AL., 1990)	AUA AND ESSIC FOR IC/BPS
Inclusion	Hunner's (mucosal) ulcer or glomerulations on cystoscopy	Pain, pressure, or discomfort for >6 weeks (AUA) >6 months (ESSIC)
	Pain associated with the bladder or urinary urgency	Lower urinary tract symptoms (frequency, urgency)
Exclusion	Age <18 years old	Other "confusable" diagnoses
	Symptomatic urethral diverticulum	(e.g., infection, cancer,
	Radiation cystitis	structural, neurological, other)
	Uterine/cervical cancer	
	Vaginal or urethral cancer	
	Cyclophoshamide cystitis	
	Tuberculous cystitis	
	Benign or malignant bladder tumors	
	Bacterial cystitis or prostatitis	
	Active genital herpes in last 3 months	
	Bladder or lower ureteral calculi	
	Vaginitis	
	Duration <9 months	
	Involuntary bladder contractions	
	Absence of nocturia	
	No urgency with bladder fill >350 cc	
	Frequency <8 times per day	
	Absence of urgency with 100 cc air or 150 cc water (fill rate 30–100 cc/min)	
	Symptoms relieved by antibiotics, urinary antiseptics, anticholinergics, or antispasmotics	

AUA, American Urological Association—guidelines in Hanno et al., 2011[ref. 72]; ESSIC, European Society for the Study of Interstitial Cystitis—guidelines in Van de Merwe et al., 2008 [ref. 105]; IC/BPS, interstitial cystitis/bladder pain syndrome.

As part of the diagnostic process, low-pressure hydrodistension is often performed and this procedure itself often proves to be therapeutic with short-term reductions in frequency and pain in more than half of the patients.[79] Patients with symptomatic improvement for 6 months or more are considered candidates for repeat hydrodistension. Other urological procedural treatments also include those related to bladder outlet obstruction (if identified[80]) and ablation/corticosteroid injection of Hunner's lesions when present.[81] In some cases anesthetic interventional procedures such as nerve blocks have been reported as efficacious: a report of a series of 13 patients by Irwin et al.[82] suggests that lumbar epidural local anesthetic blocks may have short-term efficacy in up to 75% of patients.

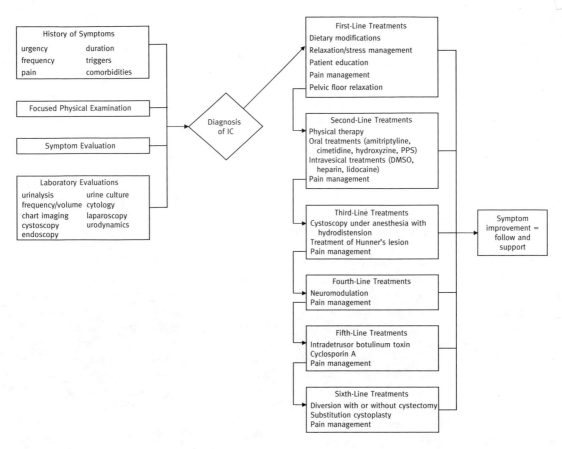

FIGURE 18.2   Diagnosis of interstitial cystitis.

Prior to interventional treatments or invasive diagnostic procedures, trials of medical therapy are now considered to be appropriate.[72] Open trials of antidepressants have produced reported success rates of 64%–90%.[83,84] Controlled multicenter trials have demonstrated benefit of amitriptyline at doses >50 mg in treatment-naïve IC/BPS patients[85] and mixed results with other antidepressants.[86] Oral antihistamines of both types (e.g., hydroxyzine, cimetidine) have been reported to produce a reduction in symptoms and have been recommended as an early treatment option.[72] The oral, renally excreted heparin-like agent pentosan polysulfate (Elmiron®) has been examined in several placebo-controlled, double-blind studies. The rationale for use of this substance is that it supplements or replaces missing protective urothelial surface substances. Combination therapies of drugs such as pentosanpolysulfate with hydroxyzine have been attempted but with mixed results to date.[87,88]

For subjects with a significant menstrual cycle exacerbation of their bladder symptoms, hormonal manipulation may prove to be beneficial.[89] Based on the hypothesis that IC/BPS is a local manifestation of a systemic autoimmune disease, immunosuppressant therapies such as systemic cyclosporine have been trialed in a controlled fashion with good success and limited toxicity.[90,91] Recommendations against use of systemic corticosteroids or long-term oral antibiotics have been given.[72] Long-term treatment with opioids is an option in patients with IC/BPS, but this treatment remains controversial for all nonmalignant processes.

Intravesical therapy with multiple agents such as local anesthetics, dimethyl sulfoxide, heparin, pentosan polysulfate, hyaluronic acid, oxybutyrin, resiniferatoxin, Bacillus Calmette-Guerin, corticosteroids, Chlorpactin (a derivative of hypochlorous acid in a buffered base), and/or bicarbonate have all been proposed as effective therapies[92–96] with success rates ranging from 50% to >90%. Notably, recent guidelines noted earlier[72] recommend against standard clinical use of resiniferatoxin or Bacillus Calmette-Guerin. Most intravescial therapies have been reported as producing short-term effects. Intravesical and pelvic intramuscular injections of botulinum toxin A have also been utilized for symptomatic relief and also been demonstrated to have short-term effects in subjects with IC/BPS refractory to other treatments.[72,97]

Neuromodulation has found an increasing role in the management of urogenital symptoms, particularly the urgency/frequency associated with IC/BPS such that it is now considered part of standard therapy.[72] Transcutaneous electrical nerve stimulation has been used in open trials and demonstrated to produce good results or remission in 26%–54% of patients.[98] Other neuromodulatory devices such as direct sacral nerve root stimulation, spinal cord stimulation, and pudendal nerve stimulation have had increasingly supportive literature related to their use.[99–102] There have been clear benefits associated with symptoms of urgency and frequency but mixed benefits in relation to pain control. Some secondary effects on other pelvic organ functions such as bowel function have also been reported.[103] Like most procedural treatments, large-scale, controlled studies are still needed to fully assess both benefits and potential complications associated with these therapeutics.

Neurolysis by percutaneous injection or surgical resection has been described as a treatment for IC/BPS, but it is an infrequently utilized therapeutic. Gillespie[104] reported that two-thirds of the 175 IC/BPS patients treated with laser obliteration of the vesicoureteric plexus bilaterally reported complete relief immediately following the procedure. The other third of patients reported partial relief. A 2-year follow-up of 45 patients in the "complete relief" group demonstrated no recurrence of symptoms.

Often considered a last resort, surgery in the form of supravesical diversions or cystectomy has also received mixed reports of efficacy. It is the last line of treatment put forward as part of the AUA algorithm for treating IC/BPS.[72] Peeker et al.[105] have reported excellent results in patients with classic (ulcerative) IC/BPS and poor results in nonulcerative IC/BPS. Webster et al.[106] reported that only 2 of their 14 patients treated surgically with urinary diversion and cystourethrectomy had symptom resolution and Baskin and Tanagho[107] have reported on patients with continued bladder pain despite the absence of a bladder. Outcomes are obviously dependent upon the surgeons involved, the selection process related to patients, and specifics of technique.

SUMMARY

IC/BPS is a disorder that mainly affects women and is associated in a unique fashion with other health issues that are more prevalent in women. It is important to note that current treatment processes are "empiric" in nature since the disease process itself has not been defined. Since it is a process of trial and error, the rational approach to the treatment of this disorder is to start simply and noninvasively, optimizing therapies that are effective for individual patients and advancing to the less simple and more invasive only when there is a lack of incremental improvement. It is important to remember, for this disorder in particular, that stress/anxiety can serve as a profound exacerbator of symptoms and so it is prudent to include treatment of known exacerbators as part of empiric trials. There is hope that one day the disease process (or more likely processes) may become more defined and allow for definitive therapies, but currently the state-of-the-art treatment is to treat in a progressive fashion with frequent reassessment.

REFERENCES

1. Hunner GL. A rare type of bladder ulcer in women: report of cases. *Boston Med Surg J* 1915;172:660–4.
2. Lifford KL, Curhan GC. Prevalence of painful bladder syndrome in older women. *Urol* 2009;73:494–8.
3. Clemens JQ, Link CL, Eggers PW, Kusek JW, Nyberg LM, Jr., McKinlay JB. Prevalence of painful bladder symptoms and effect on quality of life in black, Hispanic and white men and women. *J Urol* 2007;177:1390–4.
4. Curhan GC, Speizer FE, Hunter DJ, Curhan SG, Stampfer MJ. Epidemiology of

interstitial cystitis: a population based study. *J Urol* 1999;161:549–52.

5. Clemens JQ, Meenan RT, O'Keeffe Rosetti MC, Brown SO, Gao SY, Calhoun EA. Prevalence of interstitial cystitis symptoms in a managed care population. *J Urol* 2005;174:576–80.

6. Alagiri M, Chottiner S, Ratner V, Slade D, Hanno PM. Interstitial cystitis: unexplained associations with other chronic disease and pain syndromes. *Urol* 1997;49(Suppl 5A): 52–7.

7. Rodriguez MAB, Afari N, Buchwald D and the National Instititute of Diabetes and Digestive and Kidney Diseases Working Group on Urological Chronic Pelvic Pain. A review of the evidence for overlap between urological and non-urological unexplained clinical conditions. *J Urol* 2009;182:2123–31.

8. Butrick CW, Sanford D, Hou Q and Mahnken JD. Chronic pelvic pain syndromes: clinical, urodynamic and urothelial observations. *Int Urogynecol J Pelvic Floor Dysfunction* 2009;20: 1047–53.

9. Chung MK, Butrick CW, Chung CW. The overlap of interstitial cystitis/painful bladder syndrome and overactive bladder. *J Soc Lap Surg* 2010;14:83–90.

10. Sadler TW. *Langman's Medical Embryology*. 7th ed. Baltimore, MD: Williams & Wilkins; 1995.

11. Moore KL, Persaud TVN. *Before We Are Born: Essentials of Embryology and Birth Defects*. 4th ed. Philadelphia, PA: WB Saunders; 1993.

12. Carlson BM. *Human Embryology and Developmental Biology*. Mosby, St. Louis, MO: Mosby; 1994.

13. Palecek J. The role of dorsal column pathways in visceral pain. *Physiol Res* 2004;53(Suppl 1): S125–30.

14. Willis WD, Westlund KN. Neuroanatomy of the pain system and of the pathways that modulate pain. *J Clin Neurophysiol* 1997;14:2–31.

15. Hong D, Andren-Sandberg A. Punctate midline myelotomy: a minimally inveasive procedure for the treatment of pain in inextirpable abdominal and pelvic cancer. *J Pain Symptom Manag* 2007;33:99–109.

16. Nauta HJ, Hewitt E, Westlund KN, Willis WD. Surgical interruption of a midline dorsal column visceral pain pathway. Case report and review of the literature. *J Neurosurg* 1997;86(3):538–42.

17. Nauta HJ, Soukup VM, Fabian RH, et al. Punctate midline myelotomy for the relief of visceral cancer pain. *J Neurosurg* 2000;92:125–30.

18. Blok BFM. Central pathways controlling micturition and urinary continence. *Urol* 2002; 59(Suppl 5A):13–7.

19. Dasgupta R, Kavia RB. Fowler CJ. Cerebral mechanisms and voiding function. *BJU Int* 2007;99:731–4.

20. Slobodov G, Feloney M, Gran C, Kyker KD, Hurst RE, Culkin DJ. Abnormal expression of molecular markers for bladder impermeability and differentiation in the urothelium of patients with interstitial cystitis. *J Urol* 2004;171:1554–8.

21. Nazif O, Teichman JM, Gebhart GF. Neural upregulation in interstitial cystitis. *Urol* 2007;69:24–33.

22. Letourneau R, Sant GR, el-Mansoury M, Theoharides TC. Activation of bladder mast cells in interstitial cystitis. *Int J Tissue React* 1992;14:307–12.

23. Keay S, Seillier-Moiseiwitsch F, Zhang CO, Chai TC, Zhang J. Changes in human bladder epithelial cell gene expression associated with interstitial cystitis or antiproliferative factor treatment. *Physiol Genomics* 2003;14:107–15.

24. Randich A, Uzzell T, Cannon R, Ness TJ. Inflammation and enhanced nociceptive responses to bladder distension produced by intravesical zymosan in the rat. *BMC Urol* 2006; 6:2–8.

25. DeBerry J, Ness TJ, Robbins MT, Randich A. Inflammation-induced enhancement of the visceromotor reflex to urinary bladder distention: modulation by endogenous opioids and the effects of early-in-life experience with bladder inflammation. *J Pain* 2007;8:914–23.

26. Parsons CL, Greenberger M, Gabal L, Bidair M, Barme G. The role of urinary potassium in the pathogenesis and diagnosis of interstitial cystitis. *J Urol* 1998;159:1862–7.

27. Mukerji G, Waters J, Chessell IP, Bountra C, Agarwal SK, Anand P. Pain during ice water test distinguishes clinical bladder hypersensitivity from overactivity disorders. *BMC Urol* 2006;6:31.

28. Theoharides TC, Sant GR, El-Mansoury M, Letourneau R, Ucci AA, Jr, Meares EM, Jr. Activation of bladder mast cells in interstitial cystitis: a light and electron microscopic study. *J Urol* 1995;153:629–36.

29. Spanos C, Pang X, Ligris K, et al. Stress-induced bladder mast cell activation: implications for interstitial cystitis. *J Urol* 1997;157:669–72.

30. Dimitriadou V, Rouleau A, Trung Tuong MD, et al. Functional relationships between sensory nerve fibers and mast cells of dura mater in normal and inflammatory conditions. *Neurosci* 1997;77:829–39.

31. Farhadi A, Fields JZ, Keshavarzian A. Mucosal mast cells are pivotal elements in inflammatory bowel disease that connect the dots: stress,

intestinal hyperpermeability and inflammation. *World J Gastroenterol* 2007;13:3027–30.

32. Pang X, Boucher W, Triadafilopoulos G, Sant GR, Theoharides TC. Mast cell and substance P-positive nerve involvement in a patient with both irritable bowel syndrome and interstitial cystitis. *Urology* 1996;47:436–8.

33. Bullock AD, Becich MJ, Klutke CG, Ratliff TL. Experimental autoimmune cystitis: a potential murine model for ulcerative interstitial cystitis. *J Urol* 1992;148:1951–6.

34. Laird JM, Martinez-Caro L, Garcia-Nicas E, Cervero F. A new model of visceral pain and referred hyperalgesia in the mouse. *Pain* 2001;92:335–342.

35. Westropp JL, Buffington CA. In vivo models of interstitial cystitis. *J Urol* 2002;167:694–702.

36. Liu H-T, Tyagi P, Chancellor MB, Kuo H-C. Urinary nerve growth factor level is increased in patients with interstitial cystitis/bladder pain syndrome and decreased in responders to treatment. *Br J Urol Int* 2009;104:1476–81.

37. Sanchez Freire V, Burkhard FC, Kessler TM, Kuhn A, Draeger A, Monastyrskaya K. MicroRNAs may mediate the down regulation of neurokinin-1 receptor in chronic bladder pain syndrome. *Am J Pathol* 2010;176:288–303.

38. Keay S, Warren JW. A hypothesis for the etiology of interstitial cystitis based upon inhibition of bladder epithelial repair. *Med Hypotheses* 1998;51:79–83.

39. Keay S, Warren JW, Zhang CO, Tu LM, Gordon DA, Whitmore KE. Antiproliferative activity is present in bladder but not renal pelvic urine from interstitial cystitis patients. *J Urol* 1999;162:1487–9.

40. Zhang CO, Li ZL, Shoenfelt JL, et al. Comparison of APF activity and epithelial growth factor levels in urine from Chinese, African-American, and white American patients with interstitial cystitis. *Urol* 2003;61:897–901.

41. Ness TJ, Powell-Boone T, Cannon R, Lloyd LK, Fillingim RB. Psychophysical evidence of hypersensitivity in subjects with interstitial cystitis. *J Urol* 2005;173:1983–7.

42. Macaulay AJ, Stern RS, Holmes DM, Santon SL. Micturition and the mind: psychological factors in the etiology and treatment of urinary symptoms in women. *Br Med J (Clin Res Ed)* 1987;294:540–3.

43. Baldoni F, Ercolani M, Baldaro B, Trombini G. Stressful events and psychological symptoms in patients with functional urinary disorders. *Percept Mot Skills* 1995;80:605–6.

44. Sant GR, Kempuraj D, Marchand JE, Theoharides T. The mast cell in interstitial cystitis: role in pathophysiology and pathogenesis. *Urol* 2007;69:34–40.

45. Koziol JA, Clark DC, Gittes RF, Tan EM. The natural history of interstitial cystitis: a survey of 374 patients. *J Urol* 1993;149:465–9.

46. Rothrock NE, Lutgendorf SK, Kreder KJ, Ratliff T, Zimmerman B. Stress and symptoms in patients with interstitial cystitis: a life stress model. *Urol* 2001;57:422–7.

47. Lutgendorf SK, Kreder KJ, Rothrock NE, Ratliff TL, Zimmerman B. Stress and symptomatology in patients with interstitial cystitis: a laboratory stress model. *J Urol* 2000;164:1265–9.

48. Robbins MT, Uzzell TW, Aly S, Ness TJ. Characterization of thalamic neuronal responses to urinary bladder distention, including the effect of acute spinal lesions in the rat. *J Pain* 2006;7:218–24.

49. Robbins MT, Ness, TJ. Footshock-induced urinary bladder hypersensitivity: role of spinal corticotrophin-releasing factor receptors. *J Pain* 2008;9:991–8.

50. Bennett EJ, Tennant CC, Piesse C, Badcock CA, Kellow JE. Level of chronic life stress predicts clinical outcome in irritable bowel syndrome. *Gut* 1998;43:256–61.

51. Howell S, Poulton R, Talley NJ. The natural history of childhood abdominal pain and its association with adult irritable bowel syndrome: birth-cohort study. *Am J Gastroenterology* 2005;100:2071–8.

52. Mallen DC, Peat G, Thomas E, Croft PR. Is chronic pain in adulthood related to childhood factors? A population-based case-control study of young adults. *J Rheumatol* 2006;33:2286–90.

53. Chitkara DK, vanTilburg MAL, Blois-Martin N, Whitehead WE. Early life risk factors that contribute to irritable bowel syndrome in adults: a systematic review. *Am J Gastroenterol* 2008;103:765–74.

54. Taddio A, Katz J. The effects of early pain experience in neonates on pain responses in infancy and childhood. *Paediatr Drugs* 2005;7:245–57.

55. Hermann C, Hohmeister J, Demirakca S, Zohsel K, Flor H. Long-term alteration of pain sensitivity in school-aged children and early pain experiences. *Pain* 2006;125:278–85.

56. Walker SM, Franck LS, Fitzgerald M, Myles J, Stocks J, Marlow N. Long-term impact of neonatal intensive care and surgery on somatosensory

perception in children born extremely preterm. *Pain* 2009;141:79–87.

57. Jones CA, Nyberg L. Epidemiology of interstitial cystitis. *Urol* 1997;49:2–9.

58. Randich A, Uzzell T, DeBerry JJ, Ness TJ. Neonatal urinary bladder inflammation produces adult bladder hypersensitivity. *J Pain* 2006;7:469–79.

59. Randich A, Mebane H, Ness TJ. Ice water testing reveals hypersensitivity in adult rats that experienced neonatal bladder inflammation: implications for painful bladder yndrome/interstitial cystitis. *J Urol* 2009;182:337–42.

60. Wessely S, Nimnuan C, Sharpe M. Functional somatic syndromes: one or many? *Lancet* 1999;354:936–9.

61. Powell-Boone T, Ness TJ, Cannon R, Lloyd LK, Weigent DA, Fillingim RB. Menstrual cycle affects bladder pain sensation in subjects with interstitial cystitis. *J Urol* 2005;174:1832–6.

62. Fillingim RB, Ness TJ. Sex-related hormonal influences on pain and analgesic response. *Neurosci Biobehav Rev* 2000;24:485–501.

63. Aloisi AM. Gonadal hormones and sex differences in pain reactivity. *Clin J Pain* 2003;19:168–74.

64. Craft RM, Mogil JS, Aloisi AM. Sex differences in pain and analgesia: the role of gonadal hormones. *Eur J Pain* 2004;8:397–411.

65. Hurley RW, Adams MC. Sex, gender and pain: an overview of a complex field. *Anesth Analg* 2008;107:309–17.

66. Ji Y, Tang B, Traub RJ. Modulatory effects of estrogen and progesterone on colorectal hyperalgesia in the rat. *Pain* 2005;117:433–42.

67. Mannino CA, South SM, Quinones-Jenab V, Inturrisi CE. Estradiol replacement in ovariectomized rats is antihyperalgesic in the formalin test. *J Pain* 2007;8:334–42.

68. Spooner MF, Robichaud P, Carrier JC, Marchand S. Endogenous pain modulation during the formalin test in estrogen receptor beta knockout mice. *Neurosci* 2007;150:675–80.

69. Wein AJ, Hanno PM, Gillenwater JY. Interstitial cystitis: an introduction to the problem. In: Hanno PM, Staskin DR, eds. *Interstitial Cystitis*. New York: Springer-Verlag; 1990: 3–16.

70. Pontari MA, Hanno PM, Wein AJ. Logical and systematic approach to the evaluation and management of patients suspected of having interstitial cystitis. *Urol* 1997;49(Suppl 5A):114–20.

71. Nickel JC, Shoskes D, Irvine-Bird K. Clinical phenotyping of women with interstitial cystitis/painful bladder syndrome: a key to classification and potentially improved management. *J Urol* 2009;182:155–60.

72. Hanno PM, Burks DA, Clemens JQ, et al. AUA Guideline for the diagnosis and treatment of interstitial cystitis/bladder pain syndrome. *J Urol* 2011;185:2162–70.

73. Parsons CL, Zupkas P, Parsons JK. Intravesical potassium sensitivity in patients with interstitial cystitis and urethral syndrome. *Urol* 2001;57:428–432.

74. Parsons CL, Dell J, Stanford EJ. Increased prevalence of interstitial cystitis: previously unrecognized urologic and gynecologic cases identified using a new symptom questionnaire and intravesical potassium sensitivity. *Urol* 2002;60:573–8.

75. Bernie JE, Hagey S, Albo ME, Parsons CL. The intravesical potassium sensitivity test and urodynamics: implications in a large cohort of patients with lower urinary tract symptoms. *J Urol* 2001;166:158–61

76. Erickson DR, Xie SX, Bhavanandan VP, et al. A comparison of multiple urine markers for interstitial cystitis. *J Urol* 2002;167:2461–69.

77. Waxman JA, Sulak PJ, Kuehl TJ. Cystoscopic findings consistent with interstitial cystitis in normal women undergoing tubal ligation. *J Urol* 1998;160:1663–7

78. Shorter B, Lesser M, Moldwin RM, Kushner L. Effect of comestibles on symptoms of interstitial cystitis. *J Urol* 2007;178:145–52.

79. Aihara K, Hirayama A, Tanaka N, Fujimoto K, Yoshida K, Hirao Y. Hydrodistension under local anesthesia for patients with suspected painful bladder syndrome/interstitial cystitis: safety, diagnostic potential and therapeutic efficacy. *Int J Urol* 2009;16:947–82.

80. Cameron AP, Gajewski JB. Bladder outlet obstruction in painful bladder syndrome/interstitial cystitis. *Neurourol Urodyn* 2009;28:944–8.

81. Payne RA, O'Connor C, Kressin M, Guralnick ML. Endoscopic ablation of Hunner's lesions in interstitial cystitis patients. *Can Urol Assoc J* 2009;3:473–7.

82. Irwin PP, Hammonds WD, Galloway NTM. Lumbar epidural blockade for management of pain in interstitial cystitis. *Br J of Urol* 1993;71:413–416.

83. Hanno PM. Amitriptyline in the treatment of interstitial cystitis. *Urol Clinics of North Am* 1994;21:121–130.

84. Hertle L, van Ophoven A. Long-term results of amitriptyline treatment for interstitial cystitis. *Aktuelle Urol* 2010;41:S61–5

85. Foster HE, Jr, Hanno PM, Nickel JC, Payne CK. Effect of amitriptyline on symptoms in treatment

naïve patients with interstitial cystitis/painful bladder syndrome. *J Urol* 2010;183:1853–8.

86. Papandreou C, Skapinakis P, Giannakis D, Sofikitis N, Mavreas V. Antidepressant drugs for chronic urological pelvic pain: an evidence-based review. *Adv Urol* 2009;2009: 797031–9.

87. Sant GR, Propert KJ, Hanno PM, et al. A pilot clinical trial of oral pentosan polysulfate and oral hydroxyzine in patients with interstitial cystitis. *J Urol* 2003;170:810–5.

88. Rosenberg MT, Hazzard MA, Page SA. Patient response in a screened population for interstitial cystitis. *Compr Ther* 2006;32:248–53.

89. Lentz GM, Bavendam T, Stenchever MA, Miller JL, Smalldridge J. Hormonal manipulation in women with chronic, cyclic irritable bladder symptoms and pelvic pain. *Am J Obstet Gynecol* 2002;186:1268–71.

90. Sairanen J, Forsell T, Ruutu M. Long-term outcome of patients with interstitial cystitis treated with low dose cyclosporine A *J Urol* 2004;171:2138–41.

91. Sairanen J, Leppilahti M, Tammela TL, et al. Evaluation of health-related quality of life in patients with painful bladder syndrome/interstitial cystitis and the impact of four treatments on it. *Scand J Urol Nephrol* 2009;43:212–9.

92. Messing EM, Stamey TA. Interstitial cystitis, early diagnosis, pathology and treatment. *Urology* 1978;12:381–92.

93. Perez-Marrero R, Emerson LE, Feltis JT. A controlled study of dimethyl sulfoxide in interstitial cystitis. *J Urol* 1998;140:36–9.

94. Dawson TE, Jamison J. Intravesical treatments for painful bladder syndrome/interstitial cystitis. *Cochrane Database Syst Rev* 2007;17: CD006113.

95. Shao Y, Shen ZJ, Rui WB, Shou WL. Intravesical instillation of hyaluronic acid prolonged the effect of bladder hydrodistension in patients with severe interstitial cystitis. *Urology* 2010; 75:547–50.

96. Engelhardt PF, Morakis N, Daha LK, Esterbauer B, Riedl CR. Long-term results of intravesical hyaluronan therapy in bladder pain syndrome/interstitial cystitis. *Int Urogynecol J Pelvic Floor Dysfunct* 2011;22:401–5.

97. Tirumuru S, Al-Kurdi D, Latthe P. Intravesical botulinum toxin A injections in the treatment of painful bladder syndrome/interstitial cystitis: a systematic review. *Int Urogynecol J* 2010;21:1285–300.

98. Fall M, Lindstrom S. Transcutaneous electrical nerve stimulation in interstitial cystitis. *Urol Clinics of North Am* 1994;21:131–9.

99. Marinkovic SP, Gillen LM, Marinkovic CM. Minimum 6-year outcomes for interstitial cystitis treated with sacral neuromodulation. *Int Urogynecol J Pelvic Floor Dysfunct* 2011;22:407–12.

100. Gajewski JB and Al-Zahrani AA. The long-term efficacy of sacral neuromodulation in the management of intractable cases of bladder pain syndrome: 14 years of experience in one centre. *BJU Int* 2010;107:1258–64.

101. Fariello JY and Whitmore K. Sacral neuromodulation stimulation for IC/PBS, chronic pelvic pain and sexual dysfunction. *Int Urogynecol J Pelvic Floor Dysfunct* 2010;21:1553–8.

102. Peters KM, Killinger KA, Boguslawski BM, Boura JA. Chronic pudendal neuromodulation: expanding available treatment options for refractory urologic symptoms. *Neurourol Urodyn* 2010;29:1267–71.

103. Killinger KA, Kangas JR, Wolfert C, Boura JA, Peters KM. Secondary changes in bowel function after successful treatment of voiding symptoms with neuromodulation. *Neurourol Urodyn* 2011;30:133–7.

104. Gillespie L. Destruction of the vesicoureteric plexus for the treatment of hypersensitive bladder disorders. *Br J Urol* 1994;74:40–3.

105. Peeker R, Aldenborg F, Fall M. The treatment of interstitial cystitis with supratrigonal cystectomy and ileocystoplasty: difference in outcome between classic and nonulcer disease. *J Urol* 1998;159:1479–82.

106. Webster GD, MacDiarmid SA, Timmons SL, et al. Impact of urinary diversion procedures in the treatment of interstitial cystitis and chronic bladder pain. *Neurourol Urodyn* 1992; 11:417.

107. Baskin LS, Tanagho EA. Pelvic pain without pelvic organs. *J Urol* 1992;147:683–6.

19

CHRONIC PELVIC PAIN OF UNCERTAIN ORIGIN

Andrew Baranowski

INTRODUCTION

When considering the classification of pelvic pain, it is important to appreciate that the pain may be associated with a specific disease process of an organ or organs, but it may also occur in the absence of classical end organ pathology.[1,2] When we are dealing with a pelvic pain associated with a specific disease, there may be certain obvious differences between males and females as a result of different anatomy and physiology, which may result in sex-specific pathophysiology.[3] However, when we are dealing with the chronic pelvic pain syndrome (CPPS), many of the mechanisms will be similar in both sexes.[4–9] To understand CPPS, we must first define what constitutes CPPS. The Chronic Pelvic Pain working group of the European Association of Urology developed a classification system in 2004,[9a] which was modified in 2012.[2] The Pain of Urogenital Origin (PUGO) Taxonomy Working Group of the International Association for the Study of Pain modified this and developed the following taxonomy, which will be used in this review.

Chronic pelvic pain is defined as chronic/persistent pain perceived in structures related to the pelvis of either men or women. It is often associated with negative cognitive, behavioural, sexual, and emotional consequences

as well as with symptoms suggestive of lower urinary tract, sexual, bowel, or gynecological dysfunction. This definition applies equally to men and women. To be defined as chronic/persistent, the pain must have been continuous or recurrent for at least 6 months. The pain can be cyclical over a 6-month period, such as the cyclical pain of dysmenorrhea. If nonacute and central sensitization pain mechanisms are inferred from the history, examination, and investigations, then the pain may be regarded as chronic, irrespective of the time period. The term "perceived" indicates that the patient and clinician, to the best of their ability from the history, examination, and investigations (where appropriate) have localized the pain as being sensed within the specified anatomical pelvic area. "Dysfunction" is a term that indicates that there is a mechanistic functional disorder. For purposes of this review that term is *not* used to indicate a psychological or psychiatric disorder.

CPPS is the occurrence of chronic pelvic pain where there is no proven infection or other obvious local pathology that may account for the pain. It is often associated with negative cognitive, behavioral, sexual, and emotional consequences as well as with symptoms suggestive of lower urinary tract, sexual, bowel, or gynecological dysfunction. CPPSs are defined by a process of exclusion. In particular, there should be no evidence of local organ cancer or infection. As a consequence, early investigations by end organ specialists (e.g., gynecologists, urologists, and proctologists) should be aimed at excluding local end organ pathology. Subdivision of the CPPS into subphenotype should only occur if there is adequate evidence to support using that term and subphenotype. For instance, in nonspecific, poorly localized pelvic pain without obvious pathology, only the term CPPS should be used. If the pain can be well localized to an organ, then a more specific term (such as rectal pain syndrome) may be used. Localizing in this way may assist in the choice of specific end organ treatments. If the pain is localized to multiple organs, then the syndrome is a regional pain syndrome and the term CPPS should once more be considered.

When defining a patient, as well as defining the patient by a specific end organ phenotype, there are multiple other more general descriptors that need to be considered. These are primarily psychological (e.g., cognitive and emotional), sexual, behavioral, and functional, although others exist. Psychological and behavioral factors are well established to relate to quality-of-life issues and prognosis. The other descriptors help to classify the nature of the pain. Systemic disorders outside of the pelvis are very common in those who suffer with chronic pelvic pain. In America, a National Institutes of Health research program, the Multidisciplinary Approach to the Study of Chronic Pelvic Pain (MAPP) program, has been devised to investigate the importance of these factors and looks at all types of pelvic pain irrespective of the end organ where the pain is perceived. Moreover, it addresses systemic disorder associations, such as the co-ocurrence of fibromyalgia, facial pain, and autoimmune disorders.[9b-9d]

The debate in relation to subdividing CPPS is ongoing. As more and more information is collected suggesting that the central nervous system is involved and indeed may be the main cause of many CPPS conditions (wherever the pain is perceived—bladder, genitalia, colorectal, or myofascial), there is a general tendency to move away from end organ nomenclature. Whether this is appropriate is something that only time and good research will tell. To enable such research, it is essential to have a framework of classification to work within.

CAUSE, PREDISPOSITION, AND MAINTENANCE OF CHRONIC PELVIC PAIN SYNDROME

When considering the classification of chronic pelvic pain, it is important not to confuse cause, predisposing factors, and factors that maintain the pain with pain mechanisms, though there may be an overlap. When we are dealing with chronic pain, there may be many causes that produce the same end result. These may include trauma (including surgery), infection, and cancer; pelvic floor muscle tension[10,11]; and low-grade trauma from sitting as well.[12,13] Often in any one single patient there may be multiple potential causes that predispose the patient to chronic pain. If the cause is ongoing (specific disease-associated pain), then management should be aimed at treating the cause with symptomatic treatment of the pain as appropriate.[1] Patients will often focus on cause, especially if it has been psychologically traumatic. If the cause is no longer ongoing, then the focus needs to shift to the current mechanisms and treatment needs to be aimed at these.[1,14] Whereas a patient may need psychological support to help him or her move forward from a traumatic cause, such as a negative sexual event (NSE), to enable treatment of the ongoing pain mechanisms, there is little evidence to support that the majority of patients with pelvic pain have a past history of NSE.[15-17] However, patients who have suffered sexual trauma (rape, systematic rape, torture, and abuse) may be at greater risk of real physical pain.[18] In this situation interventions aimed at supporting the patient following the NSE are as important as well as managing the pain. Genetic predisposition[19] is likely to be a predisposing factor in certain cases. Endometriosis, as well as being associated with acute pain, may produce central nervous system sensitization and as a consequence predispose to CPPS.[5,20-22] When considering maintenance factors, we have to appreciate that the medical system can reinforce pain mechanisms through inappropriate consultations, investigation, and treatment.[23-25] Chronic pain mechanisms are now well described and these may self-maintain the pain in their own right, though physical stimuli may also play a role in perpetuating matters[9,26] (e.g., continuing with painful sex[27]).

MECHANISMS OF CHRONIC PELVIC PAIN SYNDROME

In a proportion of patients with pain perceived to be in the pelvis, *ongoing* classical visceral pain mechanisms as well as somatic mechanisms may be involved. A comparison of visceral and somatic pain features is found in Table 19.1. There may also be a peripheral neurochemistry that is particularly relevant to chronic pain[28,29] Nerve growth factor (NGF) is able to both directly activate primary afferents and also indirectly activate them (such as through bradykinin). Multiple tachykinins are implicated in both the normal control of bladder contraction and in the heightened stimulation and sensitisation of the afferent loop of the micturition reflex after inflammation. Similar mechanisms are known for the other organs. ATP released from hollow organs, such as when the bladder is distended, acts upon purine P2X3 receptors found on visceral afferents and on small-diameter DRG neurons. Once more these mechanisms may be involved in normal function and pain. Voltage-gated ion channels (tetrodotoxin-resistant sodium channel, NaV1.8) are also implicated in the visceral pain states. Central mechanisms are very important for the phenomena of the pelvic pain syndromes.[7-9] In visceral pain excitatory amino acid receptors such as N-methyl-D-aspartate (NMDA) and alpha-amino-3-hydroxy-5-methyl-4-isoxazoleeproprionic acid (AMPA) play a vital role in the production of viscero visceral, musculo visceral, and viscero muscular hyperalgesia.

SUPRASPINAL MODULATION OF PAIN PERCEPTION

It is important to appreciate that nociception is the neurological process of transmitting

Table 19.1   Differences between Visceral and Somatic Pains

CHARACTERISTIC	FEATURES OF VISCERAL PAIN	FEATURES OF SOMATIC PAIN
Stimuli associated with pain	Stretching and distension, resulting in poorly localized pain	Mechanical, thermal, chemical, and electrical stimuli, producing well-localized pain
Summation	Widespread stimulation produces a significantly magnified pain.	Widespread stimulation produces a modest increase in pain.
Primary afferents	Low-density, unmyelinated C fibers and thinly myelinated Aд are primary afferents.	Dense innervation with a wide range of nerve fibers
Primary afferent physiology	Intensity coding. As stimulation increases, afferent firing increases with an increase in sensation and ultimately pain.	Two-fiber coding; separate fibers for pain and normal sensation
Silent afferents	Approximately 50%–90% of visceral afferents are silent until the time they are switched on. These fibers are very important in the central sensitization process.	Silent afferents are present in certain areas (e.g., joints).
Autonomic involvement	Autonomic features (e.g., nausea and sweating) are frequently present.	Autonomic features are less frequent as a directly related phenomenon.

(continued)

Table 19.1(*Continued*)

CHARACTERISTIC	FEATURES OF VISCERAL PAIN	FEATURES OF SOMATIC PAIN
Central mechanisms	Play an important part in the hyperalgesias, viscera-visceral, viscera-muscular, and musculo-visceral hyperalgesias. Sensations not normally perceived become perceived and nonnoxious sensations become painful.	Responsible for the allodynia and hyperalgesia of chronic somatic pain
Referred pain	Pain perceived at a site distant to the cause of the pain is common, referred pain.	Pain is usually well localized.
Referred hyperalgesia	Referred cutaneous, muscle, and visceral hyperalgesias are common.	Hyperalgesia tends to be localized.
Abnormalities of function	Central mechanisms associated with visceral pain may be responsible for organ dysfunction such as constipation and urinary hesitance.	Somatic pain associated with somatic dysfunction, such as muscle fasciculation
Central pathways and representation	As well as classical pathways, there is evidence for a separate dorsal horn pathway and central representation.	Classical pain pathways

information to the brain centers involved in perception of information about a stimulus that has the potential to cause tissue damage. Pain is far more complex and involves not only the perception of a nociceptive event but also cognitive, emotional, behavioral, and sexual response.[30–32] Modulation of nociceptive pathways may occur throughout the whole of the neuraxis (spinal cord through to higher centers) and even in the periphery. The brain has a significant role in this neuromodulation and can both facilitate and inhibit pain perception by actions at multiple levels. The prognosis and response to treatment is thus dependent on the higher centers and psychological mechanisms.[33–35]

The midbrain periaqueductal gray (PAG) plays an important part in spinal modulation.[36] It receives inputs from those centers associated with thought and emotion. Projections from the PAG (via several relay systems) to the dorsal horn can inhibit nociceptive messages from reaching conscious perception. The PAG and its associated centers may also be involved in diffuse noxious inhibitory controls (DNIC). DNIC is when a nociceptive stimulus in an area well away from the receptive fields of a second nociceptive stimulus can prevent or reduce pain from that second area. This is thought to be the mechanism for the paradigm of counterirritation. Several neurotransmitters and neuromodulators are involved in descending pain-inhibitory pathways. The main contenders are the opioids, 5-hydroxytryptamine and noradrenaline.[37] The pathways and chemicals for the facilitatory modulation are even less well understood, but the mechanisms are well accepted.

NEUROMODULATION, PSYCHOLOGY, AND LEARNING

The main central nervous system areas associated with psychological etiologies of altered sensation (psychological neuromodulation) related to urogenital pelvic pain are those areas involved in emotion, thought, behavior, and sexual response. They may not be distinct centers but are more of a network. Some of these processes may be highly sophisticated and others fundamental in evolutionary terms. The interaction between these areas and nociception is complex. As indicated earlier, many of the areas involved in psychological neuromodulation interact with the PAG, and this is thus one mechanism by which they may influence nociceptive transmission at the spinal level. Within the spine, visceral afferent nociceptive transmission is dependent upon a system of intensity coding. That is, for the viscera, normal sensations and nociception utilize the same small peripheral afferent fibers, and the difference between a normal message and a noxious one depends upon the number of afferent signals transmitted to the dorsal horn (as opposed to the dual fiber, Aδ/C fibers for nociception, and Aβ for light touch, seen in somatic tissue). Because of this intensity coding system, it is thought that visceral pain is more prone to psychological neuromodulation at the spinal level than is seen in somatic tissue.

There is also a complex network of supratentorial interactions involving psychology that may play a significant role in nociception/pain neuromodulation at the higher level. These higher interactions may both reduce or facilitate the nociceptive signal reaching the consciousness and pain perception; they will also modulate the response to the nociceptive message and hence the pain experience. Functional magnetic resonance imaging has indicated that the psychological neuromodulation of visceral pain probably involves multiple pathways. For instance, mood and distraction probably act through different areas of the brain when reducing pain.[38] Psychological neuromodulation may act to reduce nociception within a rapid time frame but may also result in a long-term vulnerability to chronic visceral pain through long-term potentiation (learning). This involvement of higher center learning may be both at a conscious or subconscious level and is clearly established as being significant in the supratentorial neuroprocessing of nociception and pain. Long-term potentiation[39] may also occur at any level within the nervous system so that pathways for

specific stimuli or combinations of stimuli may become established, resulting in an individual being vulnerable to perceiving sensations that would not normally bother other individuals. Stress may be intrinsic or extrinsic and is considerd a phenomena that threatens to disturb the homeostasis of an organism, and it can be real (physical) or perceived (psychological). Stress induces an adaptive response that involves the endocrine, autonomic nervous, and immune systems, and these systems in turn appear to have feedback loops. Long-term potentiation is one proposed mechanism by which the nervous system learns and stress can modify the nervous system by this process so that there are long-term abnormalities or potential abnormalities within these systems. It is this process that may be responsible for the effect of early life and significant life events as potential factors associated with chronic pain syndromes.

AUTONOMIC NERVOUS SYSTEM

The role of the autonomic nervous system in chronic pain is poorly understood; however, there is good evidence that afferent fibers may develop a sensitivity to sympathetic stimulation both at the site of injury and more centrally, particularly the dorsal root ganglia and dorsal horns. In visceral pain the efferent output of the central nervous system may be influenced by central changes (once more those changes may be throughout the neuraxis); such modification of the efferent message may produce significant functional problems of the end organ and as a result stimulate peripheral nociceptors. The autonomic nervous system may also produce trophic end organ signs such as neurogenic edema, ulceration, and hemorrhage.

ENDOCRINE SYSTEM

The endocrine system is also involved in visceral function. Pain and the subsequent stress response will thus affect end organ visceral function. The hypothalamic pituitary axis (HPA) and corticotropin-releasing hormone (CRH) from the hypothalamus, which stimulates the release of adrenocorticotropic hormone from the pituitary, are key steps. An up-regulation of CRH has been implicated in several pain states such as rectal hypersensitivity to rectal disten-sion. In this model an action of CRH on mast cells has been suggested. Significant life events and in particular early life events may alter the development of the HPA and the chemicals released. Increased vulnerability to stress may occur following such events and is thought to be partly due to increased CRH gene expres-sion. A range of stress-related illnesses have been suggested—irritable bowel syndrome and bladder pain syndrome being examples. There is also evidence accumulating to suggest that the sex hormones may also modulate both nocicep-tion and pain perception.

CLINICAL PARADIGMS AND CHRONIC PELVIC PAIN

There are several different ways in which chronic pelvic pains may be sensed. [1,4,7] The first of these, "referred pain," is frequently observed and its identification is important both for diagnosis and treatment. Referral is usually from a somatic structure to another somatic structure or from a visceral structure to a somatic structure. However, there is no reason why "pain" cannot also be perceived within the vague distribution of an organ with the nociceptive signal having arisen from a somatic area. Referred pain may occur as a result of several mechanisms, but the main theory is one of convergence-projection. In the convergence-projection theory, affer-ent fibers from the viscus and the somatic site of referred pain converge onto the same second-order projection neurons. The higher centers receiving messages from these projec-tion neurons are unable to separate out the two possible sites for the origin of the nociceptive signal. Referred pain may also be experienced as hyperalgesia in somatic tissues. Hyperalgesia refers to an increased sensitivity to normally painful stimuli. In patients who have passed a renal stone, somatic muscle hyperalgesia is frequently present, even a year following the expulsion of the stone. Pain to nonpainful stimuli (allodynia) may also be present in cer-tain individuals. Somatic tissue hyperesthesia has been described to be associated with uri-nary and bilary colic, irritable bowel syndrome, endometriosis, dysmenorrhea, and recurrent bladder infection. Vulvar pain syndromes

(previous terms have included vulvar vestibu-litis and essential vulvodynia) are examples of cutaneous allodynia that in certain cases may be associated with visceral pain syndromes such as the bladder pain syndrome. Referred pain with hyperalgesia is thought to be due to central sensitization of the converging viscero-somatic neurons. Following a nociceptive insult, an acute high-frequency afferent barrage of sig-naling from a viscus produces the central sen-sitization with an increased transmission of signals to the central nervous system from the viscus. Somatic afferent fibers converging on this same sensitized central area would also be increased in their central transmission, and this combined with the convergence-projection theory results in perceived somatic pain and also the hyperalgesia response. The central sen-sitization would also stimulate efferent activity that would explain the trophic changes so often found in the somatic tissues.

Chronic pelvic pain may also be associated with visceral hyperalgesia, an increased percep-tion of stimuli applied to a viscus. The mecha-nisms behind visceral hyperalgesia are thought to be responsible for irritable bowel syndrome, bladder pain syndrome, and dysmenorrhea. The mechanisms involved will often be an acute afferent input (such as due to an infec-tion) followed by long-term central sensitiza-tion. Viscero-visceral hyperalgesia is thought to occur when two or more organs have overlap-ping sensory projections. From the pelvic pain perspective it is interesting how the bladder afferents overlap in the central nervous system with the uterine afferents and the uterine affer-ents with those from the colon.

MUSCLES AND PELVIC PAIN

In the urogenital pain syndromes, as with any pain syndrome, muscle tenderness and trigger points may be implicated as a source of pain. [40-42] Central mechanisms are of great impor-tance in the pathogenesis of these muscle hype-ralgesias. The muscles involved may be a part of the spinal, abdominal, or pelvic complex of muscles. It is not unknown for adjacent mus-cles of the lower limbs and also the thorax to become involved. Pain may be well localized to the trigger points but is more often associated with classical referral patterns. As well as trigger points, inflammation of the attachments to the bones (enthesitis) and of the bursa (bursitis) may be found.

Certain postures will affect the different muscles in different ways and as a consequence may either exacerbate the pain or reduce it. Stress has been implicated as being both an initiator of pelvic myalgia and as a maintenance factor. As a consequence, negative sexual encounters may also have a precipitating effect.[43]

PELVIC NERVES AND PAIN

It is well established that nerve injury may be associated with a range of symptoms that include dysesthesia, allodynia, hyperalgesia, and constant or intermittent pain. In some cases, the onset of pain is clearly associated with the nerve damage. However, in many cases, arriving at the diagnosis of peripheral nerve injury–generated pain can be difficult. This is particularly so for the urogenital pains. Pudendal neuralgia would be an example of a neuropathic pelvic pain.

FUNCTIONAL PROBLEMS AND PELVIC PAIN

In this chapter the term "functional" refers to the working of an organ or system and not to a psychological condition. As well as pain, many patients with urogenital pain syndromes suffer with abnormalities of organ function. Within our Pain Management Center at UCLH, approximately 30% of our patients score greater than 5 on a 1–10 score looking at interference with life for bowel problems; similar figures for bladder problems and greater than two-thirds of patients for sexual problems. The exact mechanisms involved may not be clear. It is well described that certain drugs (Table 19.2) and surgical interventions can also produce organ dysfunction.

The mechanisms, both central and peripheral, involved in the production of the pain may also be the cause of some of the functional disorders. Certainly those functions that are reliant on voluntary control may be affected by changes in sensory perception. The sensation of urge perceived with a more or less empty bladder may be associated with urinary frequency and similarly the sensation of rectal fullness may be associated with frequent attempts to defecate. Because of the crossover of the visceral central nervous system, abnormalities of sensation perceived primarily in one organ may result in functional abnormalities further afield[44] and widespread muscle spasm.[4,5,7] Abnormal visceral motor function may also occur.[45] The role of the neuro-endocrine and neuro-immune systems are poorly understood. The effect

Table 19.2   Drugs Prescribed in Pain Clinics and Some of Their Effects on Organ Function

Opioids, including tramadol	Constipation
	Urinary hesitance
	Opioid-induced hyperalgesia (a major problem with high-dose opioid)
	Reduced sexual desire (erectile dysfunction in men)
Antidepressants	Constipation
	Urinary hesitance and retention
	Reduce orgasmic sensation
	(Delay or inhibit ejaculation in men)
Anticonvulsants	(In men: carbamazepine may block testosterone production with subsequent testicular atrophy, gynaecomastia, and galactorrhoea; may inhibit ejaculation)
	Hematological and connective tissue disorders

of these conditions on fertility is also poorly understood.

PSYCHOLOGICAL CONSEQUENCES OF PELVIC PAIN

The effect of gender on illness and illness behavior is clearly established; however, there is little research on the effect of illness on gender identity and sexual psychology. One may assume that disorders of the female urogenital system will be prone to produce problems within both of these areas with a risk that the female either fails to achieve meaningful relationships or that established relationships have an increased chance of breaking down. All pain is associated with depression and cognitive-behavioral problems. The severity of the pain appears to be a significant determinant. Depression and catastrophizing are poor prognostic factors. Trip et al.'s paper[30] in men and more recent work[31,32] are key studies. Problems with work, relationships, sex, and loss of meaning of life appeared to be as equally important to the patient as well as the pain itself. For the successful management of a patient with chronic pelvic pain, a multidisciplinary team approach is essential.

GENERIC TREATMENT APPROACH

CPPS should be managed with the same general approach as is used for any of the pain syndromes. Where possible, the consultation and therapeutic procedure environment should be purpose built allowing privacy and comfort (many of these patients would prefer to stand or lie for the consultation). Anatomical models and diagrams, including drawings or photographs of genitalia that will facilitate the consultation, should be available. As well as doctors, nurses skilled in the management of this group of patients should be at hand to reinforce the discussion from the consultation. In view of the psychological consequences of urogenital pain, experienced pain management psychologists should be at hand. The full range of their skills utilized for chronic pain management will be required, but in addition to these tools, psychosexual counseling and relationship work are often required. For the sexual problems, we operate a system where the medical,

physiotherapy, and nursing staff undertake the medical management of the sexual problems but also provide medical information on normality and variants to enable the patient to place his or her sexual problems in context. Psychological interventions are instigated early and often while physical treatments are ongoing—the aim is to support and prevent psychological and sexual problem deterioration. Both the patient and the psychologist have to able to work with this model of early psychology and ongoing physical treatment.

Trigger Point and Nerve Block Therapies

Trigger points and hyperalgesic muscles should be managed as appropriate with treatment options that include drugs, stretching, paced exercise, relaxation, and injections. Injections into pelvic trigger points are no different than injections into muscles elsewhere, but they require the expertise of a specialist with skills using imaging, such as computed tomography, ultrasound, or possible procedural magnetic resonance imaging. The agent to be injected is not agreed upon, but it usually is a local anaesthetic and corticosteroid mixture. Botulinium toxin injections into some of the deeper pelvic muscles have been advocated.[46] Nerve blocks may have a role in the management of specific nerve injuries but may also serve to relax muscles. Nerve blocks may be therapeutic or diagnostic.[2,12,13,47,48]

Surgical Therapies

Surgery for the CPPS has minimal proven benefit and should not be undertaken without a good surgical reason; if the surgery is significant (e.g., cystectomy), psychological evaluation and intervention should be considered first.

Pharmacological Therapies

There is a debate about whether and when neuropathic drugs have a role in the management of CPPS.[1,2] Tricyclic and tetracyclic antidepressant drugs may have a role if there are neuropathic qualities to the pain. The best evidence is for amitriptyline. Selective serotonin reuptake inhibitors and serotonin–norepinephrine reuptake inhibitors are also considered to have a role. Venlafaxine has the strongest evidence but is troubled with cardiac side effects. Duloxetine may have an advantage where stress incontinence is a problem and there is an evidence base to support its use in widespread pain. Gabapentin and pregabalin have become very popular in the management of chronic pelvic pain, and several studies have suggested that they may have a role. Other anti-epileptics should be considered, as for the management of any neuropathic pain. Opioids should be considered, providing appropriate precautions are undertaken and guidelines are followed.

Neuromodulation

The evidence base for neuromodulation in chronic pelvic/urogenital pain is limited.[2] However, some very good guidelines do exist for the use of neuromodulation in peripheral nerve injury and complex regional pain. Hence, one would expect neuromodulation to help certain urogenital pain conditions. Case history reports support this. The main problem is achieving stimulation in the appropriate area, and whereas some specialists do claim to gain benefit by stimulating the lower thoracic region, it appears that most specialist implanters would now stimulate the sacral roots either by a lumbar retrograde or trans-sacral approach. The stimulation is thus preganglionic/ganglionic and not dorsal horn. The trans-sacral approach is easy to trial by peripheral nerve evaluation and also has the benefit of some excellent guidelines for bowel and bladder dysfunction neuromodulation. It is our policy to try transforaminal/trans-sacral neuromodulation first, and if that fails to reduce the pain, but the patient wishes to try other approaches, we then try lumbar retrograde or lumbar anterograde approaches.

FUTURE DIRECTIONS

Chronic pelvic pain syndromes are common and although they may have different features, at present the evaluation and treatment approaches are similar for all variants. With a more precise classification and careful examination of treatment approaches, it may be possible to identify those therapies most likely to benefit individual patients. However, at present, the state of the art is to have an experienced, caring clinician who interacts with the patient to provide consistent therapy that maximizes function.

REFERENCES

1. Baranowski AP, Abrams P, Fall M. *Urogenital Pain in Clinical Practice*. New York: Informa Healthcare; 2008.
2. Fall M, Baranowski AP, Elneil S, et al. EAU guidelines on chronic pelvic pain. *Eur Urol* 2012;57(1):35–48.
3. Fillingim RB, King CD, Ribeiro-Dasilva MC, Rahim-Williams B, Riley JL, 3rd. Sex, gender, and pain: a review of recent clinical and experimental findings. *J Pain* 2009;10:447–85.
4. Vecchiet L, Vecchiet J, Giamberardino MA. Referred muscle pain: clinical and pathophysiologic aspects. *Curr Rev Pain* 1999;3(6):489–98.
5. Giamberardino MA, De Laurentis S, Affaitati G, Lerza R, Lapenna D, Vecchiet L. Modulation of pain and hyperalgesia from the urinary tract by algogenic conditions of the reproductive organs in women. *Neurosci Lett* 2001;304:61–4.
6. Arendt-Nielsen L, Schipper KP, Dimcevski G, et al. Viscero-somatic reflexes in referred pain areas evoked by capsaicin stimulation of the human gut. *Eur J Pain* 2008;12:544–51.
7. Giamberardino MA, Costantini R, Affaitati G, et al. Viscero-visceral hyperalgesia: characterization in different clinical models. *Pain* 2010;151:307–22.
8. Costigan M, Woolf CJ. Pain: molecular mechanisms. *J Pain* 2000;1:35–44.
9. Latremoliere A, Woolf CJ. Central sensitization: a generator of pain hypersensitivity by central neural plasticity. *J Pain* 2009;10:895–926.
9a. Fall M, Baranowski AP, Fowler CJ, et al. EAU guidelines on chronic pelvic pain. *Eur Urol* 2004;46(6):681–9.
9b. Pasoto SG, Abrao MS, Viana VS, Bueno C, Leon EP, Bonfa E. Endometriosis and systemic lupus erythematosus: a comparative evaluation of clinical manifestations and serological autoimmune phenomena. *Am J Reprod Immunol* 2005;53:85–93.
9c. Tietjen GE, Bushnell CD, Herial NA, Utley C, White L, Hafeez F. Endometriosis is associated with prevalence of comorbid conditions in migraine. *Headache* 2007;47:1069–78.

9d. Warren JW, Wesselmann U, Morozov V, Langenberg PW. Numbers and types of non-bladder syndromes as risk factors for interstitial cystitis/painful bladder syndrome. *Urology* 2011;77:313–9.

10. Weijmar Schultz W, Basson R, et al. Women's sexual pain and its management. *J Sex Med* 2005;2:301–6.

11. Tu FF, Fitzgerald CM, Kuiken T, Farrell T, Harden RN. Comparative measurement of pelvic floor pain sensitivity in chronic pelvic pain. *Obstet Gynecol* 2007;110:1244–8.

12. Labat JJ, Riant T, Robert R, Amarenco G, Lefaucheur JP, Rigaud J. Diagnostic criteria for pudendal neuralgia by pudendal nerve entrapment (Nantes criteria). *Neurourol Urodyn* 2008;27(4):306–10.

13. Labat JJ, Robert R, Delavierre D, Sibert L, Rigaud J. [Symptomatic approach to chronic neuropathic somatic pelvic and perineal pain]. *Prog Urol* 2010;20:973–81.

14. Baranowski AP. Chronic pelvic pain. *Best Pract Res Clin Gastroenterol* 2009;23(4):593–610.

15. Raphael KG. Childhood abuse and pain in adulthood: more than a modest relationship? *Clin J Pain* 2005;21:371–3.

16. Chandler HK, Ciccone DS, Raphael KG. Localization of pain and self-reported rape in a female community sample. *Pain Med* 2006;7: 344–52.

17. Anda RF, Felitti VJ, Bremner JD, et al. The enduring effects of abuse and related adverse experiences in childhood. A convergence of evidence from neurobiology and epidemiology. *Eur Arch Psychiatry Clin Neurosci* 2006;256(3): 174–86.

18. Williams AC, Pena CR, Rice AS. Persistent pain in survivors of torture: a cohort study. *J Pain Symptom Manage* 2010;40:715–22.

19. Stamer UM, Stuber F. Genetic factors in pain and its treatment. *Curr Opin Anaesthesiol* 2007;20: 478–84.

20. Bajaj P, Madsen H, Arendt-Nielsen L. Endometriosis is associated with central sensitization: a psychophysical controlled study. *J Pain* 2003;4:372–80.

21. Berkley KJ, McAllister SL, Accius BE, Winnard KP. Endometriosis-induced vaginal hyperalgesia in the rat: effect of estropause, ovariectomy, and estradiol replacement. *Pain* 2007;132 (Suppl 1):S150–9.

22. He W, Liu X, Zhang Y, Guo SW. Generalized hyperalgesia in women with endometriosis and its resolution following a successful surgery. *Reprod Sci* 2010;17:1099–11.

23. Abrams P, Baranowski A, Berger RE, Fall M, Hanno P, Wesselmann U. A new classification is needed for pelvic pain syndromes—are existing terminologies of spurious diagnostic authority bad for patients? *J Urol* 2006;175:1989–90.

24. Baskin LS, Tanagho EA. Pelvic pain without pelvic organs. *J Urol* 1992;147(3):683–6.

25. Stones RW, Lawrence WT, Selfe SA. Lasting impressions: influence of the initial hospital consultation for chronic pelvic pain on dimensions of patient satisfaction at follow-up. *J Psychosom Res* 2006;60:163–7.

26. Woolf CJ, Doubell TP. The pathophysiology of chronic pain—increased sensitivity to low threshold A beta-fibre inputs. *Curr Opin Neurobiol* 1994;4(4):525–34.

27. Pukall CF, Smith KB, Chamberlain SM. Provoked vestibulodynia. Womens Health (Lond Engl) 2007;3(5):583–92.

28. McMahon SB. Sensitisation of gastrointestinal tract afferents. *Gut* 2004;53(Suppl 2):ii13–15.

29. Nazif O, Teichman JM, Gebhart GF. Neural upregulation in interstitial cystitis. *Urology* 2007;69:24–33.

30. Tripp DA, Nickel JC, Wang Y, et al. Catastrophizing and pain-contingent rest predict patient adjustment in men with chronic prostatitis/chronic pelvic pain syndrome. *J Pain* 2006;7:697–708.

31. Tripp DA, Nickel JC, Fitzgerald MP, Mayer R, Stechyson N, Hsieh A. Sexual functioning, catastrophizing, depression, and pain, as predictors of quality of life in women with interstitial cystitis/painful bladder syndrome. *Urology* 2009;73:987–92.

32. Nickel JC, Tripp DA, Pontari M, et al. Psychosocial phenotyping in women with interstitial cystitis/painful bladder syndrome: a case control study. *J Urol* 2010;183:167–72.

33. Elsenbruch S. Abdominal pain in irritable bowel syndrome: a review of putative psychological, neural and neuro-immune mechanisms. *Brain Behav Immun* 2011;25:386–94.

34. Vase L, Nikolajsen L, Christensen B, et al. Cognitive-emotional sensitization contributes to wind-up-like pain in phantom limb pain patients. *Pain* 2011;152:157–62.

35. Larauche M, Gourcerol G, Million M, Adelson DW, Tache Y. Repeated psychological stress-induced alterations of visceral sensitivity and colonic motor functions in mice: influence of surgery and postoperative single housing on visceromotor responses. *Stress* 2010;13(4):343–54.

36. Peyron R, Faillenot I. [Functionnal brain mapping of pain perception.]. *Med Sci (Paris)* 2011;27:82–7.
37. Bruehl S. An update on the pathophysiology of complex regional pain syndrome. *Anesthesiology* 2010;113(3):713–25.
38. Fulbright RK, Troche CJ, Skudlarski P, Gore JC, Wexler BE. Functional MR imaging of regional brain activation associated with the affective experience of pain. *AJR Am J Roentgenol* 2001;177(5):1205–10.
39. Rygh LJ, Tjolsen A, Hole K, Svendsen F. Cellular memory in spinal nociceptive circuitry. *Scand J Psychol* 2002;43(2):153–9.
40. Akermark C, Johansson C. Tenotomy of the adductor longus tendon in the treatment of chronic groin pain in athletes. *Am J Sports Med* 1992;20(6):640–3.
41. Taylor DC, Meyers WC, Moylan JA, Lohnes J, Bassett FH, Garrett WE, Jr. Abdominal musculature abnormalities as a cause of groin pain in athletes. Inguinal hernias and pubalgia. *Am J Sports Med* 1991;19(3):239–42.
42. Slocumb JC. Neurological factors in chronic pelvic pain: trigger points and the abdominal pelvic pain syndrome. *Am J Obstet Gynecol* 1984;149:536–43.
43. Savidge CJ, Slade P. Psychological aspects of chronic pelvic pain. *J Psychosom Res* 1997;42:433–44.
44. Cervero F, Laird JM. Understanding the signaling and transmission of visceral nociceptive events. *J Neurobiol* 2004;61(1):45–54.
45. Laird JM, Roza C, Cervero F. Effects of artificial calculosis on rat ureter motility: peripheral contribution to the pain of ureteric colic. *Am J Physiol* 1997;272(5 Pt 2):R1409–16.
46. Thomson AJ, Jarvis SK, Lenart M, Abbott JA, Vancaillie TG. The use of botulinum toxin type A (BOTOX) as treatment for intractable chronic pelvic pain associated with spasm of the levator ani muscles. *BJOG* 2005;112:247–9.
47. Naja MZ, Al-Tannir MA, Maaliki H, El-Rajab M, Ziade MF, Zeidan A. Nerve-stimulator-guided repeated pudendal nerve block for treatment of pudendal neuralgia. *Eur J Anaesthesiol* 2006;23:442–4.
48. Robert R, Labat JJ, Bensignor M, et al. Decompression and transposition of the pudendal nerve in pudendal neuralgia: a randomized controlled trial and long-term evaluation. *Eur Urol* 2005;47:403–8.

20

CARDIAC PAIN IN WOMEN

Eileen Handberg and Marian Limacher

INTRODUCTION

Chest pain is traditionally considered the hallmark of symptomatic coronary artery disease, which includes heart attack and stable and unstable coronary syndromes. However, for women, while many experience chest pain associated with cardiac events, many others experience something other than pain in the chest during an acute cardiac event. A full spectrum of sensations (or lack of sensations) may be associated with underlying cardiac problems, and knowledge of that spectrum is needed by both the public and health care providers. Such understanding forms the basis for devising appropriate strategies for the evaluation and management of chest pain and cardiac symptoms in women. Ultimately, the goal of determining which women have underlying cardiac conditions is to reduce the burden of cardiovascular disease on individual patients, families, and society.

This chapter reviews the epidemiology of cardiovascular disease in women, describes the cardiac conditions that elicit symptoms, identifies what differences may exist in the symptoms affecting women and men, offers suggestions for the underlying etiology for symptoms, and lists steps for addressing the diagnosis and management of cardiac symptoms.

EPIDEMIOLOGY OF CORONARY HEART DISEASE

Cardiovascular diseases pose the most significant causes of morbidity and mortality for women, accounting for more than 421,918 deaths annually in the United States, far surpassing cancer or other diseases.[1] Coronary heart disease (CHD) represents the most common type of cardiovascular disease and is caused by atherosclerosis, which is related to well-identified risk factors, including diabetes, cigarette smoking, hypertension, hypercholesterolemia, physical inactivity, and a family history of premature CHD in first-degree relatives. The spectrum of CHD includes angina (or chest pain due to myocardial ischemia), myocardial infarction (MI), ischemic cardiomyopathy, and sudden cardiac death. The incidence of MI has decreased from 1999 to 2008,[2] and overall mortality rates have decreased from 1997 to 2007 by 27.8%[1] due to utilization of evidence-based therapy and modification of risk factors.[3] However, recent trends indicate that the CHD death rates in younger women (age 35 to 54) are increasing.[1]

Estimates for the prevalence of all forms of cardiovascular disease, including CHD, hypertension, valvular heart disease, peripheral and aortic disease, heart failure, and stroke, approach 35% for women.[1] Yet this risk is not equal across racial groups. The prevalence of cardiovascular disease is higher in non-Hispanic black females (47.3%) and lower in Mexican American females (30.9%).[1] Cardiovascular disease deaths vary slightly by race, with 34.5% for whites, 35.4% for blacks, 31.1% for Hispanic or Latinos, and 34.4% of total deaths for Asian/Pacific Islander females.[1] The prevalence of CHD also increases with increasing age, rising from 9.7% of women age 20–39 to 86.7% of women age 80 or older.[1] Deaths in women due to all cardiovascular conditions comprise 51.8% of the total deaths observed annually.[1]

Over 1.1 million hospitalizations for MI occur each year, with the majority being men (721,000 vs. 410,000).[1] Yet women are much more likely to present for the evaluation of chest pain and be hospitalized for chest pain.[1] Women with chest pain symptoms often have persistent, frequent refractory chest pain that is associated with lower ratings of well-being, with more frequent reports of anxiety and/or depressive symptoms, and limitations in activities of daily living.[4]

Because of efforts of health care organizations and providers to educate the public, women are now much more aware of the presence and dangers of CHD as the leading cause of death in women. Up to 57% of women surveyed now recognize that CHD is the leading cause of death, although rates of awareness of this issue vary among racial/ethnic groups.[5,6] The Centers for Disease Control (CDC) Behavioral Risk Factor Surveillance System in 2005 assessed awareness of all five heart attack warning signs and symptoms.[7] When asked who would "call 9–1–1" as the first action to take if they thought someone was having a heart attack or stroke, a total of 86% of the 71,994 respondents indicated that they would do so. However, only 34.6% of women knew all five symptoms of heart attack (pain or discomfort in the jaw, neck, or back; feeling weak, lightheaded, or faint; chest pain or discomfort; pain or discomfort in the arms or shoulder; and shortness of breath), which was still higher than the 26.2% of men responding correctly.[7] Rates of correct responses were lower for black and Hispanic respondents. Residents of the District of Columbia, Mississippi, and Louisiana had the lowest rates for correct responses, as did those with lower levels of education.[7]

While some gains have been made, with regard to awareness of heart disease as a women's disease, with mass media education campaigns including the National Heart Lung and Blood Institute's Red Dress® campaign and American Heart Association's Go Red™ for Women program, women still are

more likely to delay presentation to the emergency department for chest pain symptoms.[7-9] Compounding the problem, women may present with complaints that do not always meet the classic definition of heart attack as described by Heberden.[10] Additionally, when diagnostic testing is performed, women are less likely to have severe obstructions in the coronary arteries, even when the chest pain symptoms are similar.[11] In many clinical trials, women are less likely to undergo the same number or types of diagnostic testing compared with men.[12-14] Consequently, women are less likely to receive interventions advocated by nationally established guidelines.[15-18] All of these factors make the case for more timely and accurate assessment of cardiac symptoms, including chest pain, in women to improve care and decrease morbidity and mortality.[19]

The economic impact of CHD is substantial. The total direct and indirect cost of cardiovascular disease and stroke in 2007 was estimated to be $286 billion,[1] with the result that atherosclerotic coronary disease is one of the top five health expenditures in the United States.[20] In 2007, approximately one-half of the total health care costs for cardiovascular disease were for women, at a cost of $108.9 billion. Nonspecific chest pain in women accounted for more than half of all hospital stays.[20] In women with nonsevere coronary disease who experience symptoms of ischemia, including chest pain, the average lifetime cost estimate of the disease is approximately $770,000, similar to the $1.0–$1.1 million lifetime expenditures for women with one-vessel to three-vessel coronary artery disease.[21]

CARDIAC PAIN

Chest pain is a common complaint of patients presenting to hospital emergency departments. In 2004, over 6 million patients presented to hospital emergency centers, second only to complaints of stomach or abdominal pain.[22] Cardiac pain in women is an important concern given its prevalence. Over 5 million women have chest pain due to coronary disease, also labeled angina pectoris.[1] Cardiac pain, like other types of pain, results in significant impairment of quality of life.[23] More important, however, is its association with morbidity and mortality due to underlying CHD.

Assessment of cardiac pain in women is not straightforward by means of its characterization, diagnosis, or treatment. Cardiac pain may be caused by any number of cardiovascular diseases, including coronary artery disease, valvular heart disease, hypertensive heart disease, arrhythmias such as atrial fibrillation, pericardial disease, and diseases of the aorta, as well as noncardiac sources such as problems involving the lungs, gastrointestinal tract, musculoskeletal systems, or other mechanisms (Table 20.1).

When defining pain as "an unpleasant sensory and emotional experience associated with actual or potential tissue damage, or described in terms of such damage,"[24] localizing pain to the chest may describe a broad range of complaints. The term "chest pain" is commonly used to reflect discomfort related to underlying cardiac disease; however, the source of chest symptoms may be other organs or systems besides the heart. For example, the chest pain of costochondritis, which is an inflammation of the cartilage of the rib cage, may cause anterior chest wall pain. The specific description of chest pain originating from ischemic myocardium due to atherosclerotic coronary disease is termed "angina pectoris" or "angina" from the Latin "angore" meaning choking/suffocation and also anxiety, fear, or terror.[25] The description of angina dates back to 1768 when William Heberden presented to the Royal College of Physicians. He described patients with angina pectoris as "They who are afflicted with it, are seized while they are walking (more especially if it be up hill, and soon after eating) with a painful and most disagreeable sensation in the breast, which seems as if it would extinguish life, if it were to increase or continue; but the moment they stand still, all this uneasiness vanishes."[10] This description has undergone only slight modification over the past century. The European Society of Cardiology defines stable angina as a "clinical syndrome characterized by discomfort in the chest, jaw, shoulder, back, or arms, typically elicited by exertion or emotional stress and relieved by rest or nitroglycerin (NTG). Less typically, discomfort may occur in the epigastric area."[26]

PHYSIOLOGY OF CHEST PAIN

Once Heberden had characterized cardiac chest pain, inquiry into the proposed mechanisms for the source of ischemic cardiac pain quickly followed. In the early 20th century, several theories emerged, including intermittent claudication, cramping of the muscle, and distention of the ventricular wall as possible explanations for the source of ischemic cardiac pain.[27] The "mechanical hypothesis" proposed by Colbeck in 1903[27] was followed many years later by a "chemical hypothesis" positing that ischemic pain was a result of the release from the myocardium of pain-producing substances brought on by ischemia.[28] Only in the last 20 years has the ability to isolate and measure cardiac nerves and receptors led to progress in better understanding the possible mechanisms of ischemic cardiac pain.[29] While the mechanical theory of Colbeck[27] has been disproven as the primary source of cardiac pain, mechanical factors may play a role in the activation of sensory receptors located in the heart.[30]

The prevailing understanding is that angina pectoris is a result of the stimulation of chemosensitive and mechanoreceptive receptors in the heart.[31] Afferent sympathetic fibers are responsible for the transmission of cardiac pain.[29] The sympathetic afferent fibers in the heart and coronary arteries lead to the upper thoracic spinal cord from T2-C8 and synapse on cells in the ascending pathways.[29,32] The perceived location of cardiac pain is a function of the visceral and somatic afferents in the central nervous system, and patients frequently experience pain in the mid portion of the sternum, the left side of the chest radiating to the left arm, the epigastric area, and into the neck region. The stimulation of fibers in the upper thoracic and lower cervical segments contributes to the pain felt in the chest and arm. The cardiac vagal afferent fibers contribute to the pain felt in the neck and the jaw. The afferent vagal fibers may also play a role in the transmission of cardiac pain.[33] Because of the spatial organization of afferent fibers in the heart, ischemic pain from different regions of the heart may be experienced in different somatic regions. However, some researchers have reported similar distributions of cardiac pain originating from different

Table 20.1   Underlying Conditions Causing Chest Pain

Cardiovascular etiologies	Acute coronary syndrome
	Unstable angina pectoris
	Acute myocardial infarction
	Stable angina pectoris
	Aortic dissection
	Aortic stenosis
	Pericarditis
	Myocarditis
	Arrhythmias
Pulmonary etiologies	Pulmonary embolism
	Pneumonia
	Pneumothorax
	Hemothorax
	Pleurisy
Gastrointestinal etiologies	Gastroesophageal reflux disease/heartburn
	Hiatal hernia
	Nutcracker esophagus
	Boerhaave syndrome
	Esophageal spasm and other disorders
	Esophageal carcinoma
	Functional dyspepsia
	Cholecystitis
	Pancreatitis
	Duodenal ulcer
	Gastritis
Chest wall etiologies	Costochondritis
	Spinal nerve conditions
	Fibromyalgia
	Rib fracture
	Herpes zoster (shingles)
	Tuberculosis
	Bornholm disease (epidemic pleurodynia/epidemic myalgia)
Psychological etiologies	Panic disorder
	Anxiety
	Depression
	Somatization disorder
	Hypochondria
Others	Hyperventilation syndrome
	DaCosta's syndrome (neurocirculatory asthenia)
	Precordial catch syndrome
	Carbon monoxide poisoning
	Sarcoidosis
	Lead poisoning

regions of the myocardium,[34,35] while others found significant differences in the spatial location of pain during coronary artery occlusion of different arteries.[36]

The chemical hypothesis was further developed by the use of adenosine to identify abnormal coronary artery function. Administration of adenosine often results in chest pain.[31] During myocardial ischemia, adenosine is rapidly formed and released into the vascular system and serves as a regulator of coronary blood flow through its dilation of coronary arteries.[37] Strong evidence exists that sympathetic afferent pathways are activated by adenosine and play a role in generation of angina pectoris through activation of membrane receptors. Surface membrane P1 receptors have two subtypes, A1 and A2, that adenosine stimulates to produce cardiac effects. Several studies suggest that A1 receptors are the primary mediators of the effects of endogenous adenosine on pain.[29,31,37,38] In response to ischemia, the heart releases a variety of chemicals, including adenosine, bradykinin, lactate, and potassium, which excite the receptors that transmit nociceptive information to the central nervous system, and substance P further sensitizes nociceptors and intensifies the pain.[29]

The temporal relationship between cardiac pain and ischemia is variable. In those who develop severe transient ischemia, chest pain only occurs after the onset of metabolic, contractile, and electrical alterations in the cardiac muscle and may take several minutes to appear (Fig. 20.1). However, some individuals who develop ischemia of milder severity still experience significant chest pain, even before these changes are seen on an electrocardiogram.[31] Cardiac pain does not always result in damage to the heart muscle, and ischemia can occur without symptoms at all. According to Crea and Gaspardone, the cause of ischemia, whether through increased demand in chronic stable angina or from an acute thrombotic occlusion, does not generally affect the characteristics of the angina.[31]

Patients with syndrome X, defined as those who present with chest pain symptoms in the absence of either electrocardiographic changes or occlusive coronary artery disease, experience sustained release of adenosine, which may be

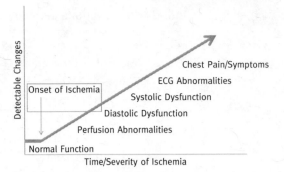

FIGURE 20.1 Manifestations of myocardial ischemia. Symptoms of chest pain or other perceptible features typically occur only after other detectable cardiac abnormalities. ECG, electrocardiogram.

enough to stimulate afferent fibers to produce pain. Syndrome X patients have been reported to have a high sensitivity to painful stimuli.[39]

CLASSIFICATION OF ANGINA PECTORIS

The diagnosis of angina is obtained by taking a careful history from the patient. Questions should include the location, quality, intensity, and duration of the pain as well as any precipitating factors, associated symptoms, and maneuvers or treatments that resulted in relief. The Canadian Cardiovascular Society classification standardizes angina based on duration and intensity[40] (Table 20.2). Because of the variability in the description of cardiac pain by women and men, other chest pain questionnaires have been developed to better discriminate cardiac pain from noncardiac causes and to be able to assess changes in chest pain over time. An early self-administered questionnaire developed by Rose and others used 19 items to classify chest pain.[41] The Rose questionnaire has been validated and utilized in many studies to classify chest pain, and it may also be used to predict coronary events, as reported in subjects enrolled in the Second Manifestations of Arterial disease study (SMART).[42] One additional validated tool is the Seattle Angina Questionnaire,[43] which captures additional domains of quality of life in addition to angina frequency. Other chest pain tools have been developed[44] to try and improve the diagnostic accuracy of chest pain

Table 20.2   Canadian Cardiovascular Society Grading of Angina Pectoris

GRADE	DESCRIPTION
Grade I	Ordinary physical activity does not cause angina, such as walking and climbing stairs. Angina with strenuous or rapid or prolonged exertion at work or recreation
Grade II	Slight limitation of ordinary activity. Walking or climbing stairs rapidly, walking uphill, walking or stair climbing after meals, or in cold, or in wind, or under emotional stress, or only during the few hours after awakening. Walking more than two blocks on the level and climbing more than one flight of ordinary stairs at a normal pace and in normal conditions
Grade III	Marked limitation of ordinary physical activity. Walking one or two blocks on the level and climbing one flight of stairs in normal conditions and at normal pace
Grade IV	Inability to carry on any physical activity without discomfort, angina syndrome may be present at rest.

Source: From Campeau L. Letter: grading of angina pectoris. *Circulation* 1976;54(3):522–3.

assessment so that appropriate care can be delivered. Application of this method has been somewhat limited because of high sensitivity (91.4%) but low specificity (28%) for coronary artery disease.[44]

ACUTE PAIN

Cardiac chest pain may either be acute or chronic, severe to mild. Acute severe cardiac pain when caused by abrupt onset myocardial ischemia or lack of blood flow to the heart muscle is labeled acute coronary syndrome (ACS). The typical chest discomfort associated with ACS is described as pressure, burning, squeezing, or smothering in the substernal region with radiation to the neck, jaw, and/or left arm. This discomfort is often associated with one or more of the following additional symptoms: diaphoresis, nausea, vomiting, dyspnea, palpitations, or lightheadedness. ACS includes a spectrum of ischemia from unstable angina, non-ST segment elevation myocardial infarction (NSTEMI) and ST segment elevation myocardial infarction (STEMI).[45,46]

The most common etiology for ACS results from coronary artery obstruction caused by a thrombus that develops at the site of disrupted atherosclerotic plaque on the intimal surface of a coronary artery. Alternatively, arterial inflammation may lead to plaque expansion and destabilization, rupture or erosion, and then subsequent formation of an occlusive thrombus. A less common cause of ACS is dynamic obstruction, which may be triggered by focal spasm of a segment of an epicardial coronary artery (also called Prinzmetal's angina). This spasm is caused by hypercontractility of vascular smooth muscle and/or by endothelial dysfunction and is usually seen in the presence of some degree of atherosclerosis. Other rarer conditions, such as coronary artery dissection, may present with acute chest pain. Additionally, some conditions that increase myocardial oxygen requirements, such as fever, increased heart rate, or excessive thyroid hormone levels, can also induce myocardial ischemia if they occur in the presence of chronic coronary arterial narrowing due to atherosclerosis. Angina pectoris can also develop when coronary arterial flow is reduced due to low blood pressure or lack of oxygen delivery due to anemia or low levels of oxygen in the blood. These conditions require rapid identification and treatment to relieve the obstruction or inciting factors and restore coronary blood flow before the heart muscle is damaged. Once damage occurs, the extent of damage and scar determines residual cardiac function and long-term outcome.[45,46] While most episodes of coronary arterial disruption and thrombus formation result in significant pain, approximately 37% of women and 27% of men with ACS report no chest pain or discomfort.[47]

CHRONIC CHEST PAIN

While many severe episodes of cardiac chest pain occur in the setting of ACS or MI with significant long-term cardiac dysfunction if not treated immediately, the spectrum of cardiac pain also includes reproducible pain that is not caused by complete coronary artery occlusion. The characteristics of classic angina, as described in men, include deep, poorly localized chest or arm discomfort that is reproducibly associated with physical exertion or emotional stress and is relieved promptly (i.e., in less than 5 min) with rest and/or the use of sublingual NTG.[41] Women may have identical symptoms but may also present with symptoms of upper back, neck, or jaw pain; nausea alone; or unexplained fatigue.[47] Some patients may have no chest discomfort but present solely with jaw, neck, ear, arm, shoulder, back, or epigastric discomfort or with dyspnea without discomfort. If the symptoms are related to exertion or stress or are relieved promptly with NTG or rest, they should be considered equivalent to angina. Unexplained shortness of breath, even without angina, is associated with an increased risk of death compared with more typical chest pain.[48] In the Women's Health Initiative, women discharged from the hospital with a diagnosis of nonspecific chest pain had up to two-fold greater risk for subsequent coronary artery disease events over the next 6 to 8 years.[49] These data are consistent with another recent report that patients, most of whom were women, discharged from rapid chest pain assessment clinics with chest pain deemed "noncardiac" accounted for nearly one-third of cardiac events during a 3-year follow-up period.[50]

Women with nonobstructive coronary artery disease but with evidence of microvascular abnormalities often have persistent chest pain that is generally considered out of proportion to the amount of disease. Despite the lack of obstructive disease, women with microvascular dysfunction utilize a lot of health care resources and have a reduced quality of life and worse outcome.[4] The characteristics of pain in women with coronary microvascular disease are often somewhat atypical and include complaints of dyspnea, occurrence at rest or with mental stress but not physical, and of debilitating severity. Interestingly, these women also have other small-vessel pain syndromes such as migraines and general pain conditions, including fibromyalgia.[51]

GENDER DIFFERENCES IN CHEST PAIN PRESENTATION

Evidence has been growing that men and women report differences in the perception and severity of pain and analgesia. Extensive research has documented that most common forms of pain are more prevalent in women and that women have a higher sensitivity to most forms of experimentally induced pain with the exception of ischemic pain.[52] Substantial data document differences between women and men in terms of their descriptions of angina pectoris.

PRESENTATION OF CHEST PAIN IN WOMEN

Evaluating women who present with chest pain may be challenging if the symptoms are not consistent with the classic description of angina.[47] Women with underlying coronary disease may be more likely to present with symptoms of fatigue, shortness of breath, and sleep disturbances.[53] Women may complain of chronic chest pain that occurs at rest, with mental stress, and during sleep.[23] Additionally, women who present with either classic or atypical chest pain symptoms are less likely than men to have underlying obstructive disease and are less likely to undergo diagnostic testing and subsequent interventions.[6,11,54] In the American College of Cardiology National Cardiovascular Registry of 375,886 patients referred for left heart catheterization, the prevalence of obstructive coronary disease was lower for women than men, across all age groups ranging from 27% to 64% for women compared with 45% to 87% in men.[54,55] Despite women being less likely to have obstructive disease, the prognosis for women once they experience an MI is worse, as women have a higher 1-year death rate and rate of reinfarction.[1]

EVALUATION OF CHEST PAIN

Women who present to emergency rooms or doctors' offices for evaluation of chest pain should be evaluated and treated based on the current ACC/AHA guidelines.[45,46] The quality and characteristics of symptoms can aid in diagnostic and management decisions, as outlined in the triage recommendations in Table 20.3.[56]

For women at intermediate risk for having significant coronary disease, management can be addressed using published algorithms (Fig. 20.2).[57] Diagnostic evaluation includes exercise stress testing with or without echocardiography or nuclear imaging, and coronary angiography. Newer imaging options exist, such as computed tomographic angiography and cardiac magnetic resonance imaging. Based on the results of these studies, the goal of therapy is to reduce the ischemic burden by reducing obstructions to flow (interventions such as percutaneous coronary interventions or coronary artery bypass grafting) or by reducing demand with pharmacological agents such as beta blockers, calcium antagonists, long-acting nitrates, and other antianginals such as ranolazine. Additional therapy for associated risk conditions such as hypertension,[58] hypercholesterolemia,[59] and anemia can also result in reductions in chest pain due to reduction in demand and/or other pleiotrophic effects of prescribed medications.

PERSISTENT CHEST PAIN

Once testing is completed, a significant percentage of women without obstructive disease continue to have chest pain. This persistent chest pain in the setting of nonobstructive disease is a prevalent issue with reports of 30%–50%.[60] A common terminology for this is microvascular angina (MVA).[61] In the NHLBI-sponsored Womens' Ischemia Syndrome Evaluation (WISE), approximately 60% of women with nonobstructive disease and chest pain were found to have measures of impaired endothelial function and reduced coronary flow reserve

Table 20.3 Recommendations for Patients and Medical Personnel in the Immediate Assessment of Cardiac Symptoms[56]

PATIENT CHIEF SYMPTOMS REQUIRING IMMEDIATE ASSESSMENT

- Chest pain, pressure, tightness, or heaviness; pain that radiates to neck, jaw, shoulders, back, or one or both arms
- Indigestion or "heartburn", nausea and/or vomiting associated with chest discomfort
- Persistent shortness of breath
- Weakness, dizziness, lightheadedness, loss of consciousness

MEDICAL PERSONNEL SHOULD DIRECT ACUTE CORONARY SYNDROME PROTOCOL ASSESSMENT FOR PATIENTS PRESENTING WITH THE FOLLOWING SIGNS AND SYMPTOMS

- Chest pain or severe epigastric pain, nontraumatic in origin, with components typical of myocardial ischemia or myocardial infarction:
  - Central/substernal compression or crushing chest pain
  - Pressure, tightness, heaviness, cramping, burning, aching sensation
  - Unexplained indigestion, belching, epigastric pain
  - Radiating pain in neck, jaw, shoulders, back, or one or both arms
- Associated dyspnea
- Associated nausea and/or vomiting
- Associated diaphoresis

Source: National Heart Attack Alert Program. *Emergency Department: Rapid Identification and Treatment of Patients with Acute Myocardial Infarction.* Bethesda, MD: US Department of Health and Human Services; 1993.

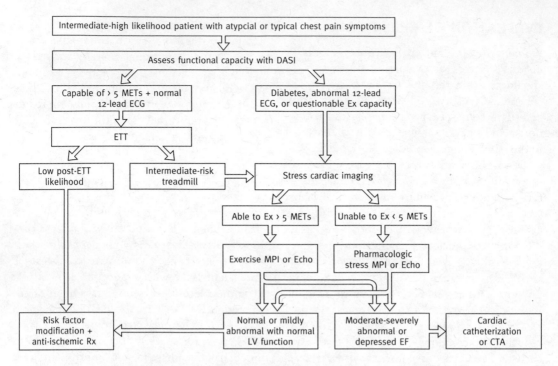

FIGURE 20.2　Algorithm for assessment of women with cardiac symptoms and intermediate risk. CTA, computed tomographic angiography; DASI, Duke Activity Status Index; ECG, electrocardiogram; Echo, echocardiogram; EF, ejection fraction; ETT, exercise treadmill test; Ex, exercise; LV, left ventricle; METs, metabolic equivalents; MPI, myocardial perfusion imaging; Rx, medication. (Reprinted with permission from Phillips LM, Mieres JH. Noninvasive assessment of coronary artery disease in women: what's next? *Curr Cardiol Rep* 2010;12[2]:147–154.)

indicating an impairment in the microcirculation.[62] While the lack of obstructive disease generally calls for a sigh of relief and move to find other noncardiac causes of chest pain, women with reduced coronary flow reserve and endothelial dysfunction have persistent chest pain and continue to seek medical attention for treatment. While previously viewed as not important, long-term follow-up of this population reveals that they are at increased risk for development of progressive obstructive disease and increased mortality.[61,63,64]

Treatment of chest pain in these women, who generally have multiple risk factors, requires a combination of current guideline-recommended treatment to reduce cardiovascular risk, including aspirin in older women, cholesterol-lowering therapy with HMG CoA reductase inhibitors commonly called statins, hypertension control, and diabetes management. Statin therapy, independent of its effects on lipid levels, has been shown to improve endothelial function.[65,66] Angiotensin-converting enzyme inhibitors, used for hypertension and heart failure, also improve endothelial function and coronary flow reserve.[67,68] Symptomatic pain relief is often achieved with conventional anti-anginal therapy—long-acting nitrates, calcium antagonists, beta blockers, and ranolazine, a newer agent approved for angina in patients with obstructive disease.[69] For persistent chest pain, other medications have been utilized with varying degrees of success, including psychiatric drugs. Tricyclic antidepressants[70] and serotonin reuptake inhibitors such as fluoxetine[71] and sertraline[72] have been shown to improve chest pain symptoms. Additionally, cognitive-behavioral therapy combined with paroxetine has been used with some success in noncardiac chest pain patients.[73] The concept of microvascular dysfunction is not universally accepted in the clinical environment, resulting in many women being referred for psychiatric, gastrointestinal, or other evaluations.[74]

SUMMARY

Women are at risk for cardiovascular disease and commonly experience chest discomfort due to underlying coronary artery disease. However, many women with chest pain have nonobstructive coronary disease and may have microvascular abnormalities. Others have noncardiac etiologies for their symptoms. Additionally, many women with significant coronary disease have no significant cardiac symptoms. The assessment and management of women with chest pain remains a challenging clinical problem. Understanding the variability of cardiac symptoms and applying the appropriate means to assess underlying etiologies of chest pain should lead to improved cardiovascular outcomes and a reduction in undiagnosed and untreated symptoms. Further research will add to the current level of understanding and guidelines for clinical practice in addressing chest pain in women.

REFERENCES

1. Roger VL, Go AS, Lloyd-Jones DM, et al. Heart disease and stroke statistics – 2011 update: a report from the American Heart Association. *Circulation* 2011;123(4):e18–209.
2. Yeh RW, Sidney S, Chandra M, Sorel M, Selby JV, Go AS. Population trends in the incidence and outcomes of acute myocardial infarction. *N Engl J Med* 2010;362(23):2155–65.
3. Ford ES, Ajani UA, Croft JB, et al. Explaining the decrease in U.S. deaths from coronary disease, 1980–2000. *N Engl J Med* 2007;356(23):2388–98.
4. Olson MB, Kelsey SF, Matthews K, et al. Symptoms, myocardial ischaemia and quality of life in women: results from the NHLBI-sponsored WISE Study. *Eur Heart J* 2003;24(16):1506–14.
5. Christian AH, Rosamond W, White AR, Mosca L. Nine-year trends and racial and ethnic disparities in women's awareness of heart disease and stroke: an American Heart Association national study. *J Womens Health (Larchmt)* 2007; 16(1):68–81.
6. Mosca L, Mochari H, Christian A, et al. National study of women's awareness, preventive action, and barriers to cardiovascular health. *Circulation* 2006;113(4):525–34.
7. Fang J, Keenan N, Dai S, Denny C. Disparities in adult awareness of heart attack warning signs and symptoms–14 states, 2005. *MMWR* 2008(57):175–9.
8. Diercks DB, Owen KP, Kontos MC, et al. Gender differences in time to presentation for myocardial infarction before and after a national women's cardiovascular awareness campaign: a temporal analysis from the Can Rapid Risk Stratification of Unstable Angina Patients Suppress ADverse Outcomes with Early Implementation (CRUSADE) and the National Cardiovascular Data Registry Acute Coronary Treatment and Intervention Outcomes Network-Get with the Guidelines (NCDR ACTION Registry-GWTG). *Am Heart J* 2010;160(1):80–7, e83.
9. Goldberg RJ, Steg PG, Sadiq I, et al. Extent of, and factors associated with, delay to hospital presentation in patients with acute coronary disease (the GRACE registry). *Am J Cardiol* 2002;89(7):791–6.
10. Heberden W. Some account of disorders of the breast. *Med Trans R Col Physicians (London)* 1772;2:59–67.
11. Bairey Merz CN, Shaw LJ, Reis SE, et al. Insights from the NHLBI-Sponsored Women's Ischemia Syndrome Evaluation (WISE) Study: Part II: gender differences in presentation, diagnosis, and outcome with regard to gender-based pathophysiology of atherosclerosis and macrovascular and microvascular coronary disease. *J Am Coll Cardiol* 2006;47(3 Suppl):S21–9.
12. Ayanian JZ, Epstein AM. Differences in the use of procedures between women and men hospitalized for coronary heart disease. *N Engl J Med* 1991;325(4):221–5.
13. Rathore SS, Wang Y, Radford MJ, Ordin DL, Krumholz HM. Sex differences in cardiac catheterization after acute myocardial infarction: the role of procedure appropriateness. *Ann Intern Med* 2002;137(6):487–93.
14. Vaitkus PT. Gender differences in the utilization of cardiac catheterization for the diagnosis of chest pain. *Am J Cardiol* 1995;75(1):79–81.
15. Kostis JB, Wilson AC, O'Dowd K, et al. Sex differences in the management and long-term outcome of acute myocardial infarction. A statewide study. MIDAS Study Group. Myocardial Infarction Data Acquisition System. *Circulation* 1994;90(4):1715–30.
16. Maynard C, Althouse R, Cerqueira M, Olsufka M, Kennedy JW. Underutilization of thrombolytic therapy in eligible women with acute myocardial infarction. *Am J Cardiol* 1991;68(5):529–30.
17. Pagley PR, Yarzebski J, Goldberg R, et al. Gender differences in the treatment of patients with acute myocardial infarction. A multihospital,

community-based perspective. *Arch Intern Med* 1993;153(5):625–9.

18. Turnbull F, Arima H, Heeley E, et al. Gender disparities in the assessment and management of cardiovascular risk in primary care: the AusHEART study. *Eur J Cardiovasc Prev Rehabil* 2011;18(3):498–503.

19. Mosca L, Benjamin EJ, Berra K, et al. Effectiveness-based guidelines for the prevention of cardiovascular disease in women—2011 update: a guideline from the American Heart Association. *J Am Coll Cardiol* 2011; 57(12):1404–23.

20. Russo CA, Andrews RM. The national hospital bill: the most expensive conditions, by payer, 2004. HCUP Statistical Brief No. 13. 2006. Available at: http://www.hcup-us.ahrq.gov/ reports/statbriefs/sb13.pdf. [accessed on June 9, 2012].

21. Shaw LJ, Merz CN, Pepine CJ, et al. The economic burden of angina in women with suspected ischemic heart disease: results from the National Institutes of Health—National Heart, Lung, and Blood Institute—sponsored Women's Ischemia Syndrome Evaluation. *Circulation* 2006; 114(9):894–904.

22. McCaig LF, Nawar EW. National Hospital Ambulatory Medical Care Survey: 2004 emergency department summary. *Adv Data* 2006; (372):1–29.

23. Pepine CJ. Angina pectoris in a contemporary population: characteristics and therapeutic implications. TIDES Investigators. *Cardiovasc Drugs Ther* 1998;12(Suppl 3):211–16.

24. Merskey H, Bogduk N. Part III. Pain terms, a current list with definitions and notes on usage. In: Merskey H, Bogduk N, eds. *Classification of Chronic Pain: Descriptions of Chronic Pain Syndromes and Definitions of Pain Terms*. 2nd ed. Seattle, WA: IASP Press; 1994: 209–14.

25. Kones R. Recent advances in the management of chronic stable angina I: approach to the patient, diagnosis, pathophysiology, risk stratification, and gender disparities. *Vasc Health Risk Manag* 2010;6:635–56.

26. Fox K, Garcia MA, Ardissino D, et al. Guidelines on the management of stable angina pectoris: executive summary: the Task Force on the Management of Stable Angina Pectoris of the European Society of Cardiology. *Eur Heart J* 2006;27(11):1341–81.

27. Colbeck EH. Angina pectoris: a criticism and a hypothesis. *Lancet* 1903;161(4151):793–5.

28. Lewis T. Pain in muscular ischemia: its relation to anginal pain. *Arch Intern Med* 1932;49:713–27.

29. Foreman RD. Mechanisms of cardiac pain. *Annu Rev Physiol* 1999;61:143–67.

30. Davies GJ, Bencivelli W, Fragasso G, et al. Sequence and magnitude of ventricular volume changes in painful and painless myocardial ischemia. *Circulation* 1988;78(2):310–9.

31. Crea F, Gaspardone A. New look to an old symptom: angina pectoris. *Circulation* 1997;96(10): 3766–73.

32. Meller ST, Gebhart GF. A critical review of the afferent pathways and the potential chemical mediators involved in cardiac pain. *Neuroscience* 1992;48(3):501–24.

33. Meller ST, Lewis SJ, Ness TJ, Brody MJ, Gebhart GF. Vagal afferent-mediated inhibition of a nociceptive reflex by intravenous serotonin in the rat. I. Characterization. *Brain Res* 1990;524(1):90–100.

34. Eriksson B, Vuorisalo D, Sylven C. Diagnostic potential of chest pain characteristics in coronary care. *J Intern Med* 1994;235(5):473–8.

35. Pasceri V, Cianflone D, Finocchiaro ML, Crea F, Maseri A. Relation between myocardial infarction site and pain location in Q-wave acute myocardial infarction. *Am J Cardiol* 1995;75(4):224–7.

36. Lichstein E, Breitbart S, Shani J, Hollander G, Greengart A. Relationship between location of chest pain and site of coronary artery occlusion. *Am Heart J* 1988;115(3):564–8.

37. Berne RM. The role of adenosine in the regulation of coronary blood flow. *Circ Res* 1980; 47(6):807–13.

38. Haneda T, Ichihara K, Abiko Y, Onodera S. Release of adenosine and lactate from human hearts during atrial pacing in patients with ischemic heart disease. *Clin Cardiol* 1989;12(2):76–82.

39. Maseri A, Crea F, Kaski JC, Crake T. Mechanisms of angina pectoris in syndrome X. *J Am Coll Cardiol* 1991;17(2):499–506.

40. Campeau L. Letter: grading of angina pectoris. *Circulation* 1976;54(3):522–3.

41. Rose G, McCartney P, Reid DD. Self-administration of a questionnaire on chest pain and intermittent claudication. *Br J Prev Soc Med* 1977;31(1):42–8.

42. Achterberg S, Soedamah-Muthu S, Cramer M, Kappelle L, van der Graaf Y, Algra A. Prognostic value of the Rose questionnaire: a validation with future coronary events in the SMART study. *Eur J Cardiovasc Prev Rehabil* 2012;19(1):5–14.

43. Spertus JA, Winder JA, Dewhurst TA, et al. Development and evaluation of the Seattle Angina Questionnaire: a new functional status measure for coronary artery disease. *J Am Coll Cardiol* 1995;25(2):333–41.

44. Wu EB, Hodson F, Chambers JB. A simple score for predicting coronary artery disease in patients with chest pain. *QJM* 2005;98(11):803–11.

45. Kushner FG, Hand M, Smith SC, Jr, et al. 2009 focused updates: ACC/AHA guidelines for the management of patients with ST-elevation myocardial infarction (updating the 2004 guideline and 2007 focused update) and ACC/AHA/SCAI guidelines on percutaneous coronary intervention (updating the 2005 guideline and 2007 focused update) a report of the American College of Cardiology Foundation/American Heart Association Task Force on Practice Guidelines. *J Am Coll Cardiol* 2009;54(23):2205–41.

46. Wright RS, Anderson JL, Adams CD, et al. 2011 ACCF/AHA Focused Update incorporated into the ACC/AHA 2007 Guidelines for the Management of Patients with Unstable Angina/Non-ST-Elevation Myocardial Infarction. A report of the American College of Cardiology Foundation/American Heart Association Task Force on Practice Guidelines developed in collaboration with the American Academy of Family Physicians, Society for Cardiovascular Angiography and Interventions, and the Society of Thoracic Surgeons. *J Am Coll Cardiol* 2011;57(19):e215–367.

47. Canto JG, Goldberg RJ, Hand MM, et al. Symptom presentation of women with acute coronary syndromes: myth vs reality. *Arch Intern Med* 2007;167(22):2405–13.

48. Abidov A, Rozanski A, Hachamovitch R, et al. Prognostic significance of dyspnea in patients referred for cardiac stress testing. *N Engl J Med* 2005;353(18):1889–98.

49. Robinson JG, Wallace R, Limacher M, et al. Elderly women diagnosed with nonspecific chest pain may be at increased cardiovascular risk. *J Womens Health (Larchmt)* 2006;15(10):1151–60.

50. Sekhri N, Feder GS, Junghans C, Hemingway H, Timmis AD. How effective are rapid access chest pain clinics? Prognosis of incident angina and non-cardiac chest pain in 8762 consecutive patients. *Heart* 2007;93(4):458–63.

51. Bairey Merz CN, Shaw LJ. Stable angina in women: lessons from the National Heart, Lung and Blood Institute-sponsored Women's Ischemia Syndrome Evaluation. *J Cardiovasc Med (Hagerstown)* 2011;12(2):85–7.

52. Fillingim RB, King CD, Ribeiro-Dasilva MC, Rahim-Williams B, Riley JL, 3rd. Sex, gender, and pain: a review of recent clinical and experimental findings. *J Pain* 2009;10(5):447–85.

53. McSweeney JC, Cody M, O'Sullivan P, Elberson K, Moser DK, Garvin BJ. Women's early warning symptoms of acute myocardial infarction. *Circulation* 2003;108(21):2619–23.

54. Shaw LJ, Shaw RE, Merz CN, et al. Impact of ethnicity and gender differences on angiographic coronary artery disease prevalence and in-hospital mortality in the American College of Cardiology-National Cardiovascular Data Registry. *Circulation* 2008;117(14):1787–801.

55. Shaw LJ, Shaw RE, Radford M, et al. Sex and ethnic differences in the prevalence of significant and severe coronary artery disease in the ACC–National Cardiovascular Data registry. *Circulation* 2004;110:SIII-800.

56. National Heart Attack Alert Program. *Emergency Department: Rapid Identification and Treatment of Patients with Acute Myocardial Infarction.* Bethesda, MD: US Department of Health and Human Services; 1993.

57. Phillips LM, Mieres JH. Noninvasive assessment of coronary artery disease in women: what's next? *Curr Cardiol Rep* 2010;12(2):147–54.

58. Chobanian AV, Bakris GL, Black HR, et al. The Seventh Report of the Joint National Committee on Prevention, Detection, Evaluation, and Treatment of High Blood Pressure: the JNC 7 report. *JAMA* 2003;289(19):2560–72.

59. Third Report of the National Cholesterol Education Program (NCEP) Expert Panel on Detection, Evaluation, and Treatment of High Blood Cholesterol in Adults (Adult Treatment Panel III) final report. *Circulation* 2002;106(25):3143–421.

60. Sharaf BL, Pepine CJ, Kerensky RA, et al. Detailed angiographic analysis of women with suspected ischemic chest pain (pilot phase data from the NHLBI-sponsored Women's Ischemia Syndrome Evaluation [WISE] Study Angiographic Core Laboratory). *Am J Cardiol* 2001;87(8):937–41, A933.

61. Vesely MR, Dilsizian V. Microvascular angina: assessment of coronary blood flow, flow reserve, and metabolism. *Curr Cardiol Rep* 2011;13(2):151–8.

62. Reis SE, Holubkov R, Lee JS, et al. Coronary flow velocity response to adenosine characterizes coronary microvascular function in women with chest pain and no obstructive coronary disease. Results from the pilot phase of the Women's Ischemia Syndrome Evaluation (WISE) study. *J Am Coll Cardiol* 1999;33(6):1469–75.

63. Pepine CJ, Anderson RD, Sharaf BL, et al. Coronary microvascular reactivity to adenosine predicts adverse outcome in women evaluated for suspected ischemia results from the National

Heart, Lung and Blood Institute WISE (Women's Ischemia Syndrome Evaluation) study. *J Am Coll Cardiol* 2010;55(25):2825–32.

64. Smilowitz NR, Sampson BA, Abrecht CR, Siegfried JS, Hochman JS, Reynolds HR. Women have less severe and extensive coronary atherosclerosis in fatal cases of ischemic heart disease: an autopsy study. *Am Heart J* 2011;161(4):681–8.

65. Caliskan M, Erdogan D, Gullu H, et al. Effects of atorvastatin on coronary flow reserve in patients with slow coronary flow. *Clin Cardiol* 2007;30(9):475–9.

66. Kayikcioglu M, Payzin S, Yavuzgil O, Kultursay H, Can LH, Soydan I. Benefits of statin treatment in cardiac syndrome-X1. *Eur Heart J* 2003;24(22):1999–2005.

67. Chen JW, Hsu NW, Wu TC, Lin SJ, Chang MS. Long-term angiotensin-converting enzyme inhibition reduces plasma asymmetric dimethylarginine and improves endothelial nitric oxide bioavailability and coronary microvascular function in patients with syndrome X. *Am J Cardiol* 2002;90(9):974–82.

68. Kaski JC, Rosano G, Gavrielides S, Chen L. Effects of angiotensin-converting enzyme inhibition on exercise-induced angina and ST segment depression in patients with microvascular angina. *J Am Coll Cardiol* 1994;23(3):652–7.

69. Phan A, Shufelt C, Merz CN. Persistent chest pain and no obstructive coronary artery disease. *JAMA* 2009;301(14):1468–74.

70. Cannon RO, 3rd, Quyyumi AA, Mincemoyer R, et al. Imipramine in patients with chest pain despite normal coronary angiograms. *N Engl J Med* 1994;330(20):1411–7.

71. Zheng AL, Qi WH, Hu DY, et al. [Effects of antidepressant therapy in patients with suspected "angina pectoris" and negative coronary angiogram complicating comorbid depression]. *Zhonghua Xin Xue Guan Bing Za Zhi* 2006;34(12):1097–1100.

72. Varia I, Logue E, O'Connor C, et al. Randomized trial of sertraline in patients with unexplained chest pain of noncardiac origin. *Am Heart J* 2000;140(3):367–72.

73. Spinhoven P, Van der Does AJ, Van Dijk E, Van Rood YR. Heart-focused anxiety as a mediating variable in the treatment of noncardiac chest pain by cognitive-behavioral therapy and paroxetine. *J Psychosom Res* 2010;69(3):227–35.

74. Rutledge T, Reis SE, Olson M, et al. Depression is associated with cardiac symptoms, mortality risk, and hospitalization among women with suspected coronary disease: the NHLBI-sponsored WISE study. *Psychosom Med* 2006;68(2):217–23.

21

MIGRAINE IN WOMEN

Satnam S. Nijjar, Jason Rosenberg , and B. Lee Peterlin

INTRODUCTION

Since the dawn of civilization, headache has troubled mankind—and in particular woman-kind. A common chief presenting complaint to emergency rooms as well as primary care outpatient clinics, headaches occur for a wide variety of reasons, ranging from benign to the acutely life threatening. The initial conundrum facing the clinician evaluating the patient with headache is as follows: is this headache benign (i.e., the symptom of an idiopathic syndrome), or is it a harbinger of a health catastrophe (i.e., a symptom of an underlying condition that requires urgent medical attention)?

To this end, The International Classification of Headache Disorders (ICHD) is a useful tool, with formal definitions and clinical pearls related to diagnosis of headaches.[1] The initial break point in the classification scheme is to distinguish second-ary headaches from primary headache disorders. Secondary headaches are caused by an underlying condition such as an infection, tumor, or hemor-rhage, where the discomfort is due to nociceptive input arising from traction, compression, inflam-mation, or invasion of pain-sensitive structures, either intracranially (e.g., meninges and cranial nerves) or pericranially (e.g., sinuses).[2]

In contrast to secondary headache disorders, primary headaches are idiopathic syndromes involving spontaneous activation of cranial pain pathways without any identifiable painful precipitant. As there is no identifiable "cause" visible on routine imaging or pathological examination, the diagnosis of primary head-ache disorders is clinical in nature, based on the consensus criteria definitions (i.e., as found in the ICHD), and only after careful consideration has been given to the possibility of an underly-ing process.

The most prevalent of the primary head-aches—migraine and tension type—are more common in women than men. Of the two, migraine carries a much higher burden of suf-fering due to its severity, frequency of misdiag-nosis, and often suboptimal management. This chapter will focus on the epidemiology, diag-nosis, comorbidity, and treatment of migraine with particular attention to the special consid-erations in women migraine sufferers.

GENERAL APPROACH TO THE PATIENT PRESENTING WITH HEADACHE

The vast majority of headache complaints pre-senting to the outpatient practitioner—in all patients, not just women—will be the result of migraine. Historical "red flags" and *any* abnor-mality on neurological screening examination

Table 21.1   The Mnemonic "SNOOP" for Headache Red Flags Prompting Workup for Secondary Headache

MNEMONIC	MEANING	EXAMPLES
S	Systemic signs or symptoms	Fever, weight loss, history of malignancy or immunosuppresion
N	Neurologic signs or symptoms	Hemiparesis, hemisensory loss, cranial nerve palsy, ataxia
O	Onset	Headache onset within seconds or "worst headache of life" (i.e., sentinel headache)
O	Old age	New onset headache >40 years of age
P	Progression of an existing headache disorder	Change in the quality, location, or frequency of existing headaches

Source: Adapted from Martin VT. Simplifying the diagnosis of migraine headache. *Adv Stud Med* 2004; 4: 200–7.

increase the likelihood for a secondary headache and should prompt additional workup. A mnemonic that is often used for headache red flags is "SNOOP," and it includes *s*ystemic signs or symptoms (e.g., immunosuppression), any associated *n*eurological symptoms or signs, headache *o*nset (e.g., onset of "worse headache of life"), *o*lder age, and *p*rogression of an existing headache disorder (e.g., change in headache quality) (see Table 21.1).[3] Intermittent self-limited headaches with complete return to baseline are seldom of medical concern, but most other presentations merit careful workup.

We generally recommend imaging in any headache patient with unusual neurological symptoms, and certainly in any with abnormal neurological findings on examination, in accordance with US Headache Consortium (USHC)[a] guidelines.[4] Imaging is usually not warranted in patients with episodic headaches fulfilling migraine criteria with normal findings on neurological examination.

MIGRAINE EPIDEMIOLOGY

Migraine affects more than 30 million adults in the United States alone.[5] The staggering numbers of patients becomes clear when set in the context of other diseases—in terms of primary care, migraine is more common than diabetes and asthma combined. For our neurology colleagues, it is more common than Alzheimer's, epilepsy, multiple sclerosis, and stroke combined.[6] Approximately 12%–15% of the general population suffers with migraine and approximately three times as many women (18%) as men (6%).[7,8] The prevalence rises further still, to 27% of the general population (30%–34.5% of women; 20.1% of men), if the definition is expanded to include probable migraine (i.e., headache lacking a single defining ICHD-II criteria).[7] Migraine prevalence is also greatest in Caucasians, intermediate in African Americans, and lowest in Asian Americans[9,10]; and a positive family history for migraine is noted in approximately 70% of patients. Thus, while the disease strikes all manners of people, the "typical" profile of a migraineur is a Caucasian woman in her 30s, in the lower quartile of socioeconomic status, and with other affected family members.

MIGRAINES ACROSS THE WOMAN'S LIFE CYCLE

Menarche/Menses

After puberty, migraine prevalence is greater in women than men. Although the exact

---

a. Comprised of seven organizations: the American Academy of Neurology (AAN), the American Headache Society (AHS), the American Academy of Family Physicians (AAFP), the American College of Emergency Physicians (AECP), American College of Physicians-American Society of Internal Medicine (ACP_ASIM), the American Osteopathic Association (AOA), and the National Headache Foundation (NHF).

mechanism is not known, it is likely that sex hormones, in particular, fluctuating levels of estrogen, play a role. Hormonal fluctuations—associated with menses, oral contraceptives, estrogen replacement therapy, and fertility medications—appear to be especially potent triggers of individual migraine attacks.[11-14] Diary studies have revealed a tendency for migraine attacks to occur close to the first day of menses, typically in those with migraine without aura.[12,13] Extrapolating from the results of such research, menstrually related migraine (MRM) has been formally defined as attacks occurring in menstruating women meeting the diagnostic criteria for migraine without aura, occurring from 2 days before to 3 days after the start of menstruation, with additional attacks at other times unrelated to menstruation. MRM is experienced by approximately 60% of women migraineurs.[1] In contrast, pure menstrual migraine, in which migraine attacks occur exclusively in the perimenstrual window, and not at other times in the cycle, are experienced by only 7%–14% of women.[13]

Pregnancy

During pregnancy, a time when estrogen levels are steadily elevated, over 60% of migraineurs improve.[15] In one study, 57% of women with migraine without aura showed a ≥50% reduction in headache frequency during the first trimester, and which further increased to 83% during the second trimester and 87% during the third trimester.[16] However, in a small number of pregnant women (~4%–8%), migraine headaches worsen. In one study, this aggravation was more common among pregnant women who had a history of migraine with aura.[17] Other studies have noted the onset of migraine for the first time in pregnancy, particularly in the first trimester.[18] While pregnancy commonly offers respite, migraine headaches generally recur within the first week postpartum (days 3–6).[19] Migraine headaches have also been reported to be associated with negative pregnancy outcomes, with increased risk for low birth weight, premature birth, and maternal hypertensive disorders (pre-eclampsia, eclampsia), as well as serious maternal vascular diseases (including stroke during pregnancy and the purpureum).[20]

The clinical significance of these worrisome findings, and any potential ramifications on treatment and prenatal care, are uncertain.

Menopause

Although after surgical menopause, that is, following bilateral oophorectomy, migraines often worsen, approximately two-thirds of women migraineurs will improve with natural menopause. Only 3.4% of women may continue to experience migraine attacks past the age of 60.[21]

MIGRAINE-RELATED DISABILITY: PERSONAL AND SOCIETAL BURDEN

Migraine is a disabling condition—when symptoms are "full blown," patients may find themselves bed bound. The World Health Organization (WHO) has ranked migraine as the twelfth leading cause of life lived with disability among women worldwide. In terms of disability-adjusted life years, a day with migraine is considered as more disabling than a day with angina or depression, and equivalent to a day with quadriplegia.[6]

Migraine-related disability has a significant economic impact on society. Direct costs (such as from outpatient visits, diagnostic testing, hospitalization, and prescriptions) have been estimated at approximately $1 billion in the United States.[22] Indirect costs, which include both absenteeism (missed work) and presenteeism (reduced productivity at work), may even more substantial.[23,24] It has been estimated that migraine costs US employers approximately $13 billion per year.[22]

Comorbidity of Migraine

Migraine is associated with a number of psychiatric disorders, including depression, anxiety, bipolar disorder, and posttraumatic stress disorder.[25,26] The occurrence of such psychiatric comorbidities results in greater disability and health care utilization.[27] Migraine is also associated with several medical disorders, including stroke, obesity, epilepsy, and temporomandibular joint disorders.[28-32] Additionally, migraineurs are more likely than controls to have risk factors for cardiovascular disease, including diabetes, hypertension, and high cholesterol.[33] Dizziness of various types is also common among migraine sufferers, even between individual attacks of headache. As many as 9% suffer from a recently defined disorder termed *migrainous vertigo*.[34] The peripheral vestibular disorders Menierre's and benign paroxysmal positional vertigo may also be more frequent in migraineurs.[35]

Migraine with aura (MA) may carry a higher risk of stroke than migraine without aura (MO), and there is literature implicating an interaction with the older, high-dose, estrogen-containing combined oral contraceptives (cOCPs).[36] Data evaluating women on older, high-dose estrogen cOCPs have demonstrated an increased risk of stroke in MA, leading the WHO and the American College of Obstetrics and Gynecology to recommend against the use of cOCP use in this population. However, more recent data suggest that the use of lower dose cOCPs in women with MA who do not smoke or have other risk factors does not independently increase the risk for stroke.[37] The population-based case-control Stroke Prevention Young Women Study found that risk of ischemic stroke was 7.0-fold higher in women who had migraine with visual aura who smoked and used cOCPs compared with women who had migraine with visual aura who were nonsmokers and non-cOCP users, and 10.0-fold higher compared with women with no migraine history who were nonsmokers and non-OC users. Although further research is needed, data suggest that low-dose cOCP use *alone* is not an independent stroke risk factor among women with MA.[37]

Women with migraine have also been found to have a higher burden of small magnetic resonance imaging (MRI) lesions in the deep white matter, independent of migraine subtype and cardiovascular risk factors.[38] The etiology and significance of such findings are not yet known.

Symptoms and Diagnosis

The International Classification of Headache Disorders (ICHD)-II criteria for migraine with and without aura are noted in Table 21.2.[1] An individual attack of migraine generally progresses in phases: prodrome, aura, headache, and postdrome. Not everyone will experience each phase, and not everyone will experience them in an individually stereotyped fashion from episode to episode. Additionally, nonfocal complaints preceding headache onset have been described in up to 60% of migraine sufferers and are known as prodromal symptoms (e.g., yawning, changes in sleep, irritability, food cravings, fatigue, or an increase in energy).[39] Symptoms may occur from hours to days prior to headache and may represent disturbance of widespread dopaminergic projections from the brainstem.

Gradually progressing, transient focal neurological deficits—auras—occur in up to 30% of migraineurs. By the ICHD-II criteria, a typical aura lasts between 5–60 minutes and occurs as gradual onset of progressive and reversible focal neurologic symptoms (see Table 21.2). Auras typically herald the onset of a migraine headache attack, but they may occur without a headache. By far the most common aura symptoms are visual.[39] Sensory auras (e.g., tingling and/or numbness) often develop over several minutes and may "march" from the hand to the face.[39] More rarely aura can involve disturbances of language (e.g., aphasia) or motor function (e.g., hemiparesis). Clinically important diagnostic features of aura are its slow, gradual progression—too slow for the typical sudden onset symptoms of an ischemic stroke or transient ischemic attack, or even seizure—and the typical occurrence of both positive (scintillation, tingling) and negative (scotoma, numbness) neurological phenomena. The physiological correlate of aura is thought to be cortical spreading depression (CSD), a complicated electrical and chemical disturbance involving sequential activation and then suppression of neuronal firing and blood flow, slowly expanding across the involved cortex in a contiguous fashion, much like a ripple in a pond.[15]

The headache phase itself is often but not always unilateral. The pain builds gradually, with peak intensity not being reached for many minutes or even hours, and often is throbbing in character. Normally innocuous stimuli and routine activities may become unpleasant, exacerbating pain. Hypersensitivity to light, sound, and/or odors is common, as is some degree of nausea. Parasympathetic involvement results

Table 21.2 International Classification of Headache Disorders (ICHD)-II Criteria for Migraine

Migraine without aura

Diagnostic criteria

A. At least five attacks fulfilling criteria B–D

B. Headache attacks lasting 4–72 hours (untreated or unsuccessfully treated)

C. Headache has at least two of the following characteristics:
   1. Unilateral location
   2. Pulsating quality
   3. Moderate or severe pain intensity
   4. Aggravation by or causing avoidance of routine physical activity (e.g., walking or climbing stairs)

D. During headache at least one of the following:
   1. Nausea and/or vomiting
   2. Photophobia and phonophobia

E. Not attributed to another disorder

Diagnostic criteria of aura

A. Aura consisting of at least one of the following, but no motor weakness:
   1. Fully reversible visual symptoms including positive features (e.g., flickering lights, spots or lines) and/or negative features (i.e., loss of vision)
   2. Fully reversible sensory symptoms including positive features (i.e., pins and needles) and/or negative features (i.e., numbness)
   3. Fully reversible dysphasic speech disturbance

B. At least two of the following:
   1. Homonymous visual symptoms and/or unilateral sensory symptoms
   2. At least one aura symptom develops gradually over ≥5 minutes and/or different aura symptoms occur in succession over ≥5 minutes
   3. Each symptom lasts ≥5 and ≤60 minutes

Source: Headache Classification Subcommittee of the International Headache Society. The international classification of headache disorders: 2nd edition. *Cephalalgia* 2004;24(suppl 1):S24–S101.

in vasodilation, often with some degree of other autonomic-related symptoms confused for "sinus" pathology—congestion, facial pressure, watery eyes, and so on. Normal cutaneous sensations may become heightened as well, a phenomenon known as allodynia. Patients may want to unclip their hair, remove jewelry, and otherwise avoid direct physical contact. For reasons poorly understood, symptoms will typically spontaneously remit in hours to a few days, and often improve following sleep or emesis, particularly in children.

When a single necessary criterion is lacking, the term "probable migraine" is used, and when severe attacks last longer than 72 hours, the episode is deemed one of status migrainosus. The final criterion "not due to an underlying disorder" deserves special attention: it is important to remember that especially in migraineurs, other conditions may provoke migraine-like headache; and it is important be alert to a significant change of headache pattern. Additional historical features reassuring for migraine include side shifting of the headache pain across attacks; history of exacerbation or provocation by menses, alcohol, or hunger; susceptibility to motion sickness; and a positive family history.

DIFFERENTIAL DIAGNOSIS

By virtue of being both prevalent and severe, migraine should be the presumptive diagnosis for any woman presenting to clinic with intermittent, recurring headache. In fact, in a prospective study by Tepper and colleagues, it was concluded that episodic, disabling primary headaches with an otherwise normal exam should be considered migraine in the absence of contradictory evidence.[2] Other primary headaches were uncommonly seen in the primary care setting and were misdiagnosed the vast majority of the time. While tension-type headaches are ubiquitous and more commonly occur in women than men, they seldom rise to the level of severity or disability that would merit a trip to the primary care provider. For the most part, tension-type headaches are featureless and mild, "just pain," and typically respond to simple nonpharmacologic measures and nonspecific analgesic treatment, as well as preventive pharmacotherapy when necessary.

Cluster headaches are rare, and they are characterized by relatively brief (15 min to 3 hours), excruciating, side-locked agitating headaches that are associated with autonomic ocular and nasal symptoms. Cluster headache attacks typically occur more than once per day for several weeks, with periods of remission and are strongly associated with smoking and alcohol consumption.[40] Once considered a primarily male disease, recent studies suggest a female:male ratio approaching 2:3.[41] While uncommon, failure to consider cluster headache in a woman could lead to a significant delay in diagnosis and treatment. An even more rare cluster-like disorder termed *paroxysmal hemicrania* is much more frequent in women than men, with five or more brief (2–30 minutes) unilateral ocular headaches occurring per day, uniquely responding to treatment with indomethacin.[42]. Due to rarity, severity, and reported occasional association with underlying lesions, we advise referral of all patients with cluster-like headaches for specialty management.

"Sinus headaches" are often a misnomer; the vast majority are in fact migraine.[43] This may explain why a number of these patients often respond to simple analgesics (found often in combination with decongestants) and triptan therapy.[44] In a study by Schreiber and colleagues, 90% of patient- or physician-diagnosed sinus headaches were actually migraines.[43]

Migraine Triggers

Patients often report various internal and external stimuli, or precipitants, of individual migraine attacks. Such precipitants are referred to as "triggers." Typical reported triggers include psychological stress—or conversely "let down" after a period of stress—change in sleep pattern, skipping meals, red wine, weather changes, certain foods (containing certain monoamines, nitrates, or nitrites), hormonal factors, and strong odors. In one study of 237 participants, the strongest migraine trigger was menstruation. Other factors such as lack of exercise, stress, and low atmospheric pressure also increased the risk of migraine (i.e., acted as migraine triggers). However, no influence was seen from chocolate, cheese, or nuts.[45]

Treatment of Migraine

Migraine is a chronic condition; it is managed rather than cured. The idea is to reduce symptoms in terms of severity, frequency, and duration, thus improving functional outcomes. For mild disease or occasional attacks, acute therapy alone may suffice. For the patient with frequent, disabling, or severe attacks, preventive therapy is emphasized, a combination of lifestyle modification and daily medication. Perhaps the most useful (and underutilized) tool in the care of the headache patient is a carefully maintained headache diary and medication record. These personalized data are of utmost importance in terms of being able to objectively assess disease activity and effects of therapies.

Acute Management

The goals for migraine management put forth by the United States Headache Consortium (USHC) are as follows: to effectively relieve attacks without recurrence, reduce the need for acute therapy, minimize adverse side effects, and optimize and restore the patients' ability to function.[46] In general, the most effective available acute treatment drug should be administered for a given headache severity, rather than starting "gently" and working up, an approach known as "stratified care." A more tailored strategy for acute treatment has been shown to improve patient outcomes and reduce disability compared with progressive "step care."[47] In practice, this typically means starting with a migraine-specific drug such as a triptan (perhaps in combination) rather than with a simple analgesic alone, especially in severe migraines. See Table 21.3 for a list of commonly used acute abortive migraine medications.

Nonspecific acute treatments include nonsteroidal anti-inflammatory drugs (NSAIDs), aspirin, acetaminophen, combinations of these with caffeine, neuroleptics (dopaminergic antiemetics such as metoclopramide and prochlorperazine), anticonvulsants, GABA agonists, antihistamines, isometheptene, dichloralphenazone, and barbiturates.[47] Evidence for treatment with nonspecific medications is mixed; however, they can be effectively used in mild to moderates cases of migraine with low disability.[48,49] Most studies examining opioid use in acute migraine have either been poorly designed or were negative. Furthermore, with chronic use opioid-induced hyperalgesia may develop and worsen pain.[50] In addition, due to high potential for barbiturates (butalbital, found in Fioricet) and opioids inducing medication overuse headaches, we recommend avoiding them. Steroids are sometimes used adjunctively; emergency room studies have shown that the use of dexamethasone up to 20 mg IV or PO can reduce the likelihood of continuation or recurrence of severe migraine symptoms 1–3 days later.[51]

Migraine-specific medications include triptans and ergots. These are both serotonin (5-HT1) agonists that have vasoconstrictive properties. Their serotonergic activity also acts to inhibit neurogenic inflammation peripherally around extracerebral intracranial arteries and to attenuate nociceptive sensitization centrally in the brainstem. Oral triptans can be divided into two groups, those with fast onset (Group 1) versus those with slower onset (Group 2). Group 1 triptans include sumatriptan, zolmitriptan, rizatriptan, almotriptan, and eletriptan, whereas group 2 triptans include naratriptan and frovatriptan.[52] A pain-free headache response can be usually obtained in 2 hours. The headache response for triptans in group 2 may take slightly longer for response but is also associated with less frequent side effects. Ergot alkaloids, such as dihydroergotamine (DHE)

Table 21.3   Medication Classes Commonly Used Acute Abortive Migraine Medication

MEDICATION CLASS	BENEFITS	LIMITATIONS
NSAIDS and combination analgesics	Available over-the-counter, good safety profile	Improper self-medication can lead to reduced efficacy, medication-overuse headache, more adverse effects, as well as gastric complications.
Barbiturate hypnotics (butalbital)	May be effective for tension-type headaches	No randomized, placebo-controlled studies have demonstrated efficacy in migraine. Adverse effects include intoxication, withdrawal symptoms, tolerance, and dependence.
DHE nasal spray	Migraine specific	Adverse effects include nausea and vasoconstrictive symptoms such as flushing. Contraindicated in patients with heart disease or hemiplegic or basilar migraine.
Triptans	Migraine specific, well tolerated with minimal sedation	Contraindicated in patients with heart disease and hemiplegic or basilar migraine.

Source: Modified from Diamond M, Cady R. Initiating and optimizing acute therapy for migraine: the role of patient-centered stratified care Am J Med 2005;118 Suppl1:18S-27S.

and ergotamine, stimulate alpha-adrenergic and 5-HT receptors and are more potent vasoconstrictors than triptans. DHE can be given in multiple different methods, including intranasally, intramuscularly, or intravenously; and an inhaled formulation is under development.[53]

To be optimally effective, triptans should be used early in an attack; advising patients to forestall use until their symptoms become severe results in lower efficacy.[54] The route of administration should be matched to the patient. For example, if there is early nausea, use a nasal or injected formulation; if the patient has limited access to water, orally dissolving may be preferable. If acute medication is needed more than once a week, preventive care should be considered. When the average combined use of acute analgesics reaches 2+ days per week, potential concern is raised for the possibility of paradoxical exacerbation of headaches (medication overuse headache, also known as "rebound") and may be a marker of inadequate prevention efforts.

There are a number of contraindications to the use of triptans and ergotamines, mostly related to concerns about vascular issues. These include patients at high risk for vascular disease, severe/uncontrolled hypertension, hemiplegic migraine, basilar-type migraine, coadministration with another triptan or ergotamine, as well as impaired liver function and previous hypersensitivity reaction. Despite these contraindications, when prescribed and used according to labeling, triptans have been demonstrated to be quite safe. The American Headache Society's position paper discusses this in great detail and does not suggest limiting triptans in those patients treated with selective serotonin reuptake inhibitors or selective norepinephrine reuptake inhibitors.[55] It is unknown whether there may be potential for interaction with peptide antagonists now in clinical trials.[56]

Preventive Lifestyle Measures and Nonmedical Therapies

"Migraine lifestyle" modification involves regularization of daily routines and, as much as is practical, avoidance of strong triggers/provoking factors, particularly in combination. Healthy eating, regular exercise, maintenance of a health body weight, minimal and regular caffeine consumption, and good sleep hygiene are emphasized. In practice, good sleeping habits are often the lowest hanging fruit in terms of easily achievable improvement. In addition, prevention may be improved by physical therapy, biofeedback, and relaxation therapy.[57]

Preventive Pharmacologic Therapy

The United States Evidence-Based Guidelines published indications for consideration of preventive therapy in migraine.[58] These include the following: (1) recurring migraine that significantly interferes with the patient's daily routine despite acute treatment; (2) failure of, contraindication to, or troublesome side effects from acute medications; (3) overuse of acute medications; (4) special circumstances, such as hemiplegic migraine or attacks with a risk of permanent neurological injury; (5) frequent headaches, or a pattern of increasing attacks over time, with the risk of developing medication overuse headache; and (6) patient preference, that is, the desire to have as few acute attacks as possible. Lipton and colleagues proposed that two most important factors to consider when assessing whether prophylactic therapy is merited are the frequency of attacks and degree of headache-related impairment.[58] Preventive therapy can be beneficial in reducing the frequency, duration, or severity of attacks, and in potentially rendering acute medications more effective.

Although multiple different classes of medications for migraine prophylaxis exist, the major groups of medications utilized include anticonvulsants (e.g., topiramate, gabapentin), tricyclic or SNRI antidepressants (e.g., amitriptyline, venlafaxine), β-adrenergic blockers (e.g., propanolol), and cardiac medications including some calcium channel antagonists (e.g., verapmail) and angiotensin receptor blockers (e.g., lisinopril). (See Table 21.4 for commonly used migraine preventive medications.) Botulinum toxin and supplemental agents (e.g., riboflavin, magnesium, coenzyme Q10, and butterbur) are also often utilized.[59,60]

Factors that should be considered in the selection of initial therapy include the efficacy of the agent in randomized controlled trials,

Table 21.4   Commonly Used Migraine Preventive Medications and Supplements

MEDICATION	DOSE	MOST COMMON SIDE EFFECTS
Anti-epileptics		
Divalproex sodium	400–600 BID	Nausea, somnolence, tremor, dizziness
Topiramate	50–200 mg Q D	Paresthesias, weight loss, altered taste, anorexia, fatigue, cognitive dysfunction
Gabapentin	900–3,600 mg BID	Somnolence, dizziness, asthenia
Supplements		
Butterbur	50–75 mg BID	Elevation of transaminases
Riboflavin	200 mg BID	Bright yellow urine
Coenzyme Q10	75 mg BID	Gastrointestinal upset
Antidepressants		
Amitriptyline	25–75 mg Q HS	Dry mouth, drowsiness, urinary retention
Venlafaxine	75–150 mg Q D	Nausea, drowsiness, urinary retention
Cardiac medications		
Propranolol	40–120 mg BID	Fatigue, postural symptoms, contraindicated in asthma
Metoprolol	25–100 mg BID	Fatigue, postural symptoms, contraindicated in asthma
Lisinopril	20 mg Q D	Cough, dizziness
Candesartan	16 mg Q D	Birth defects and fetal death
Verapamil	80–640 mg Q D (divided BID or TID)	Constipation, weight gain, peripheral edema, cardiac conduction delay

BID, twice daily; TID, three times daily. QHS once daily at bedtime

side effect profile of the medication, comorbid conditions, and the preference of the patient.[61] We suggest choosing drugs in part based on the patient's other health conditions, avoiding side effects that may worsen preexisting conditions, perhaps steering toward medications that might actually result in improvement. For example, avoid drugs that cause weight gain in the patient who is obese; consider tricyclics in a patient with insomnia. We advise clinicians to thoroughly familiarize themselves with one drug from each of the "three anti's": one antihypertensive, one antidepressant, and one anticonvulsant. Know these three drugs inside and out—their typical dosages, their interactions, their side effects (beneficial as well as detrimental), and their peculiarities—and you will

be able to manage the majority of migraineurs presenting to a general practice. A trial of gradual discontinuation of a preventive agent is reasonable to consider if a patient has been doing fantastically well for approximately 6 consecutive months.

Concerns of particular relevance to many women include chance of weight gain on medications, interactions with oral contraceptives, effect on bone loss, and potential teratogenicity.[62] It is of utmost importance for the prescribing physician to be aware of the various associated side effects and to accurately discuss these with the patient. It is advisable that the preventative drug be *both* well tolerated *and* effective; otherwise it is not worthwhile and will be abandoned.

Treatment of Menstrual Migraine

A detailed headache diary maintained by the patient is crucial for assessing and managing menstrually-related migraine (MRM). This can serve to observe cycle regularity and to identify headache predictability with respect to the peri-menstrual period. For the most part, abortive and preventative therapies are the same as for other migraineurs. However, in those patients who reliably or exclusively suffer from MRMs with predictable cycle lengths, scheduled cyclical short-term prophylaxis (STP) may be recommended.[63–78] Naproxen has been noted to be an effective STP when taken once or twice daily from 5 to 7 days before menstruation, and taken for 10 to 14 days.[65] As side effects of NSAIDs include gastrointestinal disturbance and are contraindicated in those with peptic ulcer disease, misoprostol 800 μg or omeprazole 20 to 40 mg daily may give some gastroduodenal protection.

Several studies have also demonstrated that STP is beneficial with several triptans, including sumatriptan, frovatriptan, naratriptan, and zolmitripan.[68–74] The following regimens for STP with triptans have been confirmed by large double-blind placebo-controlled trials:

- Frovatriptan 2.5 mg BID for 6 days (double loading dose on first day), starting 2 days before predicted menstrual migraine
- Naratriptan 1 mg BID for 6 days, starting 2 days before predicted menstruation
- Zolmitriptan 2.5 mg TID for 7 days, starting 2 days before predicted menstruation

Other studies have demonstrated ergotamines, hormone therapy, tamoxifen, and danzol to be effective.[79–82] Eliminating ovulatory cycles and/or the fall in estrogen prior to menses may be helpful; and a trial of continuous hormonal therapy (in particular in a patient already taking combined oral contraceptives) is worthwhile. We have had success with using the transvaginal ring preparation continuously for 4 weeks, exchanging immediately rather than using it for 3 weeks on, 1 week off. A high-dose estrogen patch (0.1 mg/24 hours) applied 2 days prior to expected menses, discontinuing after 6 days, is sometimes effective, extrapolating from earlier studies using the less desirable gel preparations.[64]

Treatment during Pregnancy and Lactation

During pregnancy and breastfeeding, nonpharmacologic therapies, such as those discussed earlier, should be emphasized. In general, medication should be avoided around time of planned conception and during the first trimester, and efforts should be put forth to discontinue drugs 2 weeks prior to delivery. The use of multiple concurrent medications should be avoided.[62] A comprehensive discussion weighing the (often uncertain) risks and benefits should be held with the patient (and documented) when pharmacologic therapy is being contemplated. In cases where the migraines themselves are disabling to the mother or threatening to the pregnancy outcome (dehydration, repeated vomiting, inadequate nutritional intake/weight gain), therapeutic nihilism should be avoided.

Pharmacotherapy for abortive purposes should be used only when necessary, ideally with drugs listed as Category B. For acute therapy in pregnancy, acetaminophen, caffeine, narcotics, metoclopramide, and prochlorperazine may be used with caution.[83] In severe acute attacks during pregnancy, a combination of intravenous hydration, intravenous/rectal proclorperazine, and prednisone have been used effectively.[83] The dopaminergic antiemetic metoclopramide is Category B, as is the 5HT3 drug ondansetron, a potentially useful rescue medication for severe nausea. Occasional use of NSAIDs can be considered in pregnancy, but not in the third trimester due to concerns of effects on fetal circulation (Category C in first two trimesters, D in third). Ergotamines are clearly contraindicated, but growing data suggest that triptans (at least sumatriptan, naratriptan, and rizatriptan) may be a reasonable option to consider without clear risk for congenital malformations when used early in pregnancy, but with potential obstetrical complications in later months.[84] Antihistamines can be used adjunctively, and opioids may be used sparingly for rescue.

Preventative medications should also only be used when necessary, weighing risks and benefits. Propanolol and verapamil are "Category C" medications and can be used with caution in low doses. For patients attempting to conceive, gabapentin can be used for prevention, although it must be discontinued by late pregnancy to avoid possible delay in the development of fetal bony growth plate. Topiramate has recently been associated with an increased rate of cleft lip and cleft palate during early exposure, and it is now Category D. Valproate should be avoided due to serious risk of teratogenicity if used early in pregnancy, as well as potential for long-term negative effects on postnatal cognitive development. Venlafaxine has mixed data, with one prospective study showing no adverse outcomes and a published registry showing increased rate of early miscarriage.[85]

In general, exposure to migraine medications via lactation typically poses less of a concern than in utero exposure. Sumatriptan is excreted minimally into breast milk and can be used safely in lactating women.[86] To minimize infant exposure, patients have traditionally been advised to pump and discard milk during the first 6–12 hours after oral administration or for at least 4 hours following injection.[87] Nonsteroidal anti-inflammatories such as ibuprofen are considered acceptably safe. Several antiemetics are excreted into breast milk, including metoclopramide at low concentrations.

Disease Progression

In some patients, migraines may progress or "transform" from an episodic disorder into a state of near constant pain, typically experienced as a low-moderate level underlying headache with superimposed "full-blown" migraines. Several potentially modifiable risk factors for chronic migraine have been identified in epidemiological studies and in some cases prospectively—baseline migraine frequency, medication overuse, caffeine consumption of over 150 mg daily (approximately one 8-ounce coffee or 4–5 cans of cola), allodynia (identifiable as skin/scalp tenderness, which tends to occur the longer a migraine persists), sleep disorders (snoring, apnea, insomnia/poor hygiene), and psychiatric conditions. We draw attention to these risk factors here because chronic migraine is much more difficult to treat and more disabling than episodic migraine; we

therefore recommend screening all episodic migraine patients for these risk factors and addressing them before the disease progresses whenever possible.

WHEN FIRST-LINE TREATMENT FAILS

Common reasons for failure of first-line therapy in prevention include overuse of acute analgesics, inadequate dosing, failure to address side effect concerns, nocebo effect (self-fulfilling patient belief that medications will be harmful), and unrealistic expectations. It should be noted that many of these are educational and behavioral issues—related to lifestyle issues, appropriate use of medications, and unaddressed risk factors. The problem is often not the disease itself but rather the setting. Before labeling a patient's headaches biologically intractable, be sure that compliance, lifestyle issues (particularly sleep), and other modifiable risk factors for progression have been addressed in a comprehensive fashion. For seemingly pharmacologically refractory patients, consider rational co-pharmacy, both for acute attacks and for preventive therapy, using medications with complementary mechanisms and differing side effect profiles. Only rarely do we find that the underlying diagnosis of migraine was incorrect, but we have certainly seen cases of intracranial hypertension, hemicrania continua, cluster headache, and psychogenic issues presenting as "intractable migraine." A neurologist or even a headache subspecialist may be required for difficult cases, where aggressive imaging, lumbar puncture, judicious use of inpatient admissions, adjunctive nerve blocks, psychological support, and "artful" use of medication may be brought to bear. Focused expertise coupled with sufficient time for education and management can often result in improvement in cases simply impossible to manage in a general practice setting.

REFERENCES

1. Headache Classification Subcommittee of the International Headache Society. The international classification of headache disorders: 2nd edition. *Cephalalgia* 2004;24(Suppl 1):9–160.

2. Tepper SJ, Dahlöf CG, Dowson A, et al. Prevalence and diagnosis of migraine in patients consulting their physician with a complaint of headache: data from the Landmark Study. *Headache* 2004;44(9):856–64.

3. Martin VT. Simplifying the diagnosis of migraine headache. Adv Stud Med 2004;4: 200–7.

4. Morey SS. Headache Consortium releases guidelines for use of CT or MRI in migraine workup [Pract Guide]. *Am Fam Physician* 2000;62: 1699–701.

5. Bigal ME, Liberman JN, Lipton RB. Age-dependent prevalence and clinical features of migraine. *Neurology* 2006;67(2):246–51.

6. World Health Organization. *The World Health Report 2001, Chapter 2*. Geneva, Switzerland: WHO 2001.

7. Bigal ME, Lipton RB. The epidemiology, burden, and comorbidities of migraine. *Neurol Clin* 2009;27(2):321–34.

8. Stewart WF, Wood C, Reed ML, Roy J, Lipton RB; AMPP Advisory Group. Cumulative lifetime migraine incidence in women and men. *Cephalalgia* 2008;28(11):1170–8.

9. Stewart WF, Lipton RB, Liberman J. Variation in migraine prevalence by race. *Neurology* 1996;47(1):52–9.

10. Stewart WF, Lipton RB, Celentano DD, Reed ML. Prevalence of migraine headache in the United States. Relation to age, income, race, and other sociodemographic factors. *JAMA* 1992;267(1):64–9.

11. MacGregor EA. "Menstrual" migraine: towards a definition. *Cephalalgia* 1996;16(1):11–21.

12. Dalton K. Progesterone suppositories and pessaries in the treatment of menstrual migraine. *Headache* 1973;12(4):151–9.

13. MacGregor EA, Chia H, Vohrah RC, Wilkinson M. Migraine and menstruation: a pilot study. *Cephalalgia* 1990;10(6):305–10.

14. MacGregor EA, Barnes D. Migraine in a specialist menopause clinic. *Climacteric* 1999;2:218–23.

15. Goadsby PJ. Migraine pathophysiology. *Headache* 2005;45(Suppl 1):S14–24.

16. Sances G, Granella F, Nappi RE, Fignon A, Ghiotto N, Polatti F, Nappi G. Course of migraine during pregnancy and postpartum: a prospective study. *Cephalalgia* 2003;23(3):197–205.

17. Granella F, Sances F, Zanferrari C, et al. Migraine without aura and reproductive life events: a clinical epidemiologic study in 1,300 women. *Headache* 1993;33:385.

18. Chancellor AM, Wroe SJ, Cull RE. Migraine occurring for the first time in pregnancy. *Headache* 1993;33:385.

19. Stein GS. Headaches in the first post partum week and their relationship to migraine. *Headache* 1981;21:201–5.

20. Chen HM, Chen SF, Chen YH, Lin HC. Increased risk of adverse pregnancy outcomes for women with migraines: a nationwide population-based study. *Cephalalgia* 2010;30:433.

21. Neri I, Granella F, Nappi R, et al. Characteristics of headache at menopause. *Maturitas* 1993;17: 31–7.

22. Hu XH, Markson LE, Lipton RB, Stewart WF, Berger ML. Burden of migraine in the United States: disability and economic costs. *Arch Intern Med* 1999;159(8):813–8.

23. Stewart WF, Lipton RB, Simon D. Work-related disability: results from the American migraine study. *Cephalalgia* 1996;16(4):231–8.

24. Von Korff M, Stewart WF, Simon DJ, Lipton RB. Migraine and reduced work performance: a population-based diary study. *Neurology* 1998;50(6):1741–5.

25. Merikangas KR, Angst J, Isler H. Migraine and psychopathology. Results of the Zurich cohort study of young adults. *Arch Gen Psychiatry* 1990;47(9):849–53.

26. Peterlin BL, Rosso AL, Sheftell FD, Libon DJ, Mossey JM, Merikangas KR. Post-traumatic stress disorder, drug abuse and migraine: new findings from the National Comorbidity Survey Replication (NCS-R). *Cephalalgia* 2011;31(2):235–44.

27. Breslau N, Davis GC. Migraine, physical health and psychiatric disorder: a prospective epidemiologic study in young adults. *J Psychiatr Res* 1993;27(2):211–21.

28. Carolei A, Marini C, De Matteis G. History of migraine and risk of cerebral ischaemia in young adults. The Italian National Research Council Study Group on Stroke in the Young. *Lancet* 1996;347(9014):1503–6.

29. Winawer MR, Hesdorffer DC. Migraine, epilepsy, and psychiatric comorbidity: partners in crime. *Neurology* 2010;74(15):1166–8.

30. Peterlin BL, Rosso AI, Rapoport AM, Scher AI. Obesity and migraine: The effect of age, gender and adipose tissue distribution. *Headache* 2010;50:52–62.

31. Vo M, Ainalem A, Qiu C, Peterlin BL, Aurora SK, Williams MA. Body mass index and adult weight gain among reproductive age women with migraine. *Headache* 2011;51(4):559–69

32. Robberstad L, Dyb G, Hagen K, Stovner LJ, Holmen TL, Zwart JA. An unfavorable lifestyle and recurrent headaches among adolescents: the HUNT study. *Neurology* 2010;75(8):712–7.

33. Bigal M, Kurth T, Santanello N, et al. Migraine and cardiovascular disease: a population-based study. *Neurology* 2010;74:628–35.

34. Neuhauser H, Lempert T. Vestibular migraine. Review. *Neurol Clin* 2009;27(2):379–91.

35. Uneri A. Migraine and benign paroxysmal positional vertigo: an outcome study of 476 patients. *Ear Nose Throat J* 2004;83(12):814–5.

36. Gillum LA, Mamidipudi SK, Johnston SC. Ischemic stroke risk with oral contraceptives: a meta-analysis. *JAMA* 2000;284:72–8.

37. MacClellan LR, Giles W, Cole J, et al. Probable migraine with visual aura and risk of ischemic stroke. The Stroke Prevention in Young Women Study. *Stroke* 2007;38:2438–45.

38. Kruit MC, van Buchem MA, Launer LJ, Terwindt GM, Ferrari MD. Migraine is associated with an increased risk of deep white matter lesions, subclinical posterior circulation infarcts and brain iron accumulation: the population-based MRI CAMERA study. *Cephalalgia* 2010;30:129–36.

39. Blau JN. Migraine prodromes separated from the aura: complete migraine. *Br Med J* 1980;281(6241):658–60.

40. Levi R, Edman GV, Ekbom K, Waldenlind E. Episodic cluster headache. II: high tobacco and alcohol consumption in males. *Headache* 1992; 32(4):184–7.

41. Manzoni GC. Male preponderance of cluster headache is progressively decreasing over the years. *Headache* 1997;37(9):588–9.

42. Boes CJ, Dodick DW. Refining the clinical spectrum of chronic paroxysmal hemicrania: a review of 74 patients. *Headache* 2002;42(8):699–708.

43. Schreiber CP, Hutchinson S, Webster CJ, Ames M, Richardson MS, Powers C. Prevalence of migraine in patients with a history of self-reported or physician-diagnosed "sinus" headache. *Arch Intern Med* 2004;164(16):1769–72.

44. Eross E, Dodick D, Eross M. The Sinus, Allergy & Migraine Study (SAMS). *Headache* 2007;47(2):213–24.

45. Wöber C, Brannath W, Schmidt K, et al. Prospective analysis of factors related to migraine attacks: the PAMINA study. *Cephalalgia* 2007;27(4):304–14.

46. Silberstein SD. Practice parameter: evidence-based guidelines for migraine headache (an evidence-based review): report of the Quality Standards Subcommittee of the American Academy of Neurology. *Neurology* 2000;55: 754–62.

47. Lipton RB, Stewart WF, Stone AM, Lainez MJA and JPC Sawyer. Stratified care versus step care strategies for migraine. The disability in

strategies of care (DISC) study: a randomized trial. *JAMA* 2000;284:2599–605.

48. Lipton RB, Bigal ME, Stewart WF. Clinical trials of acute treatments for migraine including multiple attack studies of pain, disability, and health-related quality of life. *Neurology* 2005;65(12 Suppl 4):S50–8.

49. Nijjar SS, Gordon AS, Clark MD. Entry demographics and pharmacological treatment of migraine patients referred to a tertiary care pain clinic. *Cephalalgia* 2010;30(1):87–91.

50. Hay JL, White JM, Bochner F, Somogyi AA, Semple TJ, Rounsefell B. Hyperalgesia in opioid-managed chronic pain and opioid-dependent patients. *J Pain* 2009;10(3):316–22.

51. Evans RW. Treating migraine in the emergency department. *BMJ* 2008;336(7657):1320.

52. Tepper SJ, Rapoport AM. The triptans: a summary. *CNS Drugs* 1999;12:403–17.

53. Bigal ME, Tepper SJ. Ergotamine and dihydroergotamine: a review. *Curr Pain Headache Rep* 2003;7:55–62.

54. Burstein R, Collins B, Jakubowski M. Defeating migraine pain with triptans: a race against the development of cutaneous allodynia. *Ann Neurol* 2004;55(1):19–26.

55. Evans RW, Tepper SJ, Shapiro RE, Sun-Edelstein C, Tietjen GE. The FDA alert on serotonin syndrome with use of triptans combined with selective serotonin reuptake inhibitors or selective serotonin-norepinephrine reuptake inhibitors: American Headache Society position paper. *Headache* 2010;50(6):1089–99.

56. Ho TW, Mannix LK, Fan X, et al. Randomized controlled trial of an oral CGRP receptor antagonist, MK-0974, in acute treatment of migraine. *Neurology* 2008;70:1304–1312.

57. Chaibi A, Tuchin PJ, Russell MB. Manual therapies for migraine: a systematic review. *J Headache Pain* 2011;12(2):127–33.

58. Ramadan NM, Silberstein SD, Freitag FG, et al. Evidenced-based guidelines for migraine headache in the primary care setting: pharmacological management for prevention of migraine. Available at: http://www.aan.com/professionals/practice/pdfs/gl0090.pdf. [accessed on February 2, 2006].

59. Lipton RB, Bigal ME, Diamond M, et al. Migraine prevalence, disease burden, and the need for preventive therapy. *Neurology* 2007;68(5):343–9.

60. Diener HC, Dodick DW, Aurora SK, et al. OnabotulinumtoxinA for treatment of chronic migraine: results from the double-blind, randomized, placebo-controlled phase of the PREEMPT 2 trial. *Cephalalgia* 2010;30(7): 804–14.

61. Pringsheim T, Davenport WJ, Becker WJ. Prophylaxis of migraine headache. *CMAJ* 2010;182(7):E269–76.

62. Khurana, RK. Migraine. In: *Neurologic Disease in Women*. New York: Demos Medical Publishing; 2006.

63. MacGregor EA. Prevention and treatment of menstrual migraine. *Drugs* 2010;70(14):1799–1818.

64. Guidotti M, Mauri M, Barrila C, et al. Frovatriptan vs. transdermal oestrogens or naproxen sodium for the prophylaxis of menstrual migraine. *J Headache Pain* 2007;8(5):283–8.

65. Sances G, Martignoni E, Fioroni L, et al. Naproxen sodium in menstrual migraine prophylaxis: a double-blind placebo controlled study. *Headache* 1990; 30(11):705–9.

66. Giacovazzo M, Gallo MF, Guidi V, et al. Nimesulide in the treatment of menstrual migraine. *Drugs* 1993;46(Suppl 1):140–1.

67. Von Seggern RL, Mannix LK, Adelman JU. Rofecoxib in the prevention of perimenstrual migraine: an open-label pilot trial. *Headache* 2004;44(2):160–5.

68. Silberstein SD, Berner T, Tobin J, et al. Scheduled shortterm prevention with frovatriptan for migraine occurring exclusively in association with menstruation. *Headache* 2009;49(9):1283–97.

69. Brandes JL, Poole A, Kallela M, et al. Short-term frovatriptan for the prevention of difficult-to-treat menstrual migraine attacks. *Cephalalgia* 2009;29(11):1133–48.

70. Mannix LK, Savani N, Landy S, et al. Efficacy and tolerability of naratriptan for short-term prevention of menstrually related migraine: data from two randomized, double-blind, placebo-controlled studies. *Headache* 2007;47(7): 1037–49.

71. Moschiano F, Allais G, Grazzi L, et al. Naratriptan in the short-term prophylaxis of pure menstrual migraine. *Neurol Sci* 2005; 26(Suppl 2):s162–6.

72. Newman L, Mannix LK, Landy S, et al. Naratriptan as short-term prophylaxis of menstrually associated migraine: a randomized, double-blind, placebo-controlled study. *Headache* 2001;41(3):248–56.

73. Newman LC, Lipton RB, Lay CL, et al. A pilot study of oral sumatriptan as intermittent prophylaxis of menstruationrelated migraine. *Neurology* 1998;51(1):307–9.

74. Tuchman MM, Hee A, Emeribe U, et al. Oral zolmitriptan in the short-term prevention of menstrual migraine: a randomized, placebo-controlled study. *CNS Drugs* 2008;22(10):877–86.

75. MacGregor EA, Frith A, Ellis J, et al. Prevention of menstrual attacks of migraine: a double-blind placebo-controlled crossover study. *Neurology* 2006;67:2159–63.

76. Dennerstein L, Morse C, Burrows G, et al. Menstrual migraine: a double-blind trial of percutaneous estradiol. *Gynecol Endocrinol* 1988;2:113–20.

77. Facchinetti F, Sances G, Borella P, et al. Magnesium prophylaxis of menstrual migraine: effects on intracellular magnesium. *Headache* 1991;31(5):298–301.

78. Ziaei S, Kazemnejad A, Sedighi A. The effect of vitamin E on the treatment of menstrual migraine. *Med Sci Monit* 2009;15(1):CR16–9.

79. Magos AL, Zilkha KJ, Studd JW. Treatment of menstrual migraine by oestradiol implants. *J Neurol Neurosurg Psychiatry* 1983;46(11):1044–6.

80. O'Dea JPK. Tamoxifen in the treatment of menstrual migraine. *Neurology* 1990;40:1470–1.

81. Herzog AG. Continuous bromocriptine therapy in menstrual migraine. *Neurology* 1997;48:101–2.

82. Carlton GJ, Burnett JW. Danazol and migraine. *N Engl J Med* 1984;310:721–2.

83. Silberstein SD. Migraine and pregnancy. *Neurol Clin* 1997;15:209–31.

84. Nezvalová-Henriksen K, Spigset O, Norden HME. Triptan exposure during pregnancy and the risk of major congenital malformations and adverse pregnancy outcomes: results from the Norwegian Mother and Child Cohort. *Headache* 2010;50:563–75.

85. Loder E, Marcus DA. *Migraine in Women*. Hamilton, Ontario: BC Decker; 2004.

86. American Academy of Pediatrics Committee on Drugs. Transfer of drugs and other chemicals into human milk. *Pediatrics* 2001;108(3):776–89.

87. Wojnar-Horton RE, Hackett LP, Yapp P, Dusci LJ, Paech M, Ilett KF. Distribution and excretion of sumatriptan in human milk. *Br J Clin Pharmacol* 1996;41(3):217–21.

88. Diamond M, Cady R. Initiating and optimizing acute therapy for migraine: the role of patient-centered stratified care. *Am J Med* 2005; 118(Suppl 1):18S–27S.

22

TEMPOROMANDIBULAR JOINT DISORDERS AND OROFACIAL PAIN

Asma A. Khan, William Maixner, and Pei Feng Lim

INTRODUCTION

The major theme of this book is sex differences in pain. Orofacial pain (OFP), especially temporomandibular joint disorders (TMJD), is an excellent example of this. Approximately 80% of patients seeking treatment for OFP are female, and women in the reproductive age group are more vulnerable to OFP (with the exception of trigeminal neuralgia and burning mouth syndrome).[1–3] TMJD is 1.5–2 times more prevalent in women with peak prevalence in the reproductive years (20 to 45 years of age).[4] In this chapter we first review the evidence from the preclinical studies on the modulation of trigeminal neurons by sex hormones and then build upon this foundation with clinical studies evaluating gender differences in OFP and TMJD.

PRECLINICAL STUDIES

Estrogen

Several lines of evidence indicate that the greatest difference in the excitability of trigeminal neurons between male and females occurs during proestrus when the serum estrogen levels are at their peak (Fig. 22.1).[5,6] For example, the mean number of fos-positive neurons, an indicator of neuronal activity, in the trigeminal spinal nucleus and upper cervical dorsal horn after injection of mustard oil into the TMJ region is significantly higher in proestrus females as compared to diestrus females and males.[5] There was greater enlargement of cutaneous receptive fields and enhanced sensitivity of the trigeminal system to cutaneous stimuli during proestrus as compared to metestrus and diestrus after dural activation with capsaicin.[7] The magnitude and duration of bradykinin-evoked excitation in the TMJ units in the superficial laminae at the Vc/C2 junction in proestrus females is greater than that in diestrus females.[8] Taken together, these studies suggest that sex differences in trigeminal pain are, at least in part, due to the effect of estrogen.

PRONOCICEPTIVE EFFECTS OF ESTROGEN

The neurochemical basis for the modulation of orofacial pain by estrogen may include enhanced nociceptive transmission at the level of the nociceptors and/or in the dorsal horn, decreased descending inhibitory control, and a decreased inhibition produced by the activation of G protein–coupled receptors (GPCRs) involved in mediating antinociception. Estrogen modulates a number of GPCRs, including bradykinin, opioid, noradrenergic, and γ- aminobutyric acid (GABA) receptors. 17β-Estradiol rapidly increases both the potency (eight-fold) and the efficacy (two-fold) of bradykinin to stimulate the phospholipase C-inositol triphosphate pathway in primary cultures of trigeminal neurons from ovariectomized female

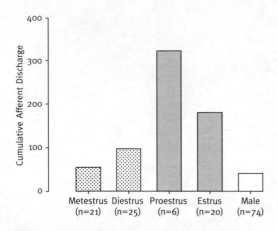

FIGURE 22.1 The effect of sex and estrous cycle on glutamate-induced afferent discharge injected in the rat masseter muscle. Data for this figure were combined from previously published studies. (Reproduced with permission from Cairns BE. *Headache* 2007;47:319–24.)

rats and has no effect in trigeminal neurons cultured from male rats.[9] In addition, behavioral experiments show that administration of 17β-estradiol to the rat hind paw rapidly enhances bradykinin-induced hyperalgesia.[9] These results suggest that 17β-estradiol acts locally, likely at membrane-associated receptors on primary sensory neuron terminals, to rapidly enhance pain sensitivity to bradykinin.

The interaction between estrogen and opioids occurs both in the peripheral and central nervous system. Trigeminal ganglion cells express low levels of mu, delta, and kappa opioid receptor mRNAs as well as the two estrogen receptors, ERα and ERβ.[10–12] Intra-articular morphine reduces muscle reflex responses to TMJ injury.[13] Intra-TMJ administration of the selective kappa-agonist U50,488 attenuates formalin-induced nociceptive behavior to a greater extent in diestrus females than in proestrus females and male rats.[14] This effect is likely the result of activation of kappa receptors local to the site of inflammation since U50,488 injection into the contralateral TMJ does not reproduce the effect and also because prior injection of the selective kappa-antagonist nor-BNI into the inflamed joint significantly diminishes the antinociceptive effect of U50,488 in males and females.

The superficial laminae at the Vc/C2 junction express a high density of μ-opioid receptors[10,15–17] and ERα-positive neurons.[18,19] This junction is thought to be a critical region for the interaction between opioid analgesia and sex hormone status in TMJD pain. In a study evaluating the interaction between estrogen and morphine, it was seen that the systemic administration of morphine reduced bradykinin-evoked activity in the Vc/C2 junction in diestrus females and in males while there was no effect in proestrus females.[20] The interaction between estrogen and opioids also occurs at other sites in the central nervous system. For example, the periaqueductal gray (PAG) contains numerous ERα[21] and μ opioid receptor-positive neurons.[17] As such, it is likely that the interaction between estrogen and opioid analgesia includes descending modulation by PAG-raphe circuits.

The α2-adrenoceptor is another GPCR that is modulated by sex hormones in the central nervous system. Activation of this receptor produces estrogen-dependent modulation of nociception in the trigeminal region.[22] Estrogen down-regulates cortical α2-adrenoceptor and decreases the coupling of the α2-adrenoceptors to G proteins.[23,24] Based on these findings, it has been postulated that the effects of estrogen on this receptor include altering the expression of the α2 gene, decreasing the coupling of the agonist bound receptor to G proteins (Gi/Go), and decreasing the binding affinity of the ligand to the receptor.[22]

In addition to modulating GPCRs, estrogen also modulates other types of receptors and ion channels. For example, estrogen is known to modulate ionotropic glutamate receptors.[25] 17 β-Estradiol up-regulates expression of the ion channel transient receptor potential V1 (TRPV1) in the hippocampus.[26] In addition, blockade of hippocampal TRPV1 attenuates the mechanical allodynia associated with an inflamed TMJ.[26]

ANTINOCICEPTIVE EFFECTS OF ESTROGEN

While most studies on orofacial pain have reported that estrogen is pronociceptive, others have reported that it has an antinociceptive effect.[27–30] Injection of formalin into the upper lip induces greater nociceptive behavior in aromatase-knockout mice (which are devoid of estrogen) than wild-type mice.[30] This increase in nociceptive behavior was noted in the interphase (6–9 minutes after formalin injection) and in the second phase (9–36 minutes after formalin injection) but not in the first phase (0–6 minutes after formalin injection). Nociceptive behavior induced by injection of formalin or glutamate into the TMJ is greater in diestrus female rats than in male and proestrus female rats (Fig. 22.2).[29] In the same study it was seen that ovariectomized female rats exhibited nociceptive behavior which was similar to that of diestrus females and higher than that of proestrus females.[29] Local or systemic administration of exogenous estrogen to the overiectomized female rats attenuates the nociceptive behavior in a dose-dependent manner.[28,29,31] The administration of the nitric oxide synthase inhibitor nitro-L-arginine or of a guanylate cyclase inhibitor (1H-{1,2,4}-oxadiasolo {4,2-a} quinoxalin-1-one) into the ipsilateral, but not into the contralateral TMJ, blocks the antinociceptive effect of estradiol. This suggests that estradiol decreases temporomandibular joint nociception in female rats through a peripheral nongenomic activation of the nitric oxide–cyclic guanosine monophosphate signaling pathway. Estrogen levels in normally cycling rats are positively correlated with N-methyl d-aspartate (NMDA)-evoked masseter afferent discharge, and the treatment of ovariectomized female rats with high-dose estrogen significantly increases NMDA evoked masseter afferent discharge.[27]

A likely explanation for these contradictory reports on the pro- and antinocicpetive effects of estrogen is that these studies are influenced by the biological behaviors observed and/or the inflammatory mediators involved. In addition, most of these studies have focused on exogenous estrogen or serum estrogen and have not considered estrogen locally synthesized in the TMJ. It is now known the estrogen can be synthesized in a number of nongonadal tissues, including cartilage and bone.[32] Proinflammatory cytokines such as tumor necrosis factor α (TNFα), interleukin-1 (IL-1) and interleukin-6 (IL-6) stimulate aromatase activity, resulting in conversion of androgens to estrogen.[33–35] Locally synthesized estrogen is thought to act predominantly at the local tissue level in a paracrine or intracrine manner,[36] and it has been hypothesized that locally synthesized estrogen may place a role in the pathogenesis of TMJD.[37]

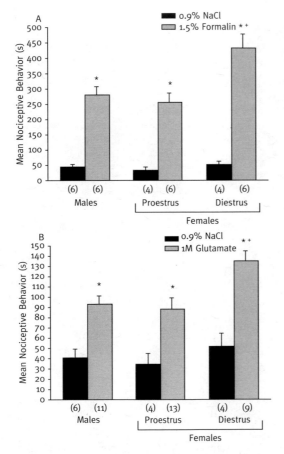

FIGURE 22.2   Effect of sex and estrous cycle on experimentally induced temporomandibular joint nociception. (*A*) Nociception induced by injection of formalin was similar in males and proestrus females and was significantly lower than that in diestrus females. (*B*) Glutamate-induced nociception was similar in males and proestrus females and was significantly lower than that in diestrus females *$p < .05$ as compared to vehicle; †$p < .05$ as compared to males and proestrus females. (Reproduced with permission from Fischer et al., *The Journal of Pain* 2008;9:630–8.)

ESTROGEN AND THE TEMPOROMANDIBULAR JOINT

In addition to its effects on the peripheral and central nervous systems, estrogen is also reported to affect the TMJ and its supporting structures. Estrogen affects bone and chondrocyte metabolism and its receptors are expressed on the mandibular condyle, articular disc, and cartilage.[38-42] Bilateral ovariectomy results in significant changes in the TMJ such as increase in the thickness of the TMJ cartilage, decrease in volumes of the subchondral bone and osteophyte formation.[43-46] Most of these changes are reversed by estrogen replacement.

Estrogen has also been reported to potentiate TMJ inflammation in a dose-dependent manner.[47,48] This effect of estrogen is mediated, at least in part, through nuclear factor κB and results in increased transcription of the proinflammatory mediators TNF-α, IL-1β, IL-6, cyclooxygenase-2 (COX-2), and inducible nitric oxide synthase (iNOS) in the synovial membrane.[47] In cultures of mandibular condylar chondrocytes estrogen increases expression of IL-1β, IL-6, and IL-8 in a dose-dependent manner, providing further evidence of its role in the pathogenesis of TMJD.[49]

Progesterone and Testosterone

A limited number of studies have evaluated the role of progesterone and testosterone in modulating trigeminal nociceptors. There is some evidence that progesterone and its metabolites affect nociceptive processing in the trigeminal system. Cyclical fluctuation of progesterone affects Complete Freund's adjuvant (CFA)-induced TMJ nociception in rats.[28] Prolonged replacement (7 days) of progesterone to ovariectomized rats reduces TMJ nociception.[29] Physiological levels of testosterone do not appear to modulate TMJ pain induced by formalin injection.[50] However, at a supraphysiological serum level, testosterone significantly attenuates formalin-induced nociception in male rats but not in females.[29]

CLINICAL STUDIES
Temporomandibular Joint Disorders

TMJD are a group of painful musculoskeletal conditions of multifactorial etiology that affect approximately 3%–15% of adults in developed nations.[2,51] It is characterized by spontaneous pain and jaw function–induced pain in the TMJ and muscles of mastication; TMJ sounds such as clicking, popping, and crepitus; and intermittent or prolonged restricted mouth opening. TMJD limits oral function (causing difficulties with chewing, speaking, and other orofacial functions), affects quality of life (leading to absence from or impairment of work or social interactions), and incurs billions of dollars in health care costs annually.[52,53] Most studies have found that TMJD is 1.5–2 times more prevalent in women in the community setting with peak prevalence in the reproductive years (20 to 45 years of age).[54] An annual incidence rate of 2%–4% is estimated for onset of the condition and approximately 0.1% for development of chronic TMJD.[55] Longitudinal studies have shown substantial variations in the time course of myofascial TMJD, with 31% of cases persisting over a 5-year period, 33% going into remission, and 36% recurring.[56] A systematic review of the literature concluded that depression, preexisting pain conditions, and female sex were risk factors most consistently associated with TMJD.[55]

Etiology

TMJD, like most other chronic pain conditions, are complex multifactorial disorders rather than a unitary or "isolated" disorder. An array of factors are thought to be involved in its etiology. The pathophysiological processes that contribute to the development and maintenance of TMJD have recently come under more intense scrutiny. Traditionally, the focus was on the anatomical variation in the masticatory system, occlusion, and pathology and trauma of the muscles and TMJs.[57] Recently, Diatchenko et al. (Fig. 22.3) proposed a conceptual model with recognition of pain sensitivity and biopsychosocial factors that control pain sensitivity as important etiological factors.[58] These are, in turn, induced and influenced by both diverse environmental factors (e.g., trauma or infection) and a complex array of multiple genetic polymorphisms. Pathological and physiological processes that involve other body regions or that produce pain in other body regions may also contribute to the etiology of TMJD by influencing endogenous pain regulatory

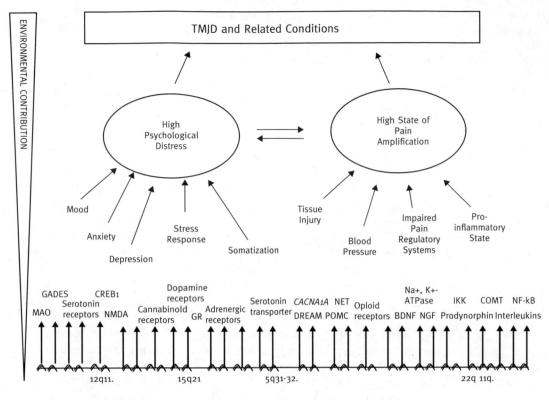

FIGURE 22.3 A conceptual model with recognition of pain sensitivity, biopsychosocial factors, environmental factors, and a complex array of multiple genetic polymorphisms as important etiological factors. These are the likely determinants of the onset and maintenance of temporomandibular joint disorder (TMJD) and related disorders. (Reproduced with permission from *Functional Pain Syndromes*, Mayer EA and Bushnell MC, eds. Seattle, WA: IASP Press.)

systems.[59,60] Conceptual models that link all of these factors are characterized as "biopsychosocial" models of TMJD.[61]

TMJD appears to be related to a general state of pain amplification. Recent data suggest that individuals who develop TMJD show altered processing of nociceptive information prior to and following the development of TMJD. Somatosensory phenotyping has revealed that individuals who exhibit enhanced perceptual responses to noxious stimuli are significantly more likely to develop TMJD than those who are less pain sensitive (risk ratio = 2.7).[62] Similar reductions in thresholds and tolerance for thermal and ischemic pain have been documented.[60] Pain sensitivity may therefore be an important predictive factor for TMJD onset and maintenance. A recent call for a mechanism-based treatment of pain syndromes is based on the hypothesis that different clinical signs and symptoms reflect different underlying pain mechanisms.[63] Somatosensory testing may therefore be important in the identification of TMJD subgroups enabling the correlation of specific individual phenotype with the likely underlying pain mechanisms thereby enhancing the treatment selection and response.

Conditions comorbid with TMJD include (but are not limited to) fibromyalgia (FM), irritable bowel syndrome (IBS), vulvar vestibulitis (VVS) (formerly known as vulvodynia), chronic headache, interstitial cystitis, and chronic tinnitus.[64–67] These complex persistent pain conditions (CPPCs), also known as functional pain syndromes, share similarity in terms of clinical pain complaints.[68] Irrespective of the peripheral pain location, CPPCs are probably regulated in a similar fashion. They overlap with respect to two intermediate phenotypes: pain amplification and psychological distress.

Individual variations in the molecular pathways that affect pain sensitivity and psychological status may produce the heterogenous signs and symptoms that result in clusters of phenotypically distinct patient subgroups, on the basis of different sets of genetic and environmental causes.[58,68] Therefore, the possibility of a pain phenotype had been suggested wherein variations between patients with TMJD may be due to different combinations of genes or environmental influences that lead to similar, though not identical, phenotypes.

No single gene or psychological characteristic can sufficiently explain the variability associated with TMJD. Therefore, the identification of gene–environment interactions, which is the population subgroup defined by genotype in which environmental influences play a relatively greater or lesser etiological role, becomes an important quest. Variations in three single-nucleotide polymorphisms (SNPs) of the gene encoding catechol-O-methyl-transferase (COMT), when combined with val[158]met, form combinations of SNPs called haplotypes. Three prevalent COMT haplotypes, labeled as low pain sensitivity (LPS), average pain sensitivity (APS), and high pain sensitivity (HPS) haplotypes based on observed associations of these haplotypes with sensitivity to experimental pain, accounted for 11% of variability in experimental pain perception in women and were predictive of TMJD risk.[69,70] During a 3-year prospective study of females who did not have TMJD when examined at baseline, the rate of TMJD onset was 2.3-fold greater for subjects who had only HPS and/or APS haplotypes compared with subjects who had one or two LPS haplotypes. Since each individual patient will experience unique environmental exposures and possess unique genetic antecedents to vulnerability to TMJD, analysis of the interactive effects of polymorphic genetic variants will yield unique patient subclusters. Although depression, perceived stress, and mood were associated with pain sensitivity and were predictive of two- to three-fold increases in risk of TMJD ($p < .05$), the magnitude of increased TMJD risk due to psychological factors remained unchanged after adjusting for COMT haplotypes.[71] However, among people with the pain-sensitive haplotypes, the risk of developing TMJD was significantly greater for subjects who reported a history of orthodontic treatment compared with subjects who did not ($p = .04$).[71] This genetic variant could potentially serve as a risk marker for TMJD in the identification of patients most likely to experience pain during orthodontic treatment. Recently, a pilot study examining the use of COMT haplotypes to serve as genetic predictors of treatment outcome identified a subgroup of TMJD patients who benefited from propranolol (a nonselective β-adrenergic receptor antagonist) therapy.[72] Treatment was most efficacious in TMJD patients without the LPS haplotype. Collectively, these translational studies have demonstrated mechanism-specific pharmacologic management of chronic pain.

The complex interactions of these risk determinants present a clear challenge to the traditional approach to diagnosis and management of TMJD. That multiple genetic pathways and environmental factors interact to produce a diverse set of symptoms with persistent pain as the primary complaint will enable the development of algorithms and methods of diagnosing, classifying, and treating patients with TMJD. The findings described earlier suggest that the pursuit of individually based interventions for TMJD is prudent and that treatments that target psychological characteristics or that compensate for decreased COMT activity would be important. Existing practices of treatment for TMJD, such as analgesics, dental-orthopedic devices, and surgery, often are made empirically, and sometimes despite evidence that some such treatments are no better than a placebo.[73] There is therefore an urgent need for a multifaceted approach to the treatment and prevention of TMJD that is based on an understanding of its etiology. In the meantime, the American Association of Dental Research published a standard of care statement in 2010 recommending that "unless there are specific and justifiable indications to the contrary, treatment of TMJD patients initially should be based on the use of conservative, reversible and evidence-based therapeutic modalities."[74] These include patient education and self-management, cognitive-behavioral therapy intervention, pharmacotherapy, physical therapy, and orthopedic appliances.[75]

Orofacial Pain

The scope of OFP includes TMJD (described in the earlier section), intraoral pain conditions, and related medical conditions that either refer pain to or cause pain in the orofacial region.[76] The intraoral dentoalveolar region, the tongue, and the extraoral or facial region are three main anatomic sites of orofacial pain. Popular diagnostic entities include trigeminal neuralgia (TN), burning mouth syndrome (BMS), and atypical odontalgia (AO). Although various authors and scientific societies, such as the American Academy of Orofacial Pain and the International Headache Society, have published comprehensive and detailed classification systems, the classification of OFP remains a work in progress.[75-78] Recent push for a mechanism-based classification of OFP has made little headway due to the controversy over which pains may be nociceptive or neuropathic in origin.[79,80] This is further complicated by the evidence of a spectrum/continuum in chronic musculoskeletal and neuropathic OFP.[81]

Approximately 80% of treatment-seeking OFP patients are female,[1-3] and women in the reproductive age group are more vulnerable, with the exception of TN and BMS, which afflict mainly elderly females. Like other chronic pains, OFP is frequently associated with sleep disturbances and elevated psychological distress, including somatization, depression, and anxiety, leading to disruption of normal social relationships.[82]

Neuropathic orofacial pains (NOP) are regarded as a heterogeneous group of entities, including deafferentation, neuralgic, posttraumatic, postsurgical, and idiopathic trigeminal neuropathies.[75] In addition, it has also been suggested that persistent inflammatory process (such as occult infection or mechanical irritation) may also produce neuropathic pain-like symptoms unaccompanied by the traditional signs of nerve damage.[83] Function brain imaging has revealed sensitization within and outside of the primary sensory pathway in patients with NOP.[84] Neurophysiological studies of the trigeminal pathway can often assist in localization of lesions involving the trigeminal complex,[85,86] while quantitative sensory testing (QST) allows quantitative measures of somesthetic function in NOP.[87] Therefore, in addition to tradition history taking and clinical examination, neurophysiologic examination and QST have been advocated for this heterogenous group. The management of NOP is largely pharmacologic, with emphasis on neuromodulating multidrug therapy,[88,89] along with psychological supportive therapy. Next, we describe three of the more common NOP affecting women, namely, TN, AO, and BMS.

TRIGEMINAL NEURALGIA

Idiopathic TN, also known as "tic douloureux," is described as a paroxysmal, lancinating, electric shock-like pain with intervening pain-free intervals. Pain attacks are usually unilateral, affecting one or more branches of the trigeminal nerve, and are frequently triggered by mild mechanical stimuli such as eating, speaking, face washing, and tooth brushing. Some patients present with a "trigger zone" upon which light touch provokes pain which appears disproportionate to the level of stimuli applied. Unique to TN, refractory periods (interval of seconds to minutes after a paroxysm during which triggering stimuli fail to elicit another bout of pain), referred paroxysmal pain (stimuli in one location evokes pain in a distant location), and remission periods[83] are commonly reported. Peak age of the disease is 50–60 years with a slight female predominance (male to female ratio is approximately 1:1.5).[90] The etiology and pathophysiology of TN is not completely understood. The "ignition" hypothesis proposed that normal nerve impulses produced epileptiform discharge of hyperexcitable demyelinated and axotomized afferent neurons resulting in the paroxysmal nature of TN pain. The controversial vascular compression theory proposes neurovascular contact or venous compression on the trigeminal root entry zone. Pharmacotherapy is the first-line treatment, and excellent pain relief has been achieved with carbamazepine, oxcarbazepine, baclofen, lamotrigine, and pimizide.[91,92] More aggressive neurosurgical treatment options include gasserian ganglion percutaneous techniques, gamma knife stereotactic radiotherapy, and microvascular decompression surgery.[93]

ATYPICAL ODONTALGIA

Atypical odontalgia (AO) is defined by continuous pain in the teeth, or in a tooth socket after extraction, in the absence of clinical and radiographic evidence of dental pathology.[94] The prevalence of AO is about 2.1% with a preponderance of females in their mid-40s. The cause of AO is unclear. Dental treatment (such as root canal treatment or extraction) has been implicated. Polycarpou et al. reported pain persistence, history of chronic pain, painful treatment in the orofacial region, and female gender as important risk factors for persistent pain after endodontic therapy.[95] The pathophysiology of AO is largely unknown, although deafferentation neuropathic pain has been suggested. It is thought that both peripheral and central sensitization play a role. This is further evidenced by the equivocal pain relief from peripheral nerve blocks and the robust pain-relieving effects of locally applied topical medicaments in most patients.[96] Like other chronic pains, patients with AO also present with elevated psychological distress, including depression and somatization. Its management is largely pharmacologic, with topical medication and supportive psychotherapy playing important roles.[96]

BURNING MOUTH SYNDROME

Oral mucosa burning can be caused by a variety of local (such as infection and irritants) and systemic (such as diabetes mellitus and iron deficiency anemia) disorders; however, "true" idiopathic BMS is defined as a burning in the tongue and/or oral mucosa in the absence of clinical and laboratory abnormalities.[9] Its prevalence ranges from 0.7% to 4.6% and is seven times more common in women than men, most frequently affecting postmenopausal females. Yet no significant differences have been reported between BMS and control subjects with menopause status and the use of hormonal replacement therapy.[98,99] BMS is frequently accompanied by impaired taste, oral dysesthesia, and xerostomia, and it is comorbid with other chronic pain conditions such as fibromyalgia. The etiogenesis and pathophysiology of BMS is largely unexplained. It is believed that BMS could represent the clinical manifestation of taste damage based on the convergence of taste sensation and pain,[100,101] and recent studies suggest trigeminal nerve degeneration as its underlying cause.[102,103] Brain hypoactivity[104] and increased sensory purinergic receptor P2X3 immunoreactivity in the trigeminal system were recently reported,[105] along with increased sensitivity to experimental pain and heighted sympathetic output.[97] The management of BMS is largely pharmacologic (excellent efficacy reported with clonazepam) along with cognitive-behavioral therapy.[106]

FUTURE DIRECTIONS

As discussed earlier in this chapter, a large number of preclinical studies have evaluated the role of sex hormones in orofacial pain. Of particular interest is the protective role of testosterone in male rats, which may explain the lower prevalence and severity of orofacial pain conditions in men. Understanding the mechanism underlying the protective effect of testosterone may help establish more successful treatments for chronic orofacial pain.

A recent study on pain after endodontic treatment reported sex-dependent differences in the analgesic effect of pentazocine.[107] Pentazocine acts as a κ-opioid receptor agonist and a partial δ-opioid receptor agonist with mixed agonist-antagonist properties at the μ-opioid receptor. In a clinical trial comparing the analgesic efficacy of a pentazocine (50 mg)/naloxone (0.5 mg) (Talwin©, Sanofi Winthrop, Morrisville, PA) to that of ibuprofen (600 mg), female patients who took pentazocine/naloxone reported significantly greater pain relief as compared to male patients who took the same medication (Fig. 22.4). Pentazocine/naloxone could be an effective analgesic in female patients who are unable to take other analgesics such as ibuprofen and acetaminophen. As compared to other opioids, it offers the additional advantage of relatively less opioid dependence and abuse potential.[108,109]

Increased awareness of the overlap between TMJD and other CPPCs will likely result in improved diagnoses and more effective pain management. As discussed earlier, TMJD and its comorbid conditions share several common features, including increased pain sensitivity,

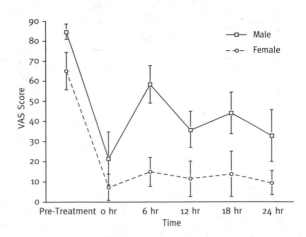

FIGURE 22.4   Postendodontic pain in male and female patients taking pentazocine (50 mg)/naloxone (0.5 mg) (Talwin©, Sanofi Winthrop, Morrisville, PA). Pain intensity was recorded on a 100 mm Visual Analog Scale (VAS) prior to and after endodontic therapy (also known as root canal treatment). After the addition of preoperative pain as a covariate, men reported higher postoperative pain intensity as compared to women. (Reproduced with permission from Ryan et al., *J Endod*. 2008;34:552–6.)

fatigue, and sleep difficulties, which often result in missed diagnosis. The OPPERA study (https://www.oppera.org/) is evaluating the genetic and environmental risk factors associated with the onset and maintenance of TMJD, and the temporal relationship between TMJD and comorbid pain conditions. Further studies are needed to address the impact of these pathways of vulnerability on the prognosis of the various treatment modalities for TMJD and other CPPCs.

REFERENCES

1. Anastassaki A, Magnusson T. Patients referred to a specialist clinic because of suspected temporomandibular disorders: a survey of 3194 patients in respect of diagnoses, treatments, and treatment outcome. *Acta Odontol Scand* 2004;62(4):183–92.
2. LeResche L. Epidemiology of temporomandibular disorders: implications for the investigation of etiologic factors. *Crit Rev Oral Biol Med* 1997;8(3):291–305.
3. White BA, Williams LA, Leben JR. Health care utilization and cost among health maintenance organization members with temporomandibular disorders. *J Orofac Pain* 2001;15(2):158–69.
4. Von Korff M, LeResche L, Dworkin S. First onset of common pain symptoms: a prospective study of depression as a risk factor. *Pain* 1993;55:251–8.
5. Bereiter DA. Sex differences in brainstem neural activation after injury to the TMJ region. *Cells Tissues Organs* 2001;169(3):226–37.
6. Arnold LM, Russell IJ, Diri EW, et al. A 14-week, randomized, double-blinded, placebo-controlled monotherapy trial of pregabalin in patients with fibromyalgia. *J Pain* 2008;9(9):792–805.
7. Martin VT, Lee J, Behbehani MM. Sensitization of the trigeminal sensory system during different stages of the rat estrous cycle: implications for menstrual migraine. *Headache* 2007;47(4):552–63.
8. Okamoto K, Hirata H, Takeshita S, Bereiter DA. Response properties of TMJ units in superficial laminae at the spinomedullary junction of female rats vary over the estrous cycle. *J Neurophysiol* 2003;89(3):1467–77.
9. Rowan MP, Berg KA, Milam SB, et al. 17beta-estradiol rapidly enhances bradykinin signaling in primary sensory neurons in vitro and in vivo. *J Pharmacol Exp Ther* 2010; 335(1):190–6.
10. Bereiter DA, Cioffi JL, Bereiter DF. Oestrogen receptor-immunoreactive neurons in the trigeminal sensory system of male and cycling female rats. *Arch Oral Biol* 2005;50(11):971–9.
11. Buzas B, Cox BM. Quantitative analysis of mu and delta opioid receptor gene expression in rat brain and peripheral ganglia using competitive polymerase chain reaction. *Neuroscience* 1997;76(2):479–89.
12. Schafer MK, Bette M, Romeo H, Schwaeble W, Weihe E. Localization of kappa-opioid receptor

mRNA in neuronal subpopulations of rat sensory ganglia and spinal cord. *Neurosci Lett* 1994; 167(1–2):137–40.

13. Bakke M, Hu JW, Sessle BJ. Morphine application to peripheral tissues modulates nociceptive jaw reflex. *Neuroreport* 1998;9(14): 3315–9.

14. Clemente JT, Parada CA, Veiga MC, Gear RW, Tambeli CH. Sexual dimorphism in the antinociception mediated by kappa opioid receptors in the rat temporomandibular joint. *Neurosci Lett* 2004;372(3):250–5.

15. Xia Y, Haddad GG. Ontogeny and distribution of opioid receptors in the rat brainstem. *Brain Res* 1991;549(2):181–93.

16. Atweh SF, Kuhar MJ. Autoradiographic localization of opiate receptors in rat brain. II. The brain stem. *Brain Res* 1977;129(1):1–12.

17. Ding YQ, Kaneko T, Nomura S, Mizuno N. Immunohistochemical localization of mu-opioid receptors in the central nervous system of the rat. *J Comp Neurol* 1996;367(3):375–402.

18. Amandusson A, Hermanson O, Blomqvist A. Colocalization of oestrogen receptor immunoreactivity and preproenkephalin mRNA expression to neurons in the superficial laminae of the spinal and medullary dorsal horn of rats. *Eur J Neurosci* 1996;8(11):2440–5.

19. Pajot J, Ressot C, Ngom I, Woda A. Gonadectomy induces site-specific differences in nociception in rats. *Pain* 2003;104(1–2):367–73.

20. Okamoto K, Tashiro A, Hirata H, Bereiter DA. Differential modulation of TMJ neurons in superficial laminae of trigeminal subnucleus caudalis/upper cervical cord junction region of male and cycling female rats by morphine. *Pain* 2005;114(1–2):203–11.

21. Shughrue PJ, Lane MV, Merchenthaler I. Comparative distribution of estrogen receptor-alpha and -beta mRNA in the rat central nervous system. *J Comp Neurol* 1997;388(4):507–25.

22. Nag S, Mokha SS. Activation of alpha2-adrenoceptors in the trigeminal region produces sex-specific modulation of nociception in the rat. *Neuroscience* 2006;142(4):1255–62.

23. Ansonoff MA, Etgen AM. Receptor phosphorylation mediates estradiol reduction of alpha2-adrenoceptor coupling to G protein in the hypothalamus of female rats. *Endocrine* 2001;14(2):165–74.

24. Karkanias GB, Li CS, Etgen AM. Estradiol reduction of alpha 2-adrenoceptor binding in female rat cortex is correlated with decreases in alpha 2A/D-adrenoceptor messenger RNA. *Neuroscience* 1997;81(3):593–7.

25. Tashiro A, Okamoto K, Bereiter DA. NMDA receptor blockade reduces temporomandibular joint-evoked activity of trigeminal subnucleus caudalis neurons in an estrogen-dependent manner. *Neuroscience* 2009;164(4):1805–12.

26. Wu YW, Bi YP, Kou XX, et al. 17-Beta-estradiol enhanced allodynia of inflammatory temporomandibular joint through upregulation of hippocampal TRPV1 in ovariectomized rats. *J Neurosci* 2010;30(26):8710–9.

27. Dong XD, Mann MK, Kumar U, et al. Sex-related differences in NMDA-evoked rat masseter muscle afferent discharge result from estrogen-mediated modulation of peripheral NMDA receptor activity. *Neuroscience* 2007; 146(2):822–32.

28. Kramer PR, Bellinger LL. The effects of cycling levels of 17beta-estradiol and progesterone on the magnitude of temporomandibular joint-induced nociception. *Endocrinology* 2009; 150(8):3680–9.

29. Fischer L, Torres-Chavez KE, Clemente-Napimoga JT, et al. The influence of sex and ovarian hormones on temporomandibular joint nociception in rats. *J Pain* 2008;9(7):630–8.

30. Multon S, Pardutz A, Mosen J, et al. Lack of estrogen increases pain in the trigeminal formalin model: a behavioural and immunocytochemical study of transgenic ArKO mice. *Pain* 2005;114(1–2):257–65.

31. Favaro-Moreira NC, Torres-Chavez KE, Fischer L, Tambeli CH. Peripheral estradiol induces temporomandibular joint antinociception in rats by activating the nitric oxide/cyclic guanosine monophosphate signaling pathway. *Neuroscience* 2009;164(2):724–32.

32. Sasano H, Ozaki M. Aromatase expression and its localization in human breast cancer. *J Steroid Biochem Mol Biol* 1997;61(3–6):293–8.

33. Nestler JE. Interleukin-1 stimulates the aromatase activity of human placental cytotrophoblasts. *Endocrinology* 1993;132(2): 566–70.

34. Macdiarmid F, Wang D, Duncan LJ, Purohit A, Ghilchick MW, Reed MJ. Stimulation of aromatase activity in breast fibroblasts by tumor necrosis factor alpha. *Mol Cell Endocrinol* 1994;106(1–2):17–21.

35. Purohit A, Ghilchik MW, Duncan L, et al. Aromatase activity and interleukin-6 production by normal and malignant breast tissues. *J Clin Endocrinol Metab* 1995;80(10):3052–8.

36. Simpson ER, Clyne C, Rubin G, et al. Aromatase—a brief overview. *Annu Rev Physiol* 2002;64:93–127.

37. Yu S, Xing X, Liang S, et al. Locally synthesized estrogen plays an important role in the development of TMD. *Med Hypotheses* 2009;72(6):720–2.

38. Aufdemorte TB, Van Sickels JE, Dolwick MF, et al. Estrogen receptors in the temporomandibular joint of the baboon (Papio cynocephalus): an autoradiographic study. *Oral Surg Oral Med Oral Pathol* 1986;61(4):307–14.

39. Abubaker AO, Raslan WF, Sotereanos GC. Estrogen and progesterone receptors in temporomandibular joint discs of symptomatic and asymptomatic persons: a preliminary study. *J Oral Maxillofac Surg* 1993;51(10):1096–1100.

40. Puri J, Hutchins B, Bellinger LL, Kramer PR. Estrogen and inflammation modulate estrogen receptor alpha expression in specific tissues of the temporomandibular joint. *Reprod Biol Endocrinol* 2009;7:155.

41. Yamada K, Nozawa-Inoue K, Kawano Y, et al. Expression of estrogen receptor alpha (ER alpha) in the rat temporomandibular joint. *Anat Rec A Discov Mol Cell Evol Biol* 2003;274(2):934–41.

42. Cheng ZN, Zhou HH. Contribution of genetic variations in estradiol biosynthesis and metabolism enzymes to osteoporosis. *Acta Pharmacol Sin* 2000;21(7):587–90.

43. Okuda T, Yasuoka T, Nakashima M, Oka N. The effect of ovariectomy on the temporomandibular joints of growing rats. *J Oral Maxillofac Surg* 1996;54(10):1201–10, discussion 10–11.

44. Yamashiro T, Takano-Yamamoto T. Differential responses of mandibular condyle and femur to oestrogen deficiency in young rats. *Arch Oral Biol* 1998;43(3):191–5.

45. Yasuoka T, Nakashima M, Okuda T, Tatematsu N. Effect of estrogen replacement on temporomandibular joint remodeling in ovariectomized rats. *J Oral Maxillofac Surg* 2000;58(2):189–96, discussion 96–7.

46. Fujita T, Kawata T, Tokimasa C, Kaku M, Kawasoko S, Tanne K. Influences of ovariectomy and orchiectomy on the remodeling of mandibular condyle in mice. *J Craniofac Genet Dev Biol* 1998;18(3):164–70.

47. Kou XX, Wu YW, Ding Y, et al. 17beta-estradiol aggravated temporomandibular joint inflammation through NF-kappaB pathway in ovariectomized rats. *Arthritis Rheum* 2011;63:1888–97.

48. Guan G, Kerins CC, Bellinger LL, Kramer PR. Estrogenic effect on swelling and monocytic receptor expression in an arthritic temporomandibular joint model. *J Steroid Biochem Mol Biol* 2005;97(3):241–50.

49. Yun KI, Chae CH, Lee CW. Effect of estrogen on the expression of cytokines of the temporomandibular joint cartilage cells of the mouse. *J Oral Maxillofac Surg* 2008;66(5):882–7.

50. Fischer L, Clemente JT, Tambeli CH. The protective role of testosterone in the development of temporomandibular joint pain. *J Pain* 2007;8(5):437–42.

51. Dworkin SF, LeResche L. Research diagnostic criteria for temporomandibular disorders: review, criteria, examinations and specifications, critique. *J Craniomandib Disord* 1992;6(4):301–55.

52. US Department of Health and Human Services. *Oral Health in America: A Report of the Surgeon General*. Rockville, MD: National Institutes of Health; 2000.

53. Lipton JA, Ship JA, Larach-Robinson D. Estimated prevalence and distribution of reported orofacial pain in the United States. *J Am Dent Assoc* 1993;124(10):115–21.

54. Von Korff M, Dworkin SF, Le Resche L, Kruger A. An epidemiologic comparison of pain complaints. *Pain* 1988;32(2):173–83.

55. Drangsholt MT, LeResche L. Temporomandibular disorder pain. In: Crombie IK, Croft PR, Linton SJ, eds. *Epidemiology of Pain*. Seattle, WA: IASP Press; 1999: 203–33.

56. Rammelsberg P, LeResche L, Dworkin S, Mancl L. Longitudinal outcome of temporomandibular disorders: a 5-year epidemiologic study of muscle disorders defined by research diagnostic criteria for temporomandibular disorders. *J Orofac Pain* 2003;17(1):9–20.

57. Macfarlane TV, Blinkhorn AS, Davies RM, Worthington HV. Association between local mechanical factors and orofacial pain: survey in the community. *J Dent* 2003;31(8):535–42.

58. Diatchenko L, Nackley AG, Slade GD, Fillingim RB, Maixner W. Idiopathic pain disorders—pathways of vulnerability. *Pain* 2006;123(3):226–30.

59. Fillingim RB, Maixner W, Kincaid S, Sigurdsson A, Harris MB. Pain sensitivity in patients with temporomandibular disorders: relationship to clinical and psychosocial factors. *Clin J Pain* 1996;12(4):260–9.

60. Maixner W. Myogenous temporomandibular disorder: a persistent pain condition associated with hyperalgesia and enhanced temporal summation of pain. In: Brune K, Handwerker HO, eds. *Hyperalgesia: Molecular Mechanisms and Clinical Implications*. Vol. 30. Seattle, WA: IASP Press; 2004: 373–86.

61. Wright AR, Gatchel RJ, Wildenstein L, Riggs R, Buschang P, Ellis E, 3rd. Biopsychosocial differences between high-risk and low-risk patients

with acute TMD-related pain. *J Am Dent Assoc* 2004;135(4):474–83.

62. Slade GD, Diatchenko L, Bhalang K, et al. Influence of psychological factors on risk of temporomandibular disorders. *J Dent Res* 2007;86(11):1120–5.

63. Jensen TS, Baron R. Translation of symptoms and signs into mechanisms in neuropathic pain. *Pain* 2003;102(1–2):1–8.

64. Yunus MB. Central sensitivity syndromes: a new paradigm and group nosology for fibromyalgia and overlapping conditions, and the related issue of disease versus illness. *Semin Arthritis Rheum* 2008;37(6):339–52.

65. Whitehead WE, Palsson OS, Levy RR, Feld AD, Turner M, Von Korff M. Comorbidity in irritable bowel syndrome. *Am J Gastroenterol* 2007;102(12):2767–6.

66. Zolnoun DA, Rohl J, Moore CG, Perinetti-Liebert C, Lamvu GM, Maixner W. Overlap between orofacial pain and vulvar vestibulitis syndrome. *Clin J Pain* 2008;24(3):187–91.

67. Ballegaard V, Thede-Schmidt-Hansen P, Svensson P, Jensen R. Are headache and temporomandibular disorders related? A blinded study. *Cephalalgia* 2008;28(8):832–41.

68. Maixner W. Temporomandibular joint disorders. In: Mayer EA, Bushnell MC, eds. *Functional Pain Syndromes: Presentation and Pathophysiology*. Seattle, WA: IASP Press; 2009: 55–70.

69. Diatchenko L, Nackley AG, Slade GD, et al. Catechol-O-methyltransferase gene polymorphisms are associated with multiple pain-evoking stimuli. *Pain* 2006;125(3):216–24.

70. Diatchenko L, Slade GD, Nackley AG, et al. Genetic basis for individual variations in pain perception and the development of a chronic pain condition. *Hum Mol Genet* 2005;14(1):135–43.

71. Slade GD, Diatchenko L, Ohrbach R, Maixner W. Orthodontic treatment, genetic factors and risk of temporomandibular disorder. *Semin Orthod* 2008;14(2):146–56.

72. Tchivileva IE, Lim PF, Smith SB, et al. Effect of catechol-O-methyltransferase polymorphism on response to propranolol therapy in chronic musculoskeletal pain: a randomized, double-blind, placebo-controlled, crossover pilot study. *Pharmacogenet Genomics* 2010;20(4):239–48.

73. List T, Axelsson S. Management of TMD: evidence from systematic reviews and meta-analyses. *J Oral Rehabil* 2010;37(6):430–51.

74. Greene CS. Managing patients with temporomandibular disorders: a new "standard of care." *Am J Orthod Dentofacial Orthop* 2010; 138(1):3–4.

75. de Leeuw R, ed. *Orofacial Pain. Guidelines for Assessment, Diagnosis, and Management*. 4th ed. Hanover Park, IL: Quintessence Publishing Co; 2008.

76. McNeill C, Dubner R, Woda A. What is pain and how do we classify orofacial pain? In: Sessle BJ, Lavigne GJ, Lund JP, Dubner R, eds. *Orofacial Pain from Basic Science to Clinical Management*. 2nd ed. Hanover Park, IL: Quintesence Publishing Co; 2008.

77. Merskey H, Bogduk N, eds. *Classification of Chronic Pain: Descriptions of Chronic Pain Syndromes and Definitions of Pain Terms*. Seattle, WA: IASP Press; 1994.

78. Woda A, Tubert-Jeannin S, Bouhassira D, et al. Towards a new taxonomy of idiopathic orofacial pain. *Pain* 2005;116(3):396–406.

79. Woolf CJ, Bennett GJ, Doherty M, et al. Towards a mechanism-based classification of pain? *Pain* 1998;77(3):227–9.

80. Zakrzewska JM. The management of orofacial pain. *Practitioner* 2004;248(1660): 508,10,14–6.

81. Bennett MI, Smith BH, Torrance N, Lee AJ. Can pain can be more or less neuropathic? Comparison of symptom assessment tools with ratings of certainty by clinicians. *Pain* 2006;122(3):289–94.

82. Benoliel R, Eliav E, Sharav Y. Self-reports of pain-related awakenings in persistent orofacial pain patients. *J Orofac Pain* 2009;23(4):330–8.

83. Bennett GJ. Neuropathic pain in the orofacial region: clinical and research challenges. *J Orofac Pain* 2004;18(4):281–6.

84. Becerra L, Morris S, Bazes S, et al. Trigeminal neuropathic pain alters responses in CNS circuits to mechanical (brush) and thermal (cold and heat) stimuli. *J Neurosci* 2006;26(42):10646–57.

85. Valls-Sole J. Neurophysiological assessment of trigeminal nerve reflexes in disorders of central and peripheral nervous system. *Clin Neurophysiol* 2005;116(10):2255–65.

86. Jaaskelainen SK, Teerijoki-Oksa T, Forssell H. Neurophysiologic and quantitative sensory testing in the diagnosis of trigeminal neuropathy and neuropathic pain. *Pain* 2005;117(3):349–57.

87. Svensson P, Graven-Nielsen T. Craniofacial muscle pain: review of mechanisms and clinical manifestations. *J Orofac Pain* 2001;15(2):117–45.

88. Dworkin RH, O'Connor AB, Backonja M, et al. Pharmacologic management of neuropathic pain: evidence-based recommendations. *Pain* 2007;132(3):237–51.

89. Attal N, Cruccu G, Baron R, et al. EFNS guidelines on the pharmacological treatment of

neuropathic pain: 2010 revision. *Eur J Neurol* 2010;17(9):1113-e88.

90. MacDonald JE. A deconstructive turn in chronic pain treatment: a redefined role for social work. *Health Soc Work* 2000;25(1):51–8.

91. Cruccu G, Gronseth G, Alksne J, et al. AAN-EFNS guidelines on trigeminal neuralgia management. *Eur J Neurol* 2008;15(10):1013–28.

92. Jorns TP, Zakrzewska JM. Evidence-based approach to the medical management of trigeminal neuralgia. *Br J Neurosurg* 2007;21(3):253–61.

93. Gronseth G, Cruccu G, Alksne J, et al. Practice parameter: the diagnostic evaluation and treatment of trigeminal neuralgia (an evidence-based review): report of the Quality Standards Subcommittee of the American Academy of Neurology and the European Federation of Neurological Societies. *Neurology* 2008;71(15):1183–90.

94. Melis M, Lobo SL, Ceneviz C, et al. Atypical odontalgia: a review of the literature. *Headache* 2003;43(10):1060–74.

95. Polycarpou N, Ng YL, Canavan D, Moles DR, Gulabivala K. Prevalence of persistent pain after endodontic treatment and factors affecting its occurrence in cases with complete radiographic healing. *Int Endod J* 2005;38(3): 169–78.

96. Heir G, Karolchek S, Kalladka M, et al. Use of topical medication in orofacial neuropathic pain: a retrospective study. *Oral Surg Oral Med Oral Pathol Oral Radiol Endod* 2008;105(4):466–9.

97. Rhodus NL, Carlson CR, Miller CS. Burning mouth (syndrome) disorder. *Quintessence Int* 2003;34(8):587–93.

98. Tarkkila L, Linna M, Tiitinen A, Lindqvist C, Meurman JH. Oral symptoms at menopause—the role of hormone replacement therapy. *Oral Surg Oral Med Oral Pathol Oral Radiol Endod* 2001;92(3):276–80.

99. Ben Aryeh H, Gottlieb I, Ish-Shalom S, David A, Szargel H, Laufer D. Oral complaints related to menopause. *Maturitas* 1996;24(3):185–9.

100. Lehman CD, Bartoshuk LM, Catalanotto FC, Kveton JF, Lowlicht RA. Effect of anesthesia of the chorda tympani nerve on taste perception in humans. *Physiol Behav* 1995; 57(5):943–51.

101. Grushka M, Epstein JB, Gorsky M. Burning mouth syndrome and other oral sensory disorders: a unifying hypothesis. *Pain Res Manag* 2003;8(3):133–5.

102. Penza P, Majorana A, Lombardi R, et al. "Burning tongue" and "burning tip": the diagnostic challenge of the burning mouth syndrome. *Clin J Pain* 2010;26(6):528–32.

103. Zidverc-Trajkovic J, Stanimirovic D, Obrenovic R, et al. Calcitonin gene-related peptide levels in saliva of patients with burning mouth syndrome. *J Oral Pathol Med* 2009;38(1): 29–33.

104. Albuquerque RJ, de Leeuw R, Carlson CR, Okeson JP, Miller CS, Andersen AH. Cerebral activation during thermal stimulation of patients who have burning mouth disorder: an fMRI study. *Pain* 2006;122(3):223–34.

105. Beneng K, Yilmaz Z, Yiangou Y, McParland H, Anand P, Renton T. Sensory purinergic receptor P2X3 is elevated in burning mouth syndrome. *Int J Oral Maxillofac Surg* 2010; 39(8):815–9.

106. Patton LL, Siegel MA, Benoliel R, De Laat A. Management of burning mouth syndrome: systematic review and management recommendations. *Oral Surg Oral Med Oral Pathol Oral Radiol Endod* 2007;103(Suppl):S39, e1–13.

107. Ryan JL, Jureidini B, Hodges JS, Baisden M, Swift JQ, Bowles WR. Gender differences in analgesia for endodontic pain. *J Endod* 2008;34(5):552–6.

108. Goldstein G. Pentazocine. *Drug Alcohol Depend* 1985;14(3–4):313–23.

109. Swift JQ, Hargreaves KM. Pentazocine analgesia: is there a niche for Talwin Nx? *Compendium* 1993;14(8):1048, 50 passim, quiz 60.

INDEX

ablation, 165
acetaminophen
    for FM treatment, 221
    for migraine treatment, 127–28, 128t, 303, 306
    pregnancy and, 127–28, 128t, 138t, 139, 142
acid-sensing ion channels (ASICs), 73, 73f
ACR. *See* American College of Rheumatology
ACS. *See* acute coronary syndrome
acupuncture, 112, 222, 222t
acute coronary syndrome (ACS), 289–90
add-back therapy, 162t, 164
addiction, 145
adjuvant therapy, as PPBCT risk factor, 189–90
adrenocorticotropic hormone, 278
affective factors. *See* cognitive/affective factors
age, as PPBCT risk factor, 188
AIs. *See* aromatase inhibitors
alfentanil, 23
allergies, 218
alpha-2 adrenergic agonists
    for FM treatment, 221
    for opioid-tolerant pregnant patients, 142
    sex hormones and, 82, 86, 88–89
alpha-2-delta ligands, 220t
American College of Rheumatology (ACR), 5, 6t, 210–11, 218
amitriptyline, 129–30, 138t, 143, 240t, 267, 280
    for FM treatment, 219, 220t
    for migraine treatment, 304, 305t
amygdala, connectivity and, 37
analgesic responses, sex differences in. *See also* sex-dependent
    genetic contributions, to pain and analgesia; sex hormones,
    in pain and analgesia; specific types of analgesia
    nonopioid analgesics
        ketamine, 54, 61, 62f
        local anesthetics, 54, 61–62
        NSAIDs, 54, 60–61
    opioids
        data interpretation, 57–60, 58f–59f
        pooled quantitative data, 54–57, 55f, 57t

overview of, 54, 62–63
anastrozole, 161t
anatomy
    brain imaging and, 35–36
    experimental pain and, 26
anesthesia, epidural, 114
angina pectoris, 8–9, 288–89, 289t
angiotensin-converting enzyme inhibitors, 292
ANLD. *See* axillary lymph node dissection
anthracycline, 187t
anticonvulsants. *See* antiepileptic drugs
antidepressants, 142–43, 238, 267, 305t
    for migraine in pregnancy, 129–30
    organ function influenced by, 279t
    TCAs, 143, 292, 304
        for CPPS treatment, 280
        for FM treatment, 219–20, 220t
    tetracyclic, 280
antiepileptic drugs, 142–43, 238, 281
    for FM treatment, 220–21
    for migraine treatment, 128–29, 303–4, 305t
    organ function influenced by, 279t
antihistamines, 267, 303, 306
anxiety, 96, 217, 250
AO. *See* atypical odontalgia
aromatase inhibitors (AIs), 161t, 164, 187t, 190
arterial spin labeling (ASL), 37
ASICs. *See* acid-sensing ion channels
ASL. *See* arterial spin labeling
aspirin, 87–88, 130, 138t, 142, 152, 303
asthma, neurogenic inflammation and, 235
atenolol, 129
atypical odontalgia (AO), 318
aura, migraine with, 300, 301t
autonomic nervous system
    CPPS and, 277
    CRPS and, 233
    IBS and, 253
axillary lymph node dissection (ANLD), 186, 187t, 189–91

testosterone and, 314
tender points, in FM, 210–12, 211f
TENS. *See* transcutaneous electrical nerve stimulation
testosterone
  OFP, TMJD and, 314
  role of, 24, 69, 82, 84, 86
tetracyclic antidepressants, 280
Δ9-tetrahydrocannabinol (THC), 85–88
thoughts. *See* cognitive/affective factors
tic douloureux. *See* trigeminal neuralgia
tizanidine, 221, 240t
TMD. *See* temporomandibular muscle and joint disorders
TMJD. *See* temporomandibular muscle and joint disorders
TN. *See* trigeminal neuralgia
TNF-⊠. *See* tumor necrosis factor alpha
topiramate, 129, 138t, 142–43, 304, 305t, 307
tramadol, 113t, 192t, 220t, 279t
transcutaneous electrical nerve stimulation (TENS), 112, 125, 131, 238–39, 240t, 268
transdermal patch, 161t
transvaginal ring, 161t
treatment biases, 99
tricyclic antidepressants (TCAs), 143, 292, 304
  for CPPS treatment, 280
  for FM treatment, 219–20, 220t
trigeminal neuralgia (TN), 317
trigger point therapies, for CPPS, 280
triptans, 303–4, 303t, 306
tumor necrosis factor alpha (TNF-α), 157, 164–65, 234
twilight sleep, 109

U50,488 analgesia, 75, 85, 312
urinary tract infections, 260t
urogenital structures, innervation of, 177–79, 177f, 260f
uterine endometrium, 158–59

valproate, 307
valproic acid, 128–29, 138t
VAPS. *See* visual analog pain scores
vascular endothelial growth factor (VEGF), 156–58
vaso-occlusive crisis, 130–31
VEGF. *See* vascular endothelial growth factor

venlafaxine, 189, 220, 281, 304, 305t, 307
verapamil, 130, 238, 240t, 304, 305t, 306
vestibulodynia, 176
vinca alkaloids, 190
visceral hyperalgesia, 278
visceral pain
  brain imaging studies on, 41t, 45–48, 47f
  from pelvic cancer, 198–99
  somatic pain different from, 275t–276t
visceral sensitivity, in IBS, 252
viscero-visceral cross-sensitization, 157
viscero-visceral hyperalgesia, 278
visual analog pain scores (VAPS), 200
vitamin C, 238–39, 240t
vulvar allodynia and hyperalgesia, 179
vulvar pain syndromes, 278
vulvar vestibulitis, 176
vulvodynia
  clinical presentations, 180–81, 181f
  definitions, 175–76
  dysesthetic, 176
  epidemiology, 176–77
  estrogen and, 178
  FM and, 179
  future directions, 181–82
  IC/BPS and, 178
  introduction to, 175
  localized provoked, 176
  oral contraceptives and, 178–79
  pathophysiological mechanisms, 179–80
  progesterone and, 178
  taxonomy, 175–76
  treatment, 180–81, 181f
  urogenital neurobiology and, 177–79, 177f

walking epidural, 116
withdrawal syndrome, 146

zolmitriptan, 306
zolpidem, 221
zonisamide, 142
zopiclone, 221